CLINICAL
GYNECOLOGIC ONCOLOGY

CLINICAL
GYNECOLOGIC ONCOLOGY

PHILIP J. DiSAIA, M.D.

Professor and Chairman, Department
of Obstetrics and Gynecology,
California College of Medicine,
University of California
Irvine Medical Center,
Irvine, California

WILLIAM T. CREASMAN, M.D.

Professor, Director of Oncology Division,
Department of Obstetrics and Gynecology,
Duke University Medical Center,
Durham, North Carolina

with **178** illustrations

The C. V. Mosby Company

ST. LOUIS • TORONTO • LONDON   1981

The C. V. Mosby Company
11830 Westline Industrial Drive, St. Louis, Missouri 63141

Library of Congress Cataloging in Publication Data

DiSaia, Philip J   1937-
  Clinical gynecologic oncology.

  Bibliography: p.
  Includes index.
  1. Generative organs, Female—Cancer. I. Creasman,
William T., 1934-   joint author. II. Title.
[DNLM: 1. Genital neoplasms, Female. WP145 D611c]
RC280.G5D46   616.99'465   80-18687
ISBN 0-8016-1314-0

GC/CB/B   9   8   7   6   5   4   3   2   03/C/371

Cognizant of our major sources of support and comfort,
we wish to dedicate this book to our loving wives,

Patti and Erble

Preface

The stimulus for the creation of this book was a recognized need for a readable text on gynecologic oncology and related subjects addressed primarily to the community physician, resident, and student involved with gynecologic cancer patients. Clinical presentation and management of these conditions have been heavily emphasized. In areas where controversy exists concerning therapy, most approaches have been discussed and we have suggested our preference. A serious attempt was made to develop a style that is easily comprehended. At the same time, most major subjects were treated in depth and supplemented with ample current literature references so that the text would provide a comprehensive resource for study by the resident and student of gynecologic oncology and serve as review material for examinations in the specialty of obstetrics and gynecology.

The beginning of each chapter contains an outline for easy reference to the content of that section. Areas of great controversy and change (for example, endometrial adenocarcinoma and its management) are treated more extensively in an effort to provide a sound foundation to the reader for changes yet to come. Other areas of gynecology that have a significant impact on the discipline of gynecologic oncology are also discussed (for example, management of the adnexal mass, malignancy in pregnancy, breast disease, and general aspects of tumor immunology). Since the practicing gynecologist often faces these problems, we felt that their inclusion in this text was quite appropriate.

Fortunately, many of the gynecologic malignancies have an associated high "cure" rate. This has been due at least in part to the development of diagnostic techniques that can identify precancerous conditions, the ability to apply highly effective therapeutic modalities that are more restricted elsewhere in the body, better understanding of disease spread patterns, and the development of more sophisticated and effective treatment in cancers that previously had a very poor prognosis. As a result, today a patient with a gynecologic cancer may look toward more successful treatment and longer survival than was previously experienced. This optimism should be realistically transferred to the patient and her family. The physician must be prepared not only to treat the malignancy in light of today's knowledge but also to deal with the patient and her family in a compassionate and honest manner. The gynecologic cancer patient needs to feel that her physician is confident and goal oriented. Although, unfortunately, some gynecologic cancers still kill many individuals, it is hoped that the information collected in this book will aid in increasing the survival rate of these patients by bringing current practical knowledge to the attention of the primary care and specialized physician.

We wish to acknowledge the advice given and contributions made by several colleagues, including Drs. Erle Henriksen, A. Robert Kagan, William M. Rich, and James Reynolds. Special thanks to Rochelle Savitt and Ellen Merritt for their diligent secretarial efforts in preparing the manuscript and to Richard Crippen and Carol Beckerman for their excellent artistic contributions to many of the figures and diagrams created for this book.

Philip J. DiSaia
William T. Creasman

Contents

CHAPTER ONE

Preinvasive disease of the cervix, vagina, and vulva

Cervical intraepithelial neoplasia
Intraepithelial neoplasia of the vagina
Intraepithelial neoplasia of the vulva

CERVICAL INTRAEPITHELIAL NEOPLASIA
Clinical profile

The unique accessibility of the cervix to cell and tissue study and to direct physical examination has permitted intensive investigation of the nature of malignant lesions of the cervix. Although our knowledge is incomplete, investigations have taught us that most of these tumors have a gradual, rather than an explosive, onset. Their preinvasive precursors may exist in a reversible phase of surface or in situ disease for some years.

According to data from the Third National Cancer Survey, published by Cramer and Cutler, the mean age of patients with carcinoma in situ was 15.6 years younger than that of patients with invasive epidermoid carcinoma, exceeding the 10-year difference found by others (Fig. 1-1). It should be kept in mind that this difference is, at best, a rough approximation of the duration of intraepithelial carcinoma in its assumed progression to clinical invasive cancer. However, data such as this serve to emphasize the essential nature of cytologic screening programs, even when performed on less than an annual basis.

Although these early phases may be asymptomatic, they are detectable by currently available methods. This concept of development of cervical malignancy has convinced many that the control of this disease is well within our grasp in the foreseeable future. We can therefore expect to eradicate most deaths due to cervical cancer by using the diagnostic and therapeutic techniques now available.

1

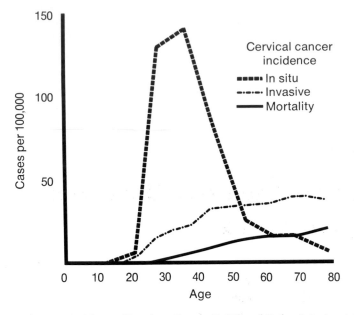

Fig. 1-1. Cervical cancer incidence. (Data from Cramer, D. W., and Cutler, S. J.: Am. J. Obstet. Gynecol. **118:**443, 1974.)

An exhaustive study by the Canadian government has confirmed that cervical cancer is a problem that can be solved. In an impressive report, Walton concluded that squamous carcinoma of the cervix lends itself to cytologic screening programs because (1) invasive squamous carcinoma of the cervix is preceded by a spectrum of disease extending over many years that may be recognized at the stages of dysplasia and carcinoma in situ; (2) in a significant proportion of patients with evidence of dysplasia or carcinoma in situ, the disease, if untreated, develops into invasive squamous carcinoma; (3) cytologic evidence of the existence of dysplasia or carcinoma in situ can be easily, safely, and economically obtained by preparing and examining smears; and (4) once dysplasia or carcinoma in situ has been identified, further progress of the disease can be prevented by simple therapeutic procedures and continuing surveillance.

There is convincing evidence, at least in Canada, that cytologic screening programs are becoming effective in reducing mortality from carcinoma of the cervix. The extent of the reduction in mortality achieved is directly related to the proportion of the population that has been screened. The prevalence of abnormalities is on the order of 0.5 to 0.7 per 1,000. It also appears that cytologic screening programs are most effective when smears are obtained by medical or specially trained paramedical personnel. In addition, smears must be correctly identified and accompanied by information as required by the pathologist, and they must be screened for abnormalities by qualified and experienced cytotechnicians under the supervision of cytopathologists. Screening programs are most effective when the frequency of exam-

Table 1-1. Cytologic report correlations

Class	Description
I	Normal
II	Atypia, usually due to inflammation
III	Dysplasia—mild, moderate, or severe
IV	Carcinoma in situ
V	Invasive cancer

ination is tailored to the degree of risk rather than when the examinations are performed on the customary annual basis. All women must be considered at risk for the development of squamous carcinoma of the cervix as soon as they become sexually active. Within the group of women at risk, a high-risk subgroup is recognized, consisting of those women who had an early onset of sexual activity, especially with multiple partners. These patients should commence annual screening at any age at which they are recognized. A woman may be assumed to be no longer at risk for the development of squamous carcinoma of the cervix when, having participated regularly in the screening program, she reaches the age of 60 without having had a smear showing significant atypia. Women who have never been sexually active have a low risk. It should be understood that there is no evidence that a cervical cytologic screening program will reduce the mortality from other gynecologic or medical conditions.

On the basis of the conclusions stated above, the following recommendations were made. In an effective screening program, smears should be obtained from all women over the age of 18 who have had sexual intercourse. If the initial smear is satisfactory and without significant atypia, a second smear should be obtained within 1 year. Provided that the initial two smears and all subsequent smears are satisfactory and without significant atypia, further smears should be obtained at approximately 3-year intervals until the age of 35 and at 5-year intervals thereafter until the age of 60. Women over the age of 60 who have had repeated satisfactory smears without significant atypia may be dropped from the screening program for squamous carcinoma of the cervix. Women who are not at high risk should be discouraged from having smears more frequently than is recommended. Women at continuing high risk should be screened annually.

The problem with these guidelines, however, is that they apply only to cervical cancer. The Papanicolaou test (Table 1-1) often brings the patient into the gynecologist's office, where she may be appropriately screened for other gynecologic malignancies and nonmalignant processes. As the age for development of cervical cancer passes, it is succeeded by the age for increasing incidence of ovarian carcinoma, which is a far more lethal process. Therefore, the recommendations of the Walton report need to be viewed in this framework, and the physician is encouraged to use considerable judgment in advising his patient.

Epidemiology and pathogenesis

The term "dysplasia" actually means "abnormality of development" and is used mainly with reference to atypical changes in the cervical epithelium. In general, the terms "dysplasia" and "basal cell hyperplasia" describe changes in the basal cells of the cervical squamous epithelium. Normally, the basal cell layer is one to two cells thick. In dysplasia, there is a proliferation of these cells, which show nuclear atypia, changes in the nuclear-cytoplasmic ratio, and often loss of polarity. Indeed, these cells have the typical appearance of neoplastic cells, but they do not invade the underlying tissues. Interestingly, maturation of some of the basal cells can occur, and often a few layers of stratified, cornified epithelium are found on the surface.

The cells making up this lesion are characterized by varying degrees of cytoplasmic maturation, whereas their nuclei are abnormally large even at high levels in the altered epithelium. The disordered growth is manifested by premature keratinization of the cells and also by abnormal differentiation of the most superficial cell layers. The ultimate cause of the abnormal reaction has not yet been established. These lesions are usually encountered during the active sexual period of life and may be found in the postmenopausal woman only in the presence of excess estrogenic effects. On gross examination the changes in dysplasia are not distinctive. There may be evidence to suggest the presence of white epithelium, and in other instances the uterine cervix may appear to be normal to the naked eye.

The term "carcinoma in situ" is applied to a lesion that has passed from the stage of hyperplasia or dysplasia to one of neoplasia, in which the laws of normal cell growth are wholly or partially lost but in which the cells have not produced invasion or metastases. The architecture of the epithelium is completely disrupted, with loss of all polarity. The division into basal, parabasal, intermediate, and superficial cornified layers is impossible, and there is complete absence of reasonable maturation.

Cervical intraepithelial neoplasia (CIN) can be divided into many categories (Table 1-2). Most of the current investigators in this area prefer to use a grading system that equates CIN I with mild dysplastic changes, CIN II with moderate dysplastic changes, and CIN III with severe dysplastic changes or overt carcinoma in situ. All of these lesions have the potential for progression to invasive cancer, but the changes in the higher-grade lesions such as CIN III progress more consistently than the milder changes, which may undergo spontaneous regression to a normal epithelium. The classification of lesions into categories CIN I through

Table 1-2. Classification of cervical intraepithelial neoplasia

CIN I	Mild dysplasia
CIN II	Moderate dysplasia
CIN III	Severe dysplasia Carcinoma in situ

Data from Richart, R. M.: Natural history of cervical intraepithelial neoplasia, Clin. Obstet. Gynecol. **10**:748, 1968.

CIN III is made by pathologists as they assess the degree of basal cell hyperplasia, cellular atypism, and loss of polarity in any particular specimen of epithelium. Since at present there is no satisfactory method for predicting which lesions will progress and which will not, the consensus is that all these lesions should be treated.

Numerous epidemiologic studies reported in the literature have established a positive association between cancer of the cervix and multiple interdependent social factors. There is a greater incidence of cervical cancer observed among blacks and Mexican-Americans, and this is undoubtedly related to their lower socioeconomic status. Increased occurrence of cancer of the cervix in multiparous women is probably related to other factors, such as age at first marriage and age at first pregnancy. This combined with the high incidence of the disease in prostitutes leads to a very firm conclusion that first coitus at an early age and multiple sexual partners definitely increase the probability of developing CIN. Even socioeconomic status is interrelated, since an association has long been noted between relative poverty and early marriage and youthful childbearing. The final common denominator appears to be not only onset of regular sexual activity before age 20 but also continued exposure to multiple sexual partners. Indeed, cervical cancer is very rare in celibate groups such as nuns, and many have labeled cancer of the cervix a "venereal disease."

More recently, the male factor in the epidemiology of this lesion has received considerable attention. It is known that the carcinogen has to be transmitted via coitus. It appears that certain males are more "carcinogenic" than others and that the carcinogenesis is related to the occupation of the male. As previously noted, most individuals from the lower socioeconomic class seem to be at a higher risk for developing cervical cancer. Cervical cancer mortality shows a strong social class gradient. Beral developed mortality ratios for cervical cancer based on social class and the husband's occupation, and a straight line correlation was established. Kessler attempted to further evaluate the role of the male in cervical carcinogenesis with an epidemiologic study. His method involved direct observation of two large groups of women; one group married to men who previously had wives who sustained cervical cancer and another group married to men without such a history. In the group married to men who had had other wives with cancer, he found 14 with cervical cancer compared with only 4 among the control group. Only 9 of these lesions were frankly invasive, several were intraepithelial disease or showed microinvasion, and two were adenocarcinoma. A corollary of the Beral study is the theory of Reid and associates. These authors have proposed that sperm act as the carcinogen in cervical neoplasia. They have found two basic types of protein, a histone and a protamine, in the ejaculate of human sperm. The ratio, although it varied widely in different males, was correlated with ranking by social class, with the lower social class having the greater proportion of protamine. The authors believe that these basic proteins found in the sperm head, particularly the protamines, may have a role in the etiology of cervical squamous carcinoma. They showed in tissue culture that sperm can actually penetrate normal mammalian cells, particularly cervical metaplastic epithelium.

Even if the carcinogen is identified, its interaction with the cervix depends on the specific female at risk. The epidemiologic data strongly suggest that the adolescent is at risk. The probable reason is that active metaplasia is occurring. Since there is active proliferation of cellular transformation from columnar to metaplastic to squamoid epithelium, the potential for interaction between the carcinogen and the cervix is increased. Once this process of metaplasia is complete, it appears that the cervix is no longer at high risk, although CIN certainly can occur in patients who are virginal until after this process has been completed. It would appear, however, that the latter patients are the exception rather than the rule.

The strikingly low incidence of cervical cancer in Jewish women demands explanation. This, along with the observation that penile cancer is also extremely rare among Jews, has led to the hypothesis that circumcision has a protective effect and that smegma of uncircumsized males plays a role in carcinogenesis. This association has been brought into considerable doubt by other studies on Moslems. Ritual circumcision is also practiced among this religious group, and studies of comparable noncircumcised groups from the same countries and localities are inconclusive for substantiating smegma as a carcinogen.

Some epidemiologic features of cervical cancer suggest that a carcinogen, such as a virus, may be carried by the male; this carcinogen may be venereally transmitted to the female. Viruses are known to produce malignancies in animals, and it is possible that they could also produce malignancies in humans. If a venereally transmitted virus is etiologically related to cervical cancer, it might be expected that the agent is a common inhabitant in the female genital tract. The number of viruses known to infect the genital tract of women is relatively small. Cytomegalovirus can be isolated from the cervix of some pregnant women, but there is no evidence supporting venereal transmission of this virus. Condyloma acuminatum is probably of viral etiology, but it has not been possible to isolate a virus from this lesion. On the other hand, herpesvirus type 2 is a common genital pathogen, and this virus is venereally transmitted. The relationship of herpesvirus type 2 to cervical cancer is under active investigation. Rawls and his associates found neutralizing antibodies to herpesvirus type 2 in the sera of a significantly greater number of women with cervical cancer than in the sera of matched controls. Firm evidence linking herpesvirus to cervical cancer is lacking.

The average age of patients with carcinoma in situ reproducibly is 10 to 15 years less than the average age of patients with invasive cancer of the cervix. In most series, the average age of patients with carcinoma in situ is 33 to 38 years and the average age of those with invasive disease, 43 to 48 years. However, there are many exceptions, and in the past 2 decades carcinoma in situ as well as invasive disease has been reported in an increasing number of patients in their late teens and early twenties. Whether all invasive carcinomas begin as in situ lesions is unknown, but Peterson reported that in one third of 127 untreated patients invasive carcinoma developed subsequently to carcinoma in situ at the end of 9 years. Masterson found that 28% of 25 untreated patients demonstrated invasive carcinoma at the end of 5 years.

Carcinoma in situ is usually asymptomatic, and on routine examination the lesion is frequently not observed. Recognition of the lesion is assisted considerably by the use of cytology and/or colposcopy. The mucous membrane sometimes bleeds easily on contact, and erosions or a superficial defect of the ectocervix is relatively common in patients with carcinoma in situ, but these findings are not pathognomonic. The diagnosis must always be confirmed by histologic sections of a biopsy specimen.

What happens to a patient with early CIN in regard to its natural history is important as it relates to management. If we could predict the eventual outcome of a given patient with an abnormal Papanicolaou smear, the problem of management would be greatly simplified. Certainly, not all patients with abnormal cervical cells develop cancer of the cervix or even progression of CIN.

Unfortunately, most of the studies performed on the natural history of this disease were carried out in the absence of today's diagnostic techniques, namely, colposcopy. Most studies used either cytologic tests or biopsy as the diagnostic tools, resulting in varying progression/regression rates. Kessler reviewed many of the studies on the biologic behavior of cervical dysplasia. The occurrence of progression of CIN lesions to either a more severe form or invasive cancer ranges from 1.4% to 60%. Of interest is the fact that the two most variant studies used cytologic tests alone to follow patients. The problems of definitive diagnosis using this technique have been studied in detail, and considerable variation has been noted even in the best of hands. When biopsies are performed, particularly if the lesion is small, the natural history of the disease may be disrupted, further complicating the evaluation of this entity. Even studies on the biologic behavior of cervical carcinoma in situ are varied, with progression to invasive cancer being reported in 0% to 35% of cases. The difference in these findings may very well be due to the length of follow-up once the diagnosis of carcinoma in situ was established. Needless to say, some patients with CIN do develop invasive cancer, whereas others, even though followed for many years, do not progress either to a more severe form of CIN or to invasive cancer.

It has become apparent from recent studies that CIN is being diagnosed at a much younger age than it was previously. In our own material, the median age for carcinoma in situ of the cervix has decreased from approximately 40 to 28 years of age. This may reflect only that screening of high-risk patients is done at an earlier time, resulting in diagnosis at a younger age. Certainly it is not at all unusual to see patients in their teens or early twenties with carcinoma in situ of the cervix. Therefore, we may be identifying the lesion early in the spectrum of disease, and a patient may continue with CIN for a prolonged period even after reaching the level of a CIN III lesion. Table 1-3 presents the transition time of intraepithelial neoplasia in our patients. Those patients who progress to carcinoma in situ do so within a very short interval. Once that level of abnormality has been reached, stabilization may occur in

Table 1-3. Transition time of intraepithelial neoplasia

	Mean years
Normal to mild-moderate dysplasia	1.62
Normal to moderate-severe dysplasia	2.20
Normal to carcinoma in situ	4.51

many of the patients. To date, there is no method for predicting which patient will remain within the CIN category and which will progress to a more severe form of CIN or to invasive cancer or in what time frame this transition will take place.

Evaluation of an abnormal cervical smear

To fully understand our recommendations for the management of an abnormal cervical smear, the following points should be noted:

1. The cervical Papanicolaou cytologic smear, or Pap test, is not a diagnostic tool but a screening mechanism. Diagnosis rests with a tissue biopsy. .
2. The Pap test is valid only for the screening of cervical neoplasia. Malignant conditions of the corpus, tubes, or ovaries are infrequently associated with positive cervical cytologic findings.
3. The Pap test must be performed with care to yield optimum accuracy. The cervix must be sampled at the squamocolumnar junction, where most lesions apparently originate. In the postmenopausal woman this junction may lie high within the endocervical canal. The sampling for every cervical smear should evaluate both the epithelium of the portio of the cervix by scraping it (usually using a wood or plastic spatula) and the epithelium of the endocervix by placing a saline-moistened cotton-tipped applicator into the canal or aspirating the contents of the canal with a bulb pipette. Both samples can be placed on the same glass slide, thus minimizing handling costs.
4. All possible explanations for the abnormal cytologic findings should be considered (Table 1-4).

The results of the recent studies on the origin and behavior of preinvasive cervical neoplasia as well as the ever increasing number of young women presenting with this disease require a reassessment of the commonly used methods of evaluating the patient with an abnormal Pap test. As a result of multiple studies of dysplasia, the belief now prevails that cervical neoplasia is a spectrum of epithelial abnormalities ranging from dysplasia to carcinoma in situ to invasive cancer. The techniques of evaluation and treatment presented here are based on the consideration that this premise is valid. The traditional manner of evaluating a patient with an abnormal Pap test suggestive of mild dysplasia or worse, or class III or worse, included repeat cytologic screening, close examination of the cervix, Schiller staining, or biopsy of nonstaining areas. If the biopsy sites showed moderate dysplasia or worse, the patient was offered a cold-knife conization to rule out invasive cancer and to confirm

Table 1-4. Causes of abnormal Pap smears   *(Keep all women for good Pap)*

Invasive cancer	Regeneration after injury (metaplasia)
Carcinoma in situ	Vaginal cancer
Dysplasia	Vulvar cancer
Condyloma acuminatum	Upper genital tract cancer (endometrium, fallopian
Inflammation, especially trichomoniasis and	tube, ovary)
chronic cervicitis	Previous radiation therapy

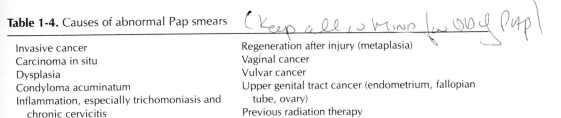

Fig. 1-2, Abnormal Pap smear. Appropriate therapy is individualized after cone biopsy (no invasion found) but is usually a choice between hysterectomy and no further therapy with a plan for careful surveillance.

histologic and cytologic findings. If conization showed severe dysplasia or carcinoma in situ, a hysterectomy was generally performed. Conization was considered therapeutic if moderate dysplasia or less was noted on pathologic review. This method is still used in many centers where colposcopy is not available.

With the advent of colposcopy, the treatment plan outlined above appeared to many to be unnecessary, expensive, and potentially hazardous. A more conservative schema and treatment plan for the patient with an abnormal Pap test has been used in many clinics during the past decade (Fig. 1-2). This schema is safe only if the steps are rigorously followed. This is particularly critical when the endocervical curettage (ECC) findings are positive, even though the lesion is completely seen. In this situation, only an expert colposcopist should proceed with local treatment; otherwise a diagnostic conization must be performed. The possibility of a coexisting unsuspected endocervical adenocarcinoma must also be considered. Omission of any of the diagnostic procedures in the evaluation may lead to the tragedy that results when invasive cancer is missed. A report by Sevin and associates of eight such cases, out of which three patients were lost, emphasizes the hazards of a less than optimal workup of patients before cryotherapy.

Not all patients need repeat cytologic screening, and its value appears to be limited to those patients whose previous cytologic examinations have been inconclusive. In performing a Pap test, one should exercise care to sample the squamocolumnar junction, or transformation zone, for it is here that the neoplastic processes begin. A thoroughly saline-moistened cotton-tipped applicator and a disposable plastic or wood spatula are commonly used for obtaining a specimen for cytology. The cotton-tipped applicator collects cells primarily from the cervical canal, whereas the spatula collects cells from the portio of the cervix. This combination of collection techniques should minimize the false-negative rate of cervical cytologic findings due to physician failures (often quoted between 5% and 15%). A report by Gad and Koch suggests that their false-negative rate can be as high as 27% and half the errors are cytotechnology failures.

This evaluation schema permits triage of patients based on the colposcopic findings (plus the results of the colposcopically directed biopsies) and the endocervical curettage findings. If the results of curettage of the canal are negative and only preinvasive neoplasia is found on directed biopsy, the patient has been adequately evaluated and treatment can begin. The method of therapy chosen depends on the patient's age, desire for fertility, and reliability for follow-up and on the histologic appearance and extent of her lesion. Cryosurgery using the double-freeze technique or destruction of the lesion with a laser beam can be performed in a number of patients who wish to retain their childbearing capacity and have disease that is more extensive than can adequately be treated with a simple office excisional biopsy. Hysterectomy, either simple vaginal or abdominal, without preceding conization is recommended for those patients who desire sterilization and have severe dysplasia or carcinoma in situ. No effort is made in the performance of the hysterectomy to excise additional vaginal cuff unless there is evidence of abnormal epithelium extending to the vagina; this occurs in less than 3% of patients. A final possibility for treatment is to perform a shallow conization or ring biopsy of the cervix.

A second major group is those patients with positive endocervical curettage findings. In our experience, roughly 15% of patients with an abnormal Pap test have positive endocervical curettage results. These women may have occult disease in the endocervical canal, and invasion carcinoma should be strongly suspected. In this group, two populations can be identified: in one, repeat colposcopy produces clear visualization of the upper limits of the disease process, and in the other, this is not possible. Since it is axiomatic that all neoplastic changes begin at the transformation zone and are contiguous with that zone, one is safe in assuming that the entire lesion has been visualized if the limits of the lesion can be identified clearly. The patient with positive endocervical curettage results in whom the entire lesion can be visualized thus presents a dilemma, which is discussed below.

As noted in the schema we have presented here for evaluation of the abnormal Pap smear, endocervical curettage is performed on all nonpregnant patients. Diagnostic conization must be seriously considered whenever endocervical curettage shows dysplastic cells or whenever colposcopic examination is unsatisfactory (the entire transformation zone is not seen). Since curettage is performed from the internal os to the external os, the lesion that extends only slightly into the canal is often picked up by the curette, resulting in a number of false-positive endocervical curettage results. Nonetheless, endocervical curettage should be performed on all patients unless they are pregnant, and if errors are made they should be made on the side of conization. Some physicians do not routinely perform endocervical curettage when the entire lesion is visible on the exocervix. Although omitting this procedure may be appropriate for a few experienced colposcopists, its inclusion as a routine step will further reduce the chances of missing a lesion in the endocervix. On occasion a previously unsuspected adenocarcinoma of the endocervix will be diagnosed, but even more frequently an early invasive squamous carcinoma will be uncovered.

In those individuals in whom the curettage findings are positive and the upper limits cannot be visualized, diagnostic conization must be performed to exclude or confirm invasive cancer. Care should be taken in performing conization to include a sufficient portion of the endocervical canal to rule out occult invasive disease high in the canal.

Kaufman and Irwin reported a series of 395 patients with CIN (126 with CIN III lesions) treated with cryosurgery and followed for 1 to 8 years. Their failure rate was less than 15% when all patients were carefully evaluated before treatment. They stressed the importance of endocervical curettage. However, their failure rate with CIN III lesions was almost 20%. Other experienced colposcopists have been discouraged by the high failure rate in the treatment of CIN III lesions with cryotherapy, even in the face of negative curettage findings. Indeed, many authors have recommended that conization be used for any patient demonstrating a CIN III lesion on cervical biopsy. We would recommend that the physician evaluate the circumstances in light of his own experience and skill with the colposcope. Our advice to all but the most experienced colposcopists would be to use conization when there is any doubt in the mind of the physician as to the true nature of the lesion. CIN III lesions limited to one quadrant of the cervix and easily demarcated colposcopically may well be treated by local therapy and close follow-up examinations of the patient (especially in the very young nulliparous woman). On the other hand, patients with diffuse involvement of the cervix (two or more quadrants) with CIN III lesions should be seriously considered for conization, even by an experienced colposcopist. Recent data would suggest that the failure rate from cryotherapy in CIN III lesions can be very high even in excellent clinics. Ostergard found a 37% failure rate among patients with CIN III lesions treated with cryotherapy and followed for 1 to 8 years.

Results such as these require that conization be considered seriously as the therapeutic modality for CIN III lesions.

Recently attention has been drawn to the fact that several patients have been reported to have invasive carcinoma of the cervix after cryosurgery. A report from Miami details eight patients who were treated by cryosurgery for various indications and subsequently were found to have invasive cancer. Only five of the patients had abnormal cervical cytologic findings, three had colposcopic examination, two had colposcopically directed biopsies, and only one had endocervical curettage. The importance of proper evaluation before outpatient treatment has been previously stated and should be apparent.

Endocervical curettage is performed from the internal os to the external os. The external os is the structure that is created by the opening of the bivalve speculum. In evaluating the patient with an abnormal Pap smear, a speculum as large as the patient can tolerate should be used. During curettage it is best to curette first the upper half of the canal and then the lower half. Short, firm motions in a circumferential pattern are the most satisfactory. Patients will experience some discomfort early in the procedure but rarely does the physician have to stop because of discomfort. It is desirable to obtain endocervical stroma in the specimen if possible. Upon completion of the curettage, all blood, mucus, and cellular debris must be collected and placed on a 2 × 2 absorbent paper towel. The material is then folded into a mound and, along with the absorbent paper towel, placed into fixative. If any neoplastic tissue is found by the pathologist in the curettings, the results are considered positive. Directed punch biopsies of the cervix are done after the curettage. Using the colposcopic findings as a guide, punch biopsy specimens are obtained with a Kevorkian-Young cervical biopsy instrument (or a similar tool that contains a basket in which the biopsy specimen may be collected). The biopsy specimens should also be placed on a small piece of paper towel or sliced cucumber with proper orientation to minimize tangential sectioning of the specimen.

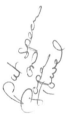

Colposcopic evaluation of the cervix in the patient with an abnormal cervical smear has dramatically altered the management of the patient afflicted during pregnancy. The schema outlined above is closely followed in pregnancy, where the transformation zone is everted, making visualization of the entire lesion almost a certainty. Cone biopsy is rarely indicated during pregnancy except when punch biopsy results suggest microinvasive cancer. This diagnosis must be confirmed by cone biopsy to allow proper management. Pregnant patients with a firm diagnosis of preinvasive or microinvasive disease of the cervix should be allowed to deliver vaginally, and further therapy can be tailored to their needs after delivery. The cervix is very vascular during pregnancy so that avoiding cone biopsy is in the best interest of both mother and fetus. *Small* biopsies of the *most* colposcopically abnormal areas are recommended in an effort to minimize bleeding in the diagnostic evaluation. When a patient is in the second or third trimester and colposcopic examination is negative for any suspicion of invasion, many colposcopists will defer all biopsies to the postpartum period. Lurain and Gallup reported on 131 pregnant patients with abnormal smears managed in this manner with excellent results and no invasive cancers missed.

Technique of colposcopy

Colposcopy was introduced by Hans Hinselman in 1925 (Hamburg, Germany) as a result of his efforts to devise a practical method of more minute and comprehensive examination of the cervix. He and others of his era believed that cervical cancer began as miniature nodules on the surface epithelium and that with increased magnification and illumination these lesions would be detectable. The meticulous examination of thousands of cases enabled him to clearly define the multiple physiologic and benign changes in the cervix as well as to correlate atypical changes with preinvasive and early invasive cancer. Unfortunately, Hinselman was primarily a clinician with very little pathology background, and this, in conjunction with the encumbrance of the tumor nodule theory, led to the development of confusing concepts and terminology associated with the use of the colposcope.

In the early 1930s, initial efforts were made to introduce colposcopy in the United States as a method of early cervical cancer detection. Owing to the cumbersome terminology present at that time, the method was generally ignored, and with the introduction of reliable cytology in the 1940s North American physicians lost interest in colposcopy. The interest was renewed in the 1950s and early 1960s, but acceptance was slow because of the competitive nature of cytologic examinations, which were more economical and easier to perform and had, for the novice, a lower false-negative rate. Over the last 2 decades the technique has gained a long-awaited popularity and has been recognized as an adjunctive technique to cytologic testing in the investigation of genital tract epithelium. The recent popularity of colposcopy has been enhanced by the discovery of a scientific basis for most morphologic changes and the acceptance of a logical and simplified terminology for these changes.

The colposcope consists, in general, of a stereoscopic, binocular microscope with low magnification. It is provided with a center illuminating device and mounted on an adjustable stand with a transformer in the base. Several levels of magnification are available, the most useful being between 8 and 18 X. A green filter is placed between the light source and the tissue to accentuate the vascular patterns and color tone differences between normal and abnormal patterns. Many instruments used in the operating rooms and offices of neurosurgeons, ophthalmologists, and otolaryngologists are essentially colposcopes. Examination of the epithelium of the female genital tract by colposcopy takes no more than a few minutes in the usual case.

Colposcopy is based on study of the transformation zone (Fig. 1-3). The transformation zone is that area of the cervix and vagina that was initially covered by columnar epithelium and through a process referred to as metaplasia has undergone replacement by squamous epithelium. The wide range and variation in the colposcopic features of this tissue make up the science of colposcopy. The inheritance of variable vascular patterns, as well as the fate of residual columnar glands and clefts, determines the great variety of patterns in this zone. It had been generally taught

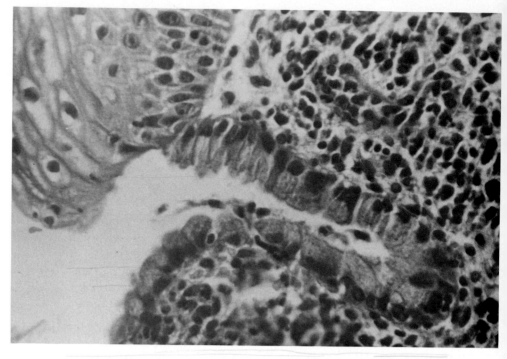

Fig. 1-3. Squamocolumnar junction (transformation zone).

that the cervix was normally covered by squamous epithelium and that the presence of endocervical columnar epithelium on the ectocervix portio was an abnormal finding. Studies by Malcolm Coppleson and his associates have established that columnar tissue can initially exist on the ectocervix in at least 70% of young women and extend onto the vaginal fornix in an additional 5% of the female population. This process of transition from columnar to squamous epithelium probably occurs throughout a woman's lifetime. However, it has been demonstrated that this normal physiologic transformation zone is most active during three periods of a woman's life, i.e., fetal development, adolescence, and during her first pregnancy. It is known that the process is enhanced by an acid pH environment and is considerably influenced by estrogen and progesterone levels.

The classification of colposcopic findings has been improved and simplified, facilitating the recognition of abnormal patterns: white epithelium (Fig. 1-4), mosaic structure (Fig. 1-5), punctation (Fig. 1-6), leukoplakia, and atypical vessels (Fig. 1-7). The term "leukoplakia" is generally reserved for the heavy, thick, white lesion that can frequently be seen with the naked eye. White epithelium, mosaic structure, and/or punctation herald atypical epithelium (CIN) and provide the target for directed biopsies. The pattern of atypical vessels is most often associated with invasive cancer, and biopsies should be performed liberally in areas with these findings. Although the abnormal colposcopic patterns reflect cytologic and histologic alterations, they are not specific enough for final diagnosis, and biopsy is necessary. The colpo-

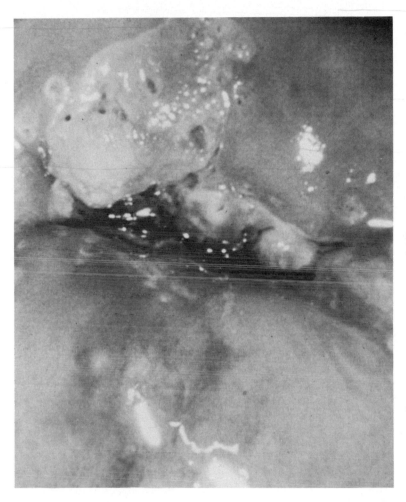

Fig. 1-4. White epithelium at cervical os (colposcopic view).

White Epithelium
MOSAIC Structure   } Colposcopic
Puctation   } Terminology
      Atypical VESSEL }

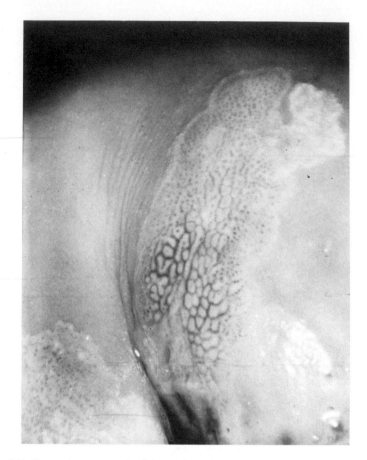

Fig. 1-5. Punctation pattern clearly seen above a mosaic structure (colposcopic view).

scope's greatest value is in directing the biopsy to the area that is most likely to yield the most significant histologic pattern.

In performing colposcopy a standard procedure is followed. First the cervix is sampled for cytologic screening, and then it is cleansed with a 3% acetic acid solution to remove the excess mucus and cellular debris. The acetic acid also accentuates the difference between normal and abnormal colposcopic patterns. The colposcope is focused on the cervix and the transformation zone, including the squamocolumnar junction, and the area is inspected in a clockwise fashion. In most instances the entire lesion can be outlined and the most atypical area can be selected for biopsy. If the lesion extends up the canal beyond the vision of the colposcopist, the patient will require a diagnostic conization to define the disease. Endocervical curettage is performed whether or not the lesion extends up the canal, and if invasive cancer is found at any time, plans for a cone biopsy are of course abandoned. This plan of investigation, which is outlined in Fig. 1-2, is based on the assumption that there are no areas of intraepithelial neoplasia higher up in the canal if indeed the upper

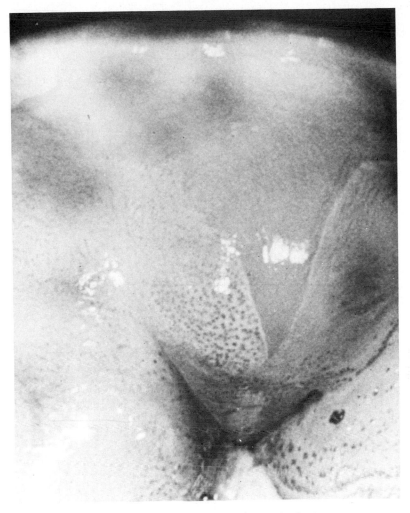

Fig. 1-6. Punctation pattern (colposcopic view).

limits of the lesion can be seen colposcopically. In other words, intraepithelial neoplasia begins at the transformation zone and extends contiguously to other areas of
the cervix such that if the upper limits can be visualized one can be assured that
additional disease is not present higher in the canal. The colposcope only suggests
an abnormality; final diagnosis must rest on a tissue examination by a pathologist.
Selected spot biopsies in the areas showing atypical colposcopic patterns, under direct colposcopic guidance and in combination with cytologic testing, give the highest
possible accuracy in the diagnosis and evaluation of the cervix. Probably the greatest
value of colposcopy is that in most instances a skilled colposcopist can establish and
differentiate invasive cancer from intraepithelial neoplasia by direct biopsy and thus
avoid the necessity of surgical conization of the cervix. This is especially valuable in

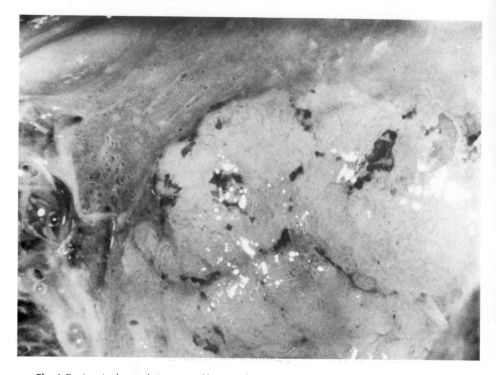

Fig. 1-7. Atypical vessels in a sea of heavy white epithelium sometimes called leukoplakia.

the young nulliparous woman desirous of childbearing in whom cone biopsy of the cervix may result in problems of impaired fertility. The avoidance of conization also is valuable in reducing the risk to the patient from anesthesia and the additional surgical procedure with its prolonged hospitalization.

Several modalities of treatment are available to the CIN patient that can be performed on an outpatient basis. If in fact these modalities are as effective as a surgical procedure accomplished in the operating room, the cost-effectiveness is of considerable importance. Electrocautery has been used for many years to eradicate cervical epithelium. It was fashionable historically to destroy the "abnormal" tissue found on the cervix after delivery. Actually, this was columnar epithelium, or the transformation zone of the cervix. Some uncontrolled studies have suggested that electrocautery decreased the appearance of CIN lesions in patients so treated. Electrocautery has been shown to be effective in the treatment of CIN. The popularity of this treatment has been more apparent in Europe and Australia than in this country. In a small controlled study, Wilbanks and associates showed that electrocautery was effective in destroying early CIN as compared with tetracycline vaginal suppositories and with a control group of patients. Ortiz and associates treated all forms of CIN with electrocautery. In CIN I and II lesions no failures were noted. In CIN III disease the failure rate was approximately 13%. Of interest is that the failure rate in those patients with carcinoma in situ did not differ whether the glands were involved

Table 1-5. Electrocautery treatment in CIN

	Failures
CIN I	11/130 (8.5%)
CIN II	6/111 (5.4%)
CIN III	11/197 (5.5%)

Data from Chanen, W., and Hollyock, V. E.: Colposcopy and the conservative management of cervical dysplasias and carcinoma in situ, Obstet. Gynecol. **43:**527, 1974.

or not. All the patients were treated on an outpatient basis. Chanen and Hollyock have used this technique extensively in Australia. Table 1-5 illustrates the excellent results they reported. An update of their experience was recently reported at the World Congress for Cervical Pathology and Colposcopy in Orlando, Florida. They treated more than 800 patients with a failure rate of only 5%. It was stated that only four patients had difficulty with cervical stenosis. Dilation and curettage (D&C) is done at the same time the electrocautery is performed. The patients are admitted to the hospital and electrocautery is performed under anesthesia in the operating room in order to burn the tissue deep enough to destroy disease that might be present in glands. Chanen and Hollyock believe that this is necessary to obtain excellent results. Electrocautery, of course, is painful if the tissue is burned deeply. If a patient needs to be anesthetized in order to obtain these results, this negates any benefits that a lesser procedure than conization would obtain. The cost of hospitalization even on an ambulatory service would be considerably higher than outpatient treatment.

Cryosurgery

During the last decade, considerable experience with cryosurgery has been obtained in the treatment of CIN. The side effects of electrocautery, mainly pain during treatment, are not present with cryosurgery, and thus it is an ideal outpatient modality as far as patient comfort is concerned. Previous data from Duke University (Table 1-6) noted that cryosurgery was effective in treating CIN I and II disease as compared with controls.

Cryosurgery is most conveniently performed within 1 week after the cessation of the last menstrual period. This practice will help avoid treating a patient with an early pregnancy and also permit the most active phase of regeneration to take place prior to the onset of the next menses. Treatment is usually performed in the office or clinic without the need for anesthesia or analgesia. Nitrous oxide is the preferred refrigerant for most purposes. A speculum as large as the patient will tolerate is used, and the blades should be fully extended. This practice provides optimum visualization of the cervix and reduces the chance of freezing vaginal epithelium. All mucus and cellular debris must be removed from the vagina and cervix with cotton balls soaked in 3% acetic acid solution. The full extent of the disease to be treated should previously have been carefully outlined colposcopically, and a cervical probe that best conforms to the anatomic configuration of the cervix should be attached to

Table 1-6. Results of cryosurgery in early cervical neoplasia

	Regression	Unchanged	Progression
Controls	6	8	7
Cryosurgery	19	1	0

the freezing gun. If the lesion is much larger than the surface area of the probe tip, the abnormal area should be subdivided and each zone individually frozen. The probe is thoroughly moistened with a water-soluble lubricant to make sure of proper heat transfer, and the probe tip at room temperature is firmly positioned on the cervix so that the greatest extent of the lesion is covered. A tenaculum is rarely necessary to stabilize the cervix and should be avoided since it can cause excess bleeding and unnecessary pain. The refrigerant should be circulated as soon as the probe has been properly positioned. Ice crystals will first form on the back of the probe tip and then spread laterally from the edge of the probe. The lateral spread of the ice-ball can be expected within 10 to 15 seconds after the refrigerant has been circulated. If timing is to be done, it should be initiated at the commencement of the lateral spread of the ice-ball. In general, it is far more important to ensure that the ice-ball extends at least 4 to 5 mm onto the colposcopically normal–appearing epithelium, and the actual duration of freezing is far less important than the extent of the freeze process. When the procedure has been timed, we have noted that the average freeze is about 2 to 3 minutes in duration. It is not necessary to know the probe tip temperature since one is guided by the extent of the visible ice-ball, which is closely related to the area of future necrosis. Often a small portion of the vagina will become attached to the probe during the freezing process with no serious sequelae. On the other hand, when a rather large area of the vagina becomes attached to the probe tip, the procedure should be discontinued and the instrument reapplied. Once the areas to be frozen have been adequately treated, the probe is defrosted and removed. At this point the cervix is carefully inspected again to be certain that the ice-ball has extended over all abnormal areas and the necessary 4 to 5 mm onto normal-appearing epithelium. Only a freeze-thaw cycle is used by some if nitrous oxide is the refrigerant. If liquid freon or carbon dioxide gas is used as the refrigerant, a freeze, partial thaw, and refreeze cycle should be employed to achieve satisfactory tissue necrosis. Our preference is to use the double-freeze technique on all patients, with adequate defrosting (3 to 5 minutes) between freezes.

Posttreatment side effects are usually few and not of a serious nature. A profuse watery discharge is noted for approximately 2 to 4 weeks after cryosurgery. This is somewhat of a nuisance to the patient but in most instances presents little problem. Coitus as well as the use of tampons is discouraged during the time of the watery discharge. The patient is asked to return in 4 months for a follow-up examination including a Pap smear. If repeat cytologic testing is done before that time, the patient may be erroneously described as having abnormal cells when in fact the reparative process mimics an abnormality. This differentiation is extremely difficult even in experienced hands. The criterion used for successful treatment is the appearance of three normal Pap smears after cryosurgery. If abnormal cytologic findings are noted at 4 months, a Pap smear is obtained in another month to 6 weeks, and if cytologic findings still remain abnormal at 6 months, one must consider the freeze procedure a failure. At that time the patient needs to be reevaluated, and other treatment or refreezing can then be considered. Other complications such as occasional spotting and cervical stenosis have been reported. Subsequent infertility in patients who have had cervical cryosurgery has not been a frequently reported finding. The endocervical glands appear to regenerate, leaving in most instances a normal endocervical canal. Patients must then be followed by means of periodic cytologic smears. The constant surveillance required when such conservative therapy is used makes it of questionable value for a patient whose family is complete.

Laser surgery

One of the most promising new developments in the treatment of CIN was the introduction of the surgical laser several years ago. As with any new modality, time and experience are needed to see if clinical reality will meet theoretical promise. The term "laser" is an abbreviation for "light amplification by stimulated emission of radiation." Conventional light produces a spontaneous emission that spreads in all directions. The wavelength of spontaneously emitted light is not precise but spreads over a certain range of the light spectrum. The main difference between laser and conventional light is that the laser produces a coherent light, a parallel beam of uniform wavelength that can be focused by a lens into an area of smaller dimensions, producing a powerful density of unprecedented magnitude.

The carbon dioxide laser, currently in clinical use, has an electrical discharge produced from a mixture of carbon dioxide, nitrogen, and helium, giving rise to an infrared invisible beam. This laser beam is continuous, unlike the pulse laser beams that were present in the initial laser instruments. The carbon dioxide laser is used in neurosurgery and otolaryngology as well as in the control of bleeding gastric ulcers and in debridement of third-degree burns. A recent 2-year study by Carter and associates at the University of Kansas concluded that laser surgery offers advantages to the patient and the surgeon and may replace cryosurgery and cauterization in outpatient treatment of CIN. In another study by Mylotte and associates, similar conclusions were reached. In addition, scanning electron microscopy documented the fact that, unlike with cryotherapy, cervices treated with the CO_2 laser were completely reepithelialized 2 weeks after laser treatment. Cryotherapy is followed by a much longer healing process. Perhaps even more significant, it would appear that with completion of the reepithelialization process, the original architecture of the cervix is fully preserved and the squamocolumnar junction remains visible. With cryotherapy, migration of the transformation zone up the endocervical canal is common, thus obscuring this critical diagnostic structure. It would also appear that recurrence rates may be as low as or lower than with cryosurgery. As with any new modality, long-term studies are needed before any cogent conclusions can be reached regarding laser surgery. Our experience would suggest two disadvantages to the technique that we have not experienced with cryosurgery. First, the process is more painful for the office patient than cryosurgery, and second, the destruction of all but the smallest lesions requires much more time from both patient and physician.

Although the preliminary data suggest that the laser can be used to destroy CIN, laser surgery must be considered experimental at this time and should be restricted to those medical centers that have established protocols for study. The cost of the instrument also would be prohibitive for most clinics, therefore restricting its use.

Conization of the cervix

After the extent of involvement of epithelium on the ectocervix has been clearly demarcated by colposcopy and/or Schiller's test, the limits of the base of the cone biopsy on the cervix can be determined. An incision that is certain to include all of the abnormal areas is made into the mucous membrane of the ectocervix. Many believe that blood loss can be lessened by injecting a dilute solution of phenylephrine (Neo-Synephrine) into the line of incision before commencing the procedure. This incision need not be circular but should have as its objective excision of all atypical epithelium. The depth of the incision as it tapers toward the endocervical

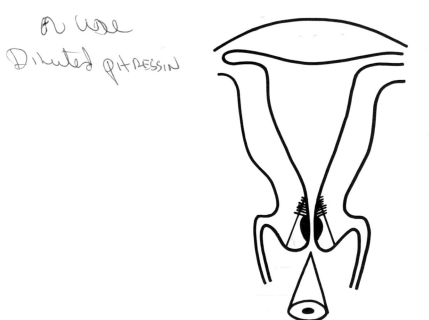

or use
Diluted pit-Ressin

Fig. 1-8. Cone biopsy for endocervical disease. Limits of the lesion were not seen colposcopically.

canal should be determined by the length of the cervical canal and the suspected depth of involvement (Fig. 1-8). Many times the entire limits of the lesion have been visualized, and a very shallow conization is sufficient (Fig. 1-9). Cervical conization need not be a fixed technical procedure for all patients, but it should always be an adequate excision of all involved areas. Bleeding from the cone bed is usually controlled by hemostatic sutures, such as anterior and posterior Sturmdorf sutures or a running-lock suture of heavy chromic material, encompassing the circumference of the cone bed. Others prefer to establish hemostasis and then leave the cone bed open to healing by secondary intention. Significant cervical stenosis, cervical incompetence, or infertility with a cervical factor are rare complications (Table 1-7) and are functions of the amount of endocervix removed.

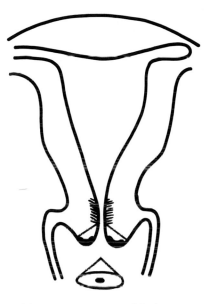

Fig. 1-9. Cone biopsy for CIN of the exocervix. Limits of the lesion were identified colposcopically.

Table 1-7. Major complications of conization

Immediate	Delayed
Hemorrhage	Bleeding (10-14 days after operation)
Uterine perforation	Cervical stenosis
Anesthetic risk	Infertility
In pregnancy:	Incompetent cervix
Rupture of membranes	
Premature labor	

Choice of therapy

Decisions as to choice of therapy for CIN depend on many factors, including the patient's attitudes and the experiences of the physician involved. Removal of the cervix or hysterectomy continues to be the definitive therapy in patients who are fully informed regarding the implications to their childbearing capacity and are in agreement in spite of the small but increased risk associated with a major operative procedure.

Patients with CIN I and II lesions who wish to maintain optimum fertility should be considered for local therapy including cryosurgery, laser surgery, and, where possible, local excision. This approach is also valid for patients with CIN III lesions that are limited to one quadrant of the cervix and can be easily outlined colposcopically. Diffuse CIN III lesions may be treated by local office therapy, but the patient and physician should be aware of the increased probability of recurrence and the necessity for posttherapy surveillance. Conization is preferred for patients with diffuse CIN III lesions regardless of whether the limits of the lesion can be clearly defined colposcopically.

In Europe (especially Scandinavia), conization has been widely used to treat patients with CIN, and some interesting data have been published. Bjerre and associates reported on 2,099 cases of women with abnormal vaginal smears in whom conization of the cervix had been performed. The frequency of complications was considered low, and cervical carcinoma in situ was diagnosed in 1,500 cases. Conization appeared to be curative in 87% of these 1,500 cases. Failure was related to whether the margins of resection were free of pathologic epithelium. If smears were repeatedly negative for the first year after conization, subsequent abnormal smears were found in only 0.4% of the cases. Kolstad and Klem reported on a series of 1,121 patients with carcinoma in situ who had been followed for 5 to 25 years. Therapeutic conization had been performed on 795 of these patients, of which 19 (2.3%) had recurrent carcinoma in situ and 7 (0.9%) developed invasive cancer. The corresponding figures for 238 patients treated by hysterectomy were, respectively, three (1.2%) and five (2.1%). The invasive lesions noted appeared several years later, and the type of initial procedure had no significant influence. Kolstad and Klem stressed that women who have had carcinoma in situ of the cervix will always be at some risk and therefore should be carefully followed for a much longer period than the conventional 5 years.

INTRAEPITHELIAL NEOPLASIA OF THE VAGINA
Clinical profile

Carcinoma in situ of the vagina has been reported sporadically in the last 3 decades, particularly in patients previously treated for cervical carcinoma in situ. The first report was apparently by Graham and Meigs in 1952. They reported on three patients with carcinoma of the vagina, two intraepithelial and one invasive, which were discovered 6, 7, and 10 years after total hysterectomy for carcinoma in situ of the cervix. Other reports have described multiple primary cancers of the vagina and

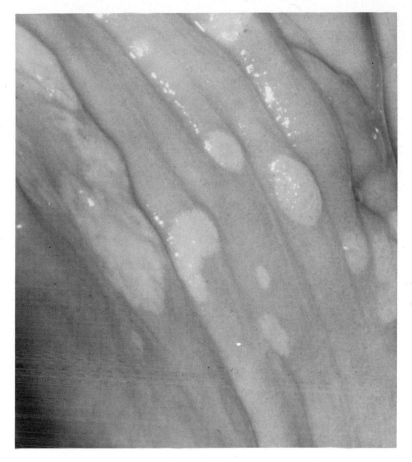

Fig. 1-10. Carcinoma in situ of the vagina (colposcopic view).

cervix and/or vulva. Several authors have commented on the "field response" of the cervix, vagina, and vulva, which suggests that the squamous epithelium of the lower genital tract may be affected in multiple sites by a similar carcinogenic trigger. Apparent extension of invasive carcinoma of the cervix to the vagina and vestibule may represent simultaneous carcinomas at sites affected by a constant carcinogenic stimulus of several end-organs in the genital tract.

Carcinoma in situ of the vagina is much less common than that of the cervix or vulva. Isolated lesions can usually be recognized colposcopically (Fig. 1-10) as white epithelium, mosaicism, and/or punctation, although some authors have described a "pink blush" appearance or a slightly granular texture. The diagnosis is usually confirmed by biopsy, and the limits of the lesion can be identified either with the colposcope or with iodine staining (Schiller stain).

Almost all lesions are asymptomatic, although an occasional patient will present with postcoital staining. An abnormal Pap smear usually initiates the diagnostic survey. Patients with abnormal squamous cytologic findings in the absence of a cervix or not explained by an adequate investigation of the cervix should be subjected to a very careful examination of the vaginal epithelium. In most series, the upper third of the vagina is most frequently involved (as is the invasive variety), and this in part relates to the association with the more common cervical lesions. TeLinde, Gusberg and Marshall, and later Parker and associates indicated that 2.0%, 1.9%, and 0.9%, respectively, had vaginal recurrences after hysterectomy for a similar lesion in the cervix. On the other hand, Ferguson and Maclure reported positive cytologic findings in 151 (20.3%) of 633 previously treated patients. This large group included invasive and in situ cancers of the cervix, which were treated by irradiation or hysterectomy. Although the long-term recurrence rate for carcinoma in situ of the vagina is uncertain, it is sufficient to merit continued careful follow-up. Incomplete excision of sufficient vaginal cuff with hysterectomy for carcinoma in situ may explain an early recurrence. The finding of carcinoma in situ in the vaginal cuff area less than 1 year after hysterectomy makes this explanation likely. It is therefore important to perform a careful preoperative evaluation of the upper vagina by Schiller tests or colposcopy at the time of hysterectomy for carcinoma in situ of the cervix. This will allow the surgeon to accurately determine the amount of upper vagina that it is necessary to remove.

It is also apparent that carcinoma in situ as well as dysplasia may develop in the vagina as a primary lesion. Still other preinvasive lesions of the vagina may appear after irradiation therapy for invasive carcinoma of the cervix. Recent data from the M. D. Anderson Hospital would suggest that these postradiation lesions are truly premalignant and can progress to invasive cancer if untreated. Approximately 25% of the patients in this series progressed to the invasive state over varying periods of follow-up without therapy. Local therapy must be executed with care because of the previous irradiation.

Diagnosis

Colposcopic examination of the vagina can be very difficult to perform. The largest possible speculum should be used and repositioned frequently to allow inspection of all surfaces. (Colposcopic findings are similar to those described for the cervix.) Our technique calls for the examination of the four walls from apex to introitus as separate and sequential steps. Biopsy specimens are taken with Kevorkian-Young alligator-jaw forceps, sometimes using a sterilized skin-hook for traction at the biopsy site. Most patients can tolerate these biopsies without local anesthesia. Lugol's solution may be helpful in delineating lesions of the vagina. In the postmenopausal patient, local use of estrogen creams for several weeks will help bring out the abnormal areas for identification by colposcopy.

Management

Local excision of the involved area has been the mainstay of therapy. Recently other therapies have been investigated, including topical application of 5-fluorouracil (5-FU) cream and laser surgery. The 5-FU cream can be kept in place with vaginal tampons or a diaphragm and should be used daily until the patient has intolerable introital irritation; results are mixed. Laser surgery is in an inconclusive stage of development. The remarks regarding use of this modality in CIN are also appropriate here. In addition, control of depth of the burn is of particular concern in the vagina because of the proximity of the bladder and rectum, although advocates of laser surgery state that it is well suited for use in the vagina, where, even in the most inaccessible regions, it can destroy minute, multifocal intraepithelial lesions without much chance of burn to the bladder or rectum. Some have advocated surface irradiation using an intravaginal applicator; however, our experience with this method of therapy has been discouraging, with a high recurrence rate and marked vaginal stenosis making follow-up therapy extremely difficult. At present, it would appear that local excision is the treatment of choice, even to the point where total vaginectomy with vaginal reconstruction using a split-thickness skin graft is performed in some younger patients.

INTRAEPITHELIAL NEOPLASIA OF THE VULVA
Clinical profile

Intraepithelial neoplasia of the vulva has been considered a problem of postmenopausal women in their fifties and sixties, but it may develop at any age. Its frequency appears to be increasing among younger women, and at least 50% of cases are asymptomatic. The most productive diagnostic technique is careful inspection of the vulva in bright light during routine pelvic examination followed by biopsy of suspicious lesions.

Physicians should be familiar with the various premalignant conditions of the vulva. As shown in Table 1-8, they range from the dysplasia that is biologically and histologically similar to dysplasia of the cervix or vagina to the more aggressive intraepithelial carcinoma or carcinoma in situ. The latter may advance quite rapidly to invasive cancer according to some authors, but in general there appears to be a slow progression spanning many years, very similar to the cervical variety. Until recently, the clinician's task was complicated by the confusing nomenclature employed to describe vulvar disease as well as by the inconsistencies in interpretation of histologic

Table 1-8. Vulvar disease

Vulvar dystrophies	Vulvar atypias
1. Hyperplastic dystrophy	1. Dysplasia, atypical hyperplasia (mild, moderate, severe)
a. Without atypia	a. Without dystrophy
b. With atypia	b. With dystrophy
2. Lichen sclerosus	Squamous cell carcinoma in situ (VIN)
3. Mixed dystrophy (lichen sclerosus with foci	Paget's disease of the vulva
of epithelial hyperplasia)	
a. Without atypia	
b. With atypia	

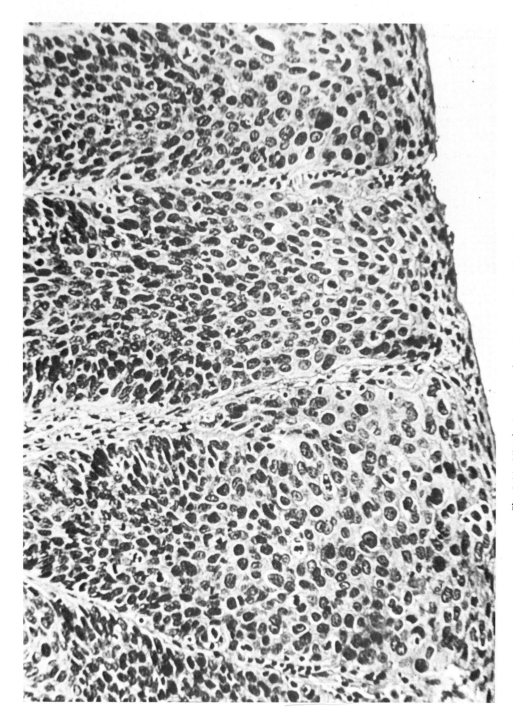

Fig. 1-11. Histologic section of carcinoma in situ of the vulva.

lesions. Fortunately, such problems provided the impetus for organizing the International Society for Study of Vulvar Disease, and establishing the now official terminology for classification of these conditions.

Cellular atypia associated with vulvar dystrophies is defined as a proliferation of squamous cells. Nuclei are enlarged and hyperchromatic, and initially show fine chromatin clumping. As the process progresses toward severe dysplasia, the chromatin clumping may be moderately coarse and irregular. There is little maturation in the cytoplasm; hence, parabasal cells almost reach the surface. When cellular atypia extends throughout more than two thirds of the thickness of the epithelium, the histologic diagnosis often proves to be carcinoma in situ (Fig. 1-11).

The milder forms of atypia present clinically as pale areas varying in density. Severe atypia and carcinoma in situ are seen as papules or macules, coalescent or discrete, single or multiple. Lesions on the cutaneous surface of the vulva usually have the appearance of lichenifield or hyperkeratotic plaques, i.e., white epithelium (Fig. 1-12). By contrast, lesions of mucous membranes are usually macular and pink or red in appearance. Vulvar lesions are hyperpigmented in 10% to 15% of patients

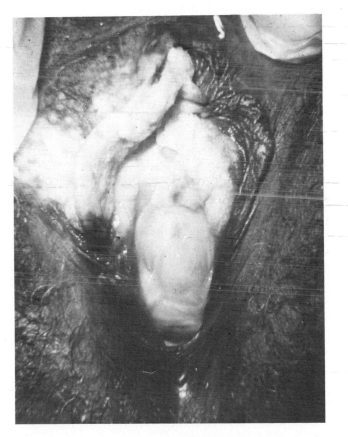

Fig. 1-12. Gross appearance of carcinoma in situ of the vulva showing heavy white epithelium.

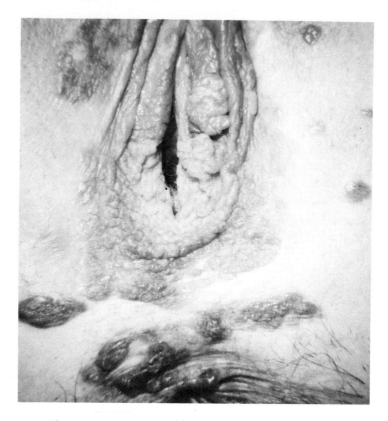

Fig. 1-13. Hyperpigmented lesions of vulvar carcinoma in situ.

(Fig. 1-13). These lesions range in color from mahogany to dark brown, and they stand out sharply when observed solely with the naked eye.

Neither age nor parity appears to be a risk factor in development of intraepithelial neoplasia of the vulva, and this has suggested a possible infectious process. Indeed, herpesvirus type 2 infection has been implicated by several investigators, but correlative data are lacking. Other suggested causes are related to the frequent association of vulvar intraepithelial neoplasia with condylomata acuminata and a proposed viral agent causing both lesions, but there is little scientific basis for this hypothesis. We have had a clinical impression that vulvar intraepithelial neoplasia is more common in patients with less pigment in their skin. The disease is asymptomatic in more than 50% of cases. In the remainder, the predominant symptom is pruritus. Presence of a distinct mass, bleeding, or discharge strongly suggests invasive disease.

Diagnosis

The value of careful inspection of the vulva during routine gynecologic examinations cannot be overstated; this remains the most productive diagnostic technique.

Colposcopy has proved quite effective in detecting multiple lesions. Once a lesion has been discovered, and the diagnosis has been confirmed histologically, colposcopic examination of the entire vulva should follow to rule out multicentric lesions. In the absence of colposcopy, lesions may be accentuated by application of 2% acetic acid solution to the vulvar skin, and inspection with bright light. Nuclear staining with 1% toluidine blue solution is also useful, although false-negative and false-positive rates are high. Colposcopy has emerged as a much more accurate technique. In general, a multifocal lesions are more common in the premenopausal patient, whereas the postmenopausal patient has a higher occurrence of unifocal disease.

The technique for the application of toluidine blue is simple: a 1% aqueous solution of the dye is applied to the external genital area and, after drying for 2 to 3 minutes, the region is washed with 1% to 2% acetic acid solution. Suspicious foci of increased nuclear activity are stained deeply (royal blue), whereas normal skin accepts little or none of the dye. Regrettably, hyperkeratotic lesions, even though neoplastic, are only lightly stained, whereas excoriations of a benign nature are often brilliant, thus explaining the high false-positive and false-negative rates.

It should be emphasized that the diagnosis of intraepithelial neoplasia of the vulva can be subtle. To avoid delay, the physician must exercise a high degree of suspicion. Vulvar biopsy should be used liberally, It is best accomplished under local anesthesia with a Keyes dermatologic punch (4- to 6-mm size). This instrument allows for removal of an adequate tissue sample and orientation for future sectioning. After obtaining the biopsy specimen, we use the Keyes punch to cut out a piece of gel foam; this is positioned in the skin defect and kept in place with a small dressing for at least 24 hours.

Adequate biopsy specimens are also obtainable with a sharp alligator-jaw instrument if one has proper traction on the skin. The problem with ordinary knife biopsies is that only superficial epithelium may be reached. If this technique is employed, one must be careful to sample deeper layers.

There have been few reports on untreated intraepithelial neoplasia of the vulva. The assumption that in situ lesions may advance to invasive carcinoma is made partly by extrapolation. This is what occurs in intraepithelial neoplasia of the cervix. The observation that diffuse carcinoma in situ may be associated with early invasive squamous cell lesions has led to the concept of "microinvasive cancer of the vulva." This entity has yet to be defined, though it appears to behave no differently than its counterpart in the cervix. Despite the uncertainties, carcinoma in situ must be approached with the anticipation that it may progress to an invasive stage.

Management

Surgical excision has been the mainstay of therapy. An important advantage is that excision allows for complete histologic assessment; lesions with microinvasive foci can thus be found. Most localized lesions are managed very effectively by wide local excision (a disease-free border of at least 5 mm) with end-to-end approximation

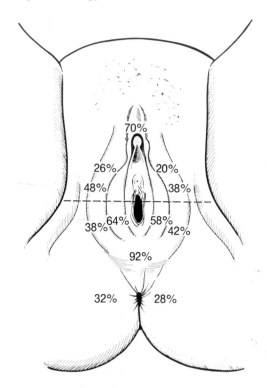

Fig. 1-14. Plot of lesion locations in 36 patients treated for multifocal carcinoma in situ of the vulva.

of the defect. The vulvar skin and mucous membrane usually have a good deal of elasticity, and cosmetic results are quite satisfactory after uncomplicated healing.

With multicentric lesions (Fig. 1-14), we usually excise the involved skin and substitute a split-thickness skin graft taken from either the buttocks or the inner aspect of the thigh. This is the skinning vulvectomy and skin graft procedure introduced by Rutledge and Sinclair in 1968 (Fig. 1-15). Its purpose is to replace the skin at risk in the vulvar site with ectopic epidermis from a donor site. We have modified the procedure in that the clitoris is always preserved and any lesions on the glans are scraped off with a scalpel blade; the epithelium of the glans regenerates without loss of sensation. Some recent reports have questioned this approach on the grounds that, at least in cases of vulvar dystrophy, the donated skin might be susceptible to a similar dystrophic process. In our experience, lesions have developed only outside the grafted area in preserved vulvar skin, but never in the graft itself. This suggests that the neoplastic potential is inherent in the original vulvar skin, and does not translate to skin from other parts of the body placed at the vulvar site.

The skinning vulvectomy and skin graft procedure preserves the subcutaneous tissue of the vulva, giving an optimal cosmetic and functional result. In more than 35 patients treated to date we have had no complaints of dyspareunia or diminished sexual responsiveness. In the elderly patient, simple vulvectomy may be preferred,

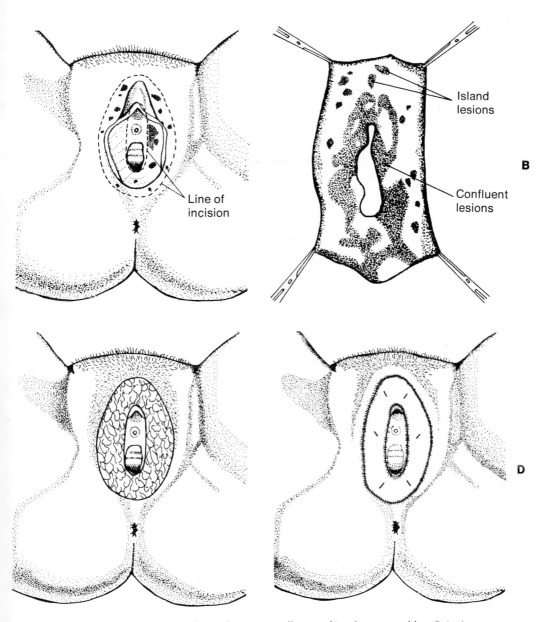

Fig. 1-15. Skinning vulvectomy and skin graft. **A,** Excise all areas of involvement en bloc. **B,** Lesions may be isolated or confluent. **C,** Preserve all subcutaneous tissue as the graft bed. **D,** Suture to graft bed.

because the skinning vulvectomy and skin graft operation requires prolonged bed rest (6 to 7 days) while the split-thickness graft adheres to the graft bed. Thus, the potential for morbidity is increased. The wishes of the patient concerning cosmetic results and sexual function must, of course, be taken into account regardless of age.

An alternative to excision of a vulvar lesion is to destroy it, principally by hot cautery, laser surgery, or cryosurgery. The disadvantage of destructive therapy is that a necrotic ulcer on the vulvar may result, and wound healing may be slow. Complete healing following cryosurgery may take up to 3 months. The treated area is often very painful for much of that time.

The Johns Hopkins group led by Donald Woodruff has reported an impressive 50% success rate with use of topical 5-FU in young patients with multicentric foci of carcinoma in situ. However, to succeed, 5-FU treatment requires denudation of the epithelium, with a significant degree of local discomfort. As a rule, medication must be applied three times daily for up to a month. Unless they are highly motivated, most patients are likely to discontinue therapy before the denudation phase is complete. In addition, with topical chemotherapy one should expect a fairly lengthy healing period, reflecting the time it takes for the agent to develop a necrotizing effect.

There have also been reports on use of nonspecific agents, such as dinitrochlorobenzene (DNCB) or dinitrofluorobenzene (DNFB), coupled with systemic sensitization of the patient with the same mitogen. Again, treatment results in a necrotic, slowly healing ulcer, and this approach has not been promising in our hands.

In summary, it is important to keep in mind that quite often these lesions develop in young women who remain asymptomatic. Early diagnosis depends on careful vulvar examination under bright light at regular intervals. Biopsy must be done on any suspicious lesions, and if the histologic report confirms intraepithelial neoplasia, an examination for multicentric foci should follow. The therapy selected depends on the extent of disease, the location of the lesions, and, not least of all, the personal desires of the patient.

BIBLIOGRAPHY
Cervical intraepithelial neoplasia

Ahlgren, M., Ingemarsson, I., Lindberg, L. G., and others: Conization as treatment of carcinoma in situ of the uterine cervix, Obstet. Gynecol. **46:**135, 1975.

Anderson, B.: Management of early cervical neoplasia, Clin. Obstet. Gynecol. **20:**815, 1977.

Ashley, D. J. B.: The biological status of carcinoma in situ of the uterine cervix, J. Obstet. Gynaecol. Br. Comm. **73:**372, 1966.

Beral, V.: Cancer of the cervix; a sexually transmitted infection? Lancet **1:**1037, 1974.

Bjerre, B., Eliasson, G., Linell, F., and others: Conization as only treatment of carcinoma in situ of the uterine cervix, Am. J. Obstet. Gynecol. **125:**143, 1976.

Carter, R., Krantz, K., Hara, G., and others: Treatment of CIN with the CO2 laser beam, Am. J. Obstet. Gynecol. **131:**831, 1979.

Catalano, L. W., Jr., and Johnson, L. D.: Herpesvirus antibody and carcinoma in situ of the cervix, J.A.M.A. **217:**447, 1971.

Chanen, W., and Hollyock, V. E.: Colposcopy and the conservative management of cervical dysplasias and carcinoma in situ, Obstet. Gynecol. **43:**527, 1974.

Coppleson, L. W., and Brown, B.: Estimation of the screening error rate from the observed detection rates in repeated cervical cytology, Am. J. Obstet. Gynecol. **119:**953, 1974.

Coppleson, L. W., and Brown, B.: Observations on a model of the biology of carcinoma of the cervix; a poor fit between observation and theory, Am. J. Obstet. Gynecol. **122**:127, 1975.

Coppleson, L. W., and Brown, B.: The prevention of carcinoma of the cervix, Am. J. Obstet. Gynecol. **125**:153, 1976.

Coppleson, M., Pixley, E., and Reid, B.: Colposcopy; a scientific and practical approach to the cervix in health and disease, Springfield, Ill., 1971, Charles C Thomas, Publisher.

Coppleson, M., and Reid, B.: Preclinical carcinoma of the cervix uteri; its nature, origin, and management, New York, 1967, Pergamon Press.

Coppleson, M., and Reid, B.: The etiology of squamous carcinoma of the cervix, editorial, Obstet. Gynecol. **32**:432, 1968.

Cramer, D. W., and Cutler, S. J.: Incidence and histopathology of malignancies of the female genital organs in the United States, Am. J. Obstet. Gynecol. **118**:443, 1974.

Creasman, W. T., and Parker, R. T.: Management of early cervical neoplasia, Clin. Obstet. Gynecol. **18**:233, 1975.

Creasman, W. T., and Rutledge, F.: Carcinoma in situ of the cervix; an analysis of 861 patients, Obstet. Gynecol. **39**:373, 1972.

Creasman, W. T., Weed, J. C., Jr., Curry, S. L., and others: Efficacy of cryosurgical treatment of severe cervical intraepithelial neoplasia, Obstet. Gynecol. **41**:501, 1973.

Delgado, G., and Smith, J. P., Diagnosis of cervical neoplasia by the nonspecialized colposcopist, Gynecol. Oncol. **3**:114, 1975.

DePetrillo, A. D., Townsend, D. E., Morrow, C. P., and others: Colposcopic evaluation of the abnormal Papanicolaou test in pregnancy, Am. J. Obstet. Gynecol. **121**:441, 1975.

DiSaia, P. J., Townsend, D. E., and Morrow, C. P.: The rationale for less than radical treatment for gynecologic malignancy in early reproductive years, Obstet. Gynecol. Surv. **29**:581, 1974.

Fluhmann, C. F.: Carcinoma in situ and the transitional zone of the cervix uteri, Obstet. Gynecol. **16**:424, 1960.

Friedell, G. H., Hertig, A. T., and Younge, P. A.: Carcinoma in situ of the uterine cervix, Springfield, Ill., 1960, Charles C. Thomas, Publisher.

Gad, C., and Koch, F.: The limitation of screening effect; a review of cervical disorders in previously screened women, Acta Cytol. **21**:719, 1978.

Gagnon, F.: The lack of occurrence of cervical carcinoma in nuns, Proc. Second Natl. Cancer Conf. **1**:625, 1952.

Galliher, H. P.: Optimal ages for Pap smear using a multistrains model of cervical cancer, Detroit, 1977, Michigan Cancer Foundation.

Gray, L. A., and Christopherson, W. M.: Treatment of cervical dysplasia, Gynecol. Oncol. **3**:149, 1975.

Gusberg, S. B., and Marshall, D.: Intraepithelial carcinoma of the cervix; a clinical reappraisal, Obstet. Gynecol. **19**:713, 1962.

Kaufman, R. H., and Irwin, J. F.: The cryosurgical therapy of cervical intraepithelial neoplasia, Am. J. Obstet. Gynecol. **131**:381, 1978.

Kessler, I. I.: Cervical cancer epidemiology in historical perspective, J. Reprod. Med. **12**:173, 1974.

Knox, E. G.: Ages and frequencies for cervical cancer screening, Br. J. Cancer **34**:444, 1976.

Kohan, S., Beckman, E. M., Bigelow, B., and others: Colposcopy and the management of cervical intraepithelial neoplasia, Gynecol. Oncol. **5**:27, 1977.

Kolstad, P., and Klem, V.: Long-term followup of 1121 cases of carcinoma in situ, Obstet. Gynecol. **48**:125, 1976.

Lurain, J. R., and Gallup, D. G.: Management of abnormal Papanicolaou smears in pregnancy, Obstet. Gynecol. **53**:484, 1979.

Masterson, J. G.: Analysis of untreated intraepithelial carcinoma of the cervix, Proceedings of the Third National Cancer Conference, Philadelphia, 1957, J. B. Lippincott Co.

Murphy, W. M., and Coleman, S. A.: The long-term course of carcinoma in situ of the uterine cervix, Cancer **38**:957, 1976.

Mylotte, M., Allen, J., and Jordan, J.: Regeneration of cervical epithelium following laser destruction of CIN, paper presented at the International Symposium on Gynecologic Oncology, Monaco, 1978.

Ortiz, R., Newton, M., and Tsai, A.: Electrocautery treatment of cervical intraepithelial neoplasia, Obstet. Gynecol. **41**:113, 1973.

Ostergard, D.: Personal communication, 1979.

Peterson, O.: Spontaneous course of cervical precancerous conditions, Am. J. Obstet. Gynecol. **72**:1063, 1956.

Rawls, W. E., Tompkins, W. A., Figueroa, M. E., and others: Herpesvirus type 2; association with carcinoma of the cervix, Science **161**:1255, 1968.

Reid, B. L., French, P. W., Singer, A., and others: Sperm basic proteins in cervical carcinogenesis; correlation with socioeconomic class, Lancet **2**:60, 1978.

Richart, R. M.: Natural history of cervical intraepithelial neoplasia, Clin. Obstet. Gynecol. **10:**748, 1968.

Saidi, M. H., White, A. J., and Weinberg, P. C.: The hazard of cryosurgery for treatment of cervical dysplasia, J. Reprod. Med. **19:**70, 1977.

Sevin, B. U., Ford, J. H., Girtanner, R. D., and others: Invasive cancer of the cervix after cryosurgery; pitfalls of conservative management, Obstet. Gynecol. **53:**465, 1979.

Shingleton, H. M., Gore, H., and Austin, J. M., Jr.: Outpatient evaluation of patients with atypical Papanicolaou smears; contribution of endocervical curettage, Am. J. Obstet. Gynecol. **126:**122, 1976.

Silbar, E. L., and Woodruff, J. D.: Evaluations of biopsy, cone and hysterectomy sequence in intraepithelial carcinoma of the cervix, Obstet. Gynecol. **27:**89, 1966.

Stafl, A., and Mattingly, R. F.: Colposcopic diagnosis of cervical neoplasia, Obstet. Gynecol. **41:**168, 1973.

Townsend, D. E., and Ostergard, D. R.: Cryocauterization for preinvasive cervical neoplasia, J. Reprod. Med. **6:**171, 1971.

Tredway, D. R., Townsend, D. E., Hovland, D. N., and Upton, R. T.: Colposcopy and cryosurgery in cervical intraepithelial neoplasia, Am. J. Obstet. Gynecol. **114:**1020, 1972.

Walton, R. J.: The task force on cervical cancer screening programs, editorial, Can. Med. Assoc. J. **114:**981, 1976.

Wilbanks, G. D., Creasman, W. T., Kaufman, L. A., and Parker, R. T.: Treatment of cervical dysplasia with electro-cautery and tetracycline suppositories, Am. J. Obstet. Gynecol. **117:**460, 1973.

Underwood, P. B., Lutz, M. H., and Fletcher, R. V., Jr.: Cryosurgery, Cancer **38:**546, 1976.

Urcuyo, R., Rome, R. M., and Nelson, J.: Some observations on the value of endocervical curettage performed as an integral part of colposcopic examination of patients with abnormal cervical cytology, Obstet. Gynecol. **128:**787, 1977.

Intraepithelial neoplasia of the vagina

Blumberg, J. M., and Ober, W. B.: Carcinoma in situ of the cervix; recurrence in the vaginal vault, Am. J. Obstet. Gynecol. **66:**421, 1952.

Carter, E. R., Salvaggio, A. T., and Jarkowski, T. L.: Squamous cell carcinoma of the vagina following vaginal hysterectomy of intraepithelial carcinoma of the cervix, Am. J. Obstet. Gynecol. **82:**401, 1961.

Copenhaver, E. H., Salzman, F. A., and Wright, K. A.: Carcinoma in situ of the vagina, Am. J. Obstet. Gynecol. **89:**962, 1964.

Cromer, J. K.: Invasive squamous-cell carcinoma of the vagina following surgery for carcinoma in situ of the cervix, Med. Ann. D.C. **34:**115, 1965.

Ferguson, J. H., and Maclure, J. G.: Intraepithelial carcinoma, dysplasia, and exfoliation of cancer cells in the vaginal mucosa, Am. J. Obstet. Gynecol. **87:**326, 1963.

Graham, J. B., and Meigs, J. V.: Recurrence of tumor after total hysterectomy for carcinoma in situ, Am. J. Obstet. Gynecol. **64:**1159, 1952.

Gusberg, S. B., and Marshall, D.: Intraepithelial carcinoma of the cervix; a clinical reappraisal, Obstet. Gynecol. **19:**713, 1962.

Koss, L. G., Melamed, M. R., and Daniel, W. W.: In situ epidermoid carcinoma of the cervix and vagina following radiotherapy for cervical cancer, Cancer **14:**353, 1961.

Marcus, S. L.: Multiple squamous cell carcinoma involving the cervix, vagina, and vulva; the theory of multicentric origin, Am. J. Obstet. Gynecol. **80:**801, 1961.

Margulis, R. R., Dustin, R. W., and Daugherty, G. D.: Carcinoma in situ of the cervix with genital tract extension, Mich. Med. **64:**251, 1965.

McPherson, H. A., Diddle, A. W., Gardner, W. H., and Williamson, P. J.: Epidermoid carcinoma of cervix, vagina, and vulva; a regional disease, Obstet. Gynecol. **21:**145, 1963.

Moran, J. P., and Robinson, H. J.: Primary carcinoma in situ of the vagina, Obstet. Gynecol. **20:**405, 1962.

Mussey, E., and Soule, E. H.: Carcinoma in situ of the cervix; a clinical review of 842 cases, Am. J. Obstet. Gynecol. **77:**957, 1959.

Newman, W., and Cromer, J. K.: The multicentric origin of carcinoma of the female anogenital tract, Surg. Gynecol. Obstet. **108:**273, 1959.

Ostergard, D. R., and Morton, D. G.: Multifocal carcinoma of the female genitals, Am. J. Obstet. Gynecol. **99:**1006, 1967.

Parker, R. T., Cuyler, W. K., Kaufman, L. A., and others: Intraepithelial cancer of the cervix, Am. J. Obstet. Gynecol. **80:**693, 1960.

Rutledge, F.: Cancer of the vagina, Am. J. Obstet. Gynecol. **97:**635, 1967.

Samuels, B., Bradburn, D. M., and Johnson, C. G.: Primary carcinoma in situ of the vagina, Am. J. Obstet. Gynecol. **82:**393, 1961.

TeLinde, R. W.: Carcinoma in situ of the cervix, Postgrad. Med. **29:**458, 1961.

Woodruff, J. D.: Treatment of recurrent carcinoma in situ in the lower genital canal, Clin. Obstet. Gynecol. **8:**757, 1965.

Intraepithelial neoplasia of the vulva

Abell, M. R., and Gosling, J. R.: Intraepithelial and infiltrative carcinoma of vulva, Bowen's type, Cancer **14:**318, 1961.

Bowen, J. T.: Precancerous dermatoses, J. Cutan. Dis. **30:**241, 1912.

Carson, T. E., Hoskins, W. J., and Wurzel, J. F.: Topical 5-fluorouracil in the treatment of carcinoma in situ of the vulva, Obstet. Gynecol. **47**(Suppl.):59, 1976.

Collins, C. G.: A clinical stain for use in selecting biopsy sites in patients with vulvar diseases, Obstet. Gynecol. **28:**158, 1966.

Friedrich. E. G., Jr.: Reversible vulvar atypia, Obstet. Gynecol. **39:**173, 1972.

Friedrich, E. G., Jr.: Vulvar carcinoma in situ in identical twins—an occupational hazard, Obstet. Gynecol. **39:**837, 1972.

Krupp, P. J., and Bohm, J. W.: 5-Fluorouracil topical treatment of in situ vulvar cancer, Obstet. Gynecol. **51:**702, 1978.

Litwin, M. S., Krementz, E. T., Mansell, P. W., and others: Topical chemotherapy of lentigo maligna with 5-fluorouracil cream, J. Surg. Oncol. **35:**721, 1975.

New nomenclature for vulva disease, Obstet. Gynecol. **47:**122, 1976.

Raaf, J. H., and others: Treatment of Bowen's disease with topical dinitrochlorobenzene and 5-fluorouracil, Cancer **37:**1633, 1976.

Richart, R. M.: A clinical staining test for the in vivo delineation of dysplasia and carcinoma in situ, Am. J. Obstet. Gynecol. **86:**703, 1963.

Rutledge, F., and Sinclair, M.: Treatment of intraepithelial carcinoma of the the vulva by skin excision and graft, Am. J. Obstet. Gynecol. **102:**806, 1968.

Woodruff, J. D., and Hildebrandt, E. E.: Carcinoma in situ of the vulva, Obstet. Gynecol. **12:**414, 1958.

Woodruff, J. D., Julian, C., Puray, T., and others: The contemporary challenge of carcinoma in situ of the vulva, Am. J. Obstet. Gynecol. **115:**677, 1973.

CHAPTER TWO

Management of the female exposed to diethylstilbestrol

Clear-cell adenocarcinoma of the genital tract
Other DES-related genital tract anomalies
Examination and treatment of the female exposed to DES
Effects on the male
Conclusions

CLEAR-CELL ADENOCARCINOMA OF THE GENITAL TRACT

Before 1965, clear-cell adenocarcinoma of the cervix in females under the age of 30 was only rarely reported and vaginal clear-cell adenocarcinoma was unknown. In April 1970, Herbst and Scully reported seven cases of primary vaginal adenocarcinoma in women between the ages of 15 and 22 years. These seven cases exceeded the number of cases in the world literature in adolescent females born before 1945. Because of this case clustering, an epidemiologic study of the patients and their families was initiated to identify associative factors. With the addition of another patient to the study, it was discovered that the mothers of seven of the eight patients with vaginal adenocarcinoma had been treated with diethylstilbestrol (DES), a nonsteroidal synthetic estrogen, in the first trimester of the relevant pregnancy. Since that time, additional cases of vaginal and cervical adenocarcinoma have been reported in patients whose mothers ingested nonsteroidal estrogen during pregnancy. DES and related drugs were used to support high-risk pregnancy and reduce fetal wastage in the mid-1940s and 1950s, but their use then declined. By 1978, 341 cases of vaginal and cervical (approximately 40% involve the cervix) adenocarcinoma had been accessioned by the registry established by Herbst. Among the cases in which a maternal history was obtainable, the proportion that were positive for medication with DES or chemically related estrogens was two out of three. Similarly, one of ten

2/3

histories has been positive for an unknown medication prescribed for a high-risk pregnancy, and one of four has been negative. In six of the cases, progestins had been administered and in another three, a steroidal estrogen.

The youngest patient was 7 years of age at the time of diagnosis, and the oldest patient was 29 years, with a peak frequency at the age of 19.5 years for those patients with a history of DES exposure (Fig. 2-1). The risk of development of these carcinomas in the DES-exposed female through the age of 24 years has been estimated to be 0.14 to 1.4 per thousand. About 68% of the individuals with clear-cell adenocarcinoma had a history of hormone exposure compared with 86% for the primary vaginal tumors.

A very careful study has been done of cases where details were available concerning the administration of DES to the mothers of afflicted daughters. A very wide variation exists in both dose and duration of DES treatment. In some cases the total dose was far less than 500 mg, and in other instances it exceeded 15,000 mg. In one case the dose was 1.5 mg daily, and in others the dose was over 200 mg daily. It has not been possible to correlate either the dose or the duration of treatment with the incidence or pattern of cancer in the cases studied. However, in all cases with accurate treatment dates, the drug was begun before the eighteenth week of pregnancy. It is not known how many exposed females there are in the United States, but estimates have placed this population at 0.5 to 2.0 million. Ninety percent of the cases have occurred in patients 14 years of age or older.

Most of the patients presented with symptoms of abnormal bleeding, but 20%

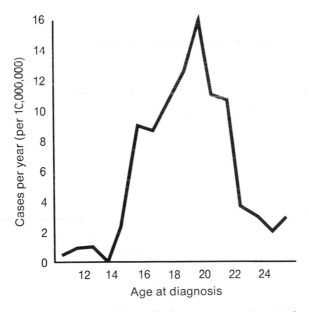

Fig. 2-1. Age-specific incidence rates of clear-cell adenocarcinoma. (From Herbst, A. L.: Intrauterine exposure to diethylstilbestrol in the human, Proceedings of Symposium on DES, 1977, Chicago, 1978, American College of Obstetricians and Gynecologists.)

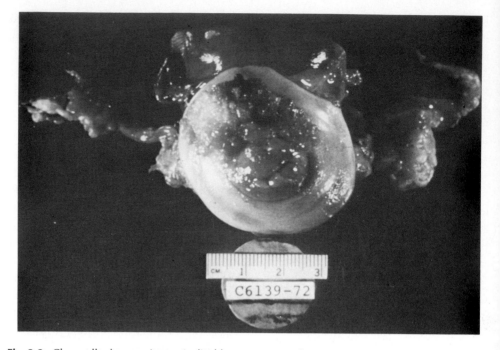

Fig. 2-2. Clear-cell adenocarcinoma (radical hysterectomy and upper vaginectomy specimen). Note involvement of cervix and anterior wall of upper vagina.

were asymptomatic and discovered on routine pelvic exam. Cytologic testing has proved useful, but a false-negative rate of up to 20% has been reported, probably because of the heavy polymorphonuclear infiltration seen with these lesions. The carcinomas may occur anywhere on the vagina or cervix, but most have been in the upper part of the vagina, particularly on the anterior wall (Fig. 2-2). Adenosis (the presence of glandular epithelium or its mucinous products in the vagina) has been found accompanying vaginal clear-cell adenocarcinoma in virtually all cases. Adenosis is benign tissue, but it may be the nonneoplastic precursor of the clear-cell adenocarcinoma in some cases, although direct transitions from adenosis to cancer have not been identified. The same observations apply to cervical eversion (ectropion, "congenital erosion") and clear-cell adenocarcinoma of the cervix. Both vaginal adenosis and cervical eversion are very common in DES-exposed females in contrast to the very rare carcinomas. Therefore, not only are these lesions benign but the premalignant potential for adenocarcinoma must be very small, if it exists at all. Both surgery and radiation have been effective in treating these tumors (Table 2-1), although most cases have been followed for less than 5 years. The optimum therapy for clear-cell carcinoma of the cervix and vagina has not been established. Incidence of lymph node metastases is fairly high, with approximately 18% in stage I and 30% or more in stage II. The neoplasm tends to remain superficial, suggesting the possi-

Table 2-1. Suggested management of clear-cell adenocarcinoma of the cervix and vagina

Stage	Surgery	Radiation
Cervix		
IB	Radical hysterectomy with clear vaginal margins and bilateral pelvic lymphadenectomy	5,000 rads W.P.* in patients with positive pelvic nodes
IIA	Radical hysterectomy with bilateral pelvic lymphadenectomy and upper vaginectomy	5,000 rads W.P. in patients with positive pelvic nodes
IIB	Consider exenteration for radiation failures	5,000 rads W.P. tandem and ovoids
III A and B	Consider exenteration for radiation failures	6,000 rads W.P. tandem and ovoids
IV	Individualize	
Vagina		
I (upper ⅓ of vagina)	Radical hysterectomy with bilateral pelvic lymphadenectomy and upper vaginectomy	5,000 rads W.P. in patients with positive pelvic nodes
I (lower ⅔ of vagina)	Radical hysterectomy with bilateral pelvic lymphadenectomy and total vaginectomy with vaginal reconstruction	5,000 rads W.P. vaginal application or interstitial implant
II	Consider exenteration for radiation failures	5,000 rads W.P. interstitial implant
III	Consider exenteration for radiation failures	6,000 rads W.P. interstitial implant
IV	Individualize	

*W.P., whole pelvis.

bility that this disease can be treated locally, especially if the lesion is small. However, one instance of pelvic node metastases has been reported in a patient with less than 3 mm of invasion. If the growth is confined to the cervix and/or upper vagina, radical hysterectomy with upper vaginectomy and pelvic lymphadenectomy is the recommended therapy with retention of the ovaries. In these young patients, avoidance of pelvicradiation is desirable in view of the increased risks of long-term morbidity (radiation-induced carcinogenesis and progressive vasculitis) in patients surviving many decades after full-dose pelvic irradiation, and the improved retention of optimal vaginal function following surgery. More extensive tumors and lesions involving the lower two thirds of the vagina are more suitable for radiation, which would include the pelvic nodes and parametrial tissues. Although some experienced surgeons have used radical hysterectomy with total vaginectomy and split-thickness skin graft vaginal reconstruction in this group of patients, we have been dissatisfied with the surgical margins (especially of the bladder) of this procedure and have followed the radiation therapy techniques of Wharton and associates from the M. D. Anderson Hospital in Houston, Texas. At our institutions, radical pelvic surgery has been reserved for radiation failures in patients with lower vaginal involvement. In 1979, Herbst and associates reported a discouraging 37% recurrence rate among 22 patients treated by conventional irradiation, but 21 of these 22 patients had large vaginal adenocarcinomas and probably would not have been good surgical candidates for vaginectomy.

Survival is stage related, and the follow-up of most of the cases is still too short for calculating a meaningful 5-year survival rate or for comparing the efficiency of various modes of therapy at this time. Although many patients have apparently been cured, of the 341 patients reported in 1978, 54 had died and an additional 29 were known to have recurrent disease. Two cases of recurrence were observed 7 years after apparently successful treatment; this emphasizes the importance of prolonged follow-up of these patients. It would appear that a higher proportion of clear-cell adenocarcinomas metastasize to the lungs and supraclavicular area than do squamous cell carcinomas of the vagina and cervix.

Recurrences of clear-cell adenocarcinoma

In a study by Herbst and associates in 1979, 346 patients were analyzed for frequency, site, and treatment of recurrent disease. Twenty of the 346 were never free of disease after initial therapy, and 19 had died at the time of the report. Fifty-eight patients had recurrences, and most of these were diagnosed within 3 years after primary tumor treatment. Sixty percent had recurrence in the pelvis with almost half of these being in the vagina. Twenty-one patients (36%) had recurrence in the lungs, and 12 (20%) had recurrence in the supraclavicular lymph nodes. Surgery and radiation have been effective in the control of pelvic recurrences in some cases. The results of chemotherapy have generally been disappointing. Isolated responses to individual cytotoxic agents have been noted, but there are no documented objective responses with the use of progestational agents. The currently recommended multiple drug therapy would include cyclophosphamide (Cytoxan), vincristine F, 5-fluorouracil, methotrexate, and/or prednisone.

OTHER DES-RELATED GENITAL TRACT ANOMALIES

Herbst and associates reported at least three nonneoplastic genital tract anomalies in young women with adenocarcinoma: cervical eversion, transverse ridges, and vaginal adenosis (presence of endocervical-like epithelium in the vagina). Cervical eversion (columnar epithelium covering portions of the exocervix) was seen frequently regardless of the cervical or vaginal origin of the adenocarcinoma. Most striking, however, was the association of adenosis. In 90% of the cases of vaginal adenocarcinoma, there was sufficient vaginal tissue to permit histologic study to confirm the presence of adenosis. As stated earlier, the high frequency of adenosis in these individuals with adenocarcinoma suggests that adenosis may play a role in the genesis of this malignancy. Vaginal adenosis has been observed in patients without a history of DES exposure, but rarely to a clinical degree. Sandberg sectioned 35 vaginas obtained at autopsy; 22 were from postpubertal women, and in nine of these (41%) he demonstrated occult glands. None of the 13 prepubertal specimens examined contained glands. However, Kurman and Scully noted six cases of vaginal adenosis among 73 prepubertal vaginal specimens obtained at autopsy.

Adenosis is more common in patients whose mothers began DES treatment early in pregnancy, and its frequency is not at all increased if DES administration began after the eighteenth week of gestation. At least 20% of females exposed to DES show an anatomic deformity of the upper vagina and cervix. This has been variously described as transverse vaginal and cervical ridge, cervical collar, vaginal hood, and cockscomb cervix. The transverse ridges and anatomic deformities found in one fifth of DES-exposed females make ascertainment of the boundaries of the vagina and cervix difficult. The cervical eversion causes the cervix grossly to have a red appearance. This coloration is due to the numerous normal-appearing blood vessels in the submucosa. By using a colposcope and applying 3% acetic acid solution, one may recognize involved areas covered with numerous papillae ("grapes") of columnar epithelium similar to those seen in the native columnar epithelium of the endocervix. The hood (Fig. 2-3) is a fold of mucous membrane surrounding the portio of the cervix; it very often disappears if the portio is pulled down with a tenaculum or displaced by the speculum. The cockscomb is an atypical peaked appearance of the

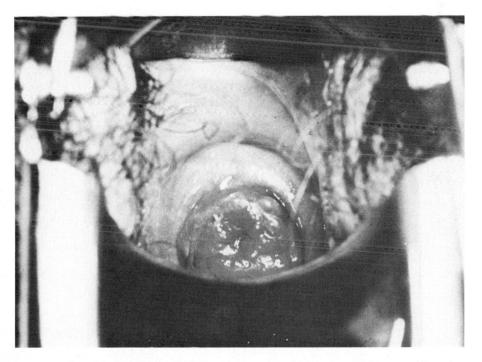

Fig. 2-3. Hood surrounding the small DES-exposed cervix, which is completely covered by columnar epithelium (pseudopolyp).

anterior lip of the cervix, whereas vaginal ridges are protruding circumferential bands in the upper vagina that may hide the cervix. A pseudopolyp formation (Fig. 2-3) has been described that occurs when the portio of the cervix is rather small and protrudes through a wide cervical hood.

The striking occurrence of vaginal adenosis and adenocarcinoma in young women whose mothers took nonsteroidal estrogens during pregnancy logically points to an embryonic explanation. The development of the müllerian system is dependent on and preceded by formation of the wolffian, or mesonephric system. The emergence of the müllerian system as the dominant structure appears unaffected by intrauterine exposure to DES when studied in animal systems. However, it is apparent that steroidal and nonsteroidal estrogens when administered during the proper stage of vaginal embryogenesis in mice can permanently prevent the transformation of müllerian epithelium into the adult type of vaginal epithelium, thus creating a situation like adenosis. The colposcopic and histologic features of vaginal adenosis strongly support the concept of persistent, untransformed müllerian columnar epithelia in the vagina as being the explanation of adenosis.

EXAMINATION AND TREATMENT OF THE FEMALE EXPOSED TO DES

Systematic examination of the female offspring exposed to DES (Table 2-2) has disclosed that at least 60% have vaginal adenosis, that is, presence of cervical-like epithelium in the vagina; a smaller portion of cases have minor anomalies of the cervix and vagina. Although the origin of clear-cell adenocarcinoma from adenosis remains to be established, these patients warrant careful observation. Some authors have suggested that DES-exposed offspring may also have an increased risk of developing squamous neoplasia because of the large number of transformation zones inherent in this condition. Although a few cases of dysplasia and carcinoma in situ associated with adenosis have been reported, the risk of developing squamous lesions remains uncertain at this time since no DES-exposed offspring have entered the age group in which squamous carcinoma is most prevalent.

Table 2-2. Examination of the DES-exposed offspring (female)

---

1. Inspect the introitus and hymen to assess the patency of the vagina.
2. Palpate the vaginal membrane with the index finger (especially noting non–Lugol staining areas), noting areas of induration of exophytic lesions.
3. Perform speculum examination with the largest speculum that can be comfortably be inserted (virginal-type speculums are often necessary). Adenosis will usually appear red and granular (strawberry surface).
4. Obtain cytologic specimens from (1) the cervical os and (2) the walls of the upper one third of the vagina.
5. Perform colposcopic examination and/or Lugol staining on the initial visit.
6. Do a biopsy of (1) indurated or exophytic areas and (2) colposcopically abnormal areas with dysplastic Pap smear.
7. Perform bimanual rectovaginal examination.

All DES-exposed females should have a gynecologic examination on a semiannual basis beginning at age 14 or menarche, whichever occurs first. In general, examinations of prepubertal individuals are not recommended, but they should be performed (usually under anesthesia) if any unusual symptoms, such as abnormal bleeding or discharge, develop. Mothers should be encouraged to instruct their daughters in the use of vaginal tampons during menses, since this will facilitate the physician's examination. Examination should include careful inspection of the cervix and any suspicious area in the vagina. Careful digital palpation of the vagina must be performed. The role of colposcopy remains in the examination of suspicious areas where biopsy may be indicated. Lugol's solution may be helpful in delineating abnormal areas. The purpose of regular examination is to permit detection of adeno-

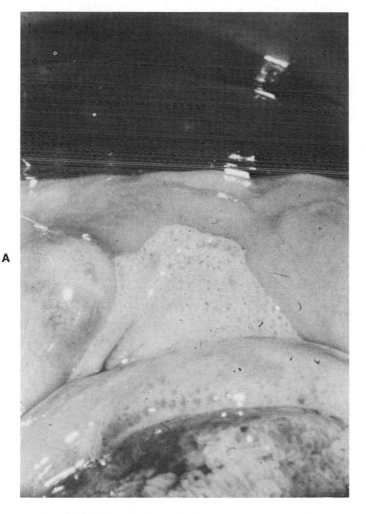

Fig. 2-4. A, Area of white epithelium of squamous metaplasia.
Continued.

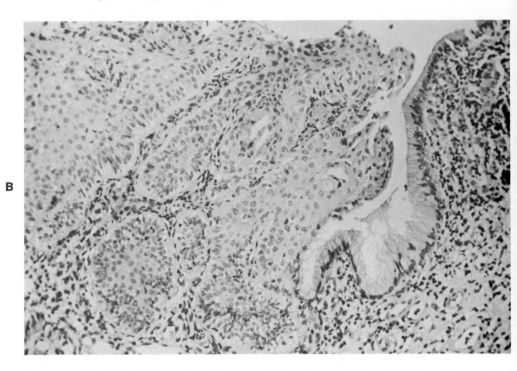

B

Fig. 2-4, cont'd. B, Histologic section of the area in **A** showing metaplasia to the left partially covering the adenosis (columnar epithelium) to the right.

carcinoma and squamous neoplasia during the earliest stages of development. Although many therapies have been attempted, there is at the present time no recommended treatment plan for vaginal adenosis. Some physicians have advised the use of jellies or foam to lower the vaginal pH and assist the reepithelialization of the mucous membrane. There are no published studies to indicate that such a practice is valid. The use of local progesterone in the vagina has been advocated by others as therapy for vaginal adenosis, but good data are similarly lacking. In most instances, the area of adenosis is physiologically transformed into squamous epithelium during a varying period of observation.

It has been postulated that squamous cell cancers may arise in the metaplastic tissue that is so extensively found in DES-exposed females. Evidence for an increase in squamous cell carcinoma does not exist at present, but this possibility provides an additional reason for close follow-up of the group. Colposcopic examination of these patients is hampered by the abnormal patterns (Fig. 2-4) seen with squamous metaplasia that can be confused with neoplastic lesions, especially by the inexperienced observer. Careful histologic confirmation is essential before any treatment is undertaken. Marked mosaic (Fig. 2-5) and punctation patterns that normally herald intraepithelial neoplasia are commonly seen in the DES-exposed female's vagina as a result of widespread metaplasia.

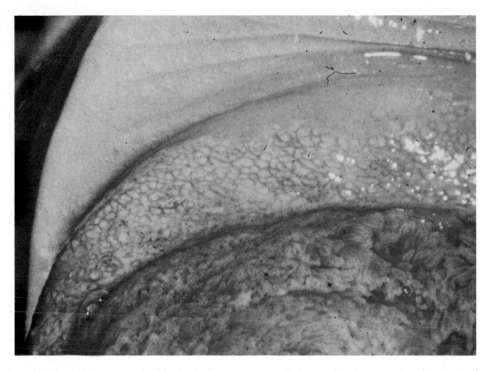

Fig. 2-5. Heavy mosaic pattern (histologically proven metaplasia) in a hood surrounding the cervix of a DES exposed offspring.

A frequently asked question regarding the care of DES-exposed women is whether oral contraceptives can be prescribed. There is no evidence that the usage of these medications is either helpful or harmful to the patient with vaginal adenosis. However, because of the uncertainty of the effects of these hormones on a disorder initiated by another hormone, many physicians prefer not to recommend oral contraceptives for their DES-exposed patients. There is a rare condition, microglandular hyperplasia of the cervix, associated with the use of oral contraceptives that can be confused with adenocarcinoma by some pathologists. It is imperative, therefore, that the pathologist be informed if the patient is taking oral contraceptives.

Many DES-exposed females have achieved pregnancy, and there appears to be no evidence of infertility being a more common problem among this group, but more studies are needed.

EFFECTS ON THE MALE

Some studies have indicated that transplacental effects of DES on human males do occur. Administration of DES during pregnancy appears to be followed by effects on the fetal male genital tract that have shown up in the form of structural and functional changes that may impair fertility. Although carcinogenesis in human males has not been reported to date, it has been demonstrated that prenatal exposure to

DES produces detectable anatomic changes in the male reproductive tract. Epididymal cysts, hypoplastic testes, cryptorchidism, and induration of the testicular capsule have all been described in greater incidence in the DES-exposed male: 30% in 289 DES-exposed males as compared with 8% in 290 controls. Blood hormone assays are essentially normal, although some studies have shown a significant decrease in sperm counts. Spermatozoa analysis revealed severely pathologic changes in 20% of 88 DES-exposed males and in 5% of 55 controls.

CONCLUSIONS

The annual increase in the occurrence of DES-related clear-cell adenocarcinoma of the vagina or cervix that began 12 years ago has continued with about the same frequency into the late 1970s. The 5-year survival rate of about 75% is better than the cumulative survival rate for either cervical or vaginal cancer. The better prognosis might be attributed to the early detection of clear-cell adenocarcinoma, since it occurs mainly in young patients exposed to DES in utero, many of whom are closely followed. This assumption is supported by data showing that 60% of clear-cell adenocarcinomas are stage I tumors, whereas approximately 35% of carcinomas of the cervix in the United States are stage I.

The potential of hormones other than DES, such as steroidal estrogens, and progestins, to cause changes of the type described in the DES-exposed female requires further investigation. Because the corpus uteri and the fallopian tubes are also müllerian duct derivative, and because müllerian-type tumors may develop in the ovary, these sites must also be marked for the development of cancer. The full impact of this problem will need additional time to be elucidated.

BIBLIOGRAPHY

Anderson, B., Watring, W. G., Edinger, D. D., Jr., and others: Development of DES-associated clear-cell carcinoma; the importance of regular screening, Obstet. Gynecol. 53:293, 1979.

Bibbo, M., Al-Naqeeb, M., Baccarini, I., and others: Follow-up study of the male and female offspring of DES treated mothers; a preliminary report, J. Reprod. Med. 15:29, 1975.

Burke, L., and Antonioli, D.: Vaginal adenosis factors influencing detection in a colposcopic evaluation, Obstet. Gynecol. 48:413, 1976.

Chambers, J., Rogers, L. W., and Julian, C. G.: Minute clear cell carcinoma of the vagina with early metastasis to pelvic lymph nodes, Am. J. Obstet. Gynecol. 131:223, 1978.

Fenoglio, C. M., Ferenczy, A., Richart, R. M., and others: Scanning and transmission electron microscopic studies of vaginal adenosis and the cervical transformation zone in progeny exposed in utero to diethylstilbestrol, Am. J. Obstet. Gynecol. 126:170, 1976.

Forsberg, J.G.: Cervicovaginal epithelium; its origin and development, Am. J. Obstet. Gynecol. 115:1025, 1973.

Gill, W. B., Schumacher, G. F. B., and Bibbo, M.: Structural and functional abnormalities in the sex organs of male offspring of mothers treated with diethstilbestrol (DES), J. Reprod. Med. 16:147, 1976.

Hart, W. R., and Norris, H. J.: Mesonephric adenocarcinomas of the cervix, Cancer 29:106, 1972.

Herbst, A. L.: Intrauterine exposure to diethylstilbestrol in the human, Proceedings of Symposium on DES, 1977, Chicago, 1978, American College of Obstetricians and Gynecologists.

Herbst, A. L., Cole, P., Colton, T., and others: Age-incidence and risk of DES-related clear cell adenocarcinoma of the vagina and cervix, Am. J. Obstet. Gynecol. 128:43, 1977.

Herbst, A. L., Norusis, M. J., Rosenow, P. J., and others: An analysis of 346 cases of clear cell adenocarcinoma of the vagina and cervix with emphasis on recurrence and survival, Gynecol. Oncol. **7**:111, 1979.

Herbst, A. L., Poskanzer, D. C., Rolloy, S. J., and others: Prenatal exposure to diethylstilbestrol; a prospective comparison of exposed female offspring with unexposed controls, N. Engl. J. Med. **292**:334, 1975.

Herbst, A. L., Robboy, S. J., Scully, R. E., and others: Clear cell adenocarcinoma of the vagina and cervix in girls; analysis of 170 registry cases, Am. J. Obstet. Gynecol. **119**:713, 1974.

Herbst, A. L., and Scully, R. E.: Adenocarcinoma of the vagina in adolescence; a report of 7 cases including 6 clear-cell carcinomas (so-called mesonephromas), Cancer **25**:745, 1970.

Herbst, A. L., Scully, R. E., and Robboy, S. J.: Problems in the examination of the DES-exposed female, Obstet. Gynecol. **46**:353, 1975.

Herbst, A. L., Ulfelder, H., and Poskanzer, D. C.: Adenocarcinoma of the vagina; association of maternal stilbestrol therapy with tumor appearance in young women, N. Engl. J. Med. **284**:878, 1971.

Kaufman, R. H., Binder, G. L., Gray, P. M., Jr., and others: Upper genital tract changes associated with exposure in utero to diethylstilbestrol, Am. J. Obstet. Gynecol. **128**:51, 1977.

Kurman, R.J., and Scully, R.E.: The incidence and histogenesis of vaginal adenosis; an autopsy study, Hum. Pathol. **5**:265, 1974.

Lanier, A. P., Noller, K. L., Decker, D. G., and others: Cancer and stilbestrol; a follow-up of 1719 persons exposed to estrogen in utero and born in 1943-1959, Mayo Clin. Proc. **48**:793, 1973.

Mattingly, R.F., and Stafl, A.: Cancer risk in DES-exposed offspring, Am. J. Obstet. Gynecol. **126**:543, 1976.

McLachlan, J. A., and Newbold, R. R.: Reproductive tract lesions in male mice exposed prenatally to diethylstilbestrol, Science **190**:991, 1975.

Ng, A. B. P., Reagan, J. W., Naji, M., and others: Natural history of vaginal adenosis in women exposed to diethylstilbestrol in utero, J. Reprod. Med. **18**:1, 1977.

Noller, K. L., Decker, D. C., Lanier, A. P., and others: Clear cell adenocarcinoma of the cervix after maternal treatment with synthetic estrogens, Mayo Clin. Proc. **47**:620, 1972.

Normura, T., and Kanzaki, T.: Induction of urogenital anomalies and some tumors in the progeny of mice receiving diethylstilbestrol during pregnancy, Cancer Res. **37**:1099, 1977.

O'Brien, P. C., Noller, K. L., Robboy, S.J., and others: Vaginal epithelial changes in young women enrolled in the National Cooperative Diethylstilbestrol Adenosis (DESAD) project, Obstet. Gynecol. **53**:300, 1979.

Poskanzer, D. C., and Herbst, A. L.: Epidemiology of vaginal adenosis and adenocarcinoma associated with exposure to stilbestrol in utero, Cancer **39**:1892, 1977.

Robboy, S. J., Herbst, A. L., and Scully, R. E.: Clear cell adenocarcinoma of the vagina and cervix in young females; analysis of 37 tumors that persisted or recurred after primary therapy, Cancer **34**:606, 1974.

Robboy, S. J., Kaufman, R. H., Prat, J., and others: Pathologic findings in young women enrolled in the National Cooperative Diethylstilbestrol Adenosis (DESAD) project, Obstet. Gynecol. **53**:1979.

Robboy, S. J., and Welch, W. R.: Microglandular hyperplasia in vaginal adenosis associated with oral contraceptives and prenatal diethylbestrol exposure, Obstet. Gynecol. **49**:430, 1977.

Roth, L. M., and Hornbuck, H. B.: Clear cell adenocarcinoma of the cervix in young women, Cancer **34**:1761, 1974.

Sandberg, E. C.: Benign cervical and vaginal changes associated with exposure to stilbestrol in utero, Am. J. Obstet. Gynecol. **125**:777, 1976.

Sandberg, E. C., Danielson, R. E., Cauwet, R. W., and others: Adenosis vaginae, Am. J. Obstet. Gynecol. **78**:1115, 1971.

Stafl, A., and Mattingly, R. F.: Vaginal adenosis; a precancerous lesion? Am. J. Obstet. Gynecol. **120**:666, 1974.

Taft, P. D., Robboy, S. J., Herbst, A. L., and others: Cytology of clear cell adenocarcinoma of the genital tract in young females; review of 95 cases from the registry, Acta Cytol. **18**:279, 1974.

Ulfelder, H., and Robboy, S. J.: The embryologic development of the human vagina, Am. J. Obstet. Gynecol. **126**:769, 1976.

Wharton, J. T., Rutledge, F. N., Gallager, H. S., and others: Treatment of clear cell adenocarcinoma in young females, Obstet. Gynecol. **45**:365, 1975.

CHAPTER THREE

Invasive cervical cancer

GENERAL OBSERVATIONS

The uterine cervix is of major interest and importance to almost every obstetrician/gynecologist. To the gynecologic oncologist it represents a very common focus for the development of malignant tissue. To the obstetrician it represents the primary barometer in the process of labor and delivery. No organ is as accessible to the obstetrician/gynecologist in terms of both diagnosis and therapy. Its accessibility led to the great strides made possible by the Pap smear, resulting in complete reversal of the prognosis in cancer of this organ. Easy access to the cervix also led to the skillful application of radiation techniques, which have resulted in some of the best overall cure rates for any malignancy found in the human.

The cause of cervical cancer is unknown, but its development seems related to multiple insults and injuries sustained by the cervix. Cervical carcinoma is virtually nonexistent in a celibate population; only one case has been reported in the litera-

50

ture. It is more prevalent in women of lower socioeconomic groups and is correlated with first coitus at an early age and with multiple sexual partners. There is no correlation with the frequency of sexual intercourse.

Herpesvirus type 2 has received attention as a possible etiologic agent for cervical cancer. When women with cytologic evidence of herpetic infection were followed prospectively, 24% developed cervical anaplasia as compared with 2% of a control group. Other studies have shown a higher incidence of antibodies to herpesvirus type 2 in the blood of cervical cancer patients than in a control group. Whether the virus is oncogenic, a carcinogen, or simply a passenger associated with a multiplicity of sexual partners is not clear at this time. Other explanations have been offered, such as a propensity for abnormal cervical epithelium to be susceptible to herpetic infection.

The cervix (L. *cervix*, neck) is a narrow cylindric segment of the uterus; it enters the vagina through the anterior vaginal wall and lies, in most instances, at right angles to it. In the average patient it measures 2 to 4 cm in length and is contiguous with the inferior aspect of the uterine corpus. The point of juncture of the uterus and the cervix is known as the isthmus; this area is marked by slight constriction of the lumen. Anteriorly, the cervix is separated from the bladder by fatty tissue and is connected laterally to the broad ligament and parametrium (through which it obtains its blood supply). The lower intravaginal portion of the cervix is a free segment that projects into the vault of the vagina and is covered with mucous membrane; the cervix opens into the vaginal cavity through the external os. The cervical canal extends from the anatomic external os to the internal os, where it joins the uterine cavity. The histologic internal os is the area where there is a transition from endocervical to endometrial glands. The intravaginal portion of the cervix (portio vaginalis, ectocervix) is covered with stratified squamous epithelium that is essentially identical to the epithelium of the vagina. The endocervical mucosa is arranged in branching folds (plicae palmatae) and is lined by cylindric epithelium. The stroma of the cervix is composed of connective tissue with stratified muscle fibers and elastic tissue. The elastic tissue is found primarily around the walls of the larger blood vessels.

The stratified squamous epithelium of the portio vaginalis is composed of several layers conventionally described as basal, parabasal, intermediate, and superficial. The basal layer consists of a single row of cells and rests on a thin basement membrane. This is the layer in which active mitosis occurs. The parabasal and intermediate layers together constitute the prickle-cell layer, which is analogous to the same layer in the epidermis. The superficial layer varies in thickness, depending on the degree of estrogen stimulation. It consists primarily of flattened cells that show an increasing degree of cytoplasmic acideophilia toward the surface. Both the thickness and the glycogen content of the epithelium increase following estrogen stimulation, accounting for the therapeutic effect of estrogens in atrophic vaginitis. The staining of glycogen in the normal epithelium of the portio vaginalis is the basis of the Schiller tests.

MICROINVASIVE CARCINOMA OF THE CERVIX

Microinvasive carcinoma of the cervix is a subject that has been associated with 2 decades of confusion. Diagnostic issues have been confused, and investigators have reported conflicting results on what appear to be the same subset of patients. The terminology used by various authors has varied greatly. Although "microinvasive carinoma" has been the term most frequently used, the subject has been considered under a dozen different headings. Indeed, some authors have used different terms within the same article and thereby have compounded the confusion. An attempt was made to eliminate some of the confusion in July 1974, when the Committee of the International Federation of Gynecology and Obstetrics reclassified these lesions as stage IA and then described them as "early stromal invasion." The definition was left vague intentionally because little agreement could be reached on a more definite description. Many authorities have taken 3 or 5 mm of invasion as the limit for

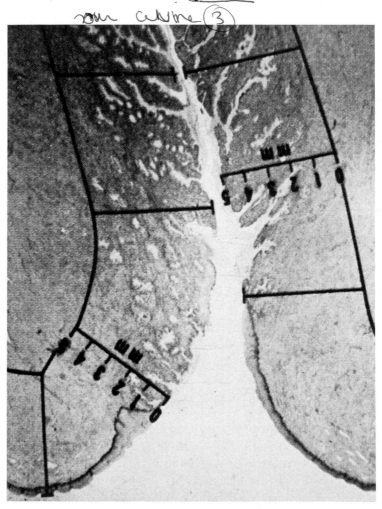

Fig. 3-1. Five-millimeter rule on a histologic section of a normal squamocolumnar junction. (Courtesy Hervy Averette, M.D., Miami, Florida.)

"microinvasive carcinoma" (Fig. 3-1). One author felt that any invasion greater than 1 mm should be considered frank invasion and that only lesions less than 1 mm are truly "microinvasive" (Fig. 3-2). In January 1974 the Society of Gynecologic Oncology (SGO) accepted the following statement on microinvasion in cancer of the cervix uteri: (1) cases of intraepithelial carcinoma with questionable invasion should be regarded as intraepithelial carcinoma and (2) a microinvasive lesion should be defined as one in which neoplastic epithelium invades the stroma in one or more places to a depth of 3 mm or less below the base of the epithelium and in which lymphatic or vascular involvement is not demonstrated. This definition was submitted for consideration by the Executive Board of the American College of Obstetricians and Gynecologists with the recommendation that it be approved and forwarded to the International Federation of Gynecology and Obstetrics.

In the opinion of most, microinvasion should be strictly defined as invasion to a

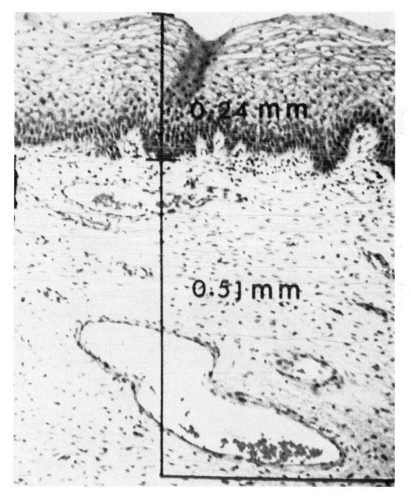

Fig. 3-2. Vascular channels within 0.5 mm of the surface epithelium shown on histologic section of a normal cervix. (Courtesy Hervy Averette, M.D., Miami, Florida.)

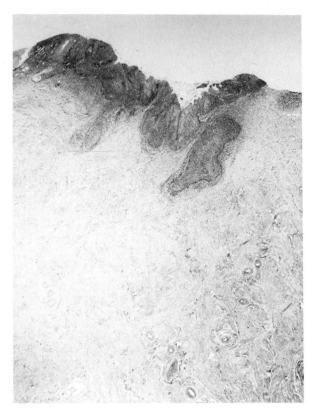

Fig. 3-3. Microinvasive (stage IA) squamous cell carcinoma of the cervix.

Volume

depth of no greater than 3 mm with no confluent tongues and no areas of lymphatic or vascular invasion (Fig. 3-3). The volume of the invasive process is the key to predicting the aggressiveness of the disease. The responsible physician must review the histologic sections himself, and if there are only a few scattered islands of invasion, the patient may be treated by simple hysterectomy. On the other hand, if there are multiple and/or confluent tongues of invasive disease (a better term for these lesions is microcarcinoma or stage IB "occult cancer") this patient should be considered at high risk for lymphatic involvement, and even though this involvement is not seen on the microscopic sections, the patient should be treated by radical hysterectomy and pelvic lymphadenectomy or pelvic irradiation including treatment of the pelvic nodes.

Creasman reported one case with a positive pelvic node among 19 patients who had invasion of 5 mm or less, giving an incidence of 5.2%. Other reports indicate an incidence of positive nodes in "microinvasion" of between 0% and 5% (Table 3-1). A review of the literature (751 collected cases) gave an overall incidence of 1.2% for lymph node metastasis. These figures include, of course, those lesions with bulky invasion relative to the 5-mm depth. One would expect that strict adherence to the

Table 3-1. Lymph node metastases in microinvasive carcinoma of the cervix

Author	Number of cases	Patients with metastases
Mussey and associates	91	2
Kolstad	177	4
Ng and Reagan	66	0
Boyes and associates	48	1
Boutselis and associates	45	0
TOTAL	427	7 (1.7%)

guidelines of the SGO (stated on p. 53) would result in a near zero incidence of lymph node metastasis.

CLINICAL PROFILE

The screening program designed to reveal preinvasive cancer of the cervix has led to the discovery of patients with truly invasive but still limited invasion of subepithelial tissues. When this invasion exceeds that of "early stromal invasion" (stage IA) but is still not clinically evident it is called stage IB (occult cancer). These lesions and anything more advanced are considered truly invasive cancer of the cervix. A substantial and well-publicized screening program must make the public and the profession more aware of cancer as the possible cause of even minimal gynecologic symptoms. All public communication of an educative nature should emphasize the prevention and cure of cancer, and a more hopeful and optimistic attitude would help motivate both patients and physicians to seek appropriate action. The need for early diagnosis rests upon the incontrovertible fact that definite cure, in actuarial terms, is readily achieved when cervical cancer is minimal but is nearly impossible if the tumor is given time to grow and spread to the pelvic wall or into adjacent structures such as the bladder and rectum. The gradient of percentage curability from early invasive cancer to late and grossly invasive disease is such a steep one that even a moderate reduction in tumor size could not fail to create a substantial improvement in curability. It is true, of course, that like other cancers, some carcinomas of the cervix grow more rapidly than others. The basis for this differential in growth rate is still beyond our knowledge, but it is not beyond our capability to prevent undue growing time. Even the relatively slow growing malignancy, if given enough time, will become incurable; and the most rapid growing tumor, if diagnosed while of still moderate dimension, is definitely curable. The sooner all patients are detected and treated, the better the chances of cure. The techniques of cytology and colposcopy have gifted the specialty of gynecology with the capability of eradicating cervical cancer. Every opportunity should be taken to disseminate modern concepts of cancer control to schools of nursing as well as other paramedical organizations, because there is still a need for more coordinated effort in this field and the burden should not be left with the physician alone.

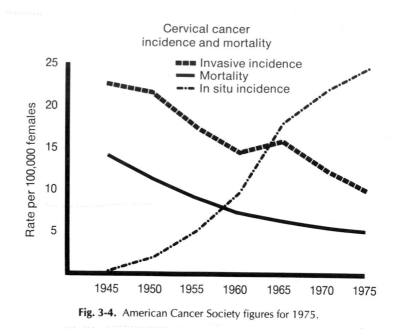

Fig. 3-4. American Cancer Society figures for 1975.

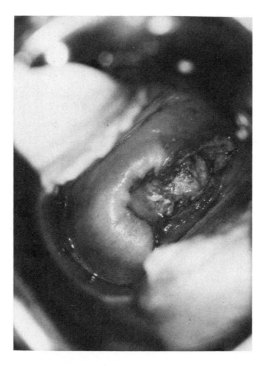

Fig. 3-5. Ulcerative squamous cell carcinoma of the cervix.

The frequency with which invasive cervical cancer occurs is not known exactly, but the best incidence data indicate a rate of approximately 10 to 12 per 100,000 per year (Fig. 3-4). The incidence appears to change from one locality to another, and it is noted to be less frequent in rural areas as compared with metropolitan areas. Cancer of the cervix is apparently less frequent in Norway and Sweden than in the United States, but it looms larger in the cancer problem in underdeveloped areas of the world than in the United States and Western Europe.

Symptoms

A typical patient with clinically obvious cervical cancer is a multiparous woman between 45 and 55 years of age who married and delivered her first child at an early age, usually before the age of 20. Probably the first symptom of early cancer of the cervix is a thin, watery, blood-tinged vaginal discharge that frequently goes unrecognized by the patient. The classic symptom is intermittent, painless, abnormal intermenstrual bleeding, often initially only spotting occurring postcoitally or after douching. As the malignancy enlarges the bleeding episodes become heavier, more frequent, and of longer duration, and the patient may also describe what seems to her to be an increase in the amount and duration of her regular menstrual flow; ultimately the bleeding becomes essentially continuous. In the postmenopausal woman the bleeding is more likely to prompt early medical attention.

Late symptoms or more advanced indicators of the disease include the development of pain referred to the flank or leg, which is usually secondary to the involvement of the ureters, pelvic wall, and/or sciatic nerve routes. Many patients complain of dysuria, hematuria, rectal bleeding, or obstipation due to bladder or rectal invasion. Distant metastasis and persistent edema of one or both lower extremities as a result of lymphatic and venous blockage by extensive pelvic wall disease are late manifestations of primary disease and frequent manifestations of recurrent disease. Massive hemorrhage and development of uremia with profound inanition may also occur as preterminal events.

Gross appearance

The gross clinical appearance of carcinoma of the cervix varies considerably and is dependent on the regional mode of involvement and the nature of the particular lesion's growth pattern. Three categories of gross lesions have traditionally been described. The most common is the exophytic lesion, which usually arises on the ectocervix and often grows to form a large friable polypoid mass that can bleed profusely. These exophytic lesions sometimes arise within the endocervical canal and distend the cervix and the endocervical canal, creating the so-called barrel-shaped lesion. A second manifestation of cervical carinoma is created by an infiltrating tumor that tends to show very little visible ulceration or exophytic mass but presents as a stony hard cervix that regresses slowly with radiation therapy. A third type of lesion is the ulcerative tumor (Fig. 3-5), which usually erodes a portion of the cervix, often replacing the cervix and a portion of the upper vaginal vault with a large crater associated with local infection and seropurulent discharge.

Routes of spread

The main routes of spread of carcinoma of the cervix are: (1) into the vaginal mucosa, extending microscopically down beyond visible or palpable disease, (2) into the myometrium of the lower uterine segment and corpus, particularly with lesions originating in the endocervix, (3) into the paracervical lymphatics and from there to the most commonly involved lymph nodes, i.e., the obturator, hypogastric, and external iliac nodes, and (4) direct extension into adjacent structures or parametria, which may reach to the obturator fascia and the wall of the true pelvis. Extension of the disease to involve the bladder or rectum can result with or without the occurrence of a vesicovaginal or rectovaginal fistula.

The prevalence of lymph node disease correlated well with the stage of the malignancy in several anatomic studies. The prevalence rate of lymph node involvement in stage I is between 15% and 20% and in stage II between 25% and 40%; in stage III it is assumed that at least 50% have positive nodes. Variations are sometimes seen with different material. The best study of lymph node involvement in

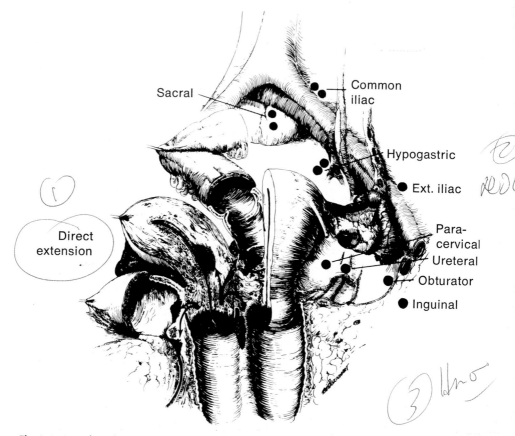

Fig. 3-6. Lymph node chains draining the cervix. (From Henriksen, E.: Am. J. Obstet. Gynecol. **58**:924, 1949.)

cervical cancer was done by Henriksen (Fig. 3-6). The nodal groups described by Henriksen were the following:

Primary group

1. The parametrial nodes, which are the small lymph nodes traversing the parametria.
2. The paracervical or ureteral nodes, located above the uterine artery where it crosses the ureter.
3. The obturator or hypogastric nodes surrounding the obturator vessels and nerves.
4. The hypogastric nodes, which course along the hypogastric vein near its junction with the external iliac vein.
5. The external iliac nodes, which are a group of from six to eight nodes that tend to be uniformly larger than the nodes of the other iliac groups.
6. The sacral nodes, which were originally included in the secondary group.

Secondary group

1. The common iliac nodes.
2. The inguinal nodes, which consist of the deep and superficial femoral lymph nodes.
3. The periaortic nodes.

Henriksen plotted the percentage of nodal involvement for both treated and untreated patients (Figs. 3-7 and 3-8). Distribution is as one would expect, with a greater number of involved nodes found in the region of the cervix and a lower percentage of distant metastases. Although the series was an autopsy study, Henriksen found that only 27% had metastasis above the aortic chain. Cervical cancer kills by local extension with ureteral obstruction in a high percentage of patients.

ADENOCARCINOMA OF THE CERVIX

Ninety-five percent of cervical cancer are of the squamous cell variety, and the remaining 5% are primarily adenocarcinomas. Adenocarcinoma arises from the cervical mucus-producing gland cells, and because of its origin within the cervix it may be present for a considerable time before it becomes clinically evident. These lesions are characteristically bulky neoplasms that expand the cervical canal and create the so-called barrel shaped lesion of the cervix. The spread pattern of these lesions is quite similar to that of squamous cancer, with direct extension accompanied by metastases to regional pelvic nodes as the primary routes of dissemination. Local recurrence is more common in these lesions, and this fact has resulted in the commonly held belief that they are more radioresistant than their squamous counterpart. It would seem more likely, however, that the bulky, expansive nature of these endocervical lesions rather than a differential in radiosensitivity accounts for the local recurrence. This problem has led many oncologists to advocate combined radiotherapy and surgery for optimum control of the central lesion.

STAGING

The staging of cancer of the cervix is a clinical appraisal, preferably confirmed with the patient under anesthesia; it cannot be changed later if findings at operation or subsequent treatment reveal further advancement of the disease.

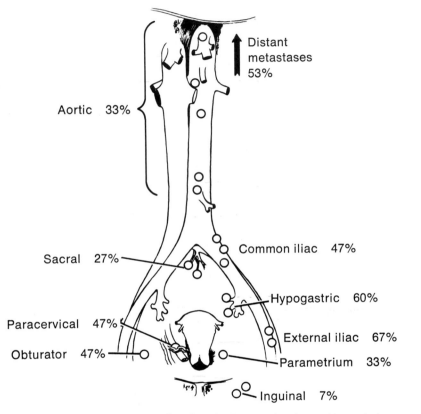

Fig. 3-7. Percent involvement of draining lymph nodes in treated patients with cervical cancer. (From Henriksen, E.: Am. J. Obstet. Gynecol. **58:**924, 1949.)

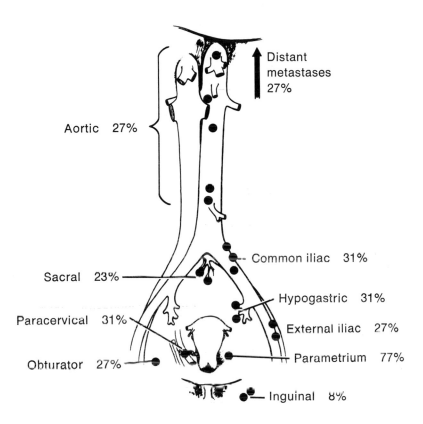

Aortic 27%

Distant metastases 27%

Common iliac 31%

Sacral 23%

Hypogastric 31%

Paracervical 31%

External iliac 27%

Obturator 27%

Parametrium 77%

Inguinal 8%

Fig. 3-8. Percent involvement of draining lymph nodes in untreated patients with cervical cancer. (From Henriksen, E.; Am. J. Obstet. Gynecol. **58:**924, 1949.)

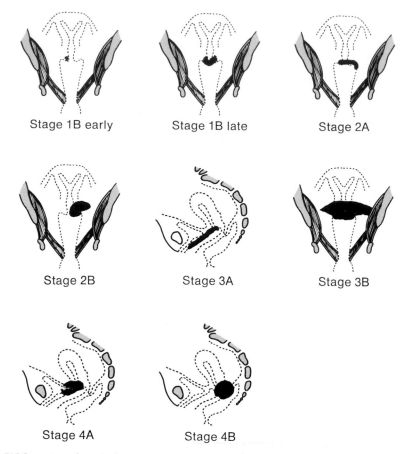

Fig. 3-9. FIGO staging of cervical cancer. (From DiSaia, P. J.: The cervix. In Romney, S. L., Gray, M. J., Little, A. B., and others, editors: Gynecology and obstetrics; health care of women, ed. 2, New York, 1978, McGraw-Hill Book Co.)

International classification of cancer of the cervix (Fig. 3-9)

Stage 0: Carcinoma in situ

Stage I: Carcinoma confined to the cervix

Stage IA: Microinvasion (early stromal invasion)

Stage IB (occult cancer): Frank invasion recognized histologically but not clinically

Stage IB: All other cancers limited to the uterus

Stage II: Involvement of the vagina but not the lower third or infiltration of the parametria but not out to the sidewall

Stage IIA: Involvement of the vagina but no evidence of parametrial involvement

Stage IIB: Infiltration of the parametria but not out to the sidewall

Stage III: Involvement of the lower third of the vagina or extension to the pelvic sidewall

Stage IIIA: Involvement of the lower third of the vagina but not out to the pelvic sidewall if the parametria are involved

Stage IIIB: Involvement of one or both parametria out to the sidewall

Stage III (urinary): Obstruction of one or both ureters on intravenous pyelogram without the other criteria for stage III disease

Stage IV: Extension outside the reproductive tract
Stage IVA: Involvement of the mucosa of the bladder or rectum
Stage IVB: Distant metastasis or disease outside the true pelvis

The following diagnostic aids are acceptable for determining a staging classification: physical examination, routine radiographs, colposcopy, cystoscopy, protosigmoidoscopy, intravenous pyelogram (IVP), and barium studies of the lower colon and rectum. Other examinations, such as lymphography, arteriography, venography, laparoscopy, and hysterography, are not recommended for staging since they are not uniformly available from institution to institution. It is important to stress that staging is a means of communicating between one institution and another. Probably more important, however, staging is a means of evaluating the treatment plans used within one institution. For these reasons, the method of staging should remain fairly constant. Staging does not limit the treatment plan, and therapy can be tailored to the architecture of the malignancy in each patient. Unfortunately, clinical staging is only of rough value in prognosis, since diseases of wide variability are often included under one subheading. This is particularly true in stage IB, where a clinically obvious 0.5-cm lesion carries the same stage as a 6-cm lesion confined to the uterus.

TREATMENT

Once the diagnosis of invasive cervical cancer is established, the question is how to best treat the patient. Specific therapeutic measures are usually governed by the age and general health of the patient, by the extent of the cancer, and by the presence and nature of any complicating abnormalities. It is thus essential to carry out a complete and careful investigation of the patient (Table 3 2), and then a joint decision regarding treatment should be made by radiotherapist and gynecologist. The choice of treatment demands clinical judgment but, apart from the occasional patient for whom only symptomatic treatment may be deemed best, this choice lies between surgery and radiotherapy. In most institutions the initial method of treatment is radiotherapy, both intracavitary radium and external x-ray therapy. The controversy between surgery and radiotherapy has existed for decades and essentially surrounds the treatment of stage I and stage IIA cervical cancer. For the most part, all stages above stage I and stage IIA are treated with radiotherapy. The 5-year survival figures from two large series, one treated with radiotherapy alone and the other with surgery, are included here. Currie reported the results of 552 radical operations for cancer of the cervix as follows:

Stage I	189 cases	86.3%
Stage IIA	103 cases	75.0%
Stage IIB	78 cases	58.9%
Other stages	41 cases	34.1%

Some of these patients with positive nodes did receive postoperative radiotherapy.

Table 3-2. Pretreatment evaluation of carcinoma of the uterine cervix

---

1. History, physical examination, and routine blood studies
2. Radiologic studies
    a. Chest film
    b. IVP
    c. Barium enema (adenocarcinomas, advanced stages, or where otherwise clinically indicated, e.g., patient with lower bowel symptoms)
3. Cystoscopy (very low yield in stage I)
4. Rectosigmoidoscopy (same indications as barium enema)

Of 2,000 patients treated with radiotherapy at M. D. Anderson Hospital and Tumor Institute, Fletcher reports the following 5-year cure rates:

Stage I	91.5%
Stage IIA	83.5%
Stage IIB	66.5%
Stage IIIA	45.0%
Stage IIIB	36.0%
Stage IV	14.0%

In general it can be stated that in early stages, comparable survival rates are obtained by both treatment techniques. The advantage of radiotherapy is that it is applicable to virtually all patients, whereas radical surgery is of necessity exclusive of certain medically inoperable patients. The selectivity of any surgical series along with the possible occurrence of immediate serious morbidity must be kept in mind when this treatment plan is selected. In many institutions, surgery for stage I and stage IIA disease is reserved for young patients in whom preservation of ovarian function is desired and the conviction is held that improved vaginal preservation will result. The modern operative mortality and the postoperative ureterovaginal fistula rate have both been recently reported at far less than 1%, making an objective decision for therapy even more difficult. Other reasons given for the selection of radical surgery over radiation include cervical cancer in pregnancy, concomitant inflammatory disease of the bowel, previous irradiation therapy for other disease, presence of pelvic inflammatory disease or an adnexal neoplasm along with the malignancy, and patient preference. Among the disadvantages of radiation therapy, one must consider the permanent injury to the tissues of the normal organ bed of the neoplasm and the possibility of second malignancies developing in this bed.

Surgical management

The use of radical hysterectomy in this country was initiated by Joe V. Meigs at Harvard University in 1944, and shortly thereafter the radical hysterectomy with pelvic lympthadenectomy was adopted by many clinics in this country because of dissatisfaction with the limitations of radiotherapy. Some had found that many lesions were not radiosensitive and some patients had metastatic disease in regional lymph nodes that were alleged to be radioresistant. Radiation injuries had been reported, and one of the overriding points in favor of surgery was that gynecologists were surgeons rather than radiotherapists and thus felt more comfortable with this treatment modality. At the time of the popularization of this procedure, modern techniques of surgery, anesthesia, antibiotics, and electrolyte balance had emerged, reducing the enormous morbidity that once attended major operative procedures in the abdomen.

Radical hysterectomy is a procedure that must be performed by a skilled technician with sufficient experience to make the morbidity very acceptable (1% to 5%). The procedure involves removal of the uterus, upper third of the vagina, entire uterosacral and uterovesicle ligaments (Fig. 3-10), and all of the parametrium on each side, along with pelvic node dissection encompassing the four major pelvic lymph node chains: ureteral, obturator, hypogastric, and iliac. Metastatic lesions to the ovaries are quite rare, and preservation of these structures is acceptable, especially in young women. The complexity of this procedure is supported by the observation that the tissues removed are in close proximity to many vital structures such as the bowel, the bladder, the ureters (Fig. 3-11), and the great vessels of the pelvis. The object of the dissection is to preserve the bladder, rectum, and ureters but remove as much of the remaining tissue of the pelvis as is feasible without incurring a significant incidence of injury to these structures.

There is no doubt that in stage I as well as the more restricted of stage II cases, surgical removal of the disease is feasible. The addition of pelvic lymphadenectomy to the operative procedure caused considerable controversy in the early part of the century. Wertheim removed nodes only if they were enlarged and then not systematically. He believed that when accessible regional nodes were involved, the inaccessible distant nodes were also involved, and removal of suspicious nodes was more for prognostic than therapeutic value. He felt that node involvement was a measure of the lethal quality of the tumor and not merely a mechanical extension of the disease. The operative procedure popularized by Meigs included meticulous pelvic lymphadenectomy Indeed, Meigs demonstrated a 42% 5-year survival rate in another series of patients with positive nodes. Lymphadenectomy now is an established part of the operative procedure for any patient with disease greater than stage IA. There has been some interest in combining a radical vaginal operation with a retroperitoneal lymphadenectomy, and the results reported by Mitra, Navratil and Kastner, and McCall are surprisingly good. The survival rate in patients with negative nodes is usually in the range of 90% or more. Patients with positive pelvic nodes usually receive postoperative whole-pelvis irradiation, although scientific evidence that this improves outcome is lacking. A small survey conducted by the SGO in 1979 revealed an unaltered incidence of recurrence with the addition of pelvic irradiation (Table 3-3). The lower incidence of pelvic recurrence in the irradiated group was countered by an increased incidence of distant metastases in the unirradiated group. A larger study is needed before firm conclusions can be reached.

The major complications of radical hysterectomy are formation of ureteral fistulae and lymphocysts, pelvic infection, and hemorrhage. All of these complications are

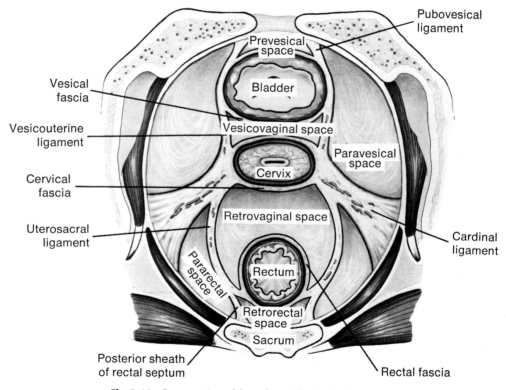

Fig. 3-10. Cross-section of the pelvis at the level of the cervix.

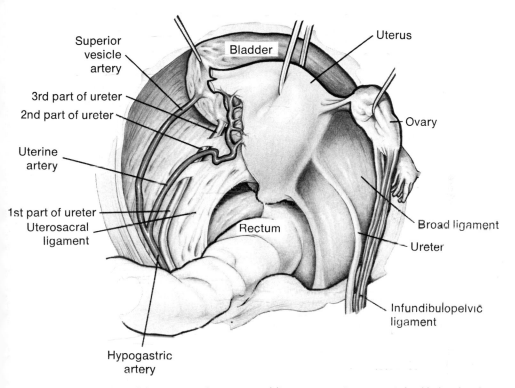

Fig. 3-11. Relationship of the ureter to the uterosacral ligaments, uterine artery, infundibulopelvic ligament, and uterus.

Table 3-3. Stage IB squamous carcinoma of cervix

	Radiotherapy		No radiotherapy	
Site of recurrence	N	% Total	N	% Total
Pelvis	5	(10.6)	27	(18.5)
Central	3	(6.4)	8	(5.5)
Pelvic wall	2	(4.2)	19	(13.0)
Distant metastases	9	(19.1)	9	(6.2)
Both	4	(8.5)	21	(14.4)
TOTAL	18/47	(38.3)	57/146	(39.0)

preventable, and the incidence is decreasing steadily. Ureteral fistulae are now infrequent (0% to 3%) primarily as a result of the imrpovement in techniques, such as avoiding excess damage to the structure itself and preserving alternate routes of blood supply. Retroperitoneal drainage of the lymphadenectomy sites by means of suction catheters has considerably reduced the incidence of lymphocysts and pelvic infection. The use of electrocautery and hemoclips has assisted the surgeon immensely with hemostasis, and postoperative hemorrhage is rare. The wide spectrum of antibiotics available today is invaluable in the prevention of pelvic infection, which had contributed significantly to fistula formation as well as adhesions and bowel complications.

Radiotherapy

Over the past 3 decades radiotherapy has emerged as a notable alternative to radical surgery primarily because of improvements in technique. The number of radiation-resistant lesions was discovered to be quite small, and radiation injury in the hands of a skilled radiotherapist is quite limited, especially with the moderate dosages used for early disease. A great deal of evidence recently has been presented that confirms the hypothesis that radiotherapy is able to destroy disease in lymph nodes as well as the primary lesion. Over the past decade radical hysterectomy has been reserved in many institutions for patients who are relatively young, lean, and in otherwise good health. In other areas of the country either radiotherapy or surgery has been used exclusively when the alternate modality is of limited availability.

Radiotherapy for cancer of the cervix was begun in 1903 in New York by Margaret Cleaves. In 1913 Abbe was able to report an 8-year cure. The Stockholm method was established in 1914, the Paris method in 1919, and the Manchester method in 1938. Radium was the first element used, and it has always been the most important element in radiotherapy of this lesion. External irradiation was used to treat the lymphatic drainage areas in the pelvis lateral to the cervix and the paracervical tissues.

Successful radiation therapy depends on:

1. Greater sensitivity of the cancer cell as compared with the cells of the normal tissue bed to ionizing radiation.

2. Greater ability of normal tissue to recuperate after irradiation.
3. A patient in reasonably good physical condition.

The maximum effect of ionizing radiation on cancer is obtained in the presence of a good and intact circulation and adequate cellular oxygenation. The preparation of the patient for a radical course of irradiation therapy should be as careful as the preparation for radical surgery. The patient's general condition should be as well maintained as possible with a high protein-vitamin and high caloric diet. Excessive blood loss should be controlled and hemoglobin maintained well above 10 grams.

Some consideration must be given to the tolerance of normal tissues of the pelvis, which are likely to receive relatively high doses during the course of treatment of cervical malignancy. The vaginal mucosa in the area of the vault tolerates between 20,000 and 25,000 rads. The rectovaginal septum is said to tolerate approximately 6,000 rads over 4 to 6 weeks without difficulty. The bladder mucosa can accept a maximum dose of 7,000 rads. The colon will tolerate in the neighborhood of 4,500 rads, but small bowel loops are less tolerant and are said to accept a maximum dose of between 4,000 and 4,200 rads. This, of course, pertains to small bowel loops within the pelvis; the tolerance of the small bowel when the entire abdomen is irradiated is limited to 2,500 rads. One of the basic principles of radiotherapy is implied here: the normal tissue tolerance of any organ is inversely related to the volume of that organ which is receiving irradiation.

External irradiation and intracavitary radium therapy must be used in various combinations (Table 3-4). Treatment plans must be tailored to each patient and her particular lesion. The size and distribution of the cancer, not the stage, should be treated. Success in curing cancer of the cervix depends on the ability of the therapy team to evaluate the lesion (as well as the geometry of the pelvis) during treatment and then make indicated changes in therapy as necessary. Intracavitary radium therapy is ideally suited to the treatment of early tumors because of the accessibility of the portio of the cervix and the cervical canal. It is possible to place radium or cesium in close proximity to the lesion and thus deliver doses that approach 15,000 to 20,000 rads. In addition, normal cervical and vaginal tissue has a particularly high tolerance to irradiation. One thus has an ideal situation for the treatment of cancer in that there are accessible lesions that lie in a bed of normal tissue (cervix and vagina) that is highly radioresistant.

Radium therapy. Radium is the isotope that has traditionally been used in the treatment of cancer of the cervix. Its greatest value lies in the fact that its half-life is some 1,620 years, and therefore it provides a very stable, durable element for therapy. In recent years both cesium and cobalt have been used for intracavitary therapy. Cesium has a half-life of 30 years and with modern technology provides a very adequate substitute for radium. Four major techniques for the application of radium in the treatment of cervical cancer have found continuing favor among gynecologists. There are three intracavitary techniques using specially designed applicators, and the fourth technique involves the application of radium in the form of needles directly into the tumor. The variations that exist between the three techniques of

Table 3-4. Suggested therapy for cervical cancer

Stage	Whole pelvis (rads)	Brachytherapy (mg-hr)	Surgery
IA true micro-invasive		—	Extrafascial hysterectomy
IB "occult"	2,000 (2,000 parametrial)	8,000 (2 applications)	Radical hysterectomy with bilateral pelvic lymphadenectomy as option
IB	4,000	6,000 (2 applications)	
IIA	4,000	6,000 (2 applications)	
IIB	4,000-5,000*	5,000-6,000 (2 applications)	Consider pelvic exenteration for tumor persistence
IIIA	5,000-6,000*	2,000-3,000 and/or interstitial implant	
IIIB	5,000-6,000*	4,000 (1 application), 5,000 (2 applications)†	
IVA	6,000	4,000 (1 application), 5,000 (2 applications)†	
IVB	500-1,000 pulse 2-4 times 1 week apart	Palliative	

*Patients with larger lesions or poor vaginal geometry merit the higher dose of external radiation.
†Two applications are suggested following whole-pelvis radiation with larger lesions or when the first application has less than optimum dosimetry.

intracavitary radium therapy are found in the Stockholm, Paris, and Manchester schools of treatment. The differences are largely in the number and length of time of applications, the size and placement of the vaginal colpostats, and radium loading. In this country, the tendency has been to use fixed radium applicators with the intrauterine tandem and vaginal colpostats originally attached to each other. Over the last 2 decades a flexible afterloading system, Fletcher-Suit, has gained increasing popularity because it provides flexibility as well as the safety of afterloading techniques.

The Paris method originally employed a daily insertion of 66.66 mg of radium divided equally between the uterus and the vagina. The radium was allowed to remain in place for 12 to 14 hours, and the period of treatment varied from 5 to 7 days. An essential feature of the Paris method, and a part of the modification of this technique, is the vaginal colpostat, consisting of two hollow corks that act as radium containers joined together by a steel spring that separates them into the lateral vaginal wall.

The Stockholm technique uses a tandem in the uterine cavity surrounded by a square radium plaque applied to the vaginal wall and portio vaginalis of the cervix. No radium is placed in the lower cervical canal, and vaginal sources are used to cover the cervical lesion. The uterine tandem and vaginal plaque are immobilized

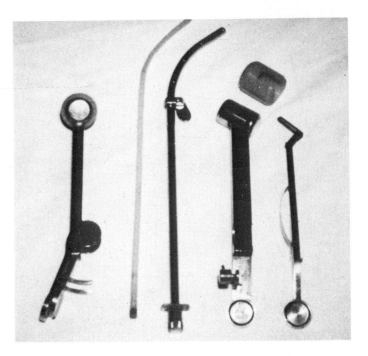

Fig. 3-12. Fletcher-Suit radium applicators: ovoids and tandem with inserts.

by packing and left in place for 12 to 36 hours. Two to three identical applications are made at weekly intervals.

The Manchester system is designed to yield constant isodose patterns regardless of the size of the uterus and vagina. The source placed in the neighborhood of the cervical canal is considered the unit strength. The remaining sources in the corpus and vagina are applied as multiples of this unit and are selected and arranged to produce equivalent isodose curves in each case and an optimum dose at preselected points in the pelvis. The applicator is shaped to allow an isodose curve that delivers radiation to the cervix in a uniform amount. The Fletcher-Suit system (Fig. 3-12) previously mentioned is a variation of the Manchester technique.

An effort is made in the two radium insertions to administer approximately 7,000 rads to the paracervical tissues as the sum of the dose from both external and intracavitary irradiation. The isodose distribution around a Manchester type of radium system is a pear-shaped structure. The maximum total dose delivered by the two radium insertions is a function of the sum dose to the bladder and rectum. The total dose received by the rectal mucosa from both radium applications usually ranges between 4,000 and 6,000 rads. The nearest bladder mucosa may receive between 5,000 and 7,000 rads. When whole-pelvis irradiation is used the radium dosage must be reduced in order to keep the total dose to the bladder and rectum within acceptable limits.

In conjunction with the development of a system of radium distribution, British

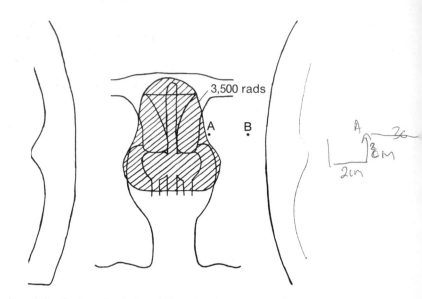

Fig. 3-13. Pear-shaped distribution of radiation delivered to tissues surrounding a typical radium application with the Manchester-type applicators. (From DiSaia, P. J.: The cervix. In Romney, S. L., Gray, M. J., Little, A. B., and others, editors: Gynecology and obstetrics; health care of women, ed. 2, New York, 1978, McGraw-Hill Book Co.)

workers have defined two anatomic areas of the parametria (Fig. 3-13) where dose designation can be correlated with clinical effect. These are situated in the proximal parametria adjacent to the cervix at the level of the internal os and in the distal parametria in the area of the iliac lymph nodes and are designated point A and point B. The description states that point A is located 2 cm from the midline of the cervical canal and 2 cm superior to the lateral vaginal fornix. The dose at point A is representative of the dose to the paracervical triangle that correlates well with the incidence of sequelae as well as with the 5-year control rate in many studies. Point B is 3 cm lateral to point A. This point together with the tissue superior to it is of significance in considering the dose to the node-bearing tissue. It is clear from what has been said relative to points A and B that they can represent important points on a curve describing the dose gradient from the radium sources to the lateral pelvic wall. This gradient is different for the various techniques. In a comparison of the physical characteristics of radiotechniques, the ratio of the dose at point A to the dose at point B should assist in defining physical differences. In addition, determining the dose at point A relative to the calculated dose at points identified as bladder trigone and rectal mucosa provides a means of assessing the relative safety of one application over another. The concepts of point A and B have been questioned by many authors, including Fletcher. They remain as imaginary points but seem to provide a framework in which therapy is planned. Again, the distribution of the disease must be the primary guide in planning therapy, and the total dose to either point A or point B is relative only to their position with regard to the disease distribution.

Whole-pelvis irradiation is usually administered in conjunction with brachy-therapy (e.g., intracavitary radium or cesium) in a dose range of 4,000 to 5,000 rads. Megavoltage machines such as cobalt, linear accelerators, and the betatron have the distinct advantage of giving greater homogeneity of dose to the pelvis. In addition, the hard, short rays of megavoltage pass through the skin without much absorption and cause very little injury, allowing virtually unlimited amounts of radiation to be delivered to pelvic depths with little if any skin irritation. Orthovoltage, because of its relatively long wavelength and low energy, has the disadvantage that doses to the skin are particularly high and, in delivering the required amount of radiation to the pelvis, may cause temporary and permanent skin changes. Thus, for pelvic irradia-tion high-energy megavoltage equipment has definite advantages over orthovoltage and even low-energy megavoltage equipment.

Interstitial therapy. In advanced carcinoma of the cervix, the associated obliter-ation of the fornices or contracture of the vagina may interfere with accurate place-ment of conventional intracavitary applicators. Poorly placed applicators fail to irra-diate the lesion and the pelvis homogeneously. Recently, Syed and others have revived a solution to this dilemma by advocating transvaginal and transperineal im-plants. The technique employs a template to guide the insertion of a group of 18-gauge hollow steel needles into the parametria transperineally. These hollow needles are subsequently "afterloaded" with iridium wires when the patient has returned to her hospital room. Theroretically this technique locates a pair of paravaginal inter-stitial colpostats in both parametria. This approach holds great promise, but long-term studies illustrating improved survival rate and reasonable morbidity are not available.

Extended field irradiation therapy. Over the past decade attempts have been made to salvage more patients with advanced cervical cancer by identifying the pres-ence of para-aortic lymph node metastases and applying extended field irradiation to the area (Fig. 3-14). The en bloc pelvic and para-aortic portals extend superiorly as far as the level of the dome of the diaphragm and inferiorly to the obturator foramen. The width of the para-aortic portion of the field is usually 8 to 10 cm, and the usual dose delivered is between 4,000 and 5,000 rads in 4 to 6 weeks. A boost of 1,000 rads is often given to the pelvic field alone. Identification of para-aortic lymph node involvement was initially attempted by use of lymphangiography, but this technique did not find general acceptance because of varied accuracy from institution to insti-tution and from radiologist to radiologist. Surgical localization of para-aortic involve-ment has been more satisfactory.

Several recent reports have discussed survival and complications in patients with carcinoma of the cervix and para-aortic metastases who received extended field ir-radiation. Piver and Barlow of Roswell Park Hospital, Buffalo, reported on 20 women with previously untreated cervical cancer who received radical irradiation to the periaortic lymph nodes and pelvis after the diagnosis of periaortic lymph node metastases had been established by surgical staging. They noted that 90% of these patients received 6,000 rads to the periaortic nodes and pelvis in 8 weeks using a

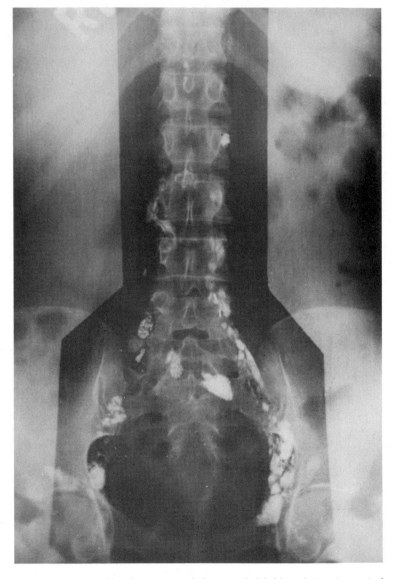

Fig. 3-14. Abdominal x-ray film showing portals for extended field irradiation in cervical cancer.

30% [directly] Complication

split-course technique. A later, updated report shows that 30% have died of complications of this therapy and 45% of recurrent disease. Only 25% of patients have survived disease-free for 16, 18, 24, and 36 months, respectively. The criticism may be that the dose is too high, yet a lesser dose might be ineffective, and four patients did survive. It is obvious that a safe, yet effective, dosage level for extended field irradiation therapy has not yet been established.

Wharton and associates of M.D. Anderson Hospital reported on 120 women who were treated with preirradiation celiotomy. Of these patients, 32 had severe bowel complications and 20 (16.6%) eventually died as a result of the surgery or of the surgery and irradiation. Four of these patients died immediately as a result of the surgical procedure. Of 64 patients with positive nodes who were irradiated, 17% are alive 13 to 38 months after treatment. No patient has survived for 5 years. Wharton and associates further reported that in 36 women with positive nodes it was possible to accurately determine the failure sites after completion of the full course of irradiation therapy. In 25 of these patients, distant metastases were the first evidence of treatment failure; 11 had disease or developed recurrence within the treatment fields; disease of the pelvic wall was found in only two patients.

The results of later studies with lower doses of radiation and modified surgical approaches cannot yet be evaluated, and thus the routine use of staging laparotomy and extended field irradiation therapy in cervical cancer is still under investigation.

Complications of radiation therapy. Morbidity resulting from properly conducted radiation therapy in patients with carcinoma of the cervix is usually minimal. Unfortunate misconceptions about the magnitude of this small radiation morbidity have several origins. Many have failed to distinguish that unnecessary adverse effects result from bad techniques and should not be extrapolated to the use of proper techniques. In addition, there has been a failure to recognize that a great deal of radiation morbidity is usually related to compromised treatment of patients with an extensive tumor in whom surgery is not applicable. Results in these patients cannot be extrapolated to the use of optimum techniques in the treatment of patients with limited malignancy. Also, it often is an unrecognized fact that a great deal of morbidity attributed to irradiation results from an uncontrolled tumor (i.e., rectovaginal-vesicovaginal fistulae). As in the case of surgery, the treatment-related morbidity can be minimized by good application, but it cannot be eliminated.

The acute treatment complications that occur during or shortly after irradiation include irritation of the rectum, small bowel, and bladder, reactions in the skin folds, and mild bone marrow suppression. Some of the transitory symptoms are tenesmus and the passage of mucus and even blood per rectum. The most frequent offending agent in proctitis is vaginal radium, particularly if physical separation (of the radioactive source) from the rectovaginal septum is less than adequate. Diarrhea and abdominal cramping characterize small intestinal irritation. Such morbidity is more frequent when a portion of intestine is fixed in the pelvis by previous surgical adhesions or other pathologic conditions. In this case, the usual offending agent is the external irradiation. In many patients, dysuria and frequency may result from blad-

Complications of Radiation

Immediate → Irritation   Rectum → Proctitis
                          SB → Diarrhea
                          Bladder → Cystitis
                          Skin
                          Bone Marrow Supp

der irritation secondary to localized high radiation dose from radium or combinations of external beam plus radium. This morbidity is more likely in patients with a preexisting abnormality such as infection or inadequate drainage with residual urine. Marked bone marrow suppression is unusual, but a mild transitory depression of the circulating white cells and occasionally of platelet levels is not uncommon. These changes are usually not severe enough to interfere with treatment. Anemia is not a consequence of properly conducted pelvic irradiation but is usually secondary to bleeding or infection and should improve during irradiation therapy.

Late irradiation sequelae including damage to the rectum, bladder, and bone are less common. The symptoms of radiation proctitis may follow an asymptomatic interval of many months to years after treatment. The changes most often are localized to the anterior rectal wall at the site of maximum dosage from radium and range from thickened, fragile mucosa to thin, atrophic mucosa or mucosal ulceration. These changes usually heal with conservative management, but on occasion a diverting colostomy is necessary for either marked fibrosis of the rectal wall or excessive bleeding from the lower bowel. It is important that these stages be recognized and not confused with tumor, since diverting procedures are curative and result in the patient returning to a state of well-being. Similarly, fibrostenotic changes in the sigmoid colon, cecum, and parts of the small intestine are occasionally seen as late complications of irradiation therapy. A typical patient with small bowel injury presents with postprandial crampy abdominal pain and anorexia. All too often these patients are classified as recurrent disease and allowed to waste away. Again, a diverting procedure with anastomosis of the small bowel (proximal to the site of the injury) to the ascending colon usually results in adequate recovery of nutritional status for the patient.

Kagan and associates have proposed a staging system for irradiation injuries following treatment for cancer of the cervix uteri that we find particularly useful. It is as follows:

R_1: Type of injury that results in complete recovery from all acute symptoms such as dysuria and hematuria, diarrhea and cramps, rectal bleeding, and hydroureter.

R_2: Type of injury in which there is incomplete recovery from urinary bleeding, edematous bladder mucosa, diarrhea, colicky pain, weight loss, persistent hydroureter, or colonic stenosis. Continuous medications as well as frequent examinations are required.

S_1: Type of injury that requires surgical intervention for a single-organ injury. This may require total cystectomy, urinary diversion, resection of an obstruced bowel segment, colostomy, or ureteral reimplantation.

S_2: Type of injury that requires more extensive surgery for injury to two or more organs.

Using this staging system we, like Kagan and his co-workers, have found a positive correlation between increasing dose and severe S_1 and S_2 injuries. There is also a definite correlation between all bladder irradiation injuries (R_1, R_2, S_1, S_2) and calculated increased bladder dose (Figs. 3-15 and 3-16).

The overall complication rate varies considerably, depending on the total dose of

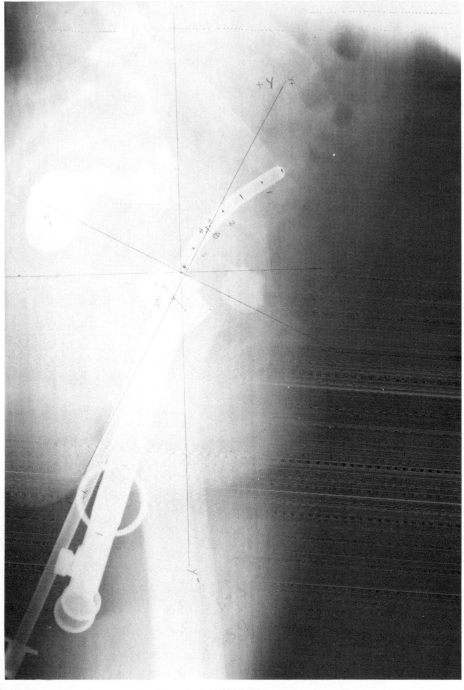

Fig. 3-15. Radium placement film (lateral). Fletcher-Suit applicator, Hypaque in the Foley catheter balloon, and contrast material in the rectum allow estimation of dose to these structures. This is a good application with reasonable distances between the radium system (tandem and ovoids) and the bladder anteriorly and the rectum posteriorly.

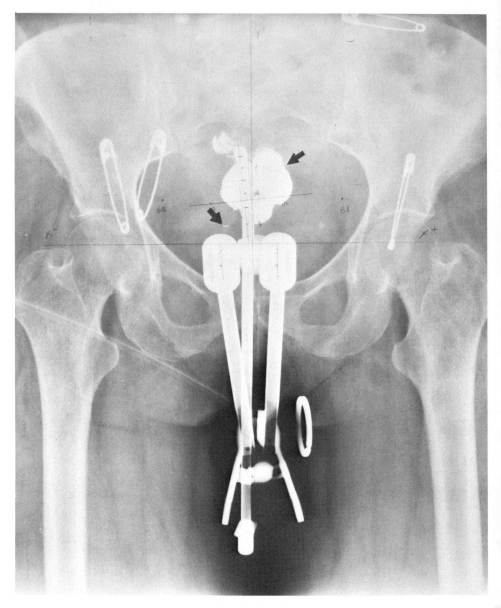

Fig. 3-16. Anteroposterior view of the system in Fig. 3-15. Arrows point to the contrast material in the rectum and stainless steel seeds placed 1 cm into the cervical tissue to identify that organ. The risk of injury from such an application would be low with average doses because of the good central positioning.

radiation used. In general, the serious morbidity of pelvic irradiation is less than 5% if the external irradiation is below 5,000 rads. Patients who receive more than 5,000 rads of external irradiation are usually those individuals with advanced disease in whom radical irradiation is a necessity. In these patients the serious complication rate approaches 10% to 20%.

Cancer of the cervix in pregnancy

Carcinoma of the cervix complicates pregnancy in approximately 0.01% of patients. In deciding on therapy for these malignant neoplasms, one must take into consideration the extent of the disease and the duration of the pregnancy. A detrimental effect of pregnancy on cancer of the cervix has not been demonstrated, anecdotal evidence to the contrary. The hypothesis found in previous literature that pregnancy accelerates the growth of the tumor has not been substantiated. It was thought that parturition was capable of squeezing viable cells into the vascular system and increasing the incidence of metastatic spread, but this has not been substantiated by recent studies. Several studies have shown that stage for stage, the outcome for the pregnant patient with cervical cancer is roughly the same as for the nonpregnant patient.

The construction of a treatment plan for the pregnant patient with cervical cancer (Table 3-5) is dependent on several factors, including stage of disease, duration of

Table 3-5. Suggested therapy for cervical cancer in pregnancy

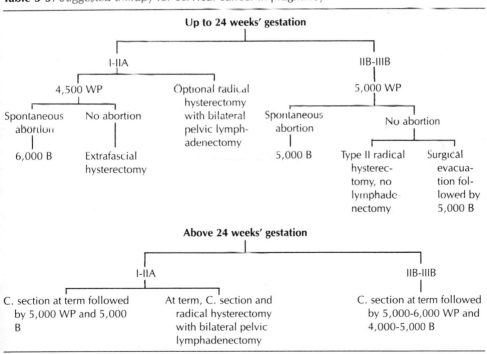

Key: WP, whole-pelvis irradiation (rads); B, brachytherapy (mg-hr), vaginal radium in two applications.

pregnancy, religious conviction of patient and family, desire of the mother for the child, and background of the physician, in addition to the medical problem itself. For stage I and early stage II lesions, a radical surgical procedure (radical hysterectomy) is acceptable therapy during any trimester. If preservation of the pregnancy is desired, a waiting period of several weeks may be required to ensure reasonable viability of the fetus. It is generally recommended that patients in the first and second trimesters not be allowed to await fetal viability, and interruption of the pregnancy is usually advised. Exceptions have been made in cases of early invasive disease in which the central lesion has been thoroughly analyzed by an excisional biopsy and found to be quite limited (e.g., stage IA).

Radiation therapy is also acceptable for patients before 24 weeks' gestation. The pregnancy is disregarded, and the patient is started on whole-pelvis irradiation. If abortion does not occur, excision of the remaining neoplasm by means of an extended (extrafascial) hysterectomy or surgical evacuation of the uterus must follow completion of the external irradiation. Once the uterus is evacuated, radiotherapy can resume. If the uterus has been removed, vaginal vault irradiation may be all that is necessary. In the event that a hysterotomy with evacuation of the uterus has been performed, standard radium techniques are applicable to the postoperative uterus and upper vagina after a 4-week waiting period.

For the patient at 24 weeks' gestation or more, therapy is usually delayed until fetal viability is reached. Cesarean section is performed when appropriate on the basis of pediatric and obstetric criteria. If a radical hysterectomy with pelvic lymphadenectomy is not performed at the time of cesarean section, whole-pelvis irradiation begins immediately after the abdominal incision is healed. Intracavitary irradiation can follow completion of the whole-pelvis irradiation. The basic treatment plan used for cancer of the cervix in a nonpregnant patient can generally be used for those patients in whom only cesarean section has been performed.

Suboptimal treatment situations

There are several situations in which patients with invasive cancer of the cervix receive suboptimal treatment. These may include (1) cancer in a cervical stump, (2) inadequate surgery, and (3) poor vaginal geometry for radium.

Cancer that occurs in a cervical stump is fortunately a diminishing problem, since supracervical hysterectomies are performed less frequently. Carcinoma occurring in a cervical stump presents a special problem, since often an optimal dose of intracavitary radium cannot be applied because there is insufficient place to insert the central tandem, which contributes significantly to the radiation dose to the central tumor as well as to the pelvic sidewall. Radical surgery is also more difficult; the bladder and rectum firmly adhere to the stump and may adhere to each other. Also, the ureters are more difficult to cleanly dissect from the parametrial tissue because of fibrosis from the previous surgery. The net result is an increase in the risk of significant surgical complications involving the ureters, bladder, and rectum. In modern gynecologic surgery, supracervical hysterectomy is rarely indicated, and only under exceptional circumstances encountered at the operating table would supracervical hysterectomy be acceptable.

Inadequate surgery usually occurs when a simple hysterectomy is performed and subsequently frank invasive cervical cancer is discovered. This situation may occur because of poor preoperative evaluation or because the surgery was performed under emergency conditions without an adequate preoperative cervical evaluation. Such a situation may occur in a patient presenting with acute abdomen from ruptured tubo-ovarian abscesses. In any event, if an extensive cancer is found in the cervix, the prognosis is poor, because optimal irradiation cannot be given with the cervix and uterus absent. An even more ominous situation occurs when a hysterectomy is performed with a "cut through" of the cancer, that is, the hysterectomy dissection passes through the cancer. The prognosis is uniformly poor in this event. In the above examples, surgical cures are not obtained, and the probability of curative radiotherapy is greatly diminished.

Adequate radiotherapy is also compromised in patients who have a vagina or cervix that cannot accommodate a complete radium application. This situation is encountered with atrophic stenotic pelvic structures. These patients are finally treated by inserting the tandem and ovoids in a compromised manner, such as inserting the ovoids singly or independently of the central tandem. In any event, standard optimal doses are usually not obtained, and the possibility of sustaining a radiation injury is increased.

SURVIVAL RESULTS

Review of the annual reports on results of treatment of carcinoma of the uterus reveals a wide dispersion of 5-year recovery rates among several stages of carcinoma of the cervix. One can find data supporting any stand one wishes to take with regard to therapy. The overall cure rate in a cumulative series of 130,111 patients (1954 to 1963) (FIGO annual report on gynecologic cancer) with stage I cancer of the cervix was 76.5%. The individual institutions reported 5-year cure rates from 69% to 90% with surgery alone and from 60% to 93% with radiotherapy alone. Differences in results may imply that one form of therapy has advantages over the other, but, considering the rather wide dispersion that in fact may be unrelated to treatment, we must maintain collective open-mindedness with regard to the efficacy of individual therapeutic regimens. The best available figures for the two methods give results that are nearly identical, and the presence of other factors affecting the samples being compared requires quite large differences to be significant. Individual physicians will probably continue to decide on the basis of personal preferences and comparison of complications and later disabilities.

RECURRENT AND ADVANCED CARCINOMA OF THE CERVIX
Clinical profile

In the United States the mortality from cervical cancer in 1945 was 15 per 100,000 female population, and this has declined to a figure that in 1975 was approxi-

Table 3-6. Interval evaluation of cervical cancer following radiotherapy (asymptomatic patient*)

Year	Frequency	Examination
1	3 months	Pelvic exam, Pap smear
	6 months	Chest film, CBC, BUN, creatinine
	1 year	IVP
2	4 months	Pelvic exam, Pap smear
	1 year	Chest films, CBC, BUN, creatinine, IVP
3	6 months	Pelvic exam, Pap smear
	1 year	Chest film

*Symptomatic patients should have appropriate examinations where indicated.

mately 6 per 100,000. It is not clear whether the mortality from cervical cancer is falling as a result of cervical cytologic screening and intervention at the in situ stage or whether cervical screening has caused an increase in the proportion of early stage cancer at diagnosis and registration. Adequate follow-up is the key to early detection of recurrence (Table 3-6).

West studied the age of registration and the age of death of women with cervical cancer in South Wales. He found that the observed age at death was very close to 59 years regardless of stage and age at diagnosis. Although the 5-year survival rate of women with localized (early stage) cervical cancer was much higher than that of women with nonlocalized (late stage) cancer, the women with localized cancer tended to be younger than those with advanced cancer. Calculations of expected age at death of the whole population suggest that more than half the advantage in survival rate shown by early stage cancers over late stage cancers is due to the diagnosis of the former in younger women.

Christopherson and associates reported that the percentage of patients diagnosed as having stage I disease increased by 78% in the population studied from 1953 to 1965. The increase was most remarkable in younger women. They concluded that the major problem in cervical cancer control was the screening of older women. Older women not only had higher incidence rates but the percentage with stage I disease decreased with each decade, reaching a low of 15% for those 70 years of age and older. These older women with cervical cancer rarely are screened and contributed heavily to the death rates. Initial advanced stage contributes heavily to the patient population with advanced recurrent cervical cancer. Therefore, these patients deserve very close posttreatment observation in an effort to detect a recurrence in its earliest possible form.

It is estimated that approximately 35% of patients with invasive cervical cancer will have recurrent or persistent disease following therapy. The diagnosis of recurrent cervical cancer is often quite difficult to establish (Table 3-7). The optimal radiation therapy that most patients receive makes cervical cytologic findings difficult to evaluate. This is especially true immediately following completion of radiation ther-

Table 3-7. Signs and symptoms of recurrent cervical cancer

Weight loss (unexplained)
Leg edema (excessive and often unilateral)
Pelvic and/or thigh-buttock pain
Serosanguineous vaginal discharge
Progressive ureteral obstruction
Supraclavicular lymph node enlargement (usually left side)
Cough
Hemoptysis
Chest pain

apy. Suit and Gallagher, using mammary carcinomas in C_3H mice, demonstrated that persistence of histologically intact cancer cells in irradiated tissue was not indicative of regrowth of tumor. Radiobiologically a viable cell is one with the capacity for sustained proliferation. A cell would be classified as nonviable if it had lost its reproductive integrity, although it could carry out diverse metabolic activities. This reproductive integrity was demonstrated by the transplantation "take" rate when histologically viable tumor cells were transplanted into a suitable recipient. It was evident from these experiments in the mouse model that relatively normal appearing cancer cells can persist for several months following radiation therapy but that these cells are "biologically doomed." Thus, cytologic evaluation of a patient immediately after radiation therapy may erroneously lead to the supposition that persistent disease exists. In addition, subsequent evaluation of the irradiated cervix is also difficult because of the distortion produced in the exfoliated cells, often called "radiation effect." Thus, histologic confirmation of recurrent cancer is essential. This can be accomplished by punch or needle biopsy of suspected areas of malignancy when they are accessible. An interval of at least 3 months should elapse following completion of radiation therapy. The clinical presentation of recurrent cervical cancer is varied and often insidious. Many patients will present with a wasting syndrome with severe loss of appetite and gradual weight loss over a period of weeks to months. This is often preceded by a period of general good health following completion of radiation therapy. Since most recurrences of cancer occur within the first 2 years following therapy, this period of good health rarely lasts more than a year, when the symptoms of cachexia become evident. Diagnostic evaluation at this time should include a chest film, IVP, CBC, BUN, creatinine clearance, and liver function tests.

The location of recurrent or persistent disease has been studied by surgeons and radiotherapists alike (Figs. 3-17 and 3-18). Following radical hysterectomy about one fourth of recurrences occur locally in the upper part of the vagina or the area previously occupied by the cervix. The location of recurrence after radiation therapy showed a 27% occurrence in the cervix, uterus, or upper vagina, 6% in the lower two thirds of the vagina, 43% in the parametrial area including the pelvic wall, 16% distant, and 8% unknown.

Often one will note the development of ureteral obstruction in a patient who had

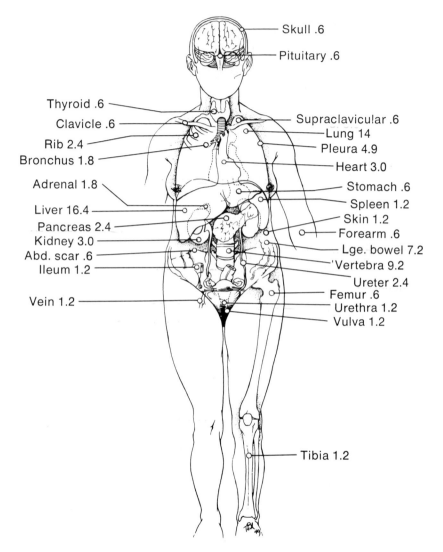

Fig. 3-17. Metastatic sites of treated patients with cervical cancer. (From Henriksen, E.: Am. J. Obstet. Gynecol. **58:**924, 1949.)

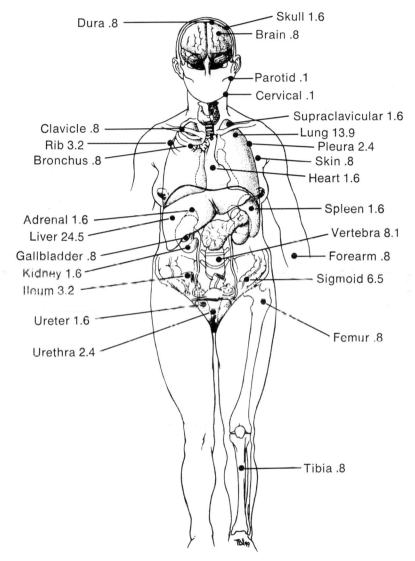

Dura .8

Skull 1.6

Brain .8

Parotid .1

Cervical .1

Supraclavicular 1.6

Clavicle .8

Lung 13.9

Rib 3.2

Pleura 2.4

Bronchus .8

Skin .8

Heart 1.6

Spleen 1.6

Adrenal 1.6

Liver 24.5

Vertebra 8.1

Gallbladder .8

Forearm .8

Kidney 1.6

Sigmoid 6.5

Ileum 3.2

Ureter 1.6

Urethra 2.4

Femur .8

Tibia .8

Fig. 3-18. Metastatic sites of untreated patients with cervical cancer. (From Henriksen, E.: Am. J. Obstet. Gynecol. **58:**924, 1949.)

a normal urinary tract before therapy. Although ureteral obstruction can be caused by radiation fibrosis, this is relatively rare and 95% of the time obstruction is due to progressive tumor. Central disease may not be evident, and a patient with ureteral obstruction following therapy in the absence of other findings should undergo exploratory laparotomy and selected biopsies to confirm the diagnosis of recurrence. Patients with ureteral obstruction in the absence of recurrent malignancy should be considered for urinary diversion.

The definition of primary healing after radiation therapy is a cervix covered with normal epithelium or an obliteration of the vaginal vault without evidence of ulceration or discharge. On rectovaginal examination the residual induration is smooth with no modularity. The cervix is no greater than 2.5 cm in width, and there is no evidence of distant metastasis. The definition of persistent disease after radiation therapy is a portion of the tumor clinically present before treatment persists or there is development of a new demonstrable tumor in the pelvis within the treatment period. The definition of recurrence after radiation therapy is a regrowth of tumor in the pelvis or distally, noted after complete healing of the cervix and vagina had been achieved.

Recurrence after surgery is defined as evidence of a tumor mass after an operative procedure in which all gross tumor was removed and the margins of the specimen were free of disease. Persistent disease after surgery is defined as either persistence of gross tumor in the operative field or local recurrence of tumor within 1 year of initial surgery. A new cancer of the cervix would be a lesion that occurs locally at least 10 years after primary therapy.

The triad of weight loss accompanied by leg edema and pelvic pain is very ominous. Leg edema is usually the result of progressive lymphatic obstruction and/or occlusion of the iliofemoral vein system. The clinician should consider the possibility of thrombophlebitis, but recurrent cancer is more likely. Patients characteristically describe pain that radiates into the upper thigh either to the anterior medial aspect of the thigh or posteriorly into the buttock. Other patients describe pain in the groin or deep-seated central pelvic pain. The appearance of vaginal bleeding or watery-foul vaginal discharge would strongly suggest central recurrence. These lesions are among the more readily detectable recurrent cervical cancers, and histologic confirmation is easily obtained.

Less than 10% of patients with recurrent cervical cancer will develop pulmonary metastatis. When this does occur patients will complain of cough, hemoptysis, and occasionally chest pain. In many instances there will be enlargement of supraclavicular lymph nodes, especially on the left side. Needle aspiration of enlarged lymph nodes can be easily accomplished and will avoid the necessity for an open biopsy of the area.

In almost every instance the diagnosis of recurrent cervical cancer must be confirmed histologically. Fluoroscopically directed needle biopsies have provided us with a tool that avoids the necessity of more elaborate operative procedures. In addition to the standard roentgenographic evaluations, such as IVP and chest film, the clinician may find more sophisticated studies such as lymphangiography and computerized axial tomography helpful in localizing deepseated areas of recurrent cervical cancer.

Bony metastases are particularly rare. In a study of 644 patients presenting with invasive cervical carcinoma, Peeples and associates were able to find only 29 cases of remote metastases. Fifteen were to the lung, and only 12 were to the bone, for an incidence of 1.8%. No bony metastases were found at initial staging and diagnosis. The earliest discovery of bone metastasis was 8 months after diagnosis. Therefore, a bone survey was not recommended as part of the staging examination for cervical cancer.

Blythe and associates reported on 55 patients treated for cervical carcinoma who developed bony metastases. Roentgenograms were diagnostic in all but two of the patients. In 15 patients, a combination of radioactive scans and roentgenograms was used to establish the diagnosis. The most common mechanism of bony involvement from carcinoma of the cervix was extension of the neoplasia from para-aortic nodes, with involvement of the adjacent vertebral bodies. Thirteen years was the longest interval from the primary diagnosis until the discovery of bony metastases. Sixty-nine percent of the patients were diagnosed within 30 months of initial therapy, and 96% of the patients died within 18 months. Thirty-six patients were treated with radiation therapy: 4 received complete relief of symptoms, 24 some relief, and 8 no relief.

Van Herik and associates examined the records of 2,107 cases of cervical cancer for recurrence after 10 years. There were 16 patients, or 0.7%, who had recurrence 10 to 26 years after initial therapy. Of these patients, 25% had bony metastasis or extension of the recurrence into bone. The finding of metastasis after 10 years correlates with the findings of Paunier and associates, who indicated that 92.5% of deaths due to carcinoma of the cervix occur in the first 5 years after diagnosis. In addition, their cumulative death rate curve was flat after 10 years.

Deaths due to cancer of the cervix occur most frequently in the first year of observation and decrease thereafter. About half of all the deaths will occur in the first year after therapy, 25% will occur in the second year, and 15% will occur in the third year, for a total of 85% by the end of the third year.

Since over three fourths of the recurrences occur in the first 2 years after initial therapy, it becomes mandatory that the posttreatment evaluation be done at frequent intervals during this critical period. The patient should be examined every 3 to 4 months, and cervical cytologic testing should be done at these visits. In addition, particular attention should be paid to the parametria on rectovaginal examination in order to detect evidence of progressive disease. For several months following the completion of radiation therapy the examiner may observe a progressive fibrosis in the parametria, creating the so-called horseshoe fibrosis. The amount of fibrosis may at times be alarming, but smoothness of the induration should be reassuring when compared with the nodular presentation of recurrent parametrial malignancy. Parametrial needle biopsies with the patient under anesthesia may be helpful when the palpatory findings are equivocal. Generous use of endocervical curettage at these follow-up visits is recommended, especially when central failure is suspected. An

IVP and chest film should be obtained biannually in the asymptomatic patient and more frequently when pelvic recurrence is suspected. Every follow-up examination should include a careful palpation of the abdomen for evidence of para-aortic enlargement, hepatomegaly, and unexplained masses. Every follow-up examination should begin with a careful palpation of the supraclavicular areas for evidence of nodal enlargement. This frequently omitted portion of the examination will sometimes reveal the only evidence of recurrent disease.

The prognosis for the patient with recurrent or advanced cervical cancer is, of course, dependent on the location of the disease. With respect to recurrent cervical cancer, the most favorable group of patients for therapy following primary irradiation are those with a central recurrence. These patients are candidates for curative radical pelvic surgery including pelvic exenteration. There will be further discussion of this group of patients later in this chapter. With the advent of sophisticated methods of radiation therapy, including improved methods of brachytherapy and supervoltage external irradiation therapy, patients with pure central recurrence have become a rarity.

Isolated lung metastases from pelvic malignancies have responded in very selected cases to lobectomy. Gallousis reported metastases to the lung from cervical cancer in 1.5% of 5,614 cases reviewed, with solitary nodules present in 25% of the cases. A surgical attack for isolated pulmonary recurrence should be considered, especially if the latent period has been greater than 3 years.

Another group of patients that deserves serious consideration is the category of individuals with radiation bowel injury. Over the past decade the limits of human tolerance to radiation therapy have been reached, with techniques for advanced disease that include large extended fields to the para-aortic area. Many patients with an advanced stage primary lesion have been treated with large doses of pelvic radiation (6,000 to 7,000 rads), often following intra-abdominal surgery. These techniques, as well as standard radiation therapy, can lead to a small but significant number of patients with chronic radiation injury to the large or small bowel. These patients will frequently present with cachexia indistinguishable from the clinical presentation of recurrent and progressive malignancy. All too often these patients will be quickly and superficially diagnosed as having recurrent disease and no further investigation initiated. Careful investigation of these patients will reveal a history of postprandial crampy abdominal pain causing anorexia and weight loss. The diagnostic evaluations discussed previously will reveal no conclusive evidence of persistent malignancy. In most instances these patients can be returned to health with appropriate bowel surgery including intestinal bypass procedures. In every patient suspected of recurrent malignancy an effort should be made to confirm this suspicion by biopsy (histologic confirmation), and patients without recurrence who have radiation bowel injury should be sought.

Management

Prognosis. Persistent or recurrent carcinoma of the cervix is a discouraging clinical entity for the clinician, with a 1-year survival rate between 10% and 15%. Treatment failures are, as expected, much more frequent in more advanced stages of the disease, and therefore most patients are not likely candidates for a second curative approach with radical pelvic surgery. Cases of curative therapy applied to isolated lung metastases or lower vaginal recurrences are reported but are rare. Unfortunately, most recurrences are suitable for palliative management only.

Irradiation therapy. With recurrent disease outside the initial treatment field, irradiation is frequently successful in providing local control and symptomatic relief. External irradiation in moderate and easily delivered doses is usually effective in relieving pain from bone metastases. A dose of 3,000 rads delivered in a 2- to 3-week period is often sufficient to relieve pain from vertebral column or long-bone metastases.

Reirradiation of pelvic recurrences of cervical cancer occurring within the previously treated field is a subject of some controversy. The results following reirradiation of patients with recurrent cervical malignancy have varied considerably. Truelsen reported a 3-year cure rate of 1.7%. Murphy and Schmitz reported a 9% salvage rate in 1956, and Nolan and associates reported on the use of cobalt 60 teleradiation with a 25% salvage rate. At the Roswell Park Memorial Institute, Murphy adopted the policy of reirradiating patients with recurrence, delivering a full or near full course for a second time. Among the highly selected series of 46 patients, 9% to 10% were living and well at the end of 5 years. Only 7 patients had a biopsy-proven recurrence before treatment. Kurohara and associates showed that the results of reirradiation depend on many factors, including site of recurrence, initial clinical stage, and initial dose of radiation therapy. Careful perusal of these reports suggests that most patients who benefited from reirradiation were individuals who received far less than optimum radiation during initial therapy. This set of circumstances has become rare in recent times, when more sophisticated radiotherapy is being delivered in many areas of the country. Therefore, reirradiation for recurrent disease is usually not a worthwile consideration.

Chemotherapy. The management of disseminated cervical cancer has not significantly improved with the progress of modern chemotherapy. There are some explanations for this observation that are worth noting. First and foremost is the fact that a large percentage of patients with recurrent disease present with tumor in a previously irradiated area and the malignant tissue is encased in a fibrotic and avascular capsule. It is therefore very difficult to obtain high blood and tissue concentrations of drug in the neoplasm, which would create the optimum situation for response. In addition, squamous cell carcinoma (constituting 95% of cervical cancers) has generally been one of the histologic varieties least responsive to most chemotherapeutic agents. Furthermore, many drugs are nephrotoxic and have limited usefulness because of the frequent occurrence of ureteral obstruction in patients with recurrent cervical cancer. Recent reports are somewhat more optimistic. Baker and associates reported on a series of 130 patients with advanced and disseminated cervical carcinoma who were treated with mitomycin C, vincristine, and bleomycin. A twice weekly schedule of bleomycin and vincristine produced a response in 60% of patients. An infusion bleomycin schedule produced a response in 39% of patients, and a once weekly vincristine-bleomycin schedule produced a 25% response rate. Responding patients lived significantly longer than nonresponding patients (30 weeks vs. 18 weeks). Complete response was defined as total disappearance of all known disease, and partial response was defined as a 50% or more decrease in the product of the perpendicular diameters of all measurable disease.

Piver and associates published their experience with Adriamycin alone or in combination in 100 patients with carcinoma of the cervix or vagina. Only 6% of the patients receiving Adriamycin alone responded. There was no improvement by the addition of bleomycin, with 6.2% of the women responding. The use of Adriamycin in conjunction with cyclophosphamide and 5-flurouracil resulted in the highest response rate (four of seven patients responding).

Cavins and Geisler reported on 37 patients with unresectable, previously irradiated epidermoid carcinoma of the cervix who were treated with one of three chemotherapy protocols: (1) moderate dose methotrexate, (2) high dose methotrexate regimen given with leucovorin rescue, and (3) Adriamycin. With methotrexate a moderate dose response rate of 50% was noted, whereas 42% responded to the higher dose regimen. The response to Adriamycin was also less than 50%.

Miyamoto and associates reported on 15 patients with a squamous type of metastatic cervical cancer treated with a sequential combination of bleomycin and mitomycin-C. Fourteen out of 15 patients (93%) responded, with complete remission in 12 (80%) and partial remission in two (13%). The metastatic disease was in most instances located outside the previous field of irradiation. During therapy one patient died of lung fibrosis, and four of the 12 complete responders had a second recurrence after 4½ months. Five patients were alive without relapse an average of over 17 months.

Day and associates from the M. D. Anderson Hospital in Houston published their results on 37 patients treated for metastatic or recurrent squamous cervical carcinoma with doxorubicin (Adriamycin) and methyl CCNU. An objective response rate of 45% was obtained, with 29% having a complete response. An increase in survival rate in responders over nonresponders was demonstrated. Patients who had received extended field irradiation before chemotherapy tolerated this combination poorly and needed dose reduction early in therapy. Recurrent anemia, anorexia, and sustained weight loss were particularly severe with this combination.

One of the more promising agents of the last decade for cervical cancer has been cis-diamminedichloroplatinum (cis-platinum). A pilot study using cis-platinum with Adriamycin conducted under the auspices of the Gynecologic Oncology Group demonstrated a near 50% response rate. Notable complete responses of disease outside previously irradiated areas were also documented. Stehman and associates studied cis-platinum as a single agent in three patients with recurrent cervical cancer and had only one responder among the two patients with lung metastases.

The Gynecologic Oncology Group studied 25 evaluable patients with recurrent squamous cell cancer of the cervix who received cis-platinum alone (50 mg/m² IV every 3 weeks) and found a favorable response rate:

Complete response	12%
Partial response	32%
Stable disease	48%
Increasing disease	8%

Six of 15 patients (40%) with disease in the pelvis responded, and five of ten patients (50%) with disease outside the pelvis showed a complete or partial response.

Intra-arterial infusion for pelvic recurrence. Morrow and associates reported on a series of 20 patients from five institutions in the Gynecologic Oncology Group who were treated with continuous pelvic arterial infusion of bleomycin for squamous cell carcinoma of the cervix recurrent after radiation therapy. All patients had documented unresectability and life expectancy of greater than 8 weeks. Bleomycin was infused through a femoral arterial catheter introduced percutaneously and threaded into the lower aorta to a position between the inferior mesenteric artery and the aortic bifurcation. A few patients were treated via bilateral hypogastric artery catheters inserted at the time of exploratory laparotomy. A continuous infusion of bleomycin (20 mg/m²/week) for a minimum of 10 weeks or a total cumulative dose of 300 mg was given by means of low-flow portable infusion pumps. Infusion was discontinued if evidence of pulmonary toxicity appeared. Of the 20 patients studied, ten had toxicity of moderate to severe degree. There were 16 evaluable patients available and no complete responses. Only two partial responses were noted among 20 patients. The mean survival time was 7 months, with a range from 1 to 19 months. The two patients exhibiting partial tumor responses survived 5 and 8 months, respectively. The authors concluded that continuous arterial infusion of bleomycin is not helpful in the management of squamous carcinoma of the cervix recurrent in the pelvis after radiation therapy.

Lifshitz and associates reported on 14 patients with histologically confirmed recurrent pelvic malignancy treated with 44 courses of intra-arterial pelvic infusion of methotrexate or vincristine. Tumor regression was observed in three of 14 patients (21.4%). In five patients there were major complications related to 28 intra-arterial catheter placements. The authors concluded that the value of intra-arterial infusion chemotherapy in gynecologic cancer is limited.

MANAGEMENT OF BILATERAL URETERAL OBSTRUCTION

The patient with bilateral ureteral obstruction and uremia secondary to the extension of cervical cancer presents a serious dilemma for the clinician. Management should be divided into two subsets of patients: (1) those who have received no prior radiation therapy and (2) those who present with recurrent disease after pelvic irradiation.

The patient who presents with bilateral ureteral obstruction from untreated cervical cancer or from recurrent pelvic disease after surgical therapy should be seriously considered for urinary diversion followed by appropriate radiation therapy. The salvage rate among this group of patients is low but realistic. Our preference has been to make a urinary conduit, anastomosing both ureters into an isolated loop of ileum (Bricker procedure). We have also used this procedure in patients who had a vesicovaginal fistula secondary to untreated cervical malignancy. The ease with which pelvic radiation therapy can be optimally delivered is facilitated when the urinary diversion is performed before the irradiation is begun. In our experience, placement of urinary stints cystoscopically as an interim relief of the obstruction has been associated with multiple problems, leading us to favor the complete urinary diversion, or Bricker procedure. The traditional urinary stints are difficult to place bilaterally, and their presence in the ureter and bladder during the weeks to months of radiation therapy invariably leads to acute and chronic urinary tract infections. In addition, our experience has failed to show a significant number of patients in whom radiation therapy results in satisfactory relief of the ureteral obstruction thus allowing avoidance of permanent diversion.

The patient who presents with bilateral ureteral obstruction following a full dose of pelvic radiation therapy is an even more complicated problem. Less than 5% of these patients will have obstruction due to radiation fibrosis, and often this group is difficult to identify. However, simple diversion of the urinary stream in this subset of patients is lifesaving, and therefore all patients must be considered as possible members of this category until recurrent malignancy is uncovered. When the presence of recurrent disease has been unequivocally established, the decision process becomes difficult and somewhat philosophical. Numerous studies have suggested that "useful life" is not achieved by urinary diversion in this subset of patients. Brin and associates reported on 47 cases (5 with cervical cancer) of ureteral obstruction secondary to advanced pelvic malignancy with very discouraging results. The average survival time was 5.3 months, with only 50% of the patients alive at 3 months and only 22.7% alive at 6 months. After the diversion, 63.8% of the survival time was spent in the hospital. Delgado also reported on a group of patients with recurrent pelvic cancer and renal failure who underwent urinary conduit diversion. His results showed no significant increase in survival time.

It has been suggested that these patients should never undergo urinary diversion, since a more preferable method of expiration (uremia) is thereby eliminated from the patient's future. It is obvious that these decisions should be made in consultation with the family and even the patient, if possible. The decision must be heavily shared by the physician, but the attitudes of the patient and family must be sought as a guide. These attitudes can, in most instances, be perceived without transferring the decision-making process entirely to the family or the patient. As more sophisticated methods of chemotherapy evolve, the option for diversion may become more suitable. There are patients who need additional time to settle personal matters, and diversion with effective chemotherapy may result in a reasonable extension of life. However, in most instances, the avoidance of uremia results in an accentuation of the other clinical manifestations of recurrent pelvic cancer (i.e., severe pelvic pain and hemorrhage). Pain control and progressive cachexia plague the physician and the patient. Episodes of massive pelvic hemorrhage are associated with difficult decisions for transfusion. An extension of the inpatient hospital stay is inevitable, and the financial impact that this may have on the patient and her family should be a consideration. Newer techniques for placement of permanent ureteral stints both via the cystoscope and percutaneously may offer another option for this difficult clinical problem in the future.

PELVIC RECURRENCE AFTER SUBOPTIMAL SURGERY

A small percentage of patients who have been treated by inadequate surgery or radical hysterectomy itself will have an isolated pelvic recurrence. These patients are candidates for radiation therapy, and this should consist of external irradiation followed by appropriate vaginal or interstitial radium therapy. In recent years vaginal recurrences have been more successfully approached by use of interstitial irradiation following optimum external irradiation. The geometry of the postsurgical vagina with recurrence is such that standard vaginal applicators are often not suitable for optimum therapy. These patients are, of course, at higher risk for radiation injury because of the antecedent radical surgery.

PELVIC EXENTERATION

Extended or ultraradical surgery in the treatment of advanced and recurrent pelvic cancer is an American invention made possible by advances in the ancillary sciences that support the surgical team. The natural history of many pelvic cancers is that they may be locally advanced but still limited to the pelvis. They thus lend themselves to radical resection, unlike most other malignancies. In 1948 Brunschwig introduced the operation of pelvic exenteration for cancer of the cervix. Since that time extensive experience with pelvic exenteration has been accumulated, and the techniques as well as patient selection have steadily improved so that now, 30 years later, this procedure has attained an important role in the treatment of gynecologic malignancies. Pelvic exenterative surgery was subjected to severe initial criticism but is now accepted as a respectable procedure that can offer life to selected patients when no other possibility of cure exists. The criticism of this procedure has been lessened by the steadily improving mortality and morbidity and a gratifying 5-year survival record. Most important, however, it has been shown that patients who survive this procedure can be rehabilitated to a useful and healthful existence.

Although pelvic exenteration has been used for a variety of pelvic malignancies, its greatest and most important role is in the treatment of advanced or recurrent carcinoma of the cervix. Total exenteration (Fig. 3-19) with removal of the pelvic viscera, including the bladder and rectosigmoid, is the procedure of choice for carcinoma of the cervix recurrent or persistent within the pelvis after irradiation. In very selected cases the procedure may be limited to either anterior exenteration (Fig. 3-20) with removal of the bladder and preservation of the rectosigmoid or posterior exenteration (Fig. 3-21) with removal of the rectosigmoid and preservation of the bladder. Cogent objections have been raised regarding these limited operations, especially in patients with carcinoma of the cervix recurrent after irradiation, because of the increased risk of an incomplete resection. In addition, those patients in

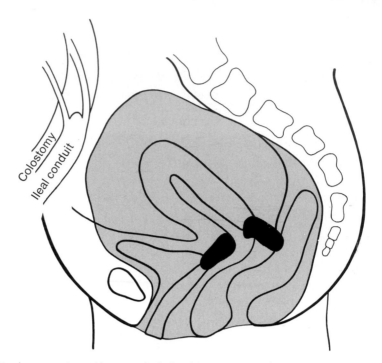

Fig. 3-19. Total exenteration with removal of all pelvic viscera. Fecal stream is diverted via colostomy, and urinary diversion is via an ileal or sigmoid conduit. (From DiSaia, P. J., and Morrow, C. P.: Calif. Med. **118**:13, Feb. 1973.)

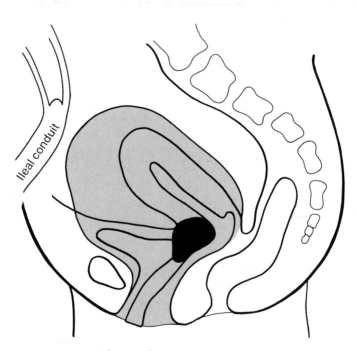

Fig. 3-20. Anterior exenteration with removal of all pelvic viscera except the rectosigmoid. Urinary stream is diverted into an ileal or sigmoid conduit. (From DiSaia, P. J., and Morrow, C. P.: Calif. Med. **118**:13, Feb. 1973.)

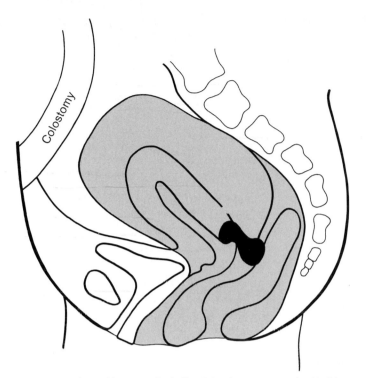

Colostomy

Fig. 3-21. Posterior exenteration with removal of all pelvic viscera except the bladder. Fecal stream is diverted via colostomy. (From DiSaia, P. J., and Morrow, C. P.: Calif. Med. **118:**13, Feb. 1973.)

whom the bladder or rectum is preserved often are victims of multiple complications and malfunctioning of the preserved organ. Consequently, some surgeons have completely abandoned subtotal exenterations, and most oncologists use them very selectively.

One of the greatest technical advances in the evolution of pelvic exenteration is the intestinal conduit for diversion of the urinary stream. Originally Brunschwig transplanted the ureters into the left colon just proximal to the colostomy, creating the so-called wet colostomy. The complication rate from this procedure, especially electrolyte imbalance and severe urinary tract infections, was unacceptable. We are indebted to Bricker for popularizing the use of an ileal segment conduit for urinary diversion. The incidence of both postoperative pyelonephritis and hypochloremic acidosis has been greatly reduced. Furthermore, the patients are dry and comfortable and therefore more easily rehabilitated. More recently, a segment of sigmoid colon rather than small bowel has been used as a urinary conduit by some surgeons in selected cases. This technique offers the additional advantage of avoiding a small-bowel anastomosis and the threat of fistula formation and obstruction attending any such procedure.

Table 3-8. M. D. Anderson Hospital central recurrence rate for carcinoma of the cervix

Stage I	1.5%
Stage IIB	5.0%
Stage IIIA	7.5%
Stage IIIB	17.0%

Patient selection

Only a small portion of the patients with recurrent cancer of the cervix are suitable for this operation (Table 3-8). Metastases outside the pelvis, whether manifested preoperatively or discovered at laparotomy, are an absolute contraindication to pelvic exenteration. The triad of unilateral leg edema, sciatic pain, and ureteral obstruction is pathognomonic of recurrent and unresectable disease in the pelvis. The triad must be complete, however, to be entirely reliable. Weight loss, cough, anemia, and other aberrations suggestive of advanced disease are not sufficient justification by themselves to discontinue efforts toward surgical management. Obesity, advanced age, and systemic disease may interdict extensive surgery in direct relation to the severity of these factors. Some patients are unsuitable for psychologic reasons, and a number of women, otherwise candidates for pelvic exenteration, elect to accept the fate of unresected recurrence.

Although the pelvic examination plays a key role in the preoperative assessment of the patient, the examiner's impression of resectability must be tempered by the knowledge that errors are common. A small central lesion with freely mobile parametria reliably demonstrates resectability; however, immobility can be due to radiation fibrosis and/or pelvic inflammatory disease (old salpingitis, inflammation from uterine perforation, etc.). Consequently, even when the disease seems inoperable on pelvic examination, if other factors are favorable, one should proceed with the investigation and exploratory laparotomy to avoid the error of a premature decision. Obviously, in many cases the finest clinical judgment must be used to avoid rejection of a potentially curable patient and also to prevent as often as possible subjection of an unsuitable patient to the anguish, fears, and false hopes of prolonged preparation for a fruitless operation.

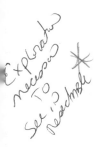

Evaluation studies before surgery include chest film, IVP, creatinine clearance, liver function tests, and assessment of the patient's hemostatic mechanism. Bilateral lower extremity lymphography has been useful in the experience of some surgeons. Bone survey and liver scan are not part of the "routine" evaluation. A blind scalene node biopsy has been advocated by Ketcham and would be a contraindication to further surgery if positive.

At laparotomy the entire abdomen and pelvis are explored for evidence of metastatic and intraperitoneal cancer (Fig. 3-22). The liver should be carefully inspected both visually and by palpation. The lymph nodes surrounding the lower aorta are the first area to be sampled if the exploration of the abdomen has revealed no evidence of disease. If a lymphangiogram has been obtained before laparotomy, it may

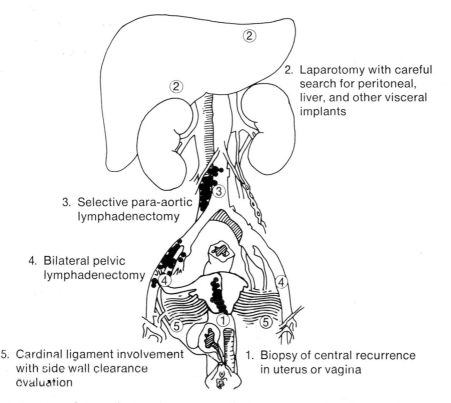

2. Laparotomy with careful
   search for peritoneal,
   liver, and other visceral
   implants

3. Selective para-aortic
   lymphadenectomy

4. Bilateral pelvic
   lymphadenectomy

5. Cardinal ligament involvement
   with side wall clearance
   evaluation

1. Biopsy of central recurrence
   in uterus or vagina

Fig. 3-22. Steps in evaluation of patient for an exenterative-type procedure. (Courtesy A. Robert Kagan, M.D., Los Angeles, California.)

be helpful in directing the surgeon to suspicious nodes in the para-aortic and pelvic area. If the lower aortic area findings are negative, a bilateral pelvic lymphadenectomy is performed. There have been virtually no survivors among those patients who have undergone pelvic exenteration with multiple positive pelvic wall nodes. Therefore, immediate frozen section analysis of the pelvic wall nodes is necessary to determine whether the resection should continue.

In Ketcham and associates' series of approximately 200 patients undergoing pelvic lymphadenectomy, a positive pelvic lymph node after radiation therapy was found in only one 5-year survivor. In a similar series by Barber from Memorial Hospital, 148 radiation failures undergoing pelvic exenteration were found to have positive nodes at the time of surgery, and only four of these patients were 5-year survivors. Creasman and Rutledge suggested a slightly more optimistic view of patients with positive lymph nodes who had undergone pelvic exenteration for recurrent cervical cancer following pelvic irradiation. However, in their series most survivors with positive nodes had only microscopic disease in the nodes. Furthermore, in nearly every case in the literature reported in detail of survival following exenteration for recurrent squamous cell carcinoma of the cervix in which there was a positive pelvic node, the nodal disease was not only microscopic but unilateral.

Strenuous efforts have been made to decrease the permanent morbidity and increase patient acceptance of pelvic exenteration by tailoring the procedure to the known extent of the patient's disease. Although it is rarely justifiable to salvage the bladder because of its natural anatomic association with the cervix, the rectosigmoid may occasionally be preserved, and at times it is feasible to perform a lower segmental resection of the rectosigmoid and reanastomosis. A temporary diverting colostomy must always be done in conjunction with this maneuver. In most patients the possibility of constructing a neovagina from a split-thickness skin graft or an isolated segment of bowel at the time of initial surgery should also be considered. With these modifications, exenteration for pelvic malignancy can frequently be performed today, leaving the patient with but one stoma and a functional vagina.

Morbidity and mortality

The morbidity and mortality directly related to exenteration occur within the first 18 months following the procedure. Many of the complications can be the sequel to any form of major surgery. These include cardiopulmonary catastrophes such as pulmonary embolism, pulmonary edema, myocardial infarction, and cerebrovascular accidents. It is evident that the length of these surgical procedures and the magnitude of blood loss definitely increase the incidence of cardiovascular complications. This category of complications usually occurs within the first week after the procedure. Then there is a period when sepsis emerges as the greatest threat to the patient's health and life. This sepsis usually originates in the pelvic cavity with occurrence of a pelvic abscess or, more commonly, diffuse pelvic cellulitis.

One of the most serious postoperative complications of exenteration is small-bowel obstruction related to the denuded pelvic floor. In the last decade several techniques have been employed in an effort to avoid the adherence of small bowel to this large raw surface, including mobilization of omentum or abdominal wall peritoneum to cover the pelvic floor. When small-bowel obstruction does occur, it is appropriately treated with conservative therapy. However, half of these patients come to reoperation, and the mortality of this group approaches 50% in some series. The risk of bowel obstruction is multiplied by pelvic infection, and both conditions predispose to the development of small-bowel fistulae, which always require reoperation and frequently precede a fatal outcome. In general, complications are far more common in patients who have recurrence after radiation therapy. Irradiated tissue is less likely to give good wound healing, and the formation of granulation tissue is severely retarded. The tendency toward fistula formation is markedly increased. Since surgical dissection is usually more difficult in the irradiated patient, longer operating times and increased blood loss often result. Both of these factors are associated with higher morbidity and mortality. Thus, the patient who has had previous radiation therapy is at much greater risk for serious complications than the nonirradiated patient and is less capable of a competent physiologic response.

The long-term morbidity from exenteration is predominantly related to urinary diversion. Once the period of susceptibility to sepsis has passed, urinary obstruction and infection become the major nonneoplastic life-threatening complications. Recurrent cancer is forever the most likely long-term life-threatening situation following the operative procedure, but the more preventable complications of the ileal conduit deserve primary attention. Many believe that these patients should be carried on chronic urinary antisepsis, perhaps for life. Pyelonephritis is common and should be treated promptly and vigorously. Periodic IVPs must be obtained to assess the collecting system for hydronephrosis. A mild degree of obstruction is frequently retained following construction of an ileal conduit, but progressive hydronephrosis will require correction to salvage renal function. It is tragic to lose a patient after exenteration because of remedial renal disease when there is no residual carcinoma.

The morbidity and mortality from radical surgery can be minimized by careful selection of patients. However, this implies a system in which some patients who may be resectable are denied an opportunity for resection in order to keep the morbidity low. This becomes a philosophical question that each physician must answer. However, the outcome of recurrent carcinoma of the cervix in a patient who is given no further treatment is clear.

Walton published a comprehensive review of the factors involved in the stress reaction of the patient after radical pelvic surgery, calling attention to the biochemical, psychologic, gastrointestinal, hepatic, and cardiac effects. He concluded that with total care, the occurrence of these stress reactions will decrease but will not disappear, since the human organism reacts in such a complex manner and derangement would occur in the weakest adaptive link to the surrounding environment.

Survival results

The 5-year cumulative survival rate after pelvic exenteration varies in the literature from 20% to 62% (Table 3-9). Reported survival rates depend greatly on the circumstances of patient selection for exenteration. For instance, patients who undergo pelvic exenteration as a primary procedure will have a 5-year survival rate 20% to 25% higher than a similar group of patients with recurrence following irradiation. (Pelvic exenteration may be performed as a primary procedure for carcinoma of the vulva extending up the vagina and into the bladder but not out to the pelvic sidewalls.) Survival rates can be improved by excluding the elderly, the obese, the heavily irradiated, and other high-risk patients. Cumulative survival rates are always improved when no patient is exenterated who has a positive pelvic node following pelvic irradiation. In general, however, both morbidity and mortality as well as the 5-year survival rate have steadily improved over the last 2 decades. Mortality in most centers is now well below 5%, and morbidity has been similarly lowered.

The survival prognosis for many patients is related to well-defined preoperative findings. The series from M. D. Anderson Hospital reported that 47% of the patients whose recurrence was symptomatic (pain or edema) but who were found resectable at the time of surgery survived 2 years. However, 73% of the patients who were symptom free at the time of laparotomy survived 2 years. Of the patients who had a

Table 3-9. Pelvic exenteration

Author	Institution	Number of patients treated	Number of operative deaths	Number surviving 5 years*
Douglas and Sweeney (1957)	New York Hospital	23	1 (4.3%)	5 (22%)
Parsons and Friedell (1964)	Harvard University	112	24 (21.4%)	24 (21.4%)
Brunschwig (1965)	Memorial Hospital	535	86 (15%)	108 (20.1%)
Bricker (1967)	Washington University	153	15 (10%)	53 (34.6%)
Krieger and Embree (1969)	Cleveland Clinics	35	4 (11%)	13 (37%)
Ketcham and associates (1970)	National Cancer Institute	162	12 (7.4%)	62 (38.2%)
Symmonds and associates (1975)	Mayo Clinic	198	16 (8%)	64 (32.3%)
Morley and Lindenauer (1976)	University of Michigan	34	1 (2.9%)	21 (62%)
Rutledge and associates (1977)	M. D. Anderson Hospital	296	40 (13.5%)	99 (33.4%)
TOTAL		1,548	199 (12.8%)	449 (29%)

* In almost every series, both the operative death rate and the 5-year survival rate were dramatically improved in the latter years of each series.

normal IVP at the time of laparotomy, 59% survived 2 years, whereas only 34% of the patients who had some IVP abnormality before laparotomy survived 2 years. Forty-six percent of the patients who had recurrence within 2 years of their primary treatment survived 2 years or more after treatment. Therefore, such factors as the status of the IVP, the presence or absence of symptoms, and the interval between primary treatment and recurrence should be considered in the preoperative assessment of the patient. One can improve the cumulative survival rate by excluding patients who have these deleterious characteristics; however, in so doing some patients who are resectable and therefore curable may be excluded.

Although lesions other than carcinoma of the cervix may be cured by pelvic exenteration, it is cervical cancer that is numerically of greatest importance. This procedure offers the only possibility for cure in patients who have pelvic recurrence after receiving optimum amounts of irradiation. With improved radiotherapy techniques, the number of patients with isolated central failure is steadily diminishing, but there remain a significant number of patients with recurrent cancer of the cervix after radiation therapy for whom the procedure offers the only chance for life. In order for the mortality and morbidity to be acceptable, the surgery should be done in medical centers by experienced surgical teams who are knowledgeable in the multidisciplinary approach to cancer therapy and can tailor the management to each patient's needs. These ultraradical surgical procedures should be done only by those individuals with adequate training and background who are willing to take on the responsibility of long-term postoperative care and rehabilitation. Each patient must be assessed individually with the risks of the procedure weighed against the possible benefits. It is encouraging that technical advances continue to reduce the operative mortality and ameliorate the postoperative morbidity associated with pelvic exenteration. Many patients can be not only cured but also rehabilitated to functional and comfortable lives; no patient should be deprived of this opportunity.

SARCOMAS OF THE CERVIX

Isolated cases of sarcomas arising in the cervix have been reported. Sarcoma botryoides is a malignancy that usually arises in the vagina but sometimes involves the cervix. Immature rhabdomyosarcoma of the cervix of the botryoid type has been reported in young women and successfully treated with radical hysterectomy. Lymphangiomas and lymphosarcomas of the reticulum cell variety are also seen rarely. Identification of these lesions requires differentiation from anaplastic carcinoma, with which they may be readily confused. These lesions are usually metastatic, and further investigation of the patient reveals multiple foci.

BIBLIOGRAPHY

Abbe, R.: The use of radium in malignant disease, Lancet 2:524, 1913.

Ashley, D. J. B.: The biological status of carcinoma in-situ of the uterine cervix, J. Obstet. Gynaecol. Br. Comm. 73:372, 1966.

Averette, H. E., Ford, J. H., Jr., Dudan, R. C., and others: Staging of cervical cancer, Clin. Obstet. Gynecol. 18:215, 1975.

Badib, A. O., Kurohara, S. S., Webster, J. H., and Pickren, J. W.: Metastasis to organs in carcinoma of the uterine cervix; influence of treatment on incidence and distribution, Cancer 21:434, 1968.

Baker, L. H., Opipari, M. I., Wilson, H., and others: Mitomycin C, vincristine, and bleomycin therapy for advanced cervical cancer, Obstet. Gynecol. 52:146, 1978.

Barber, H. R. K.: Relative prognostic significance of preoperative and operative findings in pelvic exenteration, Surg. Clin. North Am. 49(2):431, 1969.

Barber, H. R. K., and Brunschwig, A.: Gynecologic cancer complicating pregnancy, Am. J. Obstet. Gynecol. 85:156, 1963.

Barber, H. R. K., and Jones, W.: Lymphadenectomy in pelvic exenteration for recurrent cervix cancer, J.A.M.A. 215:1949, 1971.

Barron, B. A., and Richart, R. M.: A statistical model of the natural history of cervical carcinoma based on a prospective study of 557 cases, J.N.C.I. 41:1343, 1968.

Belenson, J. L., Goldberg, M. I., and Averette, H. E.: Para-aortic lymphadenectomy in gynecologic cancer, Gynecol. Oncol. 7:188, 1979.

Blythe, J. G., Ptacek, J. J., Buchsbaum, H. J., and

Latourette, H. B.: Bony metastases from carcinoma of the cervix, Cancer 36:475, 1975.

Bonfiglio, M.: The pathology of fracture of the femoral neck following irradiation, Am. J. Roentgenol. 70:449, 1953.

Bonne, V.: The results of 500 cases of Wergheim's operation for carcinoma of the cervix, J. Obstet. Gynecol. Br. Comm. 48:421, 1941.

Boronow, R. C.: Stage I cervix cancer and pelvic node metastasis, Am. J. Obstet. Gynecol. 127:135, 1977.

Bosch, A., and Marcial, V. A.: Carcinoma of the uterine cervix associated with pregnancy, Am. J. Roentgenol. 96:92, 1966.

Boutselis, J. G., Ullery, J. C., and Charmer, L.: Diagnosis and management of Stage IA (microinvasive) carcinoma of the cervix, Am. J. Obstet. Gynecol. 110:984, 1971.

Boyes, D. A., Worth, A. J., and Fidler, H. K.: The results of treatment of 4389 cases of preclinical cervical squamous carcinoma, J. Obstet. Gynaecol. Br. Comm. 77:769, 1970.

Brack, C. B., Everett, H. C., and Dickson, R.: Irradiation therapy for carcinoma of the cervix; its effect on urinary tract, Obstet Gynecol. 7:196, 1956.

Bricker, E. M.: Bladder substitution after pelvic evisceration, Surg. Clin. North Am. 30:1511, 1950.

Bricker, E. M., Butcher, H. R., and McAfee, A.: Results of pelvic exenteration, A.M.A. Arch. Surg. 73:661, 1956.

Bricker, E. M., and Modlin, J.: The role of pelvic evisceration in surgery, Surgery 30:76, 1951.

Brin, E. N., Schiff, M., and Weiss, R. M.: Palliative urinary diversion for pelvic malignancy, J. Urol. **113:**619, 1975.

Brunschwig, A.: The surgical treatment of Stage I cancer of the cervix, Cancer **13:**34, 1960.

Brunschwig, A.: What are the indications and results of pelvic exenteration? J.A.M.A. **194:**274, 1965.

Brunschwig, A.: Surgical treatment of carcinoma of the cervix, recurrent after irradiation or combination of irradiation and surgery, Am. J. Roentgenol. **99:**365, 1967

Brunschwig, A., and Pierce, V. K.: Necropsy findings in patients with carcinoma of the cervix; implications for treatment, Am. J. Obstet. Gynecol. **56:**1134, 1948.

Buchsbaum, H. J.: Extrapelvic lymph node metastases in cervical carcinoma, Am. J. Obstet. Gynecol. **133**(7):814, 1979.

Calkins, L. A.: Retreatment of carcinoma of the cervix, South. Med. J. **41:**902, 1948.

Cavins, J. A., and Geisler, H. E.: Treatment of advanced, unresectable cervical carcinoma already subjected to complete irradiation therapy, Gynecol. Oncol. **6:**256, 1978.

Chism, S. E., Park, R. C., and Keys, H. M.: Prospects for para-aortic irradiation in treatment of cancer of the cervix, Cancer **35:**1505, 1975.

Christopherson, W. M., Mendeze, W. M., Ahuza, E. M., and others: Cervical cancer control in Louisville, Kentucky, Cancer **26:**29, 1970.

Christopherson, W. M., and Parker, J. E.: A critical study of cervical biopsies including serial sectioning, Cancer **14:**213, 1961.

Christopherson, W. M., Parker, J. E., Mendeze, W. M., and Lunden, F. E.: Cervix cancer death rates and mass cytologic screening, Cancer **26:**808, 1970.

Clayton, R. S.: Carcinoma of the cervical uteri; ten-year study with comparison of results of irradiation and radical surgery, Radiology **68:**74, 1957.

Coppleson, M., Pixley, E., and Reid, B.: Colposcopy; a scientific and practical approach to the cervix in health and disease, Springfield, Ill., 1971, Charles C Thomas, Publisher.

Coppleson, M., and Reid, B.: Preclinical carcinoma of the cervix uteri; its nature, origin, and management, New York, 1967, Pergamon Press.

Coppleson, M., and Reid, B.: The etiology of squamous carcinoma of the cervix, editorial, Obstet. Gynecol. **32:**432, 1968.

Creadick, R. N.: Carcinoma of the cervical stump, Am. J. Obstet. Gynecol. **75:**565, 1958.

Creasman, W. T., and Parker, R. T.: Microinvasive carcinoma of the cervix, Clin. Obstet. Gynecol. **16:**261, 1973.

Creasman, W. T., and Rutledge, F.: Is positive pel-

vic lymphadenectomy a contraindication to radical surgery in recurrent cervical carcinoma? Gynecol. Oncol. **2:**282, 1974.

Czesnin, K., and Wronkowski, Z.: Second malignancies of the irradiated area in patients treated for uterine cervix cancer, Gynecol. Oncol. **6:**309, 1978.

Day, T. G., Jr., Wharton, J. T., Gottlieb, J. A., and Rutledge, F. N.: Chemotherapy for squamous carcinoma of the cervix; doxorubicin—methyl CCNU, Am. J. Obstet. Gynecol. **132:**545, 1978.

Delgado, G.: Urinary conduit diversion in advanced gynecologic malignancies, Gynecol. Oncol. **6:**217, 1978.

Delgado, G., Caglar, H., and Walker, P.: Survival and complications in cervical cancer treated by pelvic and extended field radiation after para-aortic lymphadenectomy, Am. J. Roentgenol. **130:**141, 1978.

Delgado, G., Smith, J. P., and Ballantyne, A. J.: Scalene node biopsy in carcinoma of the cervix; pelvic and para-aortic lymphadenectomy, Cancer **35:**784, 1975.

Douglas, R. G., and Sweeney, W. J.: Exenterative operations in the treatment of advanced pelvic cancer, Am. J. Obstet. Gynecol. **73:**1169, 1957.

El-Minawi, M. F., and Perez-Mesa, C. M.: Parametrial needle biopsy follow-up of cervical cancer, Int. J. Obstet. Gynecol. **12:**1, 1974.

Everson, T. C., and Cole, W. H.: Spontaneous regression of cancer, Philadelphia, 1966, W. B. Saunders Co.

Feder, B. H., Syed, A. M. N., and Neblett, D.: Treatment of extensive carcinoma of the cervix with the "transperineal parametrial butterfly," Int. J. Radiat. Oncol. Biol. Phys. **4:**735, 1978.

Fletcher, G. H.: The role of supervoltage therapy, Proceedings of the Conference on Research on Radiotherapy of Cancer, New York, 1961, American Cancer Society, Inc.

Fletcher, G. H.: External radiation therapy in cancer of the uterine cervix. In Lewis, G. C., and others, editors: New concepts in gynaecological oncology, Philadelphia, 1967, F. A. Davis Co.

Fletcher, G. H., and Rutledge, F. N.: Extended field technique in the management of the cancers of the uterine cervix, Am. J. Roentgenol. **114:**116, 1972.

Fletcher, G. H., Shalek, R. J., Wall, J. A., and Bloedorn, F. G.: A physical approach to the design of applicators in radium therapy of cancer of the cervix uteri, Am. J. Roentgenol. **78:**935, 1952.

Fluhmann, C. F.: The squamocolumnar transitional zone of the cervix uteri, Obstet. Gynecol. **14:**133, 1959.

Fluhmann, C. F.: Carcinoma in situ and the transitional zone of the cervix uteri, Obstet. Gynecol. **16**:424, 1960.

Fluhmann, C. F.: The cervix uteri and its diseases, Philadelphia, 1961, W. B. Saunders Co.

Fluhmann, C. F.: Involvement of clefts and tunnels in carcinoma in situ of the cervix uteri, Am. J. Obstet. Gynecol. **83**:1410, 1962.

Fluhmann, C. F., and Dickmann, Z.: The basic pattern of the glandular structures of the cervix uteri, Obstet. Gynecol. **11**:543, 1958.

Friedell, G. H., Hertig, A. T., and Younge, P. A.: Carcinoma in situ of the uterine cervix, Springfield, Ill., 1960, Charles C Thomas, Publisher.

Gagnon, F.: The lack of occurrence of cervical carcinoma in nuns, Proc. Second Natl. Cancer Conf. **1**:625, 1952.

Gallousis, S.: Isolated lung metastases from pelvic malignancies, Gynecol. Oncol. **7**:206, 1979.

Gallup, D. G., and Abell, M. R.: Invasive adenocarcinoma of the uterine cervix, Obstet. Gynecol. **49**:596, 1977.

Graham, J. B., and Abab, R. S.: Ureteral obstruction due to radiation, Am. J. Obstet. Gynecol. **99**:409, 1967.

Graham, J. B., Graham, R. M., and Hirabayashi, K.: Recurrent cancer of the cervix uteri, Surg. Gynecol. Obstet. **126**:799, 1968.

Graham, J. B., Sotto, L. S. J., and Paloucek, F. P.: Carcinoma of the cervix, Philadelphia, 1962, W. B. Saunders Co.

Graham, R., and Graham, J. B.: Mast cells and cancer of the cervix, Surg. Gynecol. Obstet. **123**:2, 1966.

Greiss, F. C., Blake, D. D., and Lock, F. R.: Complications of intensive radiation therapy for cervical carcinoma; with emphasis on supervoltage radiation and supplemental radical pelvic operation, Obstet. Gynecol. **18**:417, 1961.

Gusberg, S. B., and Corscaden, J. A.: The pathology and treatment of adenocarcinoma of the cervix, Cancer **4**:1066, 1951.

Gusberg, S. B., Fish, S. A., and Wang, Y. Y.: The growth pattern of cervical cancer, Obstet. Gynecol. **2**:557, 1953.

Gusberg, S. B., and Marshall, D.: Intraepithelial carcinoma of the cervix; a clinical reappraisal, Obstet. Gynecol. **19**:713, 1962.

Gusberg, S. B., and Moore, D. B.: Clinical pattern of intraepithelial cancer of the cervix and its pathological background, Obstet. Gynecol. **2**:1, 1953.

Gusberg, S. B., and Rudolph, J.: Individualization of treatment for cancer of the cervix, Proceedings of American College of Surgeons Meeting, Munich, 1978, American College of Surgeons.

Gusberg, S. B., Yannopoulos, K., and Cohen, C. J.: Virulence indices and lymph nodes in cancer of the cervix, Am. J. Roentgenol. **111**:273, 1971.

Guthrie, R. T., Buchsbaum, H. J., White, A. J., and Latourette, H. B.: Para-aortic lymph node irradiation in carcinoma of the uterine cervix, Cancer **34**:166, 1974.

Helper, T. K., Dockerty, M. B., and Randall, L. M.: Primary adenocarcinoma of the cervix, Am. J. Obstet. Gynecol. **63**:800, 1952.

Henderson, P. H., and Buck, C. E.: Cervical leukoplakia, Am. J. Obstet. Gynecol. **82**:887, 1961.

Henriksen, E.: The lymphatic spread of carcinoma of the cervix and of the body of the uterus; a study of 420 necropsies, Am. J. Obstet. Gynecol. **58**:924, 1949.

Henriksen, E.: The dispersion of cancer of the cervix, Radiology **54**:812, 1950.

Henriksen, E.: Distribution of metastases in Stage I carcinoma of the cervix, Am. J. Obstet. Gynecol. **80**:919, 1960.

Henriksen, E.: Pyometra associated with malignant lesions of the cervix and the uterus, Am. J. Obstet. Gynecol. **80**:919, 1960.

Hertig, A. T., and Goce, H.: Tumors of the female sex organs, part 2. In Atlas of tumor pathology, fascicle 33, Washington, D.C., 1960, Armed Forces Institute of Pathology.

Hreschyshn, M. M., Aron, B. S., Boronow, R. C., and others: Hydroxyurea or placebo combined with radiation to treat stages IIIB and IV cervical cancer confined to the pelvis, Int. J. Radiat. Oncol. Biol. Phys. **5**(3):317, 1979.

Hreshchyshyn, M. M., and Sheehan, F. R.: Lymphangiography in advanced gynecologic cancer, Obstet. Gynecol. **24**:525, 1964.

Hreshchyshyn, M. M., and Sheehan, F. R.: Collateral lymphatics in patients with gynecologic cancer, Am. J. Obstet. Gynecol. **91**:118, 1965.

Huffman, J. W.: Mesonephric remnants in the cervix, Am. J. Obstet. Gynecol. **56**:23, 1948.

Johnson, L. D., Nickerson, R. J., Easterday, C. L., and others: Epidemiologic evidence for the spectrum of change from dysplasia through carcinoma in situ to invasive cancer, Cancer **22**:901, 1968.

Kagan, A. R., Nussbaum, H., Gilbert, H., and others: A new staging system for irradiation injuries following treatment for cancer of the cervix uteri, Gynecol. Oncol. **7**:166, 1979.

Keetel, W. C., Van Voorhis, L. W., and Latourette, H. B.: Management of recurrent carcinoma of the cervix, Am. J. Obstet. Gynecol. **102**:671, 1968.

Kepp, R. K.: X-ray treatment of recurrent cervical

cancer, Deutsch. Med. Wochenschr. **78:**1391, 1953.

Ketcham, A. S.: Fifteen-year experience with pelvic exenteration, paper presented at James Ewing Society Meeting, Portland, Ore., 1971.

Ketcham, A. S., Deckers, P. J., Sugarbaker, E. V., and others: Pelvic exenteration for carcinoma of the uterine cervix; a 15-year experience, Cancer **26:**513, 1970.

Kisclaw, M., Butcher, H. R., and Bricker, E. M.: Results of the radical surgical treatment of advanced pelvic cancer, Ann. Surg. **166:**428, 1967.

Kistner, R. W., Gorbach, A. C., and Smith, G. V.: Cervical cancer in pregnancy; review of the literature with presentation of thirty additional cases, Obstet. Gynecol. **9:**554, 1957.

Kolstad, P.: Carcinoma of the cervix stage IA—diagnosis and treatment, Am. J. Obstet. Gynecol. **104:**1015, 1969.

Kottmeier, H. L.: Ten year end results; radiological treatment of carcinoma of the cervix, Acta Obstet. Gynecol. Scand. **41:**195, 1962.

Kottmeier, H. L.: Complications following radiation therapy in carcinoma of the cervix and their treatment, Am. J. Obstet. Gynecol. **88:**854, 1964.

Kottmeier, H. L.: Presentation of therapeutic results in carcinoma of the female pelvis; experience of the Annual Report on the Results of Treatment in Carcinoma of the Uterus, Vagina, and Ovary, Gynecol. Oncol. **4:**13, 1976.

Krieger, J. S., and Embree, H. K.: Pelvic exenteration, Cleve. Clin. Q. **36:**1, 1969.

Kurohara, S. S., Vongtama, V. Y., Webster, J. H., and George, F. W.: Post irradiational recurrent epidermoid carcinoma of the uterine cervix, Am. J. Roentgenol. **3:**249, 1971.

Lewis, G. C., Raventos, A., and Hale, J.: Space dose relationships for points A and B in the radium therapy of cancer of the uterine cervix, Am. J. Roentgenol. **83:**432, 1960.

Lifshitz, S., Railsback, L. D., and Buchsbaum, H. J.: Intra-arterial pelvic infusion chemotherapy in advanced gynecologic cancer, Obstet. Gynecol. **52:**476, 1978.

Liu, W., and Meigs, J. W.: Radical hysterectomy and pelvic lymphadenectomy, Am. J. Obstet. Gynecol. **69:**1, 1955,

Masterson, J. G.: Analysis of untreated intraepithelial carcinoma of the cervix, Proceedings of the Third National Cancer Conference, Philadelphia, 1957, J. B. Lippincott Co.

McGee, C. T., Cromer, D. W., and Greene, R. R.: Mesonephric carcinoma of the cervix—differentiation from endocervical adenocarcinoma, Am. J. Obstet. Gynecol. **84:**358, 1962.

Mikuta, J. J.: Invasive carcinoma of the cervix in pregnancy, South. Med. J. **60:**843, 1967.

Mitra, S.: Cancer of the cervix; prevalence, ethnology, and treatment, J. Obstet. Gynaecol. India **7:**151, 1957.

Miyamoto, T., Takabe, Y., Watanabe, M., and Terasima, T.: Effectiveness of a sequential combination of bleomycin and mitomycin-C on an advanced cervical cancer, Cancer **41:**403, 1978.

Morley, G. W., and Lindenauer, S. M.: Pelvic exenteration therapy for gynecologic malignancies; an analysis of 70 cases, Cancer **38:**581, 1976.

Morley, G. W., Lindenauer, S. M., and Young, D.: Vaginal reconstruction following pelvic exenteration, Am. J. Obstet. Gynecol. **116:**996, 1973.

Morrow, C. P., DiSaia, P. J., Mangan, C. F., and Lagasse, L. D.: Continuous pelvic arterial infusion with bleomycin for squamous carcinoma of the cervix recurrent after irradiation therapy, Cancer Treat. Rep. **61:**1403, 1977.

Morton, D. G., and Dignam, W.: The cause of death in patients treated for cervical cancer, Am. J. Obstet. Gynecol. **64:**999, 1952.

Murphy, W. T., and Schmitz, A.: The results of reirradiation of cancer of the cervix, Radiology **67:**378, 1956.

Mussey, E., Soule, E. H., and Welch, J. S.: Microinvasive carcinoma of the cervix; late results of operative treatment in 91 cases, Am. J. Obstet. Gynecol. **104:**738, 1969.

Nalick, R. H., DiSaia, P. J., Rhea, T. H., and others: Immunocompetence and prognosis in patients with gynecologic cancer, Gynecol. Oncol. **2:**81, 1974.

Nalick, R. H., DiSaia, P. J., Rhea, T. H., and others: Immunologic response in gynecologic malignancy as demonstrated by hypersensitivity reaction; clinical correlations, Am. J. Obstet. Gynecol. **118:**393, 1974.

Navratil, E., and Kastner, H.: Unsere Erfahrungen mit 997 amreichschen Operationen bie der Behandlung des invasion Zervixkarzinoms, Wien Med. Wochenschr. **116:**1012, 1966.

Nelson, J. H., Jr., Macasaet, M. A., Therese, L., and others: The incidence and significance of para-aortic lymph node metastases in late invasive carcinoma of the cervix, Am. J. Obstet. Gynecol. **118:**749, 1974.

Ng, A. B., and Reagan, J. W.: Microinvasive carcinoma of the uterine cervix, Am. J. Clin. Pathol. **52:**511, 1969.

Nolan, J. F., Anson, J. H., and Steward, M.: A radium applicator for use in the treatment of cancer of the uterine cervix, Am. J. Roentgenol. **79:**36, 1958.

Nolan, J. F., Vidal, J. A., and Anson, J. H.: Treatment of recurrent carcinoma of the uterine cervix with cobalt 60, West. J. Surg. **65**:358, 1957.

Nordqvist, S. R., Jaramillo, B., Ford, J. H., and Averette, H. E.: Selective therapy for early cancer of the cervix. I. Surgically explored nonresected cases, Gynecol. Oncol. **7**(2):248, 1979.

Nordqvist, S. R., Jaramillo, B., Sudarsanam, A., and others: Selective therapy for early cancer of the cervix. II. Surgically nonexplored cases, Gynecol. Oncol. **7**(2):257, 1979.

Novak, E. R., and Woodruff, J. D.: Gynecologic and obstetric pathology, Philadelphia, 1972, W. B. Saunders Co.

Ostergard, D. R., and Morton, D. G.: Multifocal carcinoma of the female genitals, Am. J. Obstet. Gynecol. **99**:1006, 1968.

Parker, R. T., Wilbanks, G. D., Yowell, R. K., and Carter, F. B.: Radical hysterectomy and pelvic lymphadenectomy with and without preoperative radiotherapy for cervical cancer, Am. J. Obstet. Gynecol. **99**:933, 1967.

Parsons, L., and Friedell, G. J.: Radical surgical treatment of cancer of cervix, Proc. Natl. Cancer Conf. **5**:241, 1964.

Patillo, R. A.: Immunotherapy and chemotherapy of gynecologic cancer, Am. J. Obstet. Gynecol. **124**:808, 1977.

Paunier, J. P., Delclos, L., and Fletcher, G. H.: Causes, time of death, and sites of failure in squamous-cell carcinoma of the uterine cervix on intact uterus, Radiology **88**:555, 1967.

Penn, I.: Cancer in immunosuppressed patients, Transplant Proc. **7**:553, 1975.

Peeples, W. J., Inalsingh, C. H. Huzra, T. A., and others: The occurrence of metastasis outside the abdomen and retroperitoneal space in invasive carcinoma of the cervix, Gynecol. Oncol. **4**:307, 1976.

Perez, C. A., Breaux, S., Askin, F., and others: Irradiation alone or in combination with surgery in stages IB and IIA carcinoma of the uterine cervix; a nonrandomized comparison, Cancer **43**(3): 1062, 1979.

Perez, C. A. Breaux, S., Madoc-Jones, H., and others: Correlation between radiation dose and tumor recurrence and complications in carcinoma of the uterine cervix; stages I and IIA, Int. J. Radiat. Oncol. Biol. Phys. **5**(3):373, 1979.

Peterson, O.: Spontaneous course of cervical precancerous conditions, Am. J. Obstet. Gynecol. **72**:1063, 1956.

Piver, M. S., and Barlow, J. J.: High dose irradiation to biopsy-confirmed aortic node metastases from carcinoma of the uterine cervix, Cancer **39**:1243, 1977.

Piver, M. S., Barlow, J. J., and Xynos, F. P.: Adriamycin alone or in combination in 100 patients with carcinoma of the cervix or vagina, Am. J. Obstet. Gynecol. **131**:311, 1978.

Rawls, W. E., Tompkins, W. A., Figueroa, M. E., and others: Herpesvirus type 2; association with carcinoma of the cervix, Science **16**:1255, 1968.

Reagan, J. W.: Genesis of carcinoma of the uterine cervix, Clin. Obstet. Gynecol. **10**:883, 1967.

Richart, R. M.: Natural history of cervical intraepithelial neoplasia, Clin. Obstet. Gynecol. **10**:748, 1967.

Roddick, J. W., Jr., and Miller, D. H.: Factors affecting the management of recurrent cervical carcinoma, Am. J. Obstet. Gynecol. **101**:53, 1968.

Rutledge, F. N., and Burns, B. C., Jr.: Pelvic exenteration, Am. J. Obstet. Gynecol. **91**:692, 1965.

Rutledge, F. N., and Fletcher, G. H.: Transperitoneal pelvic lymphadenectomy following supervoltage irradiation for squamous cell carcinoma of the cervix, Am. J. Obstet. Gynecol. **76**:321, 1958.

Rutledge, F. N., Gutierrez, A. G., and Fletcher, G. H.: Management of Stage I and II adenocarcinomas of the uterine cervix on intact uterus, Am. J. Roentgenol. **102**:161, 1968.

Rutledge, F. N., Smith, J. P., Wharton, J. T., and O'Quinn, A. G.: Pelvic exenteration; analysis of 296 patients, Am. J. Obstet. Gynecol. **129**:881, 1977.

Rutledge, F. N., Wharton, J. T., and Fletcher, G. H.: Clinical studies with adjunctive surgery and irradiation therapy in the treatment of carcinoma of the cervix, Cancer **38**:596, 1976.

Schellhaus, H. F.: Extraperitoneal para-aortic dissection through an upper abdominal incision, Obstet. Gynecol. **46**:444, 1975.

Schmitz, H. E., and Smith, C. J.: Radiation treatment of cervical cancer, Clin. Obstet. Gynecol. **1**:1013, 1958.

Sherman, A. I.: Cancer of the female reproductive organs, St. Louis, 1963, The C. V. Mosby Co.

Song, J.: The human uterus; morphogenesis and embryological basis for cancer, Springfield, Ill., 1964, Charles C Thomas, Publisher.

Stallworthy, J., Genital tuberculosis in the female, J. Obstet. Gynaecol. Br. Emp. **59**:729, 1952.

Stallworthy, J.: Radical surgery following radiation treatment for cervical carcinoma, Ann. R. Coll. Surg. Eng. **34**:161, 1964.

Stehman, F. B., Ballon, S. C., Lagasse, L. D., and others: Cis-platinum in advanced gynecologic malignancy, Gynecol. Oncol. **7**:349, 1979.

Stern, E., and Dixon, W. J.: Cancer of the cervix; a biometric approach to etiology, Cancer **14**:153, 1961.

Stone, M. L., Weingold, A. B., and Sall, S.: Cervical carcinoma in pregnancy, Am. J. Obstet. Gynecol. **93**:479, 1965.

Suit, H. D., and Gallagher, H. S.: Intact tumor cells in irradiated tissue, Arch. Pathol. **78**:648, 1964.

Swan, R. W., and Rutledge, F. N.: Urinary conduit in pelvic cancer patients—a report of 16 years' experience, Am. J. Obstet. Gynecol. **119**:6, 1974.

Symmonds, R. E., Pratt, J. H., and Webb, M. J.: Exenteration operations; experience with 198 patients, Am. J. Obstet. Gynecol. **121**:907, 1975.

Tak, W. K.: Interstitial therapy in gynecologic cancer, Gynecol. Oncol. **6**:429, 1978.

Townsend, D. E., and Ostergard, D. R.: Cryocauterization for preinvasive cervical neoplasia, J. Reprod. Med. **6**:171, 1971.

Tredway, D. R., Townsend, D. E., Hovland, D. N., and Upton, R. T.: Colposcopy and cryosurgery in cervical intraepithelial neoplasia, Am. J. Obstet. Gynecol. **114**:1020, 1972.

Truelsen, F.: Injury of bones by roentgen treatment of the uterine cervix, Acta Radiol. **23**:581, 1942.

Ulfelder, H., Smith, C. J., and Costello, J. B.: Invasive carcinoma of the cervix during pregnancy, Am. J. Obstet. Gynecol. **98**:424, 1967.

Van Herik, M., Decker, D. G., Lee, R. A., and Symmonds, R. E.: Late recurrence in carcinoma of the cervix, Am. J. Obstet Gynecol. **108**:1183, 1970.

Van Herik, M., and Fricke, R. E.: The results of radiation therapy for recurrent cancer of the cervix uteri, Am. J. Roentgenol. **73**:437, 1955.

Wall, J. A., Collins, V. P., Hudgins, P. T., and others: Carcinoma of the cervix, Am. J. Obstet. Gynecol. **96**:57, 1966.

Walton, L. A.: The stress of radical pelvic surgery; a review, Gynecol. Oncol. **7**:25, 1979.

West, R. R.: Cervical cancer; age at registration and age at death, Br. J. Cancer **35**:236, 1977.

Wharton, J. T., Jones, H. W. III, Day, T. G., Jr., and others: Preirradiation celiotomy and extended field irradiation for invasive carcinoma of the cervix, Am. J. Obstet. Gynecol. **118**:749, 1974.

White, W. C., and Finn, F. W.: The late complications following irradiation of pelvic viscera, Am. J. Obstet. Gynecol. **62**:65, 1951.

CHAPTER FOUR

Endometrial hyperplasia

Hyperplastic growth of the endometrium is somewhat analogous to dysplasia of the cervix. Undoubtedly some of these lesions revert to normal spontaneously or with medical therapy, some persist as hyperplasia, and a few progress to endometrial adenocarcinoma. The diagnosis of endometrial hyperplasia can only be made on pathologic examination of the endometrium, and the pathologic literature has burdened us with a variety of terms and classifications. Unfortunately, there is no reliable, commonly used method of screening asymptomatic women for endometrial hyperplasia as there is for cervical dysplasia, so most patients with endometrial hyperplasia are diagnosed because they present for medical care with symptoms—usually abnormal uterine bleeding—and endometrial samples are subsequently obtained.

Most endometrial hyperplasia is thought to result from persistent, prolonged estrogenic stimulation of the endometrium. The most common cause is a succession of anovulatory cycles, but hyperplasia may also result from excessive endogenously produced or exogenously administered estrogen (Fig. 4-1). The student is often confused in a discussion of hyperplasia because of the existing nomenclature. The terms "simple hyperplasia," "glandular hyperplasia," "cystic glandular hyperplasia," and "endometrial hyperplasia" are synonymous. Adenomatous hyperplasia

107

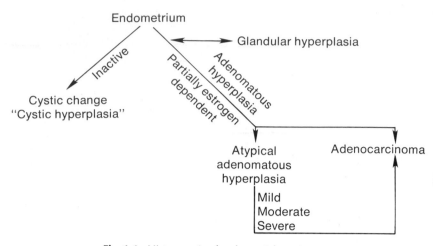

Fig. 4-1. Histogenesis of endometrial carcinoma.

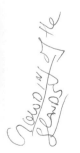

can occur with or without cytologic atypia, and this atypia may be severe enough to create difficulty in distinguishing the hyperplastic state from a well-differentiated adenocarcinoma. The process may be generalized throughout the endometrial cavity or localized to one or more areas. It may occur in any age group and is occasionally seen in teenage patients who have intermittent progesterone production and persistent estrogen stimulation without ovulation. In a like manner, it is very commonly observed during the menopause when the process of ovulation is inconsistent.

PATHOLOGIC CRITERIA

The gross appearance of the endometrial cavity containing hyperplastic tissue is quite variable. In many instances the endometrium is markedly thickened or polypoid, with large quantities of tissue being obtained at the time of uterine curettage. The gross appearance of the endometrium can be confused with the very thick and succulent endometrium removed on days 26 and 28 of the normal secretory cycle. In other patients, particularly menopausal women, the uterine curettings are scant and histologically only small foci of hyperplasia can be found. In general, endometrial hyperplasia is characterized by proliferation of both glands and stroma, resulting in the grossly thick, velvety, creamy yellow, often lobulated or pseudopolypoid appearance. In spite of the proliferation of both glands and stroma, there is focal crowding of the glands histologically. The glands are tubular or slightly convoluted and vary considerably in size and shape. Occasionally some of the glands may be cystically dilated. Secretory activity is either absent or focal and sporadic. Mitoses are present but oddly enough are not more numerous than in a proliferative endometrium. Nucleoli are prominent, and there is little or no budding of gland epithelium into the lumen.

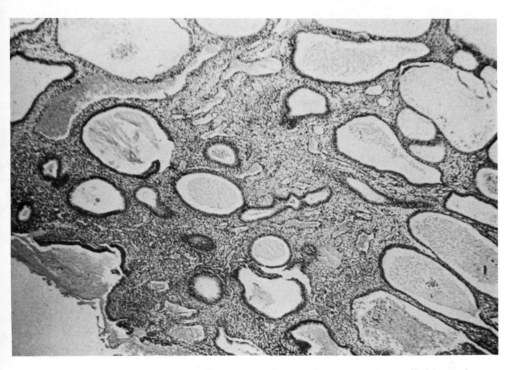

Fig. 4-2. Photomicrograph of inactive endometrium with cystic change, sometimes called "cystic hyperplasia."

"SWISS CHEESE" HYPERPLASIA

"Swiss cheese" hyperplasia is an outdated term that describes inactive endometrium with cystic change. Cystic change can be seen in virtually any endometrium to a limited extent. It is a prominent feature, however, in the endometrium of some menopausal women. This combination of inactive glands with extensive cystic change has in the past been referred to as "swiss cheese" hyperplasia. Since the endometrium in these cases is not hyperplastic but thin and atrophic, the term is a misnomer. It is our belief that this term should be reserved exclusively for patients with inactive endometrium, and a preferable designation would be inactive endometrium with cystic change (Fig. 4-2). Varying degrees of adenomatous hyperplasia may be seen concomitantly with these cystic changes, but the two histologic findings appear to be unrelated. In the opinion of most there is no premalignant potential in the patient with pure inactive endometrium with cystic change.

ADENOMATOUS HYPERPLASIA

Adenomatous hyperplasia (Fig. 4-3) is viewed with much greater concern by gynecologists and pathologists in general. It is generally accepted as a precursor of endometrial carcinoma. Mild degrees of adenomatous hyperplasia are sometimes

℗ Recursore of CA

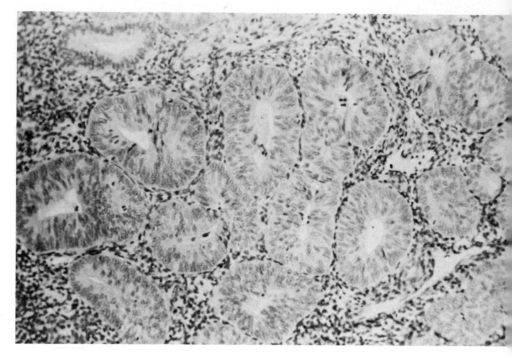

Fig. 4-3. Photomicrograph of adenomatous hyperplasia.

called glandular hyperplasia. The distinction is histologic and is based mainly on the fact that endometrial glands in adenomatous hyperplasia proliferate at the expense of the stroma. In those lesions labeled glandular hyperplasia the crowding of glands is only focal in nature, whereas in adenomatous hyperplasia crowding is quite prevalent. Indeed, the glands increase in number and complexity as the degree of hyperplasia increases, and conversely the intervening stroma diminishes in amount. The crowding of the glands may progress to a point where they are "back to back" or separated from one another by only a very delicate band of fibrous stroma. The involvement of the endometrium may be focal or quite diffuse.

ATYPICAL ADENOMATOUS HYPERPLASIA

The term "atypical" refers to the cytologic atypia occurring in adenomatous hyperplasia (Fig. 4-4). This atypia consists of nuclear enlargement, hyperchromasia, or irregularity in shape. These lesions have a great propensity for progression to adenocarcinoma and are often treated as if they were adenocarcinoma. Many pathologists and gynecologic oncologists further subdivide this category into mild, moderate, and severe atypical adenomatous hyperplasia. Severe atypical hyperplasia is characterized by anaplasia, or lessened differentiation of the glands particularly. The lining cells of the glands exhibit a pronounced variation in size, shape, cytoplasmic staining, and polarity. In a similar manner, the nuclei are usually irregularly shaped and

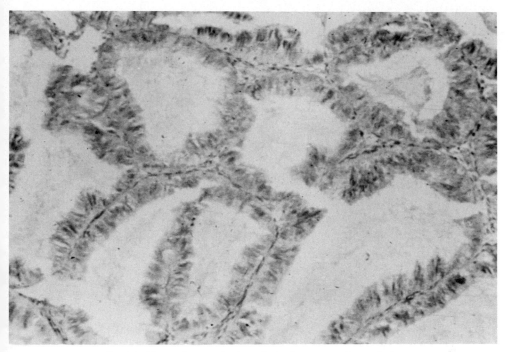

Fig. 4-4. Photomicrograph of atypical adenomatous hyperplasia.

show marked variation in size and staining qualities. There is a generalized pallor of the cells, but this may not be uniform.

Severe atypical adenomatous hyperplasia has often been labeled "carcinoma in situ" of the endometrium, or stage 0 cancer of the endometrium. This relates to the concept of most pathologists that adenocarcinoma of the endometrium begins as a focal change in the endometrial glandular epithelium. There is undoubtedly a stage that precedes endometrial stromal invasion and in which changes are limited to the endometrial glands. However, the gross appearance of the endometrium in "carcinoma in situ" is of little help since it may be normal, thin, or focally polypoid. It is doubtful whether the term "carcinoma in situ" of the endometrium is helpful, since there is no clear dividing line between severe forms of atypical adenomatous hyperplasia and this lesion described by Hertig. Our preference is to not use the term "carcinoma in situ"; we prefer the designation "severe atypical adenomatous hyperplasia."

CLINICAL PROFILE

The usual symptom associated with the progression of endometrial hyperplasia is irregular, occasionally profuse uterine bleeding. This is often accompanied by lower abdominal cramps, which are undoubtedly due to the accumulation of blood in the endometrial cavity and the expulsion of this blood along with blood clots. In

Bleeding

the young teenage patient this is usually associated with anovulatory cycles, as it is in the middle-aged perimenopausal patient. Endometrial hyperplasia has also been seen in association with other disease states such as granulosa cell tumors, ovarian thecomas, Stein-Leventhal syndrome (polycystic ovarian syndrome), and adrenocortical hyperplasia. The typical history of this group of patients reveals an interruption in cyclic menses, usually with skips and delays of menstrual flow or with prolonged periods of amenorrhea. This entire syndrome can also occur as a result of constant administration of exogenous estrogenic substances.

PREMALIGNANT POTENTIAL

It is generally agreed that patients with adenomatous hyperplasia are more likely to develop carcinoma than those with benign lesions of the endometrium, although the potential is difficult to quantitate. The usually quoted general figure of the risk of invasive cancer for patients with atypical adenomatous hyperplasia is 5% to 12%. The process appears to be relatively slow, and the progression from hyperplasia to carcinoma may take 5 or more years. In an interesting study done in 1970, Chamlian and Taylor found that endometrial hyperplasia was associated with polycystic ovarian syndromes similar to the so-called Stein-Leventhal syndrome in 24 of 97 young women with endometrial hyperplasia (25%). In 14 of these women, the lesion progressed to adenocarcinoma 1 to 14 years after the initial diagnosis of endometrial hyperplasia, in spite of the fact that 41% of the patients underwent hysterectomy at some interval after diagnosis was made.

In 1947 Gusberg morphologically defined adenomatous hyperplasia and sug-

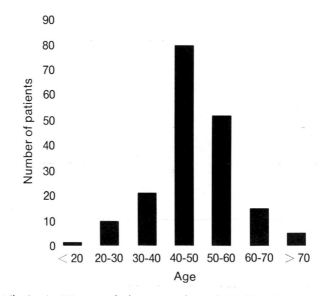

Fig. 4-5. Age distribution in 191 cases of adenomatous hyperplasia. (From Gusberg, S. B., and Kaplan, A. L.: Am. J. Obstet. Gynecol. **87:**662, 1963.)

gested that it is a precursor of endometrial carcinoma. Later, Gusberg and Kaplan did prospective follow-up studies on 191 patients with adenomatous hyperplasia diagnosed from 1934 to 1954 (Fig. 4-5). Of these, 90 were treated immediately by hysterectomy, and 20% were found to have coexisting carcinoma, while 13% had borderline lesions. This left 101 patients to be followed. In this group, 8 patients (11.8%) went on to develop endometrial cancer (mean follow-up, 5.3 years). In the control group, consisting of 202 patients (all of whom presented with postmenopausal bleeding and none of whom were shown to have hyperplasia or carcinoma on initial curettage), only one went on to develop endometrial carcinoma. Gusberg and Kaplan concluded that the cumulative risk for a patient with adenomatous hyperplasia followed for 9 to 10 years is significantly higher than for a woman without hyperplasia. Adenocarcinoma of the endometrium is considered rare during the childbearing years. When it does occur, a significant number of the cases are associated with the polycystic ovarian syndrome and anovulatory cycles. In a study by Jackson and Dockerty of 43 patients with the Stein-Leventhal syndrome, 16 (37.2%) had carcinoma of the endometrium.

MANAGEMENT

The most important features in the management of endometrial hyperplasia are the age of the patient and the histologic pattern of the hyperplastic process. Treatment of a teenage patient with glandular hyperplasia will always be conservative, whereas the postmenopausal patient with atypical adenomatous hyperplasia should, in most instances, be treated by hysterectomy and bilateral salpingo-oophorectomy. It should be kept in mind that various hyperplastic patterns may be found in nonmalignant endometrium of patients with concomitant endometrial carcinoma. Therefore, careful sampling of the endometrial cavity is a prerequisite to consideration for conservative therapy. In almost every series of endometrial hyperplasia where hysterectomy has been performed following diagnosis, there have been a significant number of patients with concomitant unrecognized invasive adenocarcinoma. The problem of sufficient sampling of the endometrium, even with D&C, is real and should be kept in mind at all times when the patient is advised on therapy. Our preference for therapy has been as follows:

1. *Teenage girl*. This patient should be treated with estrogen-progestin artificial cycles for at least 6 months. Three months after completion of this treatment period, the endometrial cavity should be resampled. If benign endometrium is found on resampling, the patient should be observed for evidence of regular menses and patterns of ovulation. In the absence of ovulation the patient should be given periodic doses of progestin (Provera, 10 mg orally each day for 10 days) to oppose the estrogen stimulation of her endometrium. This periodic use of progestin should continue until the patient has commenced an ovulatory pattern or is ready for ovulation induction and childbearing.

2. *Childbearing woman*. This patient should be treated with estrogen-progestin artificial cycles for 3 months. This period of therapy should be immediately

followed by careful sampling of the endometrium to ensure reversion to a benign pattern. The patient should then be treated with clomiphene, menotropins (Pergonal), etc. to secure ovulation induction. Should the patient not be interested in childbearing at that time, the continued use of estrogen-progestin artificial cycles is recommended.

3. *Perimenopausal woman.* This patient should be treated by either hysterectomy or large doses of progestin alone. The decision for hysterectomy would depend on the severity of the hyperplasia, the desire for sterilization, the presence of coexisting symptoms such as severe uterine bleeding, and/or the suspicion of an estrogen-secreting ovarian neoplasm. In general, our tendency is to recommend hysterectomy for patients with moderate to severe adenomatous hyperplasia and to use a trial of progestin for patients with lesser lesions and no concomitant pathologic findings. Our practice is to administer Provera (50 mg daily or 800 mg IM every 2 weeks) for at least 6 months. The endometrial cavity should be sampled by endometrial biopsy every 3 months. Patients will experience irregular bleeding and should be prepared for this so as to minimize anxiety.

4. *Postmenopausal woman.* This patient should undergo hysterectomy unless strongly contraindicated. A true postmenopausal woman (last menses 2 or more years ago) with endometrial hyperplasia is often found to have coexisting foci of invasive adenocarcinoma or concomitant estrogen-secreting ovarian neoplasms. Progestin therapy should be reserved for patients with medical problems that make them very poor operative candidates.

Progesterone and synthetic progestins have both produced reversion of adenomatous and atypical adenomatous hyperplasia to an atrophic pattern. This reversion may also be effected by induction of ovulation in women desirous of pregnancy. Some authors have advocated immediate commencement of ovulation induction in patients desirous of pregnancy and have believed that this maneuver is sufficient therapy for the endometrial hyperplasia as well. Our preference has been to continue the medical curettage (estrogen-progestin artificial cycles) for a period of up to 3 months before ovulation induction. Our preference for estrogen-progestin artificial cycles rather than progestin alone is based on ease of administration. The use of progestin alone results in irregular bleeding, which is often upsetting to the patient who is fearful of cancer. We have found the estrogen-progestin cyclic therapy to be effective in reverting the endometrium in spite of the estrogen contained in this medication, and we have been quite pleased with the smoothness of the cycles induced.

Progestins as the sole therapy eliminate in situ endometrial lesions in 62% of all cases, according to reports by Steiner and associates and Wilson and Kolsted. The incidence of invasive tumor in such patients treated with progestins is only 6%. Bonte and associates reported optimum responses with serum levels of 90 ng of medroxyprogesterone acetate (MPA) when treating both in situ and invasive endometrial cancer with progestins. MPA appears to partly inhibit hypothalamic and hypophyseal activities, especially LH production and, to a lesser extent, FSH production. Interestingly, estradiol and estrone serum levels are only slightly affected by MPA administration. At the cellular level, progestins appear to inhibit estrogen-induced RNA synthesis and thus exert their antimitotic action. Such progestin activity can partly be visualized by means of autoradiography with tagged thymidine. The cytoplasmic and nuclear receptors of estradiol and progestin, 17 β-estradiol and 20-OC-dihydroprogestin dehydrogenase, would be the primary points of impact in both normal and malignant endometrium. The end result or the local effect of progestin on neoplastic endometrial tissue is apparently differentiation, maturation, secretion, epithelial metaplasia, and atrophy.

ESTROGENS AND ENDOMETRIAL NEOPLASIA

One of the factors that has prompted a returning and increasing interest in endometrial hyperplasia and endometrial cancer has been the role of ovarian hormones, notably estrogen, in this disease. The basis for considering estrogen as an etiologic factor probably lies in the observation that hyperplasia of the endometrium is frequently associated with carcinoma, and the association of prolonged estrogen therapy and unopposed endogenous estrogens with endometrial hyperplasia has been widely recognized. The association is more suspect in the postmenopausal age group, in which 75% of cancer of the endometrium is found. It is in this age group that estrogen from any source can stimulate the endometrium unopposed by the action of progestin. In all likelihood, hyperplasia, excluding severe adenomatous hyperplasia, is not intimately related to carcinoma in the reproductive period but the same entity encountered in the postmenopausal woman is quite strongly suggestive of cancer.

The role of estrogen and its possible relationship to endometrial cancer are receiving increased attention in both the scientific and the lay press (Table 4-1). Experiments of nature have provided us with information that would implicate estrogen as a possible contributing factor to the development of endometrial cancer. It

Table 4-1. Characteristics associated with incidence of endometrial cancer

Characteristic	Effect on incidence
Delayed menopause ("bloody menopause")	↑
Hypertension	↑
Diabetes	↑
Obesity	↑
High socioeconomic status	↑
Urban residence	↑
Positive family history	↑
Polycystic ovarian syndrome	↑
Exogenous estrogen in menopause	↑
Estrogen-secreting tumor	↑
Childbearing	↓
Delayed menarche	↓

has been known for years that endometrial cancer can occur in patients with hormone-secreting tumors, particularly of the ovary. Many studies have been done on this entity since it was first reported by Novak and Yui in 1936 in the American literature. Gusberg and Kardon noted the highest correlation between endometrial cancer and the so-called feminizing ovarian tumors. They reported on 115 patients, 21% of which were found to have corpus cancer and 43% of which were found to have cancer precursors such as endometrial hyperplasia and carcinoma in situ. Still the authors were unable to draw any solid conclusions about the possible carcinogenic role of estrogen in humans. Norris and Taylor evaluated 203 patients with granulosa-theca cell tumors at the Armed Forces Institute of Pathology. They reported that only 9% of these patients had adenocarcinoma of the uterus but did not mention endometrial precursors. Mansell and Hertig reviewed 80 feminizing tumors treated at the Free Hospital in Boston between 1905 and 1953. Only 11 patients had adenocarcinoma; however, 60% of the endometria did have changes suggestive of estrogen stimulation. McDonald and associates approached the situation from another viewpoint. Between 1905 and 1975 there were 44 patients with functional ovarian tumors and endometrial cancer at the Mayo Clinic. Unfortunately, the authors do not mention how many other functional ovarian tumors or adenocarcinomas of the endometrium they noted during that time interval. They also saw 28 patients with polycystic ovarian disease and endometrial cancer. They then compared these patients with 523 adenocarcinoma patients who were seen from 1952 to 1962. The 72 patients with endometrial cancer associated with functional tumors or polycystic ovaries had a predominance of stage I, grade I lesions, less myometrial involvement, and better survival rates compared with the other 523 adenocarcinoma patients. Some authors have qualified the stromal tumors with the word "feminizing," but others have not used this designation. It is well known that granulosa cell tumors can produce androgens, although to a smaller degree than those tumors that might produce estrogen.

Another situation in which endogenous estrogen might be a contributing factor to the development of endometrial cancer is in those patients with the polycystic ovary syndrome. The incidence of endometrial cancer has been reported to be as high as 25% in those patients with the Stein-Leventhal syndrome, although in actuality this number is probably considerably smaller. If the unopposed estrogen can be alleviated in this syndrome by wedge resection or clomiphene citrate, the estrogen-stimulated endometrium and its possible premalignant changes can be reversed. Kistner has reported that progestogens can cause a regression of hyperplasia and carcinoma in situ of the endometrium.

Patients with ovarian dysgenesis (Turner syndrome) have also been reported to be at high risk for endometrial cancer because of the long-term supplemental estrogen that is given to these individuals beginning at an early age. Although several case reports have appeared recently in the literature, only 14 patients have been reported to date.

It is also well known that estrone, which makes up the largest amount of estrogen produced in the postmenopausal woman, is a result of peripheral conversion of androstenedione. There appears to be a greater conversion of androstenedione to estrone in endometrial cancer patients as compared with healthy postmenopausal women. There is also increased estrone production in the woman who is postmenopausal, older, and obese. The cause of the increased production of estrone is unknown.

In view of the relative frequency with which the uterus is stimulated by estrogen, either naturally or synthetically through the use of hormone therapy, and the relative rarity of carcinoma of the endometrium, it is obvious that the evidence of hyperestrinism as the sole etiologic explanation for endometrial cancer is unsatisfactory. We must also accept the hypothesis of the presence of a properly sensitive substrate that overreacts to estrogen stimulation. The available data from humans would suggest that in predisposed individuals, the unopposed action of estrogen substances for considerable periods will result in endometrial adenomatous hyperplasia, anaplasia, carcinoma in situ, and eventually carcinoma.

The postmenopausal ovary continues to secrete substantial amounts of androgens (testosterone and androstenedione) but virtually no estrogen. There is increasing evidence to support the concept that after menopause, most of the estrogens are derived from peripheral conversion of androgens of adrenal origin, with only a small contribution by the ovary. The origin of plasma sex hormones in postmenopausal women was further studied by determining plasma levels under basal conditions, after ACTH stimulation and dexamethasone suppression, and after hCG stimulation. The findings indicate that the adrenal cortex is the almost unique source of plasma estradiol, estrone, progesterone, and 17-OH-progesterone and the most important source of plasma dehydroepiandrosterone. The postmenopausal ovary appears to be responsible for about 50% of plasma testosterone and 30% of androstenediones, and hCG stimulation with 5,000 IU daily for 3 days hardly influences steroid secretion by postmenopausal ovaries. Removal of the ovaries frequently fails to alter the quantity of estrogen produced in postmenopausal women. Of even greater interest is the continuous presence of a small but definite amount of estrogen even after complete hypophysectomy in oophorectomized women.

Marrett reported incidence rates for invasive cancer of the uterine corpus according to stage of disease (localized, nonlocalized) based on cases reported to the Connecticut Tumor Registry between 1960 and 1975. The 1960-1964 and 1965-1969 rates were very similar for both disease stages. However, in 1970-1975 the incidence of localized corpus cancer was 26% higher than in either of the previously studied periods. Women aged 50 to 59 experienced the largest increase in localized disease, although all other age groups over 50 also had higher rates in the most recent period of diagnosis. No increases were evident in women under 50 years of age. In addition, the frequency of the diagnosis of carcinoma in situ of the endometrium increased gradually over the 16-year period, and mortality from corpus cancer declined slightly. Over the same period there was an increase in the hysterectomy rate in Connecticut, and when the corpus cancer rate was adjusted for this variable, the rate increased another 5% to 15%. Factors associated with an increased risk of endo-metrial cancer, such as overweight, nulliparity, late menopause, diabetes mellitus, hypertension, Stein-Leventhal syndrome, cancers of other sites, pelvic irradiation, and administration of estrogens, were reviewed and no evidence could be found that the prevalence of any of these, apart from estrogen use, has increased. Estrogens have been used for replacement therapy since the 1930s; by 1958, 1.6 million pre-scriptions were being filled nationally per year. This figure changed little between 1958 and 1965 but had doubled by 1966. This new higher level of use was maintained until 1971, after which time it began to increase. The increase in incidence of endo-metrial cancer that began in 1970 would lead to an estimated latency period of 4 to 8 years between initiation of drug exposure and diagnosis of cancer. Marrett cor-rectly concluded that the recent increase in the incidence of localized invasive endo-metrial cancer in women 50 years and over in Connecticut is likely to be at least partially due to the increasing use of estrogen therapy. The fact that neither mortality from corpus cancer nor nonlocalized disease incidence has increased in Connecticut since 1960 suggests that estrogen therapy may be predominantly associated with tumors that can be readily diagnosed at an early stage.

In 1941 Greene described a strain of rabbits that developed "toxemia of preg-nancy" and liver damage, whereupon such animals became infertile and developed endometrial hyperplasia and subsequent carcinoma of the endometrium depending on this so-called hyperestrinism. This was an excellent model of the infertile woman.

Cancer of the endometrium has not been produced experimentally in subhuman primates, but the studies to date have suffered from the clear species variation of endometrial response to hormonal stimulation and the lack of appropriate genetic substrate in these animals as well as the relatively short duration of most experi-ments of this type in this relatively long-lived animal. Although the development of adenocarcinoma of the endometrium in laboratory animals has been limited to the rabbit, guinea pig, and mouse, Scott and Wharton did produce adenomatous hyper-plasia in monkeys with diethylstilbestrol.

In the past decade there have been numerous retrospective studies correlating the use of exogenous estrogens in the postmenopausal woman with the increasing incidence of endometrial carcinoma. Smith and his co-workers from the University of Washington identified 317 women, aged 48 years or more, from two hospitals where they had been diagnoied as having adenocarcinoma of the endometrium be-tween 1960 and 1972. A retrospective review of the hospital's records showed that for 152 (48%) of these women, exogenous estrogen therapy had been prescribed. Of the 317 patients without endometrial carcinoma who were selected as a control group only 54 (17%) had had exogenous estrogen prescribed previously. Appropriate statistical calculations revealed a 4.5-fold increased risk of developing endometrial cancer for the women exposed to estrogen in the restrospective study. Subsequent data from these same investigators revealed that the women developing endometrial carcinoma on exogenous estrogen therapy were phenotypically quite different from the atypical obese, diabetic, hypertensive individual usually associated with this neoplasm. Indeed, most of the women developing endometrial adenocarcinoma on exogenous estrogen therapy were much more normal in appearance with nonstriking medical histories for diabetes, hypertension, etc.

Ziel and Finkle from the Kaiser Permanente Medical Center in Los Angeles published a retrospective review of their patients treated between July 1970 and December 1974. Ninety-four cases of endometrial carcinoma were discovered during that time period. The records of 54 (57%) of these individuals showed them to have received prior therapy with conjugated estrogens. Selection of 108 women as controls (2 for each case) was based on comparable age, area of residence, and duration of health plan membership. Only 29 (15%) of these women had been treated with conjugated estrogens. The risk ratio (RR) in this study was calculated to be 7.6.

The next report on this subject was published in June 1976 by Mack and associates and was conducted in a retirement community south of Los Angeles where 63 women were diagnosed between 1971 and 1975 as having endometrial carcinoma. As determined from medical records, patient interviews, or pharmacy prescription records, 56 (89%) of the patients were found to have taken some form of estrogen. These investigators selected four controls for each case. The control patients were residents of the community matched with the endometrial cancer patients for the time of entry into the community, age, and marital status. Of the group of 252 controls, 126 (50%) were found to have taken some form of estrogen, for a computed RR of 8.0.

Subsequently, there have been a number of articles in the literature that have evaluated the use of exogenous estrogen in patients with endometrial cancer. The study of McDonald and associates evaluating this relationship in Olmstead County (Rochester, Minnesota) noted 145 endometrial cancer patients over the period studied. They were compared with 417 controls. Twenty-seven percent of the endometrial cancer patients took estrogen, whereas 28% of the controls took estrogen. The RR for all exogenous estrogen was 0.9; however, it increased to 2.3 if the drug was taken for longer than 6 months. If only conjugated estrogen was considered, regardless of duration, the RR was 2.0. It is of interest that only 16 patients out of the 145 took conjugated estrogens for longer than 6 months. The authors noted that the incidence of endometrial cancer in Olmstead County had actually decreased over the last 3 decades even though estrogen use had increased from 5% to 21% during the time studied. When they evaluated their data in the manner that the previous three authors had, their RR became 2.0 as analyzed like Ziel and Finkle, 2.3 as analyzed like Smith and associates, and 0.9 as analyzed like Mack and associates.

Gray and associates evaluated their private practice experience with 205 endometrial cancer patients between 1947 and 1976 as compared with 205 controls who had had hysterectomy for benign disease. Twenty-six percent of the cancer patients took estrogen as compared with only 15% of the controls. The RR for conjugated estrogen was 3.1, but for all estrogen it was 2.1. The RR did increase with years of use but was only significant above the 10-year interval. The authors stated that the actual number of cancers due to exogenous estrogen is quite small. Only 31 of the

205 cancers could be attributed to estrogen use, even if all excess risk from estrogen leads to cancer.

Hoover and associates, in evaluating cancer of the uterine corpus after hormonal treatment for breast cancer, noted a slight increase in those women who had received estrogen after mastectomy. It was noted that in those patients who did not receive estrogen there was a 40% greater incidence of uterine cancer in that group than would be expected. Other studies have shown an increased RR for endometrial cancer in patients with breast cancer, as multiple primary cancers can occur in the same patient.

A recent study by Antunes and associates evaluated endometrial cancer patients between 1973 and 1977 in six hospitals in Baltimore. A total of 451 endometrial cancer patients were identified and compared with 888 controls. It was noted that if the controls were from the gynecologic service, the RR for estrogen use was 2.1; however, if the controls were from the nongynecologic services, the RR was 6.0. When the dosage, type of estrogen, and duration of use were considered, appropriate data were available on only 75% of the cancer patients and less than 50% of the controls. No pathologic data were presented even though the authors stated that no overestimation of the material was made. The authors believe that the difference between the two groups of patients cannot be explained, because a faster diagnosis was made in the estrogen versus the nonestrogen patient, yet only 30% of the cancer patients and 26% of the control patients were evaluated for this parameter.

In December 1975 the Obstetric Advisory Committee of the FDA reviewed these reports and concluded that "the studies provided strong evidence that postmenopausal estrogen therapy increases the risk of endometrial cancer." Based on this conclusion, the FDA has developed a revised package insert for use by patients as well as physicians that will include a clear warning of the increased risk of endometrial cancer and a "clarification" of the indications for the use of estrogen in the menopausal or postmenopausal period.

There have been several additional retrospective studies done in a manner very similar to those cited above, and similar conclusions were reached in most instances. Before the FDA position on this matter is accepted without question, a critical assessment of the reported data is necessary. All of these studies have one feature in common: the use of retrospective case control methodology. Women who had a diagnosis of endometrial carcinoma were selected as "cases" for comparison. Only then was the information gathered about prior exposure to exogenous estrogen use. Since calculation of an RR depends entirely on the different rates of estrogen exposure between the two groups, the choice of patients in the control group can obviously predetermine the results of such a study. The controls should be identical to the "cases" in every way except for the occurrence of the disease and the exposure to the ideologic factor or factors. The selection of the "controls" can introduce a so-called detection bias. Each of the studies done to date has been subjected to statistical criticisms based on the retrospective methodology. What is needed, of course, is a prospective study, but the execution of such a study would be difficult and possibly unethical. Applying different rules about the inclusion of patients as cases but not as controls is not acceptable. Imagine that a prospective comparative study is being started to evaluate the possible carcinogenicity of estrogens. The two groups of women, all with intact uteri, would be selected and then allocated to treatment or no treatment on a random basis. With the passage of time, some women in each group would undergo hysterectomy for a number of reasons. These women would have to be taken into account in the evaluation of the final results of the study. In some of the studies cited above the patients who underwent hysterectomy were specifically excluded from the control group. This and many other factors illustrate the potential pitfalls in the development of the case control methodology.

Recently, Horwitz and Feinstein have questioned the studies that have shown a large RR between endometrial cancer and exogenous estrogen. They noted a bias in the selection of controls. They evaluated their cancer patients using two sets of controls. With the conventional controls similar to the other studies, 29% of the cancer patients had taken estrogen versus 3% of the controls, for an odds ratio of 11.98. The alternative set of controls, patients who had D&C or hysterectomy, were used to equalize the forces of diagnostic surveillance that might create major detected bias. In this group of patients, an odds ratio of only 1.7 was present.

In addition, there have been several reports in the literature that have suggested no difference in estrogen use between endometrial cancer patients and controls. In 1967 Dunn and Bradbury noted that 28.6% of 56 patients with endometrial cancer took estrogen versus 27.5% of 83 control patients. The controls were those individuals who had postmenopausal bleeding but with atrophic endometrium on D&C. Pacheco and Kempers looked at a group of patients who had postmenopausal bleeding. Only 71 of 401 patients (18%) had an endometrial malignancy. Ninety-three (23%) of the patients took estrogen. Only 10% of those patients who had postmenopausal bleeding and took estrogen had cancer, whereas 18% of the patients who had postmenopausal bleeding not due to cancer took estrogen. More recently, a study from Finland evaluated 317 endometrial cancer patients followed between 1970 and 1976 compared with 304 controls. Of the cancer patients, only 9% took estrogen, whereas 19% of the controls took estrogen.

However, a great body of indirect evidence suggests that estrogen (endogenous and exogenous) can be an ideologic agent in the pathogenesis of endometrial adenocarcinoma. A very convincing study was recently reported by Sturdee and associates. In the study, vacuum curettage was performed on 348 women who had received various regimens of estrogen treatment for an average of 97 months for menopausal symptoms. Cylical unopposed oral estrogen treatment (98 cases) was associated with a 12% incidence of endometrial hyperplasia, but among the 102 women taking regimens including 10 to 13 days of progesterone there was a zero incidence of hyperplasia. Among women treated with subcutaneous estrogen implants and monthly 5-day courses of oral progestin (50 cases) there was a 28% incidence of hyperplasia, including one case of adenocarcinoma. Regular withdrawal bleeding during treatment was associated with a lower incidence of endometrial hyperplasia (6%) than unscheduled breakthrough bleeding (18%), but the one patient with carcinoma had experienced regular bleeding only.

Silverberg and Makowski, as well as others, have described the development of endometrial carcinoma in patients taking oral contraceptive agents. In virtually every instance, the agents used were of the sequential variety and progestin was administered with the estrogen only in the last 7 days of each cycle. During the first 14 days of the cycle, the patient received large doses of synthetic estrogen alone. Whether sequential agents somehow predispose their recipients to endometrial cancer or whether those women who are predisposed to develop this tumor are protected against it by the use of a combined oral contraceptive agent remains to be determined. The sequential type of oral contraceptive has been voluntarily withdrawn from the market by the various pharmaceutical companies producing it, so this question may remain moot.

Benefits of estrogen replacement

Estrogen replacement therapy is usually beneficial for women experiencing involuntary hot flashes and sweats as well as symptoms attributable to atrophy of the vagina or the urethra and to bladder trigone. Vasomotor symptoms including hot flashes and sweats are quite distinct and are troublesome to between 20% and 60% of postmenopausal women. Double-blind studies have established that estrogen therapy is beneficial in treating these symptoms. Emotional problems associated with these symptoms are best treated with supportive therapy and, if necessary, with other drugs. Menopausal symptoms respond to low doses of estrogen (i.e., 0.625 mg of conjugated estrogens). Estrogen deficiency results in a gradual reduction and eventual loss of the cornified epithelial layer of the vagina. Though not as marked, changes occur in the urethra and bladder epithelium as well. The results are increasing dryness in the vagina and, when deficiency is severe, vaginal irritation, pruritus vulvae, and urethritis.

A fair amount of evidence indicates that estrogen replacement does not prevent cardiovascular disease. However, estrogen's beneficial effects in preventing or treating postmenopausal osteoporosis are becoming better recognized. Approximately 25% of all white women over the age of 60 have spinal compression fractures resulting from osteoporosis. The risk of hip fracture is 20% by the age of 90, and hip fractures are about 2½ times as common in women as in men. An increased rate of loss of both cortical and cancellous bone is associated with the menopause. In a follow-up study of 82 postmenopausal women 5 to 10 years after their first examination, Meema and associates concluded that (1) menopausal women as a group lost bone, and the beginning of this loss is less related to age than to loss of ovarian function, (2) the rate of loss was not significantly correlated with age, and (3) the bone loss was prevented by estrogen administration (i.e., 0.625 mg of conjugated estrogens). A similar beneficial effect of estrogen administration was shown by Lindsay and associates (Fig. 4-6) in a short-term double-blind study of changes in metacarpal bone in oophorectomized women given an average daily dose of 25 mg of mestranol.

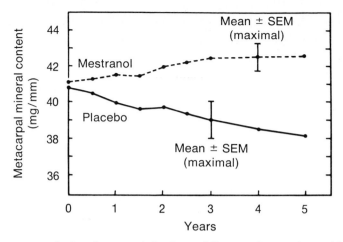

Fig. 4-6. Mean metacarpal mineral content during 5-year follow-up of group observed from 3 years after bilateral oophorectomy (zero time). (From Lindsay, R., Hart, D. M., Aitken, J. M., and others: Lancet 1:1038, 1976.)

Nachtigall and associates conducted a 10-year double-blind prospective study to evaluate the effects of estrogen replacement therapy. They took a sample population consisting of 84 pairs of randomly chosen postmenopausal patients who were matched for age and diagnosis. Half of the patients received conjugated estrogens and cyclic progesterone while the other half received placebo. The estrogen-treated patients whose therapy was started within 3 years of menopause showed improvement or no increase in osteoporosis. The control patients demonstrated an increase in osteoporosis. A subsequent report by the same authors showed that there was no statistically significant difference in the incidence of thrombophlebitis, myocardial infarction, or uterine cancer in the two groups. Indeed, there was a lower incidence of breast cancer in the treated group. Estrogen-treated patients did show a higher incidence of cholelithiasis. The low number of cases precludes drawing any real conclusions from the data on diseases of low frequency. The study does exclude a high incidence of complications from estrogens.

At present there is no evidence that there is an increased risk of breast carcinoma in postmenopausal women taking estrogen. In one study, 735 women were followed for an average of 15 years after they began taking estrogens. Overall, 21 cases of breast carcinoma were found; 18 were expected. Hoover and associates reported on 1,891 menopausal women treated with conjugated estrogen. The women were followed for an average of 12 years. In the treated group, 49 cases of breast carcinoma were observed; 39 were expected on the basis of the incidence in the general population. This difference was not statistically significant. The study's findings indicate that menopausal estrogen use does not protect against breast cancer, but neither does it appear to increase the risk of breast cancer markedly. However, with breast carcinoma, as with endometrial carcinoma, the possible association of estrogen use with increased risk remains and requires constant evaluation.

The questionable association of estrogen use with carcinoma of either the endometrium or the breast is not the only concern for those prescribing or receiving estrogen therapy. Estrogens are contraindicated in patients with acute liver disease, thromboembolic disease, undiagnosed vaginal bleeding, and breast malignancy or other estrogen-dependent neoplasms. The onset of hypertension in a previously normotensive individual and abnormal carbohydrate and/or lipid metabolism are also of concern.

How to use estrogens

In each instance, before estrogen therapy is begun a complete evaluation of the woman, including a complete history and physical examination with appropriate laboratory studies, should be done to discern any factors that may put the individual at an increased adverse risk. Any history of abnormal bleeding requires a histologic evaluation of the endometrium before initiation of estrogen therapy, and many authors have recommended that an endometrial evaluation be done even in the asymptomatic patient. Our feeling is that this is unnecessary in the patient with a normal pelvic examination and a history of an uneventful menopause. It is recommended that patients be started on 0.625 mg of conjugated estrogens or its equivalent (Table 4-2). The exception to this would be young women who have been surgically castrated, who must be started at a higher dose (1.25 mg/day) in order to adequately relieve symptoms. Doses should be increased only in the face of very severe and intolerable symptoms. Estrogen should be administered in cyclic fashion, allowing 5 to 7 days each month when no drug is ingested. In each case, before estrogen therapy is instituted the benefits and risks of this therapy should be weighed for each patient and discussed thoroughly. Some authorities have recommended cyclic progestin therapy (the last 7 to 10 days of each monthly cycle) in addition to the exogenous estrogen to prevent excessive endometrial proliferation. There is consid-

Table 4-2. Comparative physiologic doses of common estrogen preparations

Estrogen	Dose (mg)
Ethinyl estradiol	0.02
Diethylstilbestrol	0.25
Conjugated estrogens	0.625
Estrone	1.25

Table 4-3. Surveillance of patients receiving exogenous estrogens (performed every 6 months)

Blood pressure
Breast examination
Pelvic examination
Endometrial sampling if there is abnormal bleeding

erable merit in this recommendation if the patient and physician will accept periodic menses even late in the postmenopausal period. Many elderly patients are annoyed with the inconvenience of periodic vaginal bleeding. In situations where estrogen is contraindicated (e.g., endometrial carcinoma), menopausal symptoms may be adequately relieved by daily ingestion of progestins such as megestrol acetate (Megace, 20 mg daily) or medroxyprogesterone (Provera, 10 to 20 mg daily). Although vasomotor symptoms are consistently relieved with the use of progestins, patients may complain of vaginal dryness and increased appetite with weight gain. Patients receiving exogenous estrogen therapy should be examined every 6 to 12 months for changes in uterine size, excessive breast stimulation, and elevated blood pressure (Table 4-3). *Any patient who has any uterine bleeding in the postmenopausal period should be suspected of having endometrial carcinoma until adequate endometrial sampling has proved otherwise.*

BIBLIOGRAPHY

Aitken, J. M., Hart, P. M., Anderson, J. B., and others: Osteoporosis after oophorectomy for non-malignant disease in premenopausal women, Br. Med. J. **2:**325, 1973.

Alffram, P. A.: An epidemiologic study of cervical and trochanteric fractures of the femur in an urban population, Acta Orthop. Scand. (Suppl.) **65:**1, 1964.

Antunes, C. M. F., Stolley, P. D., Rosenshein, N. B., and others: Endometrial cancer and estrogen use; report of a large case-control study, N. Engl. J. Med. **300:**9, 1979.

Bonte, J., Decoster, J. M., Ide, P., and Billiet, G.: Hormonoprophyaxis and hormonotherapy in the treatment of endometrial adenocarcinoma by means of medroxyprogesterone acetate, Gynecol. Oncol. **6:**60, 1978.

Chamlian, D. L., and Taylor, H. B.: Endometrial hyperplasia in young women, Obstet. Gynecol. **36:**659, 1970.

Cramer, D. W., Cutler, S. J., and Christine, B.: Trends in the incidence of endometrial cancer in the United States, Gynecol. Oncol. **2:**120, 1974.

Cutler, S. J., and Young, J. L., Jr.: Third national cancer survey; incidence data, National Cancer Institute Monograph 41, Bethesda, Md., March 1975.

Dunn, L. J., and Bradbury, R. D.: Endocrine factors in endometrial carcinoma; a preliminary report, Am. J. Obstet. Gynecol. **97:**1465, 1967.

Emge, L. A.: Endometrial cancer and feminizing tumors of the ovary, Obstet. Gynecol. **1:**511, 1953.

Fechner, R. E., and Kaufman, R. H.: Endometrial adenocarcinoma in Stein-Leventhal syndrome, Cancer **34:**444, 1974.

Federal Drug Administration: FDA drug bulletin, Washington, D.C., 1976, FDA.

Fremont-Smith, M., Meigs, J. V., Graham, R. M., and others: Cancer of the endometrium and prolonged estrogen therapy, J.A.M.A. **131:**805, 1946.

Gordon, G. S., and Greenberg, B. G.: Exogenous estrogen and endometrial cancer—an invited review, Postgrad. Med. **59:**67, 1976.

Gordon, G. S., Picchi, J., and Roof, B. S.: Antifracture efficacy of long-term estrogens for osteoporosis, Trans. Assoc. Am. Physicians **86:**326, 1973.

Gray, L. A., Christopherson, W. M., and Hoover, R. N.: Estrogens and endometrial carcinoma, Obstet. Gynecol. **49:**385, 1977.

Greene, H. S. N.: Uterine adenomata in the rabbit; susceptibility as a function of constitutional factors, J. Exp. Med. **73:**273, 1941.

Gusberg, S. B.: Precursors of corpus carcinoma, estrogens, and adenomatous hyperplasia, Am. J. Obstet. Gynecol. **54:**905, 1947.

Gusberg, S. B., and Hall, R. E.: Precursors of corpus cancer. III. The appearance of cancer of the endometrium in estrogenically conditioned patients, Obstet. Gynecol. **17:**397, 1961.

Gusberg, S. B., and Kaplan, A. L.: Precursors of corpus cancer, Am. J. Obstet. Gynecol. **87:**662, 1963.

Gusberg, S. B., and Kardon, P.: Proliferative endometrial response to thecal granulosa cell tumors, Am. J. Obstet. Gynecol. **3:**633, 1971.

Gusberg, S. B., Moore, D. B., and Martin, F.: Precursors of corpus cancer. II. A clinical and pathological study of adenomatous hyperplasia, Am. J. Obstet. Gynecol. **68:**1472, 1954.

Hammond, C. B., Jelovsek, F. R., Lee, K. L., and others: Effects of long-term estrogen replacement therapy. I. Metabolic effects, Am. J. Obstet. Gynecol. **133:**525, 1979.

Hoover, R., Gray, L. A., Cole, P., and MacMahon, B.: Menopausal estrogens and breast cancer, N. Engl. J. Med. **295:**401, 1976.

Horwitz, R. I., and Feinstein, A. R.: Alternative analytic methods for case-control studies of estrogens and endometrial cancer, N. Engl. J. Med. **299:**1089, 1978.

Horwitz, R. I., and Feinstein, A. R.: Susceptibility bias and the estrogen-endometrial cancer controversy (meeting abstract), Clin. Res. **27**(2):222A, 1979.

Horwitz, R. I., Feinstein, A. R., and Stremiau, J. R.: The influence of patient availability and discrepant sources of data on the odds ratio in case-control studies of estrogens and endometrial cancer (meeting abstract), Clin. Res. **27**(2):222A, 1979.

Ingram, J. M., Jr., and Novak, E.: Endometrial carcinoma associated with feminizing ovarian tumors, Am. J. Obstet. Gynecol. **61:**774, 1951.

Jackson, R. L., and Dockerty, M. B.: The Stein-Leventhal syndrome analysis of 43 cases with special reference to association with endometrial carcinoma, Am. J. Obstet. Gynecol. **73:**161, 1957.

Kistner, R. W.: Histological effects of progestins on hyperplasia and carcinoma in situ of the endometrium, Cancer **12:**1106, 1959.

Larsen, J. A.: Estrogens and endometrial carcinoma, Obstet. Gynecol. **3:**551, 1954.

Lindsay, R., Hart, D. M., Aitken, J. M., and others: Long term prevention of post-menopausal osteoporosis by oestrogen; evidence for an increased bone mass after delayed onset of oestrogen treatment, Lancet **1:**1038, 1976.

Lyon, F. A.: The development of adenocarcinoma of the endometrium in young women receiving long-term sequential oral contraception, Am. J. Obstet. Gynecol. **123:**299, 1975.

Lyon, F. A., and Frisch, M. J.: Endometrial abnormalities occurring in young women on long-term sequential oral contraception, Obstet. Gynecol. **47:**639, 1976.

MacDonald, P. C., and Siiteri, P. K.: The relationship between the extraglandular production of estrone and the occurrence of endometrial neoplasia, Gynecol. Oncol. **2:**259, 1974.

Mack, T. M., Pike, M. C., Henderson, B. E., and others: Estrogens and endometrial cancer in a retirement community, N. Engl. J. Med. **294:**1262, 1976.

Mansell, H., and Hertig, A. T.: Granulosa-theca cell tumor and endometrial carcinoma; a study of their relationship and survey of 80 cases, Obstet. Gynecol. **6:**385, 1955.

Mantel, N., and Haenszel, W.: Statistical aspects of the analysis of data from retrospective studies of disease, J. Natl. Cancer Inst. **22:**719, 1959.

Markush, R. E., and Turner, S. L.: Epidemiology of exogenous estrogens, H.S.M.H.A. Health Rep. **86:**74, 1971.

Marrett, L. D., Elwood, J. M., Epid, S. M., and others: Recent trends in the incidence and mortality of cancer of the uterine corpus in Connecticut, Gynecol. Oncol. **6:**183, 1978.

McDonald, T. W., Annegers, J. F., O'Fallon, W. M., and others: Exogenous estrogen and endometrial carcinoma; case control and incidence study, Am. J. Obstet. Gynceol. **49:**385, 1977.

Meema, S., Bunker, M. L., and Meema, H. E.: Preventive effect of estrogen on postmenopausal bone loss; a follow-up study, Arch. Intern. Med. **135:**1436, 1975.

Merriam, J. C., Jr., Easterday, C. L., McKay, D. G., and Hertig, A. T.: Experimental production of endometrial cancer in the rabbit, Obstet. Gynecol. **16:**253, 1960.

Nachtigall, L. E., Nachtigall, R. H., Nachtigall, R. D., and Beckman, E. M.: Estrogen replacement therapy I: a 10-year prospective study in the relationship to osteoporosis, Obstet. Gynecol. **53:**277, 1979.

Nachtigall, L. E., Nachtigall, R. H., Nachtigall, R. D., and Beckman, E. M.: Estrogen replacement therapy II: a prospective study in the relationship to carcinoma and cardiovascular and metabolic problems, Obstet. Gynecol. **54:**74, 1979.

Norris, H. J., and Taylor, H. B.: Prognosis of granulosa-theca tumors of the ovary, Cancer **21:**255, 1968.

Novak, E. R., and Woodruff, J. B.: Gynecologic and obstetric pathology, ed. 7, Philadelphia, 1974, W. B. Saunders Co., p. 190.

Pacheco, J. C., and Kempers, R. D.: Etiology of postmenopausal bleeding, Obstet. Gynecol. **32:**40, 1968.

Riggs, B. L., Jowsey, J., Goldsmith, R. S., and others: Short and long term effects of estrogen and synthetic anabolic hormone in postmenopausal osteoporosis, J. Clin. Invest. **51:**1659, 1972.

Rosenwaks, Z., Wentz, A. C., Jones, G. S., and others: Endometrial pathology and estrogens, Obstet. Gynecol. **53:**403, 1979.

Schmidt, A. M., Whitehorn, W. V., and Martin, E. W.: Estrogens and endometrial cancer, FDA Drug Bull. **6:**18, 1976.

Scott, R. B., and Wharton, L. R., Jr.: The effects of excessive amounts of diethylstilbestrol on experimental endometriosis in monkeys, Am. J. Obstet. Gynecol. **69:**573, 1955.

Sheehan, E. G., and Tucker, A. W.: Carcinoma of the endometrium, J.S.C. Med. Assoc. **45:**239, 1949.

Silverberg, S. Q., and Makowski, E. L.: Endometrial carcinoma in young women taking oral contraceptives, Obstet. Gynecol. **46:**503, 1975.

Sirota, D. K., and Marinoff, S. C.: Endometrial carcinoma in Turner's syndrome following prolonged treatment with diethylstilbestrol, Mt. Sinai J. Med. **42:**586, 1975.

Smith, D. C., Prentic, R., Thompson, D. J., and others: Estrogens and endometrial cancer in a retirement community, N. Engl. J. Med. **293:**1164, 1975.

Sommers, S. C., Hertig, A. T., and Bengloff, H.: Genesis of endometrial carcinoma, Cancer **2:**957, 1949.

Steiner, G. J., Kistner, R. W., and Craig, J. M.: Histological effects of progestin on hyperplasia and carcinoma in situ of the endometrium—further observations, Metabolism **14:**356, 1965.

Sturdee, D. W., Wade-Evans, T., Paterson, M. E., and others: Relations between bleeding pattern, endometrial histology, and oestrogen treatment in menopausal women, Br. Med. J. **1:**1575, 1978.

Weiss, N. S., Szekely, D. R., and Austin, D. F.: Increasing incidence of endometrial cancer in the United States, N. Engl. J. Med. **294:**1259, 1976.

Whitehead, M. I., McQueen, J., Beard, R. J., and others: The effects of cylical oestrogen therapy and sequential oestrogen progestogen therapy on the endometrium of postmenopausal women, Acta Obstet. Gynecol. Scand. (Suppl.) **65:**91, 1977.

Wilson, P. A., and Kolstad, P.: Hormonal treatment of preinvasive and invasive carcinoma of the corpus uteri. In Endometrial cancer, London, 1973, William Heinemann Medical Books Ltd.

Wood, G. P., and Boronow, R. C.: Endometrial adenocarcinoma and the polycystic ovary syndrome, Am. J. Obstet. Gynecol. **124:**140, 1976.

Ziel, H. K., and Finkle, W. D.: Increased risk of endometrial carcinoma among users of conjugated estrogens, N. Engl. J. Med. **293:**1167, 1975.

CHAPTER FIVE

Adenocarcinoma of the uterus

Epidemiology
Diagnosis
Prognostic factors
Treatment
Recurrence

Cancer of the uterine corpus is the most common malignancy seen in the female pelvis today. It is estimated by the American Cancer Society that approximately 37,000 women will develop uterine cancer this year in the United States. This malignancy is twice as common as carcinoma of the ovary and the cervix. The increased frequency of carcinoma of the endometrium has been apparent only during the last several years. In reviewing the predicted incidence for the 1970s, the American Cancer Society has noted a 1½-fold increase in the number of patients with endometrial cancer. During that time, the predicted deaths from this malignancy have actually decreased slightly. In 1978 Greenblatt and Stoddard suggested several reasons for the apparent increase in endometrial cancer: (1) greater availability of medical care so that more women with endometrial cancer are detected, (2) an increase in the number of women who reach the critical age for development of endometrial cancer, (3) a broadening of criteria for the diagnosis of endometrial cancer by the inclusion of severe dysplasia, atypical adenomatous hyperplasia, carcinoma in situ, and so-called well-differentiated endometrial cancers in the cancer registry as adenocarcinoma, and (4) a worldwide increase in endometrial cancer, possibly due to environmental and unknown factors. The increased use of estrogen has been implicated; however, Norway and Czechoslovakia report a 50% to 60% increase in endometrial cancer despite the fact that estrogens are rarely prescribed or are not generally available there. Regardless of the reason for the increased number of women with corpus cancer, this malignancy has become an important factor in the care of the female patient.

EPIDEMIOLOGY

Endometrial cancer may be found during the reproductive and menopausal years. The median age for cancer of the uterine corpus is 61 years, with the largest number of patients noted between the ages of 50 and 59 years. Approximately 5% of patients will have adenocarcinoma before the age of 40, and 20% to 25% will be diagnosed before the menopause.

Multiple risk factors for endometrial cancer have been identified, and Mac-Mahon divides these into three categories: variants of normal anatomy or physiology, frank abnormality or disease, and exposure to external carcinogens. Obesity, nulliparty, and late menopause are all variants of normal anatomy or physiology that are classically associated with endometrial carcinoma. These three factors are evaluated in regard to the possible risk of developing endometrial cancer (Table 5-1). If a patient is nulliparous and obese and reaches menopause at age 52 or later, there appears to be a fivefold increase in the risk of endometrial cancer over the patient who does not satisfy these criteria (Table 5-2).

Diabetes mellitus and hypertension are frequently associated with endometrial cancer. Kaplan and Cole report a relative risk of 2.8 associated with a history of diabetes after controlling for age, body weight, and socioeconomic status. High blood pressure is prevalent in the elderly, obese patient but does not appear to be a significant risk factor by itself, even though 25% of endometrial cancer patients have hypertension or arteriosclerotic heart disease.

Table 5-1. Endometrial cancer risk factors

Risk factors		Risk
Obesity	Overweight	
	21-50 lb	3×
	>50 lb	10×
Nulliparity	Compared with	
	1 child	2×
	5 or more children	3×
Late menopause	Age	
	>52 yr	2.4×

Table 5-2. Multiple risk factors in endometrial cancer

	Risk	
Nulliparous Top 15% in weight Menopause at 52 yr	5× more than	Parous Lower ⅔ in weight Menopause at <49 yr

DIAGNOSIS

The postmenopausal patient with uterine bleeding must be evaluated for endometrial cancer, although only 20% of these patients will have a genital malignancy. As the patient's age increases after the menopause, there is a progressively increasing probability that her uterine bleeding is due to endometrial cancer. Perimenopausal patients may have abnormal uterine bleeding indicative of endometrial cancer but may not be evaluated because the patient or her physician may interpret her new bleeding pattern as due to "menopause." During this time in a woman's life, the menstrual periods should become lighter and lighter and further and further apart. Any other bleeding pattern should be evaluated with carcinoma of the endometrium in mind.

A high index of suspicion must be maintained if the diagnosis of endometrial cancer is to be made in the young patient. Prolonged and heavy menstrual periods as well as intermenstrual spotting may indicate that the cause is cancer, and endometrial sampling is advised. Most of the young patients who develop endometrial cancer are obese and, in many instances, massively overweight, often with anovulatory menstrual cycles. Sequential oral contraceptives have also been incriminated in young patients with endometrial cancer but should no longer be of concern since these agents are no longer commercially available.

Historically, the fractional D&C has been the definitive diagnostic procedure used in ruling out endometrial cancer. In the 1920s, Kelly advocated the use of what amounts to an outpatient curettage in order to obtain adequate endometrial tissue for diagnostic study. Since then, many individuals have advocated the routine use of the endometrial biopsy as an office procedure in order to make a definitive diagnosis and save the patient from hospitalization. Several studies have indicated that the accuracy of the endometrial biopsy in detecting endometrial cancer is approximately 90%. Hofmeister noted that 17% of the endometrial carcinomas diagnosed by routine office biopsy occurred in asymptomatic perimenopausal women. Unfortunately, in his study, where the endometrial biopsy was used, several patients may have been missed, because not all of these individuals had a subsequent D&C. Other procedures have been developed to be used on an outpatient basis not only for diagnosis but also for screening. Those techniques using endometrial cytology to make the diagnosis of endometrial cancer have been less successful than when tissue itself is evaluated.

Cytologic detection of endometrial cancer by routine cervical Pap smear has generally been poor in comparison with its efficacy in diagnosing early cervical disease. Several studies in the literature indicate that only one third to one half of the patients with adenocarcinoma of the endometrium have an abnormal Pap smear on routine cervical screening. The main reason for the poor detection with the cervical Pap smear is that cells are not removed directly from the lesion as they are on the cervix. When a cytologic preparation is obtained directly from the endometrial cavity, malignant cells are present in higher numbers than if routine cervical or vaginal smears are obtained.

Several commercial apparatus are available for sampling the endometrial cavity on an outpatient basis. Those techniques that obtain only a cytologic preparation are generally inadequate if used alone. Devices that remove tissue for histologic evaluation have generally been good if tissue is obtained from the endometrial cavity. In the symptomatic patient in whom inadequate or no tissue is obtained for pathologic evaluation, a D&C must be done. For many years at our institutions, a small curette such as a Duncan or Kevorkian has been used successfully for endometrial biopsies.

The use of multiple diagnostic techniques to increase the capability of outpatient diagnosis appears to be most helpful. The use of cytologic and histologic methods will increase the detection rate of patients with endometrial cancer. If diagnosis of endometrial cancer can be made on an outpatient basis, the patient is saved from hospitalization and a minor surgical procedure. Endocervical curettage at the same time is mandatory, and it rules out cervical involvement and obviates the need for fractional curettage. Any cytologic or histologic abnormality short of invasive cancer mandates a formal fractional curettage to rule out a small focus of invasive disease. All patients with persistent symptoms despite normal cytologic tests and biopsy should submit to fractional curettage as well.

PROGNOSTIC FACTORS

After a tissue diagnosis of endometrial malignancy is established, the patient should have a thorough diagnostic evaluation for the completion of clinical staging before the institution of therapy. The International Federation of Gynecologists and Obstetricians (FIGO) classification for endometrial carcinoma is presented in Table 5-3. Approximately 75% of patients with endometrial cancer present with stage I disease (Table 5-4). Endocervical curettage should be performed in any patient who has not had a fractional curettage. Routine hematologic studies and clotting profiles are obtained on all patients. Presurgical metastatic evaluation should include a chest film, intravenous urogram, and metabolic profiles. Sigmoidoscopy and barium ene-

Table 5-3. FIGO classification of endometrial carcinoma

Stage I	The carcinoma is confined to the corpus	
	Stage IA: The length of the uterine cavity is 8 cm or less	
	Stage IB: The length of the uterine cavity is more than 8 cm	
	Stage I cases should be subgrouped with regard to the histologic type of adenocarcinoma as follows:	
	G1: Highly differentiated adenomatous carcinoma	
	G2: Differentiated adenomatous carcinoma with partly solid areas	
	G3: Predominantly solid or entirely undifferentiated carcinoma	
Stage II	The carcinoma involves the corpus and cervix	
Stage III	The carcinoma extends outside the corpus but not outside the true pelvis (it may involve the vaginal wall or the parametrium but not the bladder or the rectum)	
Stage IV	The carcinoma involves the bladder or rectum or extends outside the pelvis	

Modified from Manual for staging of cancer 1978, Chicago, 1978, American Joint Committee for Cancer Staging and End Results Reporting.

Table 5-4. Distribution of endometrial carcinoma by stage

Stage	Patients (%)
I	10,699 (73.8)
II	1,980 (13.6)
III	1,355 (9.3)
IV	472 (3.3)

From Kottmeier, H., and Kolstad, P., editors: Annual report on the results of treatment in carcinoma of the uterus, vagina, and ovary, vol. 16, Stockholm, 1976, FIGO.

Table 5-5. Prognostic factors in endometrial adenocarcinoma

Histologic differentiation	Myometrial invasion
Uterine size	Peritoneal cytology
Stage of disease	Lymph node metastasis

mas have been reserved for patients who demonstrate palpable disease outside of the uterus or in whom symptoms of bowel disease have been recognized. Brain, liver, and bone scans have been used only in those patients suspected of having extant disease.

Pretreatment evaluation of patients with malignant neoplasms coupled with clinical pathologic experience should allow the physician to individualize therapy for the best results. Multiple factors have been identified for endometrial carcinoma that appear to have significant predictive value for these patients (Table 5-5). FIGO, in developing the recent classification for endometrial cancer, has taken into consideration two factors in the substage category within stage I (Table 5-3). Essentially all reports in the literature agree that differentiation (grade) of the tumor is an important prognostic consideration, but there are differing opinions concerning the predictive value of size of the uterus.

Histologic differentiation

The degree of histologic differentiation of endometrial cancer has long been accepted as one of the most sensitive indicators of prognosis (Fig. 5-1). In his extensive review of this subject, Jones evaluated survival rate in regard to grade from 15 reports in the literature (Table 5-6). As the tumor loses its differentiation, the chance of survival decreases. Grade of tumor also correlates with other factors of prognosis. Table 5-7 shows the relationship between differentiation of the tumor and depth of myometrial invasion as reported by Cheon. As the tumor becomes less differentiated, the chances of deep myometrial involvement increase. One should remember, however, that exceptions can occur; patients with a well-differentiated lesion can have deep myometrial invasion, whereas patients with a poorly differentiated malignancy might have only endometrial or superficial myometrial involvement.

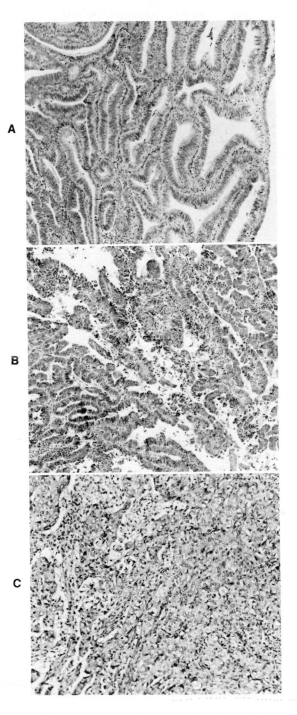

Fig. 5-1. Histologic patterns of differentiation in endometrial carcinoma. **A**, Well differentiated (G1). **B**, Moderately differentiated (G2). **C**, Poorly differentiated (G3). (From McCarty, K. S., Jr., Barton, T. K., Fetter, B. F., and others: Am. J. Pathol. **96:**171, 1979.)

Table 5-6. Relationship between tumor differentiation and 5-year survival rate

Grade	Survival rate
I	1,267/1,558 (81%)
II	1,124/1,515 (74%)
III	462/917 (50%)

Data from Jones, H. W.: Treatment of adenocarcinoma of the endometrium, Obstet. Gynecol. Surv. **30:**147, 1975.

Table 5-7. Correlation of differentiation and myometrial invasion

Myometrial invasion	Grade		
	1	2	3
None	58%	51%	38%
Superficial	30%	28%	16%
Deep	12%	20%	46%

Modified from Cheon, H. K.: Prognosis of endometrial carcinoma, Obstet. Gynecol. **34:**680, 1969.

Uterine size

The size of the uterus as determined by the uterine sound has been incorporated into the substaging as recommended by FIGO. Although most studies that have evaluated this factor in regard to survival agree that those patients with a larger uterine cavity have a poor survival rate, there are some reports that would suggest that uterine size is not a prognostic factor in endometrial cancer. Jones evaluated the relationship between uterine size and survival rate (Table 5-8). It is well recognized that all enlarged uteri are not due to an increasing amount of cancer. Fibromyomas and adenomyosis may contribute to this enlargement. In evaluating the hysterectomy specimens of 100 patients with endometrial cancer, Javert found that the uterus was enlarged in half, but in only eight was cancer the cause.

The pretreatment staging of patients with malignant neoplasia is designed to have prognostic value by determining the size and extent of tumor. Survival rate in regard to stage of disease has been consistent, and Table 5-9 demonstrates the 5-year survival rate as reported by FIGO from the 46 reporting institutions worldwide for the period 1962 to 1968. Prognosis for women with cervical involvement (stage II) is much worse than for earlier lesions. The importance of documentation of endocervical involvement by fractional curettage or endocervical curettage is apparent by the drop in survival rate. Location of the tumor within the endometrial cavity could be significant, since tumors low in the cavity may be expected to involve the cervix earlier than fundal lesions. It would appear that the extent of disease within the endocervix is also of importance. Surwit and associates recently noted that in patients with stromal invasion of the cervix, the survival rate was much lower at 3 years (47%) than in those patients in whom involvement was limited to the endocervical glands or in whom no stroma was present in the endocervical curettage specimen (74%).

Table 5-8. Relationship between uterine size and 5-year survival rate

Uterine size	Survival rate
Normal	1,010/1,183 (84.5%)
Enlarged	385/578 (66.6%)

Data from Jones, H. W.: Treatment of adenocarcinoma of the endometrium, Obstet. Gynecol. Surv. **30:**147, 1975.

Table 5-9. Survival in endometrial cancer—5-year rate

Stage	Patients (%)
I	7,695/10,699 (71.9)
II	984/1,980 (49.7)
III	416/1,355 (30.7)
IV	44/472 (9.3)

From Kottmeier, H., and Kolstad, P., editors: Annual report on the results of treatment in carcinoma of the uterus, vagina, and ovary, vol. 16, Stockholm, 1976, FIGO.

Table 5-10. Relationship between depth of myometrial invasion and 5-year survival rate

Myometrial invasion	Survival rate
None	736/910 (80%)
Superficial	827/971 (85%)
Deep	376/621 (60%)

Data from Jones, H. W.: Treatment of adenocarcinoma of the endometrium, Obstet. Gynecol. Surv. **30:**147, 1975.

Table 5-11. Five-year survival rate in relation to histologic grade and extent

Myometrial invasion	Grade		
	1	2	3 and 4
None	95%	93%	63%
Superficial	92%	72%	50%
Deep	33%	37%	18%

Modified from Ng, A. B., and Reagan, J. W.: Incidence and prognosis of endometrial carcinoma by histologic grade and extent, Obstet. Gynecol. **35:**437, 1970.

Myometrial invasion

The degree of myometrial invasion is a consistent indicator of tumor virulence. The literature as reviewed by Jones demonstrates a decrease in survival rate as myometrial penetration increases (Table 5-10). Lutz and associates determined that the depth of myometrial penetration was not as important as the proximity of the invading tumor to the uterine serosa. Patients whose tumor invaded to within 5 mm of the serosa had a 65% 5-year survival rate, whereas patients whose tumors were more than 10 mm from the serosa had a 97% survival rate at 5 years.

The depth of myometrial invasion is associated with the other prognostic factors, such as the grade of the tumor. As noted by Ng and Reagan (Table 5-11), the 5-year survival rate for patients with a poorly differentiated lesion and deep myometrial invasion is very poor in contrast to the patient who has a well-differentiated lesion but no myometrial invasion. This suggests that virulence of the tumor may vary considerably, and as a result, therapy should depend on the individual prognostic factors.

Peritoneal cytology

The importance of cytologic samples of peritoneal fluids or washings has been recognized as a prognostic and staging factor in pelvic malignancies. Creasman and Rutledge reported positive washings in 12% of corpus cancer patients, although most of the patients with positive washings did have gross metastatic disease outside the uterus. We routinely obtain peritoneal cytologic specimens in all of our patients undergoing surgery for endometrial cancer. Approximately 15% of patients with stage I carcinoma of the endometrium will have malignant cells in their peritoneal cytologic specimen. This finding can occur in a significant number of patients even without gross disease outside the uterus. These latter patients are at risk for developing recurrences in the peritoneal cavity.

Once the peritoneal cavity is opened, an assessment of the amount of peritoneal fluid in the pelvis is made. If none is present, 100 to 125 ml of normal saline solution is injected into the pelvis. This can be done easily with an asepto syringe. The saline solution is admixed in the pelvis and then withdrawn with the syringe. The fluid is sent for cytologic evaluation.

Lymph node metastasis

A total abdominal hysterectomy and bilateral salpingo-oophorectomy have been the hallmarks of therapy for endometrial cancer. As a result, the significant incidence of lymph node metastases has been somewhat disregarded (Fig. 5-2). Although the remote as well as the recent literature has indicated that a significant number of women with endometrial cancer, even stage I, will have lymph node disease, these potential metastatic sites have not been routinely included in the treatment plan. In 1973 Morrow and associates reviewed the recent literature and noted that in a collected series of 369 patients with stage I carcinoma of the endometrium, 39 had metastasis to the pelvic noded area. In 1976 Creasman and associates reported on an

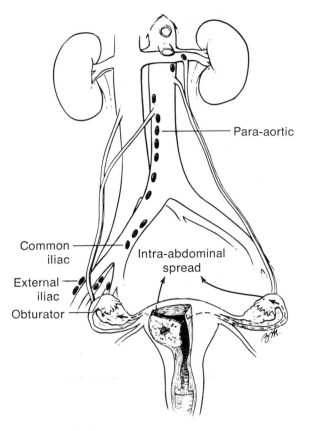

Para-aortic

Common
iliac

Intra-abdominal
spread

External
iliac

Obturator

Fig. 5-2. Spread pattern of endometrial cancer with particular emphasis on potential lymph node spread. Pelvic as well as para-aortic nodes are at risk, even in stage I disease.

Table 5-12. Incidence of pelvic node metastases

	Positive nodes/patients
Stage I	55/509 (10.8%)

Data collected by Morrow and others (1973) from Liu and Meigs (1955), Lefevre (1956), Schwartz and Brunschwig (1957), Roberts (1961), Hawksworth (1964), Rickford (1968), Lees (1969), and Lewis and others (1970); and data from Creasman and others (1976).

additional 140 patients, 16 of whom had positive pelvic nodes (Table 5-12). Therefore, in this relatively large group of patients with clinical stage I carcinoma of the endometrium, almost 11% had metastases to the pelvic lymph node area. In the study by Morrow and associates only 31% of those patients with stage I disease and positive pelvic nodes survived 5 years, and most of these had been treated with postoperative radiation. In the study by Creasman and associates, 102 of the patients

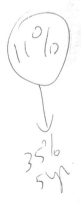

Table 5-13. Stage vs. positive pelvic and aortic nodes

Stage	Pelvic	Aortic
IA	9 (7.5%)	7 (5.8%)
IB	14 (16.0%)	9 (10.3%)

Table 5-14. Grade vs. positive pelvic and aortic nodes

Grade	Pelvic	Aortic
G1	2 (2.2%)	1 (1.1%)
G2	8 (10.1%)	4 (5.0%)
G3	13 (34.2%)	11 (28.9%)

also had the para-aortic fat pad removed for histologic evaluation, and it was found that ten of these patients (9.8%) had metastasis to the para-aortic area.

The occurrence of lymph node metastasis in patients with stage II carcinoma of the endometrium is considerably higher than in patients with stage I disease. Morrow and associates identified 85 patients in whom the pelvic lymph nodes were evaluated, and 31 (36.5%) had disease in the pelvic nodes.

Correlation of multiple prognostic factors

In 1976 Creasman and associates reported a preliminary study of 140 patients concerning the metastatic lymph node potential in adenocarcinoma of the endometrium. This study was undertaken by the gynecologic oncology divisions at the University of Mississippi, the University of Southern California, and the Duke University Medical Center under the aegis of the Gynecologic Oncology Group (GOG). This study continues as a groupwide protocol of the GOG. In an analysis of 206 patients with clinical stage I cancer of the endometrium, 23 patients (11.2%) had metastasis to one or more pelvic lymph nodes. Only 75% of the patients had para-aortic node sampling; however, 16 (10%) of those sampled had disease in the para-aortic area. When the size of the uterus was evaluated in regard to pelvic and para-aortic node metasis, a correlation was present (Table 5-13). When the grade of the tumor was compared to pelvic or para-aortic node metastasis, again an excellent correlation was noted (Table 5-14). Likewise, when the depth of invasion was correlated with nodal metastasis, the chance of having regional node metastasis increased with the depth of myometrial invasion (Table 5-15). When the six substages of stage I carcinoma were evaluated for nodal metastasis, within stage IA as well as IB lesions metastasis again increased as the tumor became less differentiated (Table 5-16). This relationship is also present when the depth of invasion is evaluated within each grade of the tumor in that as the depth of invasion increases within each grade, the chances of nodal metastasis also increase.

Table 5-15. Maximum invasion and node metastasis

Maximum invasion	Pelvic	Aortic
Endometrium only	2 (2.5%)	1 (1.2%)
Superficial muscle	7 (8.4%)	6 (7.2%)
Intermediate muscle	2 (13.3%)	1 (6.6%)
Deep muscle	13 (46.4%)	8 (28.5%)

Table 5-16. Stage and grade vs. pelvic and aortic node metastases

Stage	Pelvic (%)	Aortic (%)
IA, G1	1.7	1.7
IA, G2	9.3	6.9
IA, G3	22.2	16.6
IB, G1	3.2	0.0
IB, G2	11.1	2.7
IB, G3	45.0	40.0

TREATMENT

What is considered optimal therapy in patients with carcinoma of the endometrium, particularly stage I, still remains controversial. According to the last annual report published by FIGO, diverse therapy for patients with stage I endometrial cancer is apparent (Table 5-17). Thomas Cullen, as early as 1900, stated that the treatment of choice in patients with endometrial cancer was abdominal hysterectomy with removal of the adnexa. This remains the mainstay of therapy for this malignancy today. For much of this century, a relatively large number of patients with endometrial cancer were considered inoperable, and as radium and external radiation became available, alternative methods of treatment were developed. Because the surgery has become more applicable to patients who are older or have serious medical illness, the number of inoperable patients with this malignancy has decreased considerably, particularly in recent years. In fact, the previous classification for this malignancy, which included "inoperable" patients, has been changed, and these patients are no longer considered in a separate category.

Since the first part of the twentieth century, when radium became available, it has been evaluated in the treatment of endometrial cancer not only singly but as an adjunct to surgery. In 1916 Kelly reported a large series of patients with uterine cancer who had been treated with radium; however, he believed that surgical treatment was still an important part of the overall therapy. During the ensuing years, many studies have been reported evaluating the role of radium and/or external radiation with or without adjunctive hysterectomy. Heyman, during the 1930s, made an important contribution with his technique of packing the uterus with multiple

Table 5-17. Summary of therapy for stage I

	Patients
Hysterectomy*	4,409 (41.2%)
Preoperative radiation	2,752 (25.7%)
Radiation only	3,534 (33.1%)

From Kottmeier, H., and Kolstad, P., editors: Annual report on the results of treatment in carcinoma of the uterus, vagina, and ovary, vol. 16, Stockholm, 1976, FIGO.
*With or without postoperative radiation.

capsules of radium before hysterectomy. His results showed approximately a 60% 5-year survival rate in stage I carcinoma.

During the 1940s, renewed interest in radical surgery for the treatment of endometrial carcinoma became apparent. Javert was one of the earliest proponents using radical hysterectomy and pelvic lymphadenectomy for this malignancy. He believed that the preoperative radiation added nothing to the surgical procedure. Rutledge, in his excellent review (1974) of the role of radical hysterectomy in adenocarcinoma of the endometrium, concluded that in stage I cancer of the uterus, radical hysterectomy and pelvic lymphadenectomy have a limited role and probably are not indicated. The information from the lymphadenectomy, however, can give considerable insight into the disease process of the individual patient. In those individuals who were treated by radical hysterectomy and pelvic lymphadenectomy and had positive nodes, a poorer survival rate was noted than in those with negative nodes even if preoperative radiation was given.

For the last several decades, considerable interest has been shown in the use of preoperative radiation in the management of endometrial cancer. Several reports were presented indicating that those patients who were treated with preoperative radiation had less histologically defined disease in the uterus at the time of hysterectomy, and these patients did much better than those who had tumor identified in the uterus. Also, reports tend to indicate that those patients treated with preoperative radiation had less vaginal recurrence than if surgery only was done. Considerable data were collected, and in the thorough review article by Jones, in which he extensively reviewed the literature of the 1950s, 60s, and 70s, he noted that the 5-year survival rate for patients treated with surgery only was essentially the same as for those who were treated with radiation plus surgery (Table 5-18). Unfortunately, the vast majority of these reports were not evaluated in regard to the grade of the tumor or myometrial involvement. It is anticipated that many of the patients who were found to have a poorly differentiated lesion were more likely to be treated in the combined group and, as a result, would prejudice the overall survival rate in the combined therapy category. Data are available to suggest that patients treated with postoperative radiation in the form of vaginal radium had as good a 5-year survival rate as those who were treated with preoperative radiation or who had surgery only. As a result, some investigators have suggested that postoperative radiation should

Table 5-18. Comparison of the 5-year survival results with surgery alone and radiation plus surgery in the treatment of endometrial carcinoma

	Surgery only	Combined therapy
Survival rate	1,794/2,392 (75%)	2,886/3,679 (78%)

Data from Jones, H. W.: Treatment of adenocarcinoma of the endometrium, Obstet. Gynecol. Surv. **30:**147, 1975.

be given to those individuals who are found to have poorly differentiated carcinomas or deep myometrial invasion in the uterine specimen.

More recently, a considerable amount of data has been collected to evaluate vaginal recurrence and survival rate in regard to whether surgery alone or combined therapy with mainly preoperative radium or surgery was used. Data have also been evaluated in regard to the grade of the tumor (Table 5-19) and, in some instances, the depth of myometrial involvement (Table 5-20). In those patients who had pre- or postoperative radiation, there did appear to be a lower incidence of vaginal vault recurrences, although there does not appear to be much difference in the grade 1 and 2 lesions. Vaginal vault recurrence did not appear to affect survival. The survival rate was similar in those treated by surgery only in comparison with those treated by radiation plus surgery, particularly in the grade 1 and 2 lesions. Those individuals with poorly differentiated adenocarcinoma treated with combined therapy had a slightly better survival rate, although most studies showed no statistical difference between these patients and those treated with surgery only. In the only prospective randomized study done to date that evaluates the role of external pelvic radiation and radium versus radium alone in addition to surgery in stage I carcinoma of the endometrium, Onsrud and associates noted no difference in survival rate between the two groups of patients. Those patients who received pelvic radiation had an 88% 5-year survival rate, whereas those who did not receive external radiation had a 90% survival rate. When recurrence and survival were evaluated in regard to histologic grade and myometrial involvement, no difference was noted. In those patients who did receive external radiation, there was less recurrence in the pelvis, but a larger number of individuals had distant recurrences. Those who did not receive external radiation had a higher number of recurrences locally in the pelvis.

Most authorities, even those who are advocates of preoperative radiation, agree that in stage I, grade 1 lesions the procedure of choice is total abdominal hysterectomy and bilateral salpingo-oophorectomy alone. If extensive disease is present in the uterus or if metastasis outside the uterus is noted, appropriate radiation, progestins, and/or chemotherapy is given.

There is no agreement on treatment of patients with grade 2 or 3 disease, as noted by the various modalities advocated in the literature. Some authors prefer preoperative radium either by Heyman packing plus vaginal ovoid or by tandem and ovoids if the uterus is small. A total abdominal hysterectomy with bilateral salpingo-oophorectomy is performed 6 weeks later. More recently, Underwood and associates

Table 5-19. Survival rate in stage I carcinoma of the endometrium with regard to grade and treatment

	G1		G2		G3	
	S	S + R	S	S + R	S	S + R
Wharam and associates	80/82	14/14	63/69	60/69	5/9	15/26
Frick and associates	78/88	78/86	7/10	25/36	3/5	9/14
Salazar and associates	10/12	10/11	13/14	38/42	12/17	67/81
TOTAL	168/182	102/111	83/93	123/147	20/31	91/121
	(92.3%)	(91.8%)	(89.2%)	(83.6%)	(64.5%)	(75.2%)

Key: S = surgery, R = radiation therapy.

Table 5-20. Survival rate in stage I carcinoma of the endometrium with regard to depth of invasion and treatment

Residual	Surgery only	Surgery + radiation
No tumor	11/12 (91.6%)	27/28 (96.4%)
Endometrium + inner muscle	69/80 (86.2%)	49/64 (76.5%)
Mid or outer muscle	8/11 (72.7%)	36/44 (81.8%)

Modified from Frick, H. C., Munnell, E. W., Richart, R. M., and others: Carcinoma of endometrium, Am. J. Obstet. Gynecol. **115:**663, 1973.

have recommended that the hysterectomy be done immediately after the radium is removed. If deep myometrial or extant disease is present, external radiation (4,000 to 5,000 rads to the appropriate areas) is given. Underwood and associates have shown that depth of myometrial invasion is best determined by measuring the tumor-free area from serosa inward. If there is less than 5 mm of tumor-free area, they advocate external radiation (4,000 to 5,000 rads to the whole pelvis) during the postoperative period, because these patients will have a high risk for developing recurrence. If there is less than 10 mm of tumor-free area, surgery alone appears adequate. Treatment of patients with 5 to 10 mm of tumor-free area is unresolved at the present time, although recurrence appears to be greater than disease with less than 10 mm of tumor-free area. Because depth of myometrial invasion can be destroyed by radium if the surgery is performed 4 to 6 weeks later, Underwood and associates prefer to do surgery immediately after the radium has been removed.

Many authors suggest that patients with an enlarged uterus or poorly differentiated carcinoma should be treated preoperatively with external radiation (4,000 to 5,000 rads to the whole pelvis) followed by radium and then 6 weeks later a total abdominal hysterectomy and bilateral salpingo-oophorectomy (Fig. 5-3). In grade 3 neoplasias, a significant number of patients will have disease outside the treatment field. Because there can be a significant delay between diagnosis and final surgery, it may be more applicable to do surgery first and then radiation postoperatively.

Small uterus   Uterine tandem (3,000 mg-hr)
                      Vaginal ovoids (7,000 rads surface)

                                    ↓

                      Immediate TAH, BSO

                                    ↓

                      Deep muscle involvement

                                    ↓

                      4,000 rads whole pelvis

Moderately
large uterus,   Heyman packing or tandem (2,500 mg-hr) ⎫ Two times,
G1   Vaginal ovoids (4,000 rads surface)   ⎬ 2-3 weeks apart
                                                              ⎭

                                    ↓

                      Immediate TAH, BSO

Large uterus or
anaplastic tumor   4,000 rads whole pelvis

                                    ↓

                      Heyman packing or tandem (2,500 mg-hr)
                      Vaginal ovoids (4,000 rads surface)

                                    ↓

                      6 weeks later TAH, BSO

Fig. 5-3. Suggested radiotherapy in endometrial cancer. (TAH, total abdominal hysterectomy; BSO, bilateral salpingo-oophorectomy.)

Suggested treatment

Treatment must take into account potential spread patterns (Fig. 5-2), but predictability of spread can be determined to a large degree by evaluation of prognostic factors. It is suggested that radiation therapy for adenocarcinoma of the endometrium should be used primarily in those patients with poor prognostic factors. Therefore, it would seem prudent to evaluate these factors and then apply radiation therapy selectively after surgery. The grade of the tumor can be determined before surgery; however, determination of the depth of myometrial invasion awaits hysterectomy. Some patients with well-differentiated lesions can have deep myometrial involvement, and it appears that in this small group of patients the recurrence rate is higher and the survival rate lower than with a lesion of the same grade but limited invasion.

Prognostic factors and survival data have recently been reviewed in our study, about which only prognostic factors have previously been reported. Preliminary

Table 5-21. Endometrial cancer: grade 1

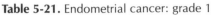

Low lymph node metastasis (2%)
Infrequent deep myometrial invasion (4%)
Low recurrence rate (3%)
Two out of three recurrences had positive washings

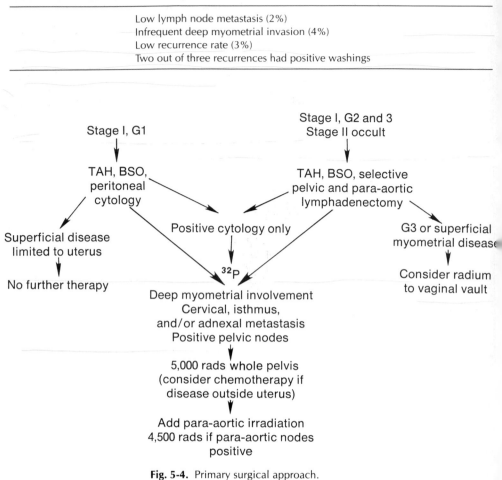

Fig. 5-4. Primary surgical approach.

evaluation of this data would suggest several important factors that would allow therapy to be planned selectively. In grade 1 disease, lymph node metastasis, deep myometrial invasion, and recurrences are infrequent. When malignant peritoneal cytologic findings are detected, recurrence appears high (Table 5-21). In our opinion, the treatment of choice is a total abdominal hysterectomy and bilateral salpingo-oophorectomy without preoperative radiation (Fig. 5-4). Peritoneal cytologic specimens should be obtained immediately on opening of the peritoneal cavity. In most instances, subsequent radiation therapy would not be necessary unless there are malignant cells in the peritoneal washings, adnexal metastases, involvement of the cervix or isthmus, or significant myometrial invasion (Fig. 5-5).

In patients with grade 2 disease, lymph node metastasis, deep myometrial invasion, and recurrences are more frequent. If nodal disease is present, recurrence is

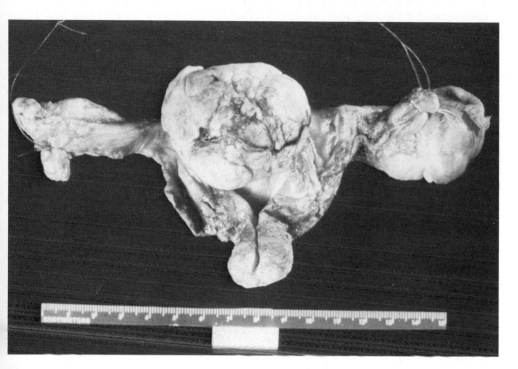

Fig. 5-5. Total abdominal hysterectomy (TAH) and bilateral salpingo-oophorectomy (BSO) showing a large polypoid adenocarcinoma of the endometrium with deep myometrial invasion.

Table 5-22. Endometrial cancer: grade 2

Moderate lymph node metastasis (12%)
Moderate deep myometrial invasion (17%)
Moderate recurrence rate (7%)
Twelve times greater recurrence if there are positive nodes (3% vs. 36%)
Two out of six recurrences had positive washings only

Table 5-23. Endometrial cancer: grade 3

High lymph node metastasis (25%)
Increased deep myometrial invasion (30%)
High recurrence rate (25%)
Fourfold increase in recurrence if there are positive nodes, even with radiation therapy (13% vs. 55%)
A large number of recurrences had positive washings only (27%)

extremely high even when radiation therapy is given (Table 5-22). When grade 3 disease is present, lymph node metastasis, deep myometrial invasion, and recurrences are quite prevalent (Table 5-23). Therefore, in patients with stage I, grade 2 and 3 carcinomas of the endometrium, a total abdominal hysterectomy, bilateral salpingo-oophorectomy, and selective pelvic and para-aortic lymphadenectomy, along with the collection of peritoneal cytologic specimens, should be considered for primary therapy (Fig. 5-4). In both grade 2 and 3 disease, significant lymph node metastasis is possible and, if identified, should be treated appropriately with external radiation. Adjunctive chemotherapy may also be advantageous, because a significant number of these patients with disease outside the uterus will have recurrence even if appropriate radiation therapy is given. Malignant cells present in peritoneal cytologic specimens should be indicative of metastatic disease and treated appropriately. The role of intraperitoneal radioisotopes is being evaluated, but a definite statement concerning their efficacy cannot be made at this time.

The hysterectomy should be extrafascial, and removal of the upper vagina does not appear to decrease vault recurrences. Peritoneal cytologic specimens should be obtained immediately on opening of the peritoneal cavity (see description of the technique earlier in this chapter.) If ascites is present, appropriate samples of fluid should be sent for cytologic evaluation. When selected lymphadenectomy is performed, the retroperitoneal spaces in the pelvis are opened in routine fashion. The vessels are outlined, and any enlarged lymph nodes are removed separately and sent for histologic evaluation. If no enlarged lymph nodes are present, the lymph node-bearing tissue along the external iliacs from the bifurcation to the inguinal ligament is removed. The obturator fossa anterior to the obturator nerve is cleaned of lymphoid tissue. Any enlarged lymph nodes along the common iliacs are also removed. No attempts to dissect behind or between the major vessels are made. The use of Hemovac drains in the retroperitoneal space has decreased the incidence of lymphocysts. The para-aortic node sampling is approached by retracting the small intestine into the upper abdomen and incising the peritoneum over the upper common iliac artery and lower aorta. The main vessels are outlined, and the ureter is retracted laterally. The tissue overlying the vena cava and the aorta is removed en bloc beginning at the bifurcation of the aorta and extending caudad. The upper limit of the dissection (unless enlarged nodes are noted above this area) is usually the second and third portion of the duodenum as it crosses the main vessels retroperitoneally. Hemostasis can usually be accomplished with hemoclips. Using this technique, one should have a total of 15 to 20 lymph nodes available for histologic evaluation.

Patients with stage II carcinoma of the endometrium, because of extension of disease into the endocervix, will have a greater propensity for lymph node metastasis. Therapy should encompass likely metastatic sites and can be performed in several fashions. Primary surgery in the form of radical hysterectomy and pelvic lymphadenectomy would appear to be acceptable therapy, and if positive nodes are present, adjunctive radiation therapy may be added. Others prefer to use external radiation in a dose of 4,000 to 5,000 rads to the whole pelvis with at least one radium application before simple hysterectomy and bilateral salpingo-oophorectomy, which are usually performed 6 weeks after radiation therapy has been completed. A third method of treatment, which we prefer particularly if no visible disease is present on the cervix and no suspicion of parametrial disease exists, is as outlined for those patients with stage I, grade 2 and 3 disease (Fig. 5-4). External radiation in the range of 4,000 to 5,000 rads can then be given postoperatively if disease is limited to the uterus. If metastases are present in the lymph nodes, adjuvant chemotherapy should be considered following radiotherapy.

Treatment of patients with stage III and IV disease must be individualized; however, in most instances hormonal treatment and/or chemotherapy must be used in addition to surgery and radiation therapy.

RECURRENCE

Even though the number of deaths due to endometrial carcinoma is lower than with malignancies of the cervix and the ovary, the mortality is still significant, particularly in view of the number of patients with carcinoma of the uterus seen initially with stage I disease. Some recurrences, particularly those that occur in the vaginal vault, can be treated successfully with either surgery or radiation therapy, or a combination of the two. Many of these patients do extremely well and are long-term survivors. Unfortunately, many of the recurrences are seen outside the confines of the upper vagina and therefore are not amenable to surgery or radiation therapy. Radiation therapy may be of limited value in other patients, particularly if it has been used as part of primary therapy. Therefore, hormonal treatment or chemotherapy may be the treatment of choice in many patients with recurrent carcinoma of the endometrium.

Progestins have been used for over 20 years, and the objective responsiveness of recurrent carcinoma of the endometrium to these hormones has been substantiated. Approximately one third of all patients with recurrent carcinoma of the endometrium will respond to the hormone, although those patients with a well-differentiated tumor have a higher response rate than those with a moderately or poorly differentiated lesion (Table 5-24). More recently, considerable interest has been shown in the presence of specific estrogen-progesterone receptors in neoplastic human uterine tissue (Fig. 5-6). These receptors are definitely present and vary from tumor to tumor. It has been shown that there are a greater number of both estrogen and progesterone receptors in well-differentiated lesions as compared with poorly differentiated ones (Table 5-25). In a small group of patients, it was noted that about one third of those with recurrent cancer had a positive receptor site analysis to both estrogen and progesterone. The receptor data may therefore correlate with clinical findings of responsiveness to progesterones in those patients with recurrent cancer. Preliminary data suggest an excellent correlation (Table 5-26). Obviously, considerable additional data are needed to verify these findings; however, the prospects are excellent. If direct correlation can be substantiated, the receptor site analysis can guide the types of progestin or chemotherapy given for recurrent endometrial can-

Table 5-24. Response to progestins in regard to differentiation of tumor

Tumor grade	Objective response
G1	30/58 (51.7%)
G3	7/45 (15.5%)

Data from Kohorn, E. I.: Gestagens and endometrial carcinoma, Gynecol. Oncol. **4**:398, 1976.

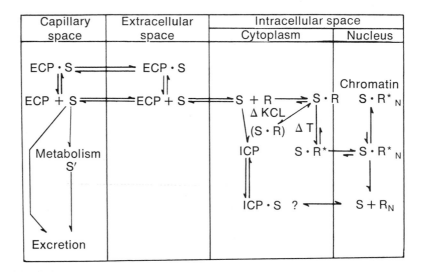

Fig. 5-6. Interrelationship of steroid receptor proteins in the capillary, extracellular, intracellular cytoplasmic, and nuclear spaces. Extracellular proteins (ECP), metabolism (S′), and excretion all influence the availability of steroids (S) for the target cell. Intracellular proteins (ICP) compete for steroid binding with the specific cytoplasmic receptor (R) at many levels. Although the 8S [(S•R)] is an important marker for the identification of the steroid receptor complex, there is no evidence that it is an obligatory intermediate in vivo. The steroid receptor undergoes a critical temperature-dependent (Δ T) modification (S•R) required for its translocation to the nucleus (S•R*$_N$) and binding to chromatin. Little is known concerning the release of the nuclear receptor (R$_N$) or the free steroid. (From McCarty, K. S., Jr., Barton, T. K., Fetter, B. F., and others: Am. J. Pathol. **96**:171, 1979.)

cer. If receptor site analysis is positive for both estrogen and progesterone, the patient's chances of responding to progestins are extremely good even if she has a poorly differentiated lesion. On the other hand, if receptor site analysis is negative, the data would suggest that the patient's response to progestins may be extremely low, making it more advisable to go directly to cytotoxic agents without wasting time on progestin therapy.

Progestin therapy may be administered in several different ways. We prefer Depo-Provera, 400 mg IM at weekly intervals. Oral Provera in the range of 150 mg/ day or Megace, 160 mg/day, are other recommended progestins. Progestins are continued indefinitely if an objective response is obtained. If progression of disease is noted, progestins should be discontinued and chemotherapy considered.

Table 5-25. Correlation of tumor differentiation with receptor content

Differentiation	E_2 and P_R positive
Well	20/34 (83%)
Moderate	14/24 (58%)
Poor	5/16 (31%)

From McCarty, K. S., Jr., Barton, K. W., Fetter, B. F., and others: Correlation of estrogen and progesterone receptors with histologic differentiation in endometrial carcinoma, Am. J. Pathol. **97:**171, 1979.

Table 5-26. Response to progestin therapy in regards to receptor content

Receptor content	Progestin response
Positive	5/5
Negative	1/8

From Creasman, W. T., and others: Clinical correlates of estrogen and progesterone binding protein in human endometrial adenocarcinoma, Obstet. Gynecol. **55:**363, 1980.

Since one third of the patients with recurrent carcinoma of the endometrium responded to progestins and because hormone therapy is essentially nontoxic, evaluations of cytotoxic agents have not been pursued until recently. Recent data would suggest that doxorubicin (Adriamycin) is an effective agent in adenocarcinoma of the endometrium, with approximately a 35% response rate in those individuals not responding to progestins. Combination chemotherapy may be more effective; however, further evaluation must be made. Other active drugs appear to be alkylating agents and 5-fluorouracil.

BIBLIOGRAPHY

Abate, S. D., Edwards, C. L., and Vellias, F.: A comparative study of the endometrial jet-washing technique and endometrial biopsy, Am. J. Clin. Pathol. **58:**118, 1972.

Anderson, B., Marchant, D. J., Munzenrider, J. E., and others: Routine noninvasive hysterography in the evaluation and treatment of endometrial carcinoma, Gynecol. Oncol. **4:**354, 1976.

Antunes, C. M. F., Stolley, P. D., Rosensheim, N. B., and others: Endometrial cancer and estrogen use (report of a large case-control study), N. Engl. J. Med. **300:**9, 1979.

Arneson, A.: Clinical results and histological changes following irradiation treatment of cancer of the corpus uteri, Am. J. Roentgenol. **36:**461, 1936.

Badib, A. O., Vongtama, V., Kurohara, S. S., and Webster, J. H.: Radiotherapy in the treatment of sarcomas of the corpus uteri, Cancer **24:**724, 1969.

Bruchner, H. W., and Deppe, G.: Combination chemotherapy of advanced endometrial adenocarcinoma with Adriamycin, cyclophosphamide, 5-fluorouracil, and medroxyprogesterone acetate, Obstet. Gynecol. **50:**105, 1977.

Butler, E. B., Monahan, P. B., and Warrell, D. W.: Kuper brush in the diagnosis of endometrial lesions, Lancet **2:**1390, 1971.

Cancer statistics, 1979, CA **29:**6, 1979.

Caspi, E., Perpinial, S., and Reif, A.: Incidence of malignancy in Jewish women with postmenopausal bleeding, Isr. J. Med. Sci. **13:**299, 1977.

Chatfield, W. R., and Bremner, A. D.: Intrauterine sponge biopsy, Obstet. Gynecol. **39:**323, 1972.

Cheon, H. K.: Prognosis of endometrial carcinoma, Obstet. Gynecol. **34:**680, 1969.

Cohen, C. J., and Deppe, G.: Endometrial carcinoma and oral contraceptive agents, Obstet. Gynecol. **49:**390, 1977.

Cohen, C. J., Deppe, G., and Bruchner, H. W.: Treatment of advanced adenocarcinoma of the endometrium with melphalan, 5-fluorouracil, and medroxyprogesterone acetate; a preliminary study, Obstet. Gynecol. **50:**415, 1977.

Cohen, C. J., and Gusberg, S. B.: Screening for endometrial cancer, Clin. Obstet. Gynecol. **18:**27, 1975.

Creasman, W. T., Boronow, R. C., Morrow, C. P., and others: Adenocarcinoma of the endometrium; its metastatic lymph node potential; a preliminary report, Gynecol. Oncol. **4:**239, 1976.

Creasman, W. T., McCarty, K. S., Sr., and Mc-Carty, K. S., Jr.: Clinical correlation of estrogen, progesterone binding proteins in human endometrial adenocarcinoma, Obstet. Gynecol. **55:**363, 1980.

Creasman, W. T., and Rutledge, F. N.: The prognostic value of peritoneal cytology in gynecologic malignant disease, Am. J. Obstet. Gynecol. **110:**773, 1971.

Creasman, W. T., and Weed, J. C., Jr.: Screening techniques in endometrial cancer, Cancer **38:**436, 1976.

Cullen, T. H.: Cancer of the uterus, Philadelphia, 1900, W. B. Saunders Co.

Damon, A.: Host factors in cancer of the breast and uterine cervix and corpus, J. Natl. Cancer Inst. **24:**483, 1960.

De Muelenaere, G. F. G. O.: Prognostic factors in endometrial carcinoma, S. Afr. Med. J. **49:**1695, 1975.

Dunn, L. J., and Bradbury, J. T.: Endocrine factors in endometrial carcinoma, Am. J. Obstet. Gynecol. **97:**465, 1967.

Frick, H. C., Munnell, E. W., Richart, R. M., and others: Carcinoma of endometrium, Am. J. Obstet. Gynecol. **115:**663, 1973.

Geisler, H. E.: The use of megestrol acetate in the treatment of advanced malignant lesions of the endometrium, Gynecol. Oncol. **1:**340, 1973.

Gordon, J., Reagan, J. W., Finkle, W. D., and Ziel, H. K.: Estrogen and endometrium carcinoma; an independent pathology review supporting original risk estimate, N. Engl. J. Med. **297:**500, 1977.

Gray, L. A., Christopherson, W. M., and Hoover, R. N.: Estrogens and endometrial carcinoma, Obstet. Gynecol. **49:**385, 1977.

Greenblatt, R. B., and Stoddard, L. B.: The estrogen-cancer controversy, J. Am. Geriatr. Soc. **26:**1, 1978.

Gusberg, S. B., and Kardon, P.: Proliferative endometrial response to thecal granulosa cell tumors, Am. J. Obstet. Gynecol. **3:**633, 1971.

Healy, W., and Brown, R.: Experience with surgical and radiation therapy in carcinoma of the corpus uteri, Am. J. Obstet. Gynecol. **38:**1, 1939.

Heyman, J.: The so-called Stockholm method and the results of treatment of uterine cancer with Radiumhemmet, Acta Radiol. **16:**129, 1935.

Hofmeister, F. J.: Endometrial biopsy; another look, Am. J. Obstet. Gynecol. **118:**733, 1974.

Hoover, R., Everson, R., Fraumeni, J. F., and Myers, M. H.: Cancer of the uterine corpus after hormonal treatment for breast cancer, Lancet **1:**885, 1976.

Horwitz, R. I., and Feinstein, A. F.: Alternative analytic methods for case-control studies of estrogens and endometrial cancer, N. Engl. J. Med. **299:**1090, 1978.

Husslein, H., Brietenecker, G., and Tatra, G.: Premalignant and malignant uterine changes in immunosuppressed renal transplant recipients, Acta Obstet. Gynecol. Scand. **57:**73, 1978.

Javert, C., and Douglas, R.: Treatment of endometrial carcinoma, Am. J. Roentgenol. **75:**580, 1956.

Javert, C. T.: The spread of benign and malignant endometrium in the lymphatic system with a note on co-existing vascular involvement, Am. J. Obstet. Gynecol. **64:**780, 1952.

Johnsson, J. E., and Norman, O.: Relation between prognosis in early carcinoma of the uterine body and hysterographically assessed localization and size of tumor, Gynecol. Oncol. **7:**71, 1979.

Jones, H. W.: Treatment of adenocarcinoma of the endometrium, Obstet. Gynecol. Surv. **30:**147, 1975.

Kademian, M. T., Buehler, D. A., and Wirtanen, G. W.: Bipedal lymphangiography in malignancies of the uterine corpus, Am. J. Roentgenol. **129:**903, 1977.

Kaplan, S. D., and Cole, P.: Epidemiology of cancer of the endometrium, in press.

Kelley, H. W., Miles, P. A., Buster, J. E., and Seragg, W. H.: Adenocarcinoma of the endometrium in women taking sequential oral contraceptives, Obstet. Gynecol. **47:**200, 1972.

Kelly, H.: Radium therapy and cancer of the uterus, Trans. Am. Gynecol. Soc. **41:**532, 1916.

Kelly, R. N., and Baker, W. H.: The effect of 17-alpha-hydroxyprogesterone caproate on metastatic endometrial cancer. In Conference on Experimental and Clinical Cancer Chemotherapy, monograph 9, Bethesda, Md., 1960, National Cancer Institute.

Kennedy, B. J.: Progestins in the treatment of carcinoma of the endometrium, Surg. Gynecol. Obstet. **127:**103, 1968.

Kistner, R. W.: Histologic effects of progestin of hyperplasia and carcinoma in situ of the endometrium, Cancer **12:**116, 1959.

Kistner, R. W.: The effects of progesteronal agents on hyperplasia and carcinoma in situ of the endometrium, Int. J. Gynaecol. Obstet. **8:**561, 1970.

Kohorn, E. I.: Gestagens and endometrial carcinoma, Gynecol. Oncol. **4:**398, 1976.

Kottmeier, H., and Kolstad, P., editors: Annual report on the results of treatment of carcinoma of the uterus, vagina, and ovary, vol. 16, Stockholm, 1976, FIGO.

Lauritzen, C.: Oestrogens and endometrial cancer; a point of view, Clin. Obstet. Gynecol. **4:**145, 1977.

Lees, D.: An evaluation of treatment in carcinoma of the body of the uterus, J. Obstet. Gynaecol. Br. Comm. **76:**615, 1969.

Lefevre, H.: Node dissection in cancer of the endometrium, Surg. Gynecol. Obstet. **102:**649, 1956.

Lewis, B., Stallworthy, J. A., and Cowdell, R.: Adenocarcinoma of the body of the uterus, J. Obstet. Gynaecol. Br. Comm. **77:**343, 1970.

Lutz, M. H., Underwood, P. B., Jr., Kreutner, A., Jr., and Miller, M. C.: Endometrial carcinoma; a new method of classification of therapeutic and prognostic significance, Gynecol. Oncol. **6:**83, 1978.

Mack, T. M., Pike, M. C., Henderson, B. C., and others: Estrogens and endometrial cancer in a retirement community, N. Engl. J. Med. **294:**1262, 1976.

MacMahon, B.: Risk factors for endometrial cancer, Gynecol. Oncol. **2:**122, 1974.

Mahle, A.: The morphological histology of adenocarcinoma of the body of the uterus in relationship to longevity, Surg. Gynecol. Obstet. **36:**385, 1923.

Malkasian, G. D., Decker, D. G., Mussey, E., and Johnson, C. E.: Progestogen treatment of recurrent endometrial carcinoma, Am. J. Obstet. Gynecol. **110:**15, 1971.

Mansell, H., and Hertig, A. T.: Granulosa-theca cell tumor and endometrial carcinoma; a study of their relationship and survey of 80 cases, Obstet. Gynecol. **6:**385, 1955.

Masubuchi, K., and Nemoto, H.: Epidemiologic studies on uterine cancer at Cancer Institute Hospital, Tokyo, Japan, Cancer **30:**268, 1972.

Mattingly, R. F.: Malignant tumors of the uterus. In Mattingly, R. F.: TeLinde's operative gynecology, ed. 5, Philadelphia, 1977, J. B. Lippincott Co.

McCarty, K. S., Jr., Barton, T. K., Peete, C. H., Jr., and Creasman, W. T.: Gonadal dysgenesis with adenocarcinoma of the endometrium; electron microscopic and steroid receptor analyses with a review of the literature, Cancer **42:**510, 1978.

McDonald, T. W., Annegers, J. F., O'Fallon, W. M., and others: Exogenous estrogen and endometrial carcinoma; case-control and incidence study, Am. J. Obstet. Gynecol. **127:**572, 1977.

McDonald, T. W., Malkasian, G. D., and Gaffey, T. A.: Endometrial cancer associated with feminizing ovarian tumors and polycystic ovarian disease, Obstet. Gynecol. **94:**654, 1977.

Milan, A. R., Markley, R. L., Fisher, R. S., and others: Endometrial cytology; using the Milan-Markley technique, Obstet. Gynecol. **48:**111, 1976.

Monson, R. R., MacMahon, B., and Austin, J. H.: Postoperative irradiation and carcinoma of the endometrium, Cancer **31:**630, 1973.

Morrow, C. P., DiSaia, P. J., and Townsend, D. E.: Current management of endometrial carcinoma, Obstet. Gynecol. **42:**399, 1973.

Ng, A. B., and Reagan, J. W.: Incidence and prognosis of endometrial carcinoma by histologic grade and extent, Obstet. Gynecol. **35:**437, 1970.

Ng, A. B., Reagan, J. W., Hawliczek, S., and Wentz, W. B.: Significance of endometrial cells in the detection of endometrial carcinoma and its precursors, Acta Cytol. **18:**356, 1974.

Nolan, J. F., and Huen, A.: Prognosis in endometrial cancer, Gynecol. Oncol. **4:**384, 1976.

Norris, H. J., and Taylor, H. B.: Prognosis of granulosa thecal tumor of the ovary, Cancer **21:**255, 1968.

Novak, E., and Yui, E.: Relationship of endometrial hyperplasia to adenocarcinoma of the endometrium, Am. J. Obstet. Gynecol. **32:**674, 1936.

Onsrud, M., Kolstad, P, and Normann, T.: Postoperative external pelvic irradiation in carcinoma of the corpus stage I; a controlled clinical trial, Gynecol. Oncol. **4:**222, 1976.

Ostor, A. G., Fortune, D. W., Evans, J. H., and Kneale, B. L.: Endometrial carcinoma in gonadal dysgenesis with and without estrogen therapy, Gynecol. Oncol. **6:**316, 1978.

Pacheco, J. C., and Kempers, R. D.: Etiology of postmenopausal bleeding, Obstet. Gynecol. **32:**40, 1968.

Plentyl, A. A., and Friedman, E. A.: Lymphatic system of the female genitalia; the morphologic basis of oncologic diagnosis and therapy, Philadelphia, 1971, W. B. Saunders Co.

Rauramo, L.: Estrogen replacement therapy and endometrial carcinoma, Front. Horm. Res. **5:**117, 1978.

Rozier, J. C., and Underwood, P. B.: Use of progestational agents in endometrial adenocarcinoma, Obstet. Gynecol. **44:**60, 1974.

Rutledge, F., Tan, S., and Fletcher, G.: Vaginal metastases from adenocarcinoma of the corpus uteri, Am. J. Obstet. Gynecol. **75:**157, 1958.

Rutledge, F. N.: The role of radical hysterectomy in adenocarcinoma of the endometrium, Gynecol. Oncol. **2:**331, 1974.

Salazar, O. M., Bonfiglio, T. A., Patten, S. F., and others: Uterine sarcomas; natural history, treatment and prognosis, Cancer **42:**1152, 1978.

Sall, S., Sonnenblick, B., and Stone, M. L.: Factors affecting survival of patients with endometrial adenocarcinoma, Am. J. Obstet. Gynecol. **107:**116, 1970.

Sandstrom, R. E., Welch, W. R., and Green, T. H., Jr.: Adenocarcinoma of the endometrium in pregnancy, Obstet. Gynecol. **53**(3 Suppl.): 73S, 1979.

Schwartz, P. E., Kohorn, E. I., Knowlton, A. H., and Morris, J. Mch.: Routine use of hysterography in endometrium carcinoma and postmenopausal bleeding, Obstet. Gynecol. **45:**378, 1975.

Segaloff, A.: Steroids in carcinogenesis, J. Steroid Biochem. **6:**171, 1975.

Silverberg, E., and Halleb, A.: Cancer statistics, 1971, CA **21:**13, 1971.

Silverberg, S. G., and Makowski, E. L.: Endometrial carcinoma in young women taking oral contraceptive agents, Obstet. Gynecol. **46:**503, 1975.

Smith, D. C., Prentice, R., Thompson, D. J., and Herrmann, W. L.: Association of exogenous estrogen and endometrial carcinoma, N. Engl. J. Med. **293:**1164, 1975.

Steert, H.: Cancer of the endometrium in young women, Surg. Gynecol. Obstet. **88:**332, 1949.

Surwit, E. A., Fowler, W. C., Jr., Rogoff, E. E., and others: Stage II carcinoma of the endometrium, Int. J. Radiat. Oncol. Biol. Phys. **5:**323, 1979.

Szekely, D. R., Weiss, N. S., and Schweid, A.: Incidence of endometrial carcinoma in Kings County, Washington; a standardized histologic review, brief communication, J. Natl. Cancer Inst. **60:**985, 1978.

Tak, W. K., Anderson, B., Vardi, J. R., and others: Myometrial invasion and hysterography in endometrial carcinoma, Obstet. Gynecol. **50:**159, 1977.

Thigpen, J. T., Buchsbaum, H. J., Mangan, C., and Blessing, J. A.: Phase II trial of Adriamycin in treatment of advanced or recurrent endometrial carcinoma, Cancer Treat. Rep. **63:**21, 1979.

Underwood, P. B., Lutz, M. H., Krentner, A., and others: Carcinoma of the endometrium; radiation followed immediately by operation, Am. J. Obstet. Gynecol. **128:**86, 1977.

Weiss, N. S.: Noncontraceptive estrogens and abnormalities of endometrial proliferation, Ann. Intern. Med. **88:**410, 1978.

Wharam, M. D., Phillips, T. L., and Bagshaw, M. A.: The role of radiation therapy in clinical stage I carcinoma of the endometrium, Am. J. Roentgenol. **1:**1081, 1976.

Wolff, J. P., Goldfarb, E., Rumeau-Rouquette, C., and Breart, G.: The value of hysterogram for the prognosis of endometrial cancer, Gynecol. Oncol. **3:**103, 1975.

Wynder, E. L., Escher, G. C., and Mantel, N.: An epidemiological investigation of cancer of the endometrium, Cancer **19:**489, 1966.

Ziel, H. K., and Finkle, W. D.: Increased risk of endometrial carcinoma among users of conjugated estrogens, N. Engl. J. Med. **293:**1167, 1975.

CHAPTER SIX

Sarcoma of the uterus

Classification
Clinical profile
Leiomyosarcoma
Mixed mullerian sarcoma
Endometrial stromal sarcoma
Treatment

Sarcomas of the uterus are rare. This is fortunate since the prognosis is quite poor. The incidence of this tumor comprises only about 3% to 5% of all uterine tumors. These tumors arise primarily from two tissues: (1) endometrial sarcomas from the endometrial glands and stroma and (2) leiomyosarcomas from the uterine muscle itself. Other sarcomas, such as angiosarcoma and fibrosarcoma, arise in supporting tissues and are very rare. As a result, the experience even in a large cancer referral institution is still quite limited. To a certain degree, this has led to a lack of unanimity in regard to certain criteria of diagnosis as well as definitive therapy.

CLASSIFICATION

Ober in 1959 suggested a classification of uterine sarcomas that attempted to develop a categorization of these tumors by their cell type and site of origin. (Table 6-1). The tumors that are pure are composed of one cell type only, whereas those that are mixed are composed of more than one cell type. Homologous tumors contain tissue elements entirely indigenous to the uterus, whereas heterologous are defined as those tumors that contain tissue elements foreign to the uterus. Numerous modifications of this classification have been made for various reasons. The Gynecologic Oncology Group (GOG) has accepted the histologic evaluation noted in Table 6-2. This was done since the vast majority of sarcomas will fall into the four main histo-

Table 6-1. Ober classification of uterine sarcomas

	Homologous	Heterologous
Pure	Stromal sarcoma (endolymphatic stromal myosis) Leiomyosarcoma Angiosarcoma Fibrosarcoma	Rhabdomyosarcoma Chondrosarcoma Osteosarcoma Liposarcoma
Mixed	Carcinosarcoma	Mixed mullerian tumors (mixed mesodermal tumor)

Table 6-2. Classification of uterine sarcomas endorsed by the Gynecologic Oncology Group

Leiomyosarcomas
Endometrial stromal sarcomas
Mixed homologous mullerian sarcomas
(carcinosarcoma)
Mixed heterologous mullerian sarcomas
(mixed mesodermal sarcoma)
Other uterine sarcomas

logic categories and data can be accumulated more rapidly so that definitive statements concerning diagnosis and therapy can be made.

CLINICAL PROFILE

The mean age of patients with a leiomyosarcoma (LMS) is the mid-fifties, 10 years younger than those individuals with mixed mesodermal sarcoma (MMS) and endometrial stromal sarcoma (ESS). An abdominal mass and/or pain is a frequent complaint and finding. A rapidly enlarging uterus is a common entity. Particularly in the premenopausal patient, diagnosis of a myomatous uterus is commonly made preoperatively. In any rapidly enlarging uterus, especially in the postmenopausal patient, sarcomas must be considered (Figs. 6-1 and 6-2). Menorrhagia or perimenopausal bleeding may occur in the younger patient. One must consider sarcomas when the patient presents with vaginal bleeding and a relatively large, friable polypoid mass extending through a dilated cervix into the vagina. This is particularly true in the postmenopausal patient. Associated clinical findings include obesity and hypertension in a third of the patients. A history of prior pelvic irradiation is noted in 5% to 10% of sarcoma patients.

In patients with these symptoms, a histologic evaluation is mandatory. If there is a tumor mass presenting at the cervix, tissue is readily available for biopsy. A large polypoid mass may extend into the endometrial cavity, and the diagnosis can be readily made based on either endometrial biopsy or curettage specimens (Figs. 6-3 and 6-4). The diagnosis is more difficult to make preoperatively in patients with LMS

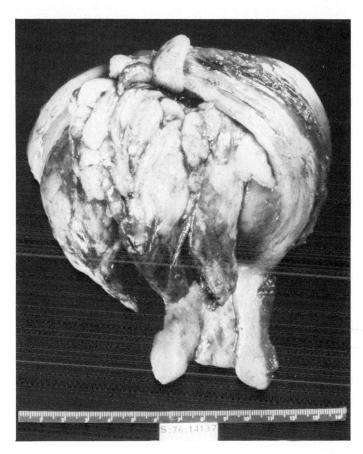

Fig. 6-1. Large uterus with tumor filling the endometrial cavity. (Courtesy Department of Pathology, Duke University Medical Center.)

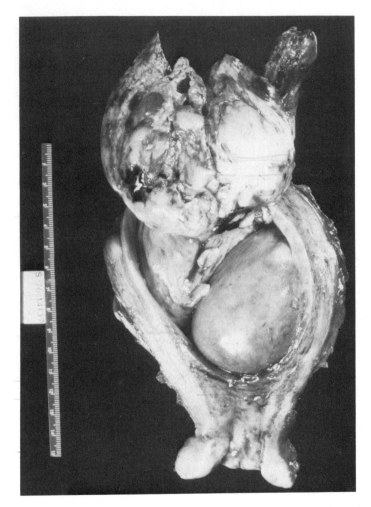

Fig. 6-2. Same uterus as shown in Fig. 6-1 with the polypoid mass pulled out of the endometrial cavity. Significant myometrial involvement is apparent. Sarcoma extended to within 3 mm of the serosal surface. (Courtesy Department of Pathology, Duke University Medical Center.)

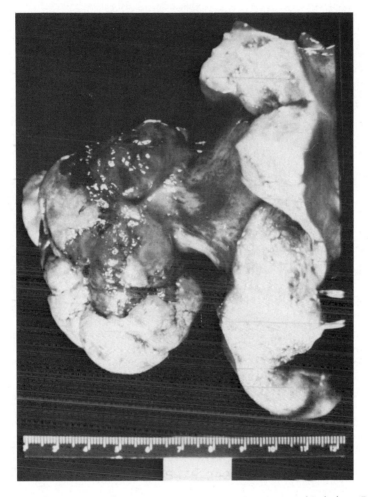

Fig. 6-3. Large polyp that contains a leiomyosarcoma. (Courtesy Department of Pathology, Duke University Medical Center.)

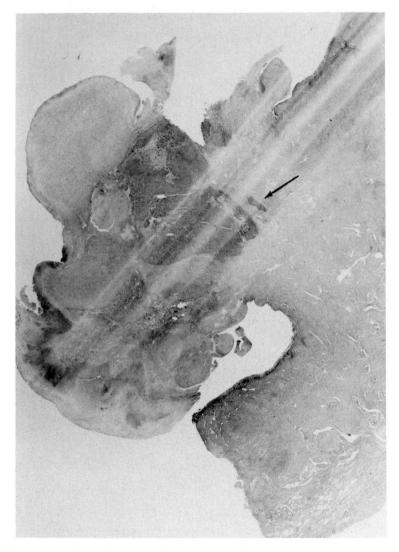

Fig. 6-4. Whole-mount histologic section of tumor presented in Fig. 6-3. Tumor was limited to the polyp. (Courtesy Department of Pathology, Duke University Medical Center.)

because biopsy is difficult and many lesions are incidentally found within a benign myoma. Some authors have reported that a LMS may be present in the submucosa of the uterus in one third of patients, but even at that, biopsy is not easily accomplished. Although advanced disease accounts in part for the poor prognosis of sarcoma, an appreciable number of these patients will have stage I disease (see corpus cancer staging in Table 5-3). As many as 50% of all sarcomas are stage I disease.

LEIOMYOSARCOMA

The older literature would indicate that LMS is the most common sarcoma of the uterus; however, in an evaluation of the recent data from the GOG, the MMS represented about 40% of all cases, whereas LMS was seen in only 16% of 74 patients. Other recent reports have also noted the preponderance of mixed mesodermal lesions. As indicated by its name, LMS may be associated with a myoma of the uterus, and the diagnosis may not be established until the hysterectomy specimen has been evaluated histologically.

There is considerable discussion concerning the histologic criteria necessary for the diagnosis of LMS. The categories of cellular leiomyoma and bizarre leiomyoma add to the confusion of this entity but are considered to be benign. These two entities are distinguished from a true LMS mainly by the mitotic count of the tumor. Although cellular myoma and bizarre leimomyoma may appear at first sight to be malignant, in histologic evaluation they contain less than five mitoses per ten high-power field (HPF), and with surgery only the prognosis is excellent. Taylor and Norris felt that mitotic count was extremely important in that if fewer than ten mitoses per ten HPF were identified, then the lesion was benign regardless of the degree of cellular atypia. If greater than ten mitoses per ten HPF were present, the prognosis was extremely grave. More recently, Norris stated that tumors with less than five mitoses per ten HPF very rarely can metastasize.

Kempson and Bari feel that the mitotic count is important but state that prognosis is poor if greater than five mitoses per ten HPF are identified. Their experience with tumors containing five to nine mitoses per ten HPF indicates that they usually behave aggressively and will metastasize. These authors believe that the degree of cellular atypism is of limited value by itself in determining the malignancy of smooth muscle tumors. In those tumors with higher mitotic counts, there were usually a greater number of markedly atypical cells. This atypia was also seen in those tumors with five to nine mitoses per ten HPF. Tumors with less than five mitoses per ten HPF were thought to be benign regardless of the atypism of the cells. None of Kempson and Bari's patients with zero to four mitoses per ten HPF had disease outside the uterus, whereas distant disease was a common finding if greater than five mitoses per ten HPF were noted.

On the other hand, Silverberg feels that the mitotic count alone cannot be used as a strict histologic criteria because he has had patients with less than ten mitoses per ten HPF who have succumbed to their disease. He believes that the grade of the tumor, which reflects the cytologic atypia, is a better criterion than mitotic count alone. Essentially all investigators emphasized the gravity of the situation if intravascular invasion or disease outside the uterus is found. Silverberg feels that the single most important prognostic indicator is the menopausal status of the patient. Those individuals who are premenopausal when the diagnosis is made tend to have a much better prognosis than those who are postmenopausal, even when criteria such as blood vessel invasion, growth pattern, grade, and mitotic counts are taken into consideration. LMSs occur in younger patients and tend to be more localized when first diagnosed and probably exhibit a slower growth pattern than do MMSs or ESSs.

MIXED MULLERIAN SARCOMA

A better term for mixed mullerian sarcomas may be malignant mixed mullerian tumors. This includes the homologous malignant mixed mullerian tumors and the heterologous malignant mixed mullerian tumors. Carcinoma and sarcoma must both be identified. Tumors should not be placed in the heterologous group unless there is definitive histologic evidence of tissue not normally found in the uterus, such as bone, cartilage, or skeletal muscle.

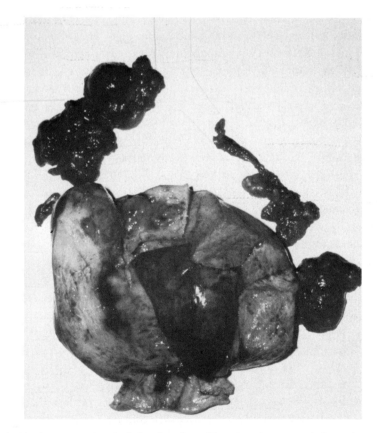

Fig. 6-5. Uterine sarcoma with obviously enlarged lymph nodes, particularly on the right side.

These tumors are aggressive. They spread early to regional lymph nodes and adjacent tissue (Fig. 6-5). In a study by DiSaia and associates from the M. D. Anderson Hospital, 101 patients were evaluated and more than 60% of these patients had disease outside the uterine corpus at the time the diagnosis was originally established. Microscopic invasion of blood vessels and lymphatic channels is frequent. As a result, hematogenous spread, particularly to the lung and liver, is common. An appreciable number of patients may have a uterine polypoid growth pattern, which may be associated with myomas. Tumor hemorrhage and necrosis are common.

If heterologous elements are present and these are rhabdomyoblasts or osteoblasts, the prognosis is very poor according to Kempson and Bari. Their only survivors were patients whose tumor contained chondrosarcoma as the heterologous element. Patients with heterologous elements tended to have more advanced disease both locally and distant than did those with homologous tumors. The survival rate was better in the homologous group, but only when disease was limited superficially in the uterus.

ENDOMETRIAL STROMAL SARCOMA   ESS

Although individual reports have suggested that ESS has a better prognosis than other sarcomas, an analysis of the literature indicates that ESS is just as aggressive and survival rate no better. The endometrial stromal tumors are the rarest of the sarcomas. They are usually considered in two groups: endolymphatic stromal myosis and ESS. The former is an infiltrating stromal lesion that usually follows an indolent course. Endolymphatic stromal myosis is usually considered a low-grade stromal sarcoma. This lesion can have an infiltrating growth pattern, and on cut surface, tissue can project out in a wormlike fashion. These wormlike projections may be found in the blood vessels of the broad ligament. Microscopically, there is little or no cellular atypia and very few, if any, mitoses. Although metastasis can occur, the clinical course is usually indolent, and surgery only is usually adequate treatment. Endolymphatic stromal myosis may recur but does so after a long interval. On the other hand, ESSs infiltrate the myometrium to a greater degree and have a more aggressive course with frequent metastasis and poor prognosis. Since these two lesions are similar, differentiation is important. Norris and Taylor separated the two tumors by the number of mitoses per ten HPF. They feel that those tumors with ten or more mitoses per ten HPF should be categorized as ESS and those with fewer mitoses as endolymphatic stromal myosis. Kempson and Bari in a review of their material noted that ten tumors contained more than 20 mitoses per ten HPF and nine of the ten patients died of their disease. Seven patients had tumors that contained five or fewer mitoses per ten HPF, and none have developed a recurrence. No tumors were seen with mitotic counts between six and 20 per ten HPF. Pleomorphism was present in both groups of patients. Both tumors are composed of stromal cells with a slight amount of cytoplasm. They infiltrate and separate the muscle fibers of the uterus. Tumor is found frequently within lymphatic spaces.

TREATMENT

Total abdominal hysterectomy and bilateral salpingo-oophorectomy have been considered to be the hallmark of therapy in uterine sarcomas. Some authorities have advocated the addition of bilateral pelvic lymphadenectomy, especially in the low-grade lesions, since local pelvic spread is common and the value of adjuvant therapy is in doubt or untested. The use of radiation either given preoperatively as intracavitary and/or external irradiation or given postoperatively with external irradiation and/or vaginal radium has been advocated by many centers. Some authors including radiotherapists are now questioning the efficacy of adjunctive radiotherapy. True, there are patients who have received preoperative radiation and have no residual sarcoma present in the uterine specimen; however, the spread pattern and sites of recurrences detract from the possible benefits of radiation therapy.

When radiation therapy is given, 5,000 to 6,000 rads to the pelvis have been advocated. Preoperative intracavitary radium is given in a dose of about 5,000 mg-hr. Postoperative radium has been given to deliver 4,000 rads to the vaginal surface. If surgery is not anticipated, the amount of radiation, particularly brachytherapy, has been increased. Perez and associates noted fewer central recurrences if the amount of external radiation was 5,000 rads or greater, although the difference was not statistically significant.

Results of therapy unless analyzed critically may leave one with erroneous conclusions. Patients with MMS have a poorer survival rate than patients with LMS or stromal sarcomas (Table 6-3). However, when cell type is compared stage for stage, no difference in survival rate is noted (Table 6-4). Patients with LMS tend to have an earlier stage of disease than do those with MMS. Some data would suggest that those patients treated with radiation therapy plus surgery have a better survival rate than do those treated with surgery alone. Unfortunately, a randomized prospective study has not been done to answer this question. Collected data would, however, allow us to draw some conclusions. Salazar and associates, in presenting their material as well as a review of the literature of over 900 patients, noted that in stage I disease there is no statistically significant difference between surgery alone and surgery plus irradiation in LMS, MMS, or ESS. This is also true of patients with more advanced disease. Those patients who were treated with radiation therapy alone did considerably worse than those treated with surgery alone or surgery plus irradiation (Table 6-5).

What then is the possible role of radiation therapy in the management of uterine sarcomas? It would appear that those patients who were treated with radiation did have a greater degree of local (pelvic) tumor control than did those patients treated with surgery only. This factor unfortunately was not reflected in an increased survival rate. In those patients treated with radiation alone, recurrences occurred in the vast majority, indicating that radiation therapy did not control these tumors.

Site and time of recurrence are important in our treatment consideration. In a pilot study, the GOG evaluated the surgical pathologic spread patterns of sarcomas of the uterus. In those patients with disease limited to the uterus, a significant num-

Table 6-3. Uterine sarcomas: survival rate in terms of pathology*

	Survival rate	
Cell type†	2 years	5 years
MMS	29%	22%
LMS	56%	38%
ESS	38%	39%

Modified from Salazar, O. M., Bonfiglio, T. A., Patten, S. F., and others: Uterine sarcomas; natural history, treatment and prognosis, Cancer **42:**1152, 1978.
*Based on 525 patients available for analysis at 2 years and 871 patients available for analysis at 5 years.
†MS = mixed mesodermal sarcoma, LMS = leiomyosarcoma, ESS = endometrial stromal sarcoma.

Table 6-4. Uterine sarcomas: survival rate in terms of stage and pathology*

	5-year survival rate	
Cell type†	Stage I	Stage II-IV
MMS	50%	12%
LMS	56%	7%
ESS	55%	12%

Modified from Salazar, O. M., Bonfiglio, T. A., Patten, S. F., and others: Uterine sarcomas; natural history, treatment and prognosis, Cancer **42:**1152, 1978.
*Based on 208 patients available for analysis in stage I and 187 patients in stage II-IV.
†MMS = mixed mesodermal sarcoma, LMS = leiomyosarcoma, ESS = endometrial stromal sarcoma.

Table 6-5. Uterine sarcomas: survival rate in terms of stage, treatment, and pathology*

Stage	Cell type†(N)	5-year survival rate‡		
		S	S + R	R
I	MMS (63)	52%	48%	29%
	LMS (55)	58%	75%	33%
	ESS (24)	47%	88%	50%
II-IV	MMS (48)	5%	16%	0%
	LMS (33)	0%	13%	0%
	ESS (18)	0%	33%	0%

Modified from Salazar, O. M., Bonfiglio, T. A., Patten, S. F., and others: Uterine sarcomas; natural history, treatment and prognosis, Cancer **42:**1152, 1978.
*Based on 142 patients with stage I disease (62% treated with S only, 30% treated with S + R, and 8% treated with R only) and 99 patients with stage II-IV disease (33% treated with S only, 46% treated with S + R, and 21% treated with R only).
†MMS = mixed mesodermal sarcoma, LMS = leiomyosarcoma, ESS = endometrial stromal sarcoma.
‡S = surgery, S + R = surgery + radiation, R = radiation.

Table 6-6. Uterine sarcomas: failure sites

	Failure sites		
Cell type* (N)	Pelvis	Pelvis + distant	Distant
LMS (81)	14%	60%	26%
MMS (97)	13%	54%	39%
ESS (37)	14%	51%	35%

Modified from Salazar, O. M., Bonfiglio, T. A., Patten, S. F., and others: Uterine sarcomas; natural history, treatment and prognosis, Cancer **42:**1152, 1978.
*LMS = leiomyosarcoma, MMS = mixed mullerian sarcoma, ESS = endometrial stromal sarcoma.

ber (16%) were found to have metastasis to the regional lymph nodes. As in endometrial cancer, it was noted that survival was related to this factor as well as to the depth of myometrial invasion and whether the lower uterine segment or cervix was involved. It would also appear that patients with malignant cells in the peritoneal cytologic specimen also have an extremely poor prognosis and must be considered the same as the individual who has extant disease outside the uterus. The failure rate is considerably higher in MMS and ESS than in LMS, but this is probably related to initial earlier stage disease in LMS. The average failure time is considerably shorter in those patients with MSS and ESS than with LMS. In fact, LMS may have a very long tumor-free interval. Unfortunately, when recurrence appears, isolated pelvic occurrence is very rare. In the study by Salazar and associates, only 4% of the recurrences were confined to the pelvis. Their collection of data from the literature indicated the prevalence of distant metastasis (Table 6-6). Since the main failure site is distant from the pelvis, the use of adjunctive local radiation is ineffective in increasing the overall survival rate.

We prefer to treat sarcomas primarily by surgery. A peritoneal cytologic specimen is obtained immediately on opening of the peritoneal cavity. A total abdominal hysterectomy and bilateral salpingo-oophorectomy are performed if possible. Selective pelvic and para-aortic lymphadenectomy is performed as described in Chapter 5. Postoperatively, adjunctive chemotherapy in the form of doxorubicin (Adriamycin) is given.

Adjunctive therapy

Since there is such a poor survival rate with standard therapy, chemotherapy has been evaluated in an adjuvant setting. The use of vincristine, actinomycin D, and cytoxan has been recommended by some investigators not only in the adjuvant setting but also in the treatment of recurrent disease. Other investigators are questioning whether this regimen is of benefit. More recently, the use of Adriamycin in those patients with recurrent disease has proved to be beneficial. In 51 patients with recurrent sarcoma, Omura and Blessing, reporting the GOG experience, noted a 27% response (complete and partial) to Adriamycin. The addition of DTIC did not increase response. Adriamycin appears to be the most important drug in the treatment of sarcomas of the uterus today, and other drugs are being tested in combination with it. The GOG is currently evaluating the role of adjunctive Adriamycin in patients who have had hysterectomy for early stage disease. Definitive statements concerning its efficacy cannot be made at this time.

Lehrner and associates have reported a complete response in a patient with metastatic (spinal cord, femur, and lung) ESS with surgery, radiation, and chemotherapy using Adriamycin, vincristine, cyclophosphamide, and megestrol acetate. Further evaluation of chemotherapy in this high-risk group of patients must be made.

BIBLIOGRAPHY

Badib, A. O., Vongtama, V., Kurohara, S. S., and Webster, J. H.: Radiotherapy in the treatment of sarcomas of the corpus uteri, Cancer **2**:724, 1969.

Baggish, M. S.: Mesenchymal tumors of the uterus, Clin. Obstet. Gynecol. **17**:51, 1974.

Burns, B., Curry, R. H., and Bell, M. E. A.: Morphologic features of prognostic significance in uterine smooth muscle tumors; a review of 84 cases, Am. J. Obstet. Gynecol. **135**:109, 1979.

Christopherson, W. M., Williamson, E. O., and Gray, L. A.: Leiomyosarcomas of the uterus, Cancer **29**:1512, 1972.

DiSaia, P. J., Castro, J. R., and Rutledge, F. N.: Mixed mesodermal sarcoma of the uterus, Am. J. Roentgenol. **117**:632, 1973.

DiSaia, P. J., Morrow, C. P., Boronow, R., and others: Endometrial sarcoma; lymphatic spread pattern, Am. J. Obstet. Gynecol. **130**:104, 1978.

Gilbert, H. A., Kagan, A. R., Lagasse, L., and others: The value of radiation therapy in uterine sarcoma, Obstet. Gynecol. **45**:84, 1975.

Kempson, R. L., and Bari, W.: Uterine sarcomas; classification, diagnosis, and prognosis, Hum. Pathol. **1**:331, 1970.

Lehrner, L. M., Miles, P. A., and Enck, R. E.: Complete remission of widely metastatic endometrial stromal sarcoma following combination chemotherapy, Cancer **43**:1189, 1979.

Norris, H. J., and Taylor, H. B.: Mesenchymal tumors of the uterus. I. A clinical and pathological study of 53 endometrial stromal tumors, Cancer **19**:755, 1966.

Ober, W. B.: Uterine sarcomas; histogenesis and taxonomy, Ann. N.Y. Acad. Sci. **75**:568, 1959.

Omura, G. A., and Blessing, J. A.: Chemotherapy of stage III, IV, and recurrent uterine sarcomas; a randomized trial of Adriamycin versus Adriamycin + DTIC, AACR Abstract No. 103, Proceedings of AACR/ASCO, April 1978.

Perez, C. A., Askin, F., Baglan, R. J., and others: Effects of irradiation on mixed mullerian tumors of the uterus, Cancer **43**:1274, 1979.

Saksela, E., Lampinen, V., and Procopé, B.: Malignant mesenchymal tumors of the uterine corpus, Am. J. Obstet. Gynecol. **120**:452, 1974.

Salazar, O. M., Bonfiglio, T. A., Patten, S. F., and others: Uterine sarcomas, analysis of failures with special emphasis on the use of adjuvant radiation therapy, Cancer **42**:1161, 1978.

Salazar, O. M., Bonfiglio, T. A., Patten, S. F., and others: Uterine sarcomas; natural history, treatment and prognosis, Cancer **42**:1152, 1978.

Silverberg, S. G.: Leiomyosarcoma of the uterus, Obstet. Gynecol. **38**:613, 1971.

Taylor, H. B., and Norris, H. J.: Mesenchymal tumors of the uterus. IV. Diagnosis and prognosis of leiomyosarcomas, Arch. Pathol. **82**:40, 1966.

White, T. H., Glover, J. S., Peete, C. H., Jr., and Parker, R. T.: A 34-year clinical study of uterine sarcoma, including experience with chemotherapy, Obstet. Gynecol. **25**:657, 1965.

CHAPTER SEVEN

Gestational trophoblastic neoplasia

Hydatidiform mole
Gestational trophoblastic neoplasia
    Diagnosis and evaluation
    Nonmetastatic trophoblastic disease
    Good prognosis metastatic trophoblastic neoplasia
    Poor prognosis metastatic trophoblastic neoplasia
    Recurrence

The antecedent of gestational trophoblastic neoplasia has been known since antiquity. Hippocrates, 4 centuries before the birth of Christ, described the hydatidiform mole as dropsy of the uterus and attributed it to unhealthy water. In the thirteenth century, the tombstone of Countess Henneberg noted that at 40 years of age she had delivered 365 children, half of which were christened John and half Elizabeth. William Smellie, in 1700, was the first to use the terms "hydatidid" and "mole." In the early nineteenth century, Velpeau and Boivin recognized the hydatidiform mole as cystic dilatation of the chorionic villi. In 1895, Felix Marchand demonstrated that the hydatidiform mole, and less commonly a normal pregnancy or abortion, preceded the development of choriocarcinoma. He described proliferation of the syncytium and the cytotrophoblast of the villi in molar pregnancies. In the early part of the twentieth century Fels, Ehrhart, Roessler, and Zondek demonstrated that an excess of chorionic gonadotrophic hormones could be identified in the urine of patients with a hydatidiform mole.

Gestational trophoblastic neoplasia (GTN) is the term that is now commonly applied to choriocarcinoma and related tumors. It appeared to be more appropriate because it is indicative of the spectrum of trophoblastic diseases (hydatidiform mole, invasive mole, and choriocarcinoma). Before the mid-1950s, the prognosis of these diseases, particularly the end stage (choriocarcinoma), was very dismal. Even though

166

Hertz in the late 1940s had demonstrated that fetal tissues require a large amount of folic acid and could be inhibited by the antifolic compound methotrexate, it was not until 1956 that Li and associates reported the first complete and sustained remission of a patient with metastatic choriocarcinoma by using methotrexate. Since then, a considerable amount of knowledge and experience has been obtained, and GTN is recognized today as the most curable gynecologic malignancy. Several reasons are apparent for this change of events: (1) a sensitive marker is produced by the tumor— human chorionic gonadotrophins (hCG)—and the amount of hormone present is directly related to the number of viable tumor cells; (2) this malignancy is extremely sensitive to various chemotherapeutic agents; (3) one can identify high-risk factors in this disease process and thereby individualize treatment; and (4) the aggressive use of multiple modalities is possible, such as single or multiple agent chemotherapy regimens, radiation, and surgery.

HYDATIDIFORM MOLE

In the United States, the hydatidiform mole occurs in one out of 1,200 pregnancies. In other areas of the world this entity occurs much more frequently, particularly the Far East, where it is reported in as many as one out of 120 pregnancies. Spontaneous remission is common in 80% to 85% of all patients with a hydatidiform mole. Molar pregnancies tend to occur in older patients and are seen infrequently in teenagers. There appears to be no difference in parity among patients with molar pregnancies compared with normal pregnancies. Age and parity do not appear to affect the clinical outcome of an individual with a hydatidiform mole. Gestational age at the time of diagnosis of the hydatidiform mole does not appear to influence subsequent sequelae.

Symptoms

Essentially all patients with hydatidiform mole have delayed menses for varying periods, and most patients are considered to be pregnant. Vaginal bleeding occurs in essentially all patients, usually during the first trimester. The bleeding may be a dark brown discharge or bright red in quantities sufficient to lead to anemia requiring blood transfusion. Nausea and vomiting are reported to occur in almost one third of patients with hydatidiform mole, although Curry and associates, in a report on a large number of patients with hydatidiform mole, noted only 14% of 347 patients with this symptom. This symptom, of course, can be confused with nausea and vomiting accompanying a normal pregnancy. Preeclampsia occurring in the first trimester of pregnancy has been said to be almost pathognomonic of a hydatidiform mole, although this occurred in only 12% of the patients in the study by Curry and associates. Hypothyroidism occurs rarely but when present can precipitate a medical emergency. Laboratory manifestations of hyperthyroidism can occur in as many as 10% of patients; however, clinical manifestations occurred in less than 1% of Curry and associates' patients. Hyperthyroidism in molar pregnancy is due to the production of thyrotrophin by molar tissue. Clinical manifestations of hyperthyroidism dis-

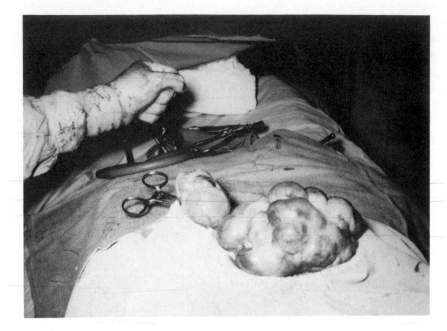

Fig. 7-1. Thecal luteal cysts that are markedly enlarged. The cysts are due to the increased hCG production from the molar pregnancy. Thecal luteal cysts will resolve spontaneously as the hCG titer drops.

appear once the molar pregnancy is treated. Antithyroid therapy may be indicated for a short period.

Classically, a patient with a hydatidiform mole is said to have a uterine size excessive for gestational age, and this is found in about 50% of patients with a mole; however, approximately one third of patients will have a uterus that is smaller than expected for gestational age. Thecal luteal cysts of the ovary may be quite large and are due to the excessive hCG produced by the molar pregnancy (Fig. 7-1). About 15% of patients with an intact molar pregnancy will have enlarged thecal luteal cysts. Patients with an associated thecal luteal cyst appear to have a higher incidence of developing malignant sequelae of trophoblastic disease. The combination of enlarged ovaries and large for gestational age uteri has an extremely high risk for malignant sequelae of trophoblastic disease and required subsequent therapy (57%).

Diagnosis

In many patients with a hydatidiform mole the first evidence to suggest this entity is the passage of vesicular tissue (Fig. 7-2). Several techniques are available to substantiate diagnosis of a mole when pathologic material is not available for analysis. A quantitative pregnancy test of greater than 1,000,000 IU/L along with an enlarged uterus and vaginal bleeding would suggest a diagnosis of hydatidiform mole. A single hCG determination, however, is not diagnostic. Occasionally a single high hCG titer may be seen with a normal single or multiple pregnancy and should not be

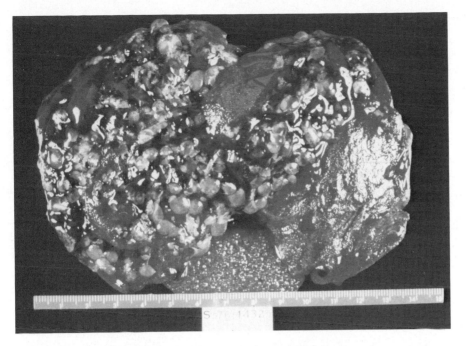

Fig. 7-2. Typical enlarged cystic villi are apparent in this molar pregnancy. (Courtesy Department of Pathology, Duke University Medical Center.)

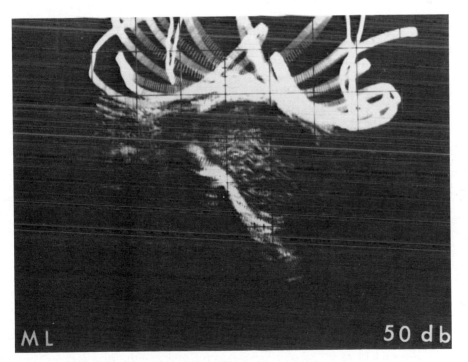

Fig. 7-3. Gray scale ultrasound of a patient with a hydatidiform mole. The echo pattern, or "snowflake" effect, is typical of a molar pregnancy. (Courtesy A. F. Haney, M.D., Durham, North Carolina.)

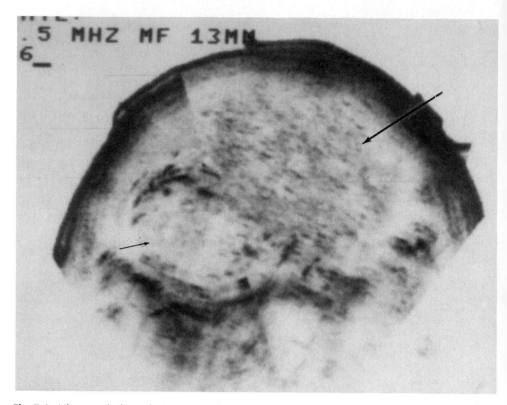

Fig. 7-4. Ultrasound of a molar pregnancy (large arrow) coexistent with a fetus (small arrow). (Courtesy Julius Butler, M.D., Minneapolis, Minnesota.)

used as the determining factor in making a diagnosis of hydatidiform mole. Conversely, a "normal" hCG titer for an anticipated gestational age can be seen with a mole.

Amniography can be used to make a definitive diagnosis of a hydatidiform mole. The uterus should be at least 14 weeks in size. A needle is inserted percutaneously into the uterus, and radiopaque dye is injected into the uterine cavity. Very little, if any, amniotic fluid is obtained on aspiration of the uterine cavity. An x-ray film demonstrating the characteristic honeycomb pattern substantiates the diagnosis of a mole.

In a smaller uterus or if an equivocal amniogram is present, ultrasonography is available and can be very specific for differentiating between a normal pregnancy and a hydatidiform mole. In a molar pregnancy, the characteristic ultrasound notes multiple echoes, which are formed by the interface between the molar villi and the surrounding tissue without the normal gestational sac or fetus present (Fig. 7-3). With the newer and more refined ultrasonic techniques, the diagnosis of a molar pregnancy can be substantiated in essentially all of these types of pregnancies. In rare instances, a fetus may be coexistent with a mole (Figs. 7-4 and 7-5).

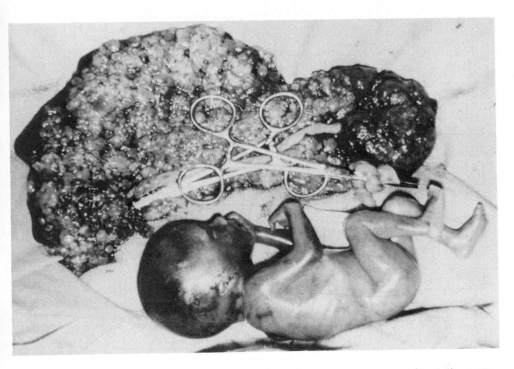

Fig. 7-5. Molar pregnancy and fetus as noted on ultrasound in Fig. 7-4. (Courtesy Julius Butler, M.D., Minneapolis, Minnesota.)

Evacuation

Several techniques have been used in the past to evacuate a molar pregnancy. These have included a D&C (routine and suction), hysterotomy, hysterectomy, and various induction techniques. Before the use of suction curettage, hysterotomy was frequently used on those uteri that were greater than 12 to 14 weeks in size. At the present time, suction curettage is the method of choice for evacuation of a mole, and the role of hysterotomy is extremely limited unless major hemorrhage is present. Suction curettage can be carried out even when the uterus is larger than 20 weeks in size. Blood loss has been moderate. We recommend that all patients with molar pregnancy have evacuation carried out by suction D&C, with a laparotomy set-up available for those individuals with a large uterus. After a moderate amount of the tissue has been removed, intravenous oxytocin (Pitocin) is begun. When the suction curettage has been completed and involution has begun to occur, a sharp curettement is then performed, and this tissue is submitted separately for pathologic evaluation.

A primary hysterectomy may be selected as the method for evacuation if the patient is not desirous of future pregnancies. If at the time of hysterectomy thecal luteal cysts are encountered, the ovaries should be left in situ since these will regress to normal as the hCG diminishes to a normal level. One must remember that even if hysterectomy is used as the method of evacuation, these patients must be followed in the same manner as if other evacuation techniques had been used.

Follow-up of molar pregnancy

Since hCG is produced by molar pregnancies and is a very sensitive marker of trophoblastic cells present in the body, the patient who has had a mole evacuated must be followed very closely by this parameter. This can be done *only* with a sensitive bioassay or radioimmunoassay. Pregnancy tests using either biologic or immulogic materials are inadequate. These tests require a urinary hCG concentration of at least 500 to 1,000 IU/L of urine to give a positive test. As many as 25% of patients with GTN have been found to have urinary hCG concentrations that are elevated but less than the value that can be detected by the urinary pregnancy test. Therefore, a negative pregnancy test in the postmole patient is of no value, and these patients *must* be followed with the radioimmunoassay for hCG.

After evacuation, the patient should have serial radioimmune beta-hCG determinations at 1- to 2-week intervals until there are two normal determinations. This would indicate a spontaneous remission and should occur in approximately 80% of the patients. The hCG titer should then be repeated bimonthly for at least 1 year. It is imperative that the patient use some type of contraception during this year, since a subsequent normal pregnancy cannot be differentiated from GTN by the hCG determination. Unless otherwise contraindicated, oral contraceptives may be used. Regular pelvic examinations should be performed at 2-week intervals until the hCG titers return to normal levels. During the first year, repeat examinations at 3-month intervals should be performed. A chest film is recommended at 2- to 4-week intervals until spontaneous remission and then at 6-month intervals for 1 year (Table 7-1). In the patient who has gone into spontaneous remission with negative titers, examinations, and chest films for 1 year and who is desirous of further pregnancies, contraceptives can now be stopped. Molar pregnancies occur in only about 1% of subsequent pregnancies, and many patients with a history of molar pregnancy have subsequently had normal gestations without difficulty.

Table 7-1. Management of hydatidiform mole

1. hCG determination (radioimmunoassay or bioassay) every 1-2 weeks until negative 2 times
   a. Then bimonthly for 1 year
   b. Contraception for 1 year
2. Physical exam including pelvic every 2 weeks until remission
   a. Then every 3 months for 1 year
3. Chest film every 2-4 weeks until remission
   a. Then every 6 months for 1 year
4. Chemotherapy started immediately if:
   a. hCG titer rises or plateaus during follow-up
   b. Metastases are detected at any time

If the hCG titer plateaus or rises during the observation period, this is indicative of persistent or recurrent GTN, and the patient must be evaluated and started on chemotherapy. Any obvious metastases found on clinical examination or chest film also dictate the immediate use of chemotherapy. Some investigators have previously suggested that if the hCG titers are not within the normal range by 60 days after evacuation of the mole, then chemotherapy should be started. Subsequent data would indicate that those patients with a dropping hCG titer, even though not negative after 60 days, may continue to be followed. As long as there is not a plateauing or rising hCG titer, chemotherapy is not indicated at 60 days.

Prophylactic chemotherapy

Goldstein and associates have suggested that actinomycin D can decrease the possibility of a patient with a hydatidiform mole developing subsequent malignancy. Since 80% of the patients with molar pregnancy will go into a spontaneous remission and not require any therapy, it does not seem appropriate to treat all patients. This is particularly true since serial sensitive hCG determinations can identify the 20% who will develop malignant sequelae. The toxicity from prophylactic chemotherapy may be severe, and deaths have been noted in patients receiving prophylactic chemotherapy.

GESTATIONAL TROPHOBLASTIC NEOPLASIA

The hydatidiform mole precedes malignant trophoblastic disease in approximately 50% of patients. There is an antecedent normal pregnancy in 25% of patients and an abortion or ectopic pregnancy in the other 25%. There may or may not be persistent uterine bleeding after the antecedent pregnancy. If the malignant trophoblastic neoplasia appears within a relatively short time after pregnancy, then the index of suspicion is relatively high. Unfortunately, in many instances the preceding pregnancy occurred years before, and malignant gestational trophoblastic neoplasia is usually not considered in the differential diagnosis. Essentially all types of symptoms have been described in patients with this disease entity. Lesions have been noted in the lower genital tract, and unfortunately many of these lesions when biopsied have been reported as "anaplastic malignant disease." Metastatic disease can be found in the gastrointestinal tract and the genitourinary system as well as in the liver, lung, and brain. Patients have had thoracotomies and craniotomies performed for diagnostic purposes, and only when the histologic evaluation suggested trophoblastic neoplasia were diagnostic hCG determinations obtained. Here again, a high index of suspicion can prevent these invasive diagnostic procedures, which in most instances are unnecessary. A quantitative pregnancy test if positive is diagnostic but if negative does not rule out disease. The serum beta-hCG determination is relatively fast, simple, inexpensive, and diagnostic.

In a patient with abnormal uterine bleeding, a D&C may or may not be of benefit. If malignant trophoblastic disease is identified pathologically, then of course this is of help. Unfortunately, disease may be deep in the myometrium and unobtainable

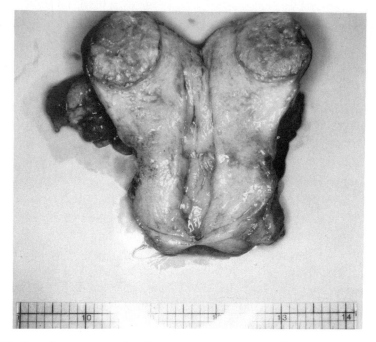

Fig. 7-6. Choriocarcinoma present deep in myometrium. A D&C would not identify residual disease.

by curettage (Fig. 7-6). In other instances, patients with GTN may have no localized disease in the uterus but only metastatic disease.

Diagnosis and evaluation

In 1973 Hammond and associates suggested a new categorization for GTN. To a certain degree, this has eliminated the old terminology of chorioadenoma destruens and choriocarcinoma, because those designations tended to identify separate and distinct entities of what is truly a spectrum of disease. This new classification (Table 7-2) treats GTN as a spectrum of neoplasia and allows identification of high-risk factors in this disease process, and by so doing, one is able to individualize therapy and thereby treat a specific patient more applicably.

Once a diagnosis of GTN has been suggested or established, proper evaluation must be performed. Table 7-3 lists the minimum workup suggested for these patients. Obvious identification of foci of disease should be established if at all possible. Since GTN can metastasize to the liver, lung, and brain, quite commonly these areas are evaluated in depth. In the past, EEG and brain scan were routinely used; however, with the addition of the CAT scan, this now appears to be the diagnostic procedure of choice. Once these tests have been obtained, categorization of disease can be performed and specific therapy begun.

Table 7-2. Classification of gestational trophoblastic neoplasia

I. Nonmetastatic disease: no evidence of disease outside of uterus
II. Metastatic disease: any disease outside of uterus
   A. Good prognosis metastatic disease
     1. Short duration (last pregnancy <4 months)
     2. Low pretreatment hCG titer (<100,000 IU/24 hr or <40,000 mIU/ml)
     3. No metastasis to brain or liver
     4. No significant prior chemotherapy
   B. Poor prognosis metastatic disease
     1. Long duration (last pregnancy >4 months)
     2. High pretreatment hCG titer (>100,000 IU/24 hr or >40,000 mIU/ml)
     3. Brain or liver metastasis
     4. Significant prior chemotherapy

Table 7-3. Workup of gestational trophoblastic neoplasia

History and physical exam
Chest film
Liver and brain scan
IVP
EEG
Hematologic survey
Serum chemistries
Pretreatment hCG titer
CAT scan
Ultrasound of pelvis

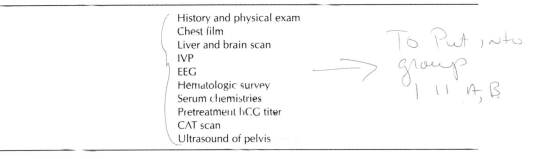

Nonmetastatic trophoblastic disease

Nonmetastatic trophoblastic disease is the first part of the spectrum of GTN and is the most common (Table 7-2). By definition, disease is limited to the uterus, with this designation usually arrived at as an exclusion diagnosis since metastasis cannot be identified. Particularly if subsequent fertility is desired, a pelvic arteriogram can be performed and disease identified within the uterus. This may be a guide, especially if chemotherapy is unsuccessful.

Patients with nonmetastatic trophoblastic disease can be treated with single-agent chemotherapy (Table 7-4). For years, the use of methotrexate as primary therapy has been the treatment of choice at the Southeastern Regional Center for Trophoblastic Disease. If patients have abnormal liver function, methotrexate should not be used since this agent is metabolized in the liver. Other investigators have used actinomycin D as primary therapy with equally good results. They believe that the toxicity from actinomycin D is less than that from methotrexate. Alternate chemotherapy with methotrexate and actinomycin D has been reported. This regi-

Table 7-4. Single-agent chemotherapy

1. Methotrexate 20-25 mg IM every day for 5 days
   (repeat every 7 days if possible)
2. Actinomycin D 10-12 µg/kg IV every day for 5 days
   (repeat every 7 days if possible)
3. Methotrexate 1 mg/kg IM on days 1, 3, 5, and 7
   Folinic acid 0.1 mg/kg IM on days 2, 4, 6, and 8
   (repeat every 7 days if possible)

Table 7-5. Management of single-agent chemotherapy

A. Chemotherapy as noted in Table 7-4
   1. Repeated at 7-10 day intervals depending on toxicity
   2. Contraception begun (oral if not contraindicated)
B. Drug continued as above until:
   1. hCG titer is normal   x3
C. Chemotherapy changed if:
   1. Titer rises (tenfold or more)
   2. Titer plateaus
   3. Evidence of new metastasis
D. Laboratory values—chemotherapy not repeated unless:
   1. WBC >3,000/cu mm
   2. Polys >1,500/cu mm
   3. Platelets >100,000/cu mm
   4. BUN, SGOT, SGPT essentially normal
E. Other toxicity mandating postponement of chemotherapy
   1. Severe oral or gastrointestinal ulceration
   2. Febrile course (usually present only with leukopenia)
F. Remission defined as three consecutive normal weekly
   hCG titers

Table 7-6. Remission and follow-up in gestational trophoblastic neoplasia

1. Three consecutive normal weekly
   hCG assays (1-3 courses after
   normal)
2. hCG titers every 2 weeks for 3
   months
   Then monthly for 3 months
   Then every 2 months for 6 months
   Then every 6 months
3. Frequent chest film and pelvic exam
4. Contraception for 1 year

men has been used in the hope of decreasing chemotherapy toxicity. More recently, the use of high-dose methotrexate with folinic acid rescue has been tested with excellent results. The advantage of this regimen is that toxicity is extremely low. The methotrexate–folinic acid regimen has recently been adopted as the treatment of choice in this disease by the Southeastern Trophoblastic Center.

Therapy should be repeated at 7-day intervals if at all possible. Criteria as noted in Table 7-5 must be strictly adhered to so that toxicity will not become life-threatening. Severe oral mucosal ulcerations can occur from single-agent methotrexate and be so severe that oral intake is impossible. This type of toxicity would preclude frequently repeated courses. It has not been seen with the methotrexate–folinic acid regimen. The therapy should be continued until negative hCG titers are obtained. A remission is defined as three consecutive normal weekly hCG titers. However, if a patient's hCG titer rises or if there is a titer plateau after two courses of chemotherapy, then an alternative drug should be tried. Evidence of new metastasis while the patient is being treated is also an indication for changing the chemotherapy. Once the hCG titers have returned to normal levels, appropriate follow-up is mandatory. This is outlined in Table 7-6. It is important that some type of contraception be used for at least 1 year after remission. Unless otherwise contraindicated, oral contraceptives can be used. If a patient has remained in remission for longer than 1 year and desires further childbearing, this can now be allowed.

Treatment of nonmetastatic GTN has been 100% successful. A total of 139 patients with this disease entity so treated at the Southeastern Trophoblastic Center have entered into remission (Tables 7-7 and 7-16). In those patients treated with chemotherapy, 106 of 122 have entered into remission. In nine patients who failed to go into remission, a hysterectomy was performed followed by remission. Seven patients had pelvic infusion performed in an attempt to save fertility, and in three of these success was obtained. The other four were treated successfully by tertiary hysterectomy (Table 7-7). In those patients who no longer desire fertility, it has been suggested that a primary hysterectomy performed during the first course of chemotherapy can shorten the treatment period. In 17 patients so treated, remission was obtained in a shorter period and with fewer courses of chemotherapy (Table 7-8).

Table 7-7. Role of therapy in nonmetastatic gestational trophoblastic neoplasia

Therapy	Remission	
Chemotherapy only	106/122	
Chemotherapy + hysterectomy (2°)	9/9	122/122
Chemotherapy + pelvic infusion	3/7	
Chemotherapy + pelvic infusion + hysterectomy (3°)	4/7	
Chemotherapy + 1° hysterectomy	17/17	
TOTAL	139/139 (100%)	

Data from Hammond, C. B., Weed, J. C., Jr., and Currie, J. L.: The role of operation in the current therapy of gestational trophoblastic disease, Am. J. Obstet. Gynecol. **136:**844, 1980.

Table 7-8. Role of therapy in nonmetastatic gestational trophoblastic neoplasia

Therapy	Patients	Days hospitalized	Number of courses of chemotherapy
Chemotherapy + 1° hysterectomy	17	32.8	2.2
Chemotherapy only (cure)	106	50.8	4.0
Chemotherapy + 2° surgery	16	121.2	8.3

Data from Hammond, C. B., Weed, J. C., Jr., and Currie, J. L.: The role of operation in the current therapy of gestational trophoblastic disease, Am. J. Obstet. Gynecol. **136:**844, 1980.

Table 7-9. Fertility in nonmetastatic gestational trophoblastic neoplasia

Desired fertility	109/122 (89%)
Subsequent pregnancies (47 patients)	57
Normal infants	45 (2 sets of twins)
Spontaneous abortion	7
Therapeutic abortion	3
Mole	2

Data from Hammond, C. B., Weed, J. C., Jr., and Currie, J. L.: The role of operation in the current therapy of gestational trophoblastic disease, Am. J. Obstet. Gynecol. **136:**844, 1980.

Those patients who required secondary surgery in addition to chemotherapy were more difficult to place into remission, requiring more courses of chemotherapy and a considerably longer period of hospitalization. An attempt to preserve fertility was the reason for the delay in subsequent surgery. Of those patients desiring fertility, 89% went into remission with preservation of the uterus (Table 7-9). Fifty-seven subsequent pregnancies in 47 patients occurred. There were two subsequent molar pregnancies. It should be remembered that in order to substantiate remission, patients who have either primary or secondary hysterectomy must be followed in exactly the same manner as those who are treated primarily with chemotherapy.

Good prognosis metastatic trophoblastic neoplasia

Patients with GTN who on evaluation are found to have metastatic disease are categorized as good prognosis when none of the following are present: (1) brain or liver metastasis; (2) urinary hCG titer greater than 100,000 IU/24 hr or serum beta-hCG titer greater than 40,000 mIU/ml; (3) previous chemotherapy; and (4) symptoms (antecedent pregnancy) greater than 4 months. Recently, it has been suggested by the Southeastern Trophoblastic Center that those patients who had an antecedent term pregnancy and developed GTN should be placed in the poor prognosis category. There is no general agreement in the literature concerning this. In a recent publication, three fourths of the patients who had an antecedent full-term pregnancy were categorized as poor prognosis using the above four criteria. The five patients who were categorized as having good prognosis disease following full-term pregnancy were successfully treated with chemotherapy and/or surgery. This issue remains unresolved.

Table 7-10. Role of therapy in good prognosis metastatic gestational trophoblastic neoplasia

Therapy	Remission	
Chemotherapy only	35/40 ⎫	
Chemotherapy + hysterectomy (2°)	5/5 ⎬	40/40
Chemotherapy + 1° hysterectomy	15/15	
TOTAL	55/55 (100%)	

Data from Hammond, C. B., Weed, J. C., Jr., and Currie, J. L.: The role of operation in the current therapy of gestational trophoblastic disease, Am. J. Obstet. Gynecol. **136**:844, 1980.

Therapy for good prognosis metastatic GTN can be the same as described for nonmetastatic disease (Table 7-4). The regimen of methotrexate and folinic acid is still believed to be investigational for this disease entity by the physicians at the Southeastern Trophoblastic Center. It would appear that it may be very applicable but further evaluation is needed. Methotrexate is considered the drug of choice in good prognosis metastatic patients, and they are treated with 20 to 25 mg given intramuscularly every day for 5 days and repeated after a 7-day drug-free interval if toxicity so allows. Liver and kidney function as well as the hemopoietic survey must be evaluated, and therapy should not be instituted unless these values are adequate. Once negative titers have been achieved, one additional course is routinely given. Should resistance to methotrexate occur manifested either by rising or plateauing titers or by the development of new metastasis, or if negative titers are not achieved by the fifth course of methotrexate, then the patients are switched to actinomycin D. If resistance to both drugs develops, the patient should then be started on a multiagent protocol such as methotrexate, actinomycin D, and chlorambucil (MAC) or the modified Bagshawe protocol (MBP) (Table 7-13). If there is no evidence of metastatic disease and titers are still elevated, a uterine site for the disease should be vigorously sought (such as identifying foci in the uterus by pelvic arteriography). In those individuals desiring further fertility, pelvic artery infusion may be considered, or hysterectomy may be performed if future fertility is not desired.

Fifty-five patients with good prognosis metastatic GTN have been treated at the Southeastern Trophoblastic Center (Table 7-10). Forty patients were treated with chemotherapy only, of which 35 were placed into remission. The other five had secondary hysterectomy, with clearing of their disease. An additional 15 patients had chemotherapy and hysterectomy performed primarily, all of whom were placed into remission. Those patients who had chemotherapy and primary hysterectomy went into remission in a shorter time and with fewer courses of chemotherapy than those patients treated with chemotherapy alone or chemotherapy plus secondary surgery. When compared with the nonmetastatic GTN patients, more courses of chemotherapy were required in good prognosis metastatic GTN patients treated in like manner, with the exception of those who had chemotherapy plus secondary surgery. The efficacy of primary surgery is apparent, although this finding is probably related to extent of disease within the good prognosis metastatic GTN category.

II β

Poor prognosis metastatic trophoblastic neoplasia

Patients who have been categorized as having poor prognosis metastatic GTN (Table 7-11) present the physician and the medical team with a real challenge. Many of these patients have been previously treated with chemotherapy and have been resistant to that treatment while accumulating considerable toxicity and depleting bone marrow reserves. Multiple-agent chemotherapy is recommended in this disease, and a multiple-modality approach is necessary in many of these patients. These individuals should be treated in centers that have special interests and expertise in this disease. Most of these patients require prolonged hospitalization for up to several months. They will have life-threatening toxicity from therapy and in some instances require specialized care such as total parenteral nutrition and other life support measures during periods of minimal host resistance.

Before 1969, patients with this disease entity were treated by single-agent therapy, and in the first seven patients so treated, only one was placed into remission. Beginning in 1969, patients with poor prognosis GTN were started initially on triple chemotherapy as outlined in Table 7-12. Triple chemotherapy (MAC) is repeated at 12 to 14 days, depending on the toxicity and using the parameters established for single-agent therapy (Table 7-5). Cerebral or hepatic metastases are treated concurrently with 2,000 to 3,000 rads (in 10 days) to the whole brain or liver. If the hCG titer rises or plateaus after two courses of MAC, the chemotherapy is changed. Currently, the modified Bagshawe protocol (MBP) is used (Table 7-13). This therapy is repeated at 7- to 14-day intervals and has been successful even in those patients who have not been placed into remission by MAC. Six of seven patients in whom MBP was used as second-line therapy have gone into remission, although adjunctive surgery was also used in some of these individuals. If this second-line therapy is unsuccessful, patients are then treated with velban, bleomycin, and cis-platinum. This third-line regimen is given at weekly intervals or as bone marrow toxicity permits. In these resistant cases of poor prognosis GTN, adjunctive modalities must be used in addition to chemotherapy. These can include hysterectomy, resection of metastasis, or irradiation of nonresectable lesions. Complete remission is documented only after three consecutive normal weekly hCG titers. Individuals with poor prognosis metastatic GTN should have one to three courses of chemotherapy after a negative titer is first noted. After the individual is placed into remission, follow-up is the same as for hydatidiform mole and nonmetastatic or good prognosis metastatic GTN.

The Southeastern Trophoblastic Center has recently reported on 63 patients with poor prognosis GTN. The remission rate for these patients is 66% (Table 7-14). Those patients who were treated by chemotherapy with concurrent radiation therapy have the best prognosis, with 87% of these going into remission. If primary or secondary surgery is needed, the prognosis does worsen. These patients require longer hospitalization as well as more courses of chemotherapy to place them into remission than do those patients with nonmetastatic or good prognosis metastatic disease.

Table 7-11. Poor prognosis metastatic gestational trophoblastic neoplasia

> Brain or liver metastasis
> Urinary hCG >100,000 IU/24 hr or serum
>   beta-hCG >40,000 mIU/ml
> Unsuccessful prior chemotherapy
> Symptoms greater than 4 months
> Gestational trophoblastic neoplasia after
>   term pregnancy (?)

Table 7-12. Treatment of poor prognosis gestational trophoblastic neoplasia

> Methotrexate 15 mg IM every day for 5 days
> Actinomycin D 10-12 µg/kg IV every day for
>   5 days   } Every 12-14 days   _MAC_
> Chlorambucil 10 mg PO every day for 5 days
> Brain or liver radiation therapy 2,000-3,000
>   rads

[handwritten notes: ① Hydroxurea ④ methtrex ② Actnom D ⑤ cytoxan ③ Vincristin ⑥ Folic acid ⑦ adriamycin]

Table 7-13. Modified Bagshawe chemotherapy*

Day	Hour	Treatment
1	0600	Hydroxyurea 500 mg PO
	1200	Hydroxyurea 500 mg PO
	1800	Hydroxyurea 500 mg PO
	1900	Actinomycin D 200 µg IV
	2400	Hydroxyurea 500 mg PO
2	0700	Vincristine 1 mg/m² IV
	1900	Methotrexate 100 mg/m² IV
		Methotrexate 200 mg/m²
		infused over 12 hr
		Actinomycin D 200 µg IV
3	1900	Actinomycin D 200 µg IV
		Cytoxan 500 mg/m² IV
		Folinic acid 14 mg IM
4	0100	Folinic acid 14 mg IM
	0700	Folinic acid 14mg IM
	1300	Folinic acid 14 mg IM
	1900	Folinic acid 14 mg IM
		Actinomycin D 500 µg IV
5	0100	Folinic acid 14 mg IM
	1900	Actinomycin D 500 µg IV
6	No treatment	
7	No treatment	
8	1900	Cytoxan 500 mg/m² IV
		Adriamycin 30 mg/m² IV

[handwritten: HU 500 gm PO Act D 200]

*Currently used at the Southeastern Regional Center for Trophoblastic Disease.

Table 7-14. Role of therapy in poor prognosis metastatic gestational trophoblastic neoplasia

Therapy	Remission
Chemotherapy ± radiation therapy	20/23 (87%)
Chemotherapy + 1° surgery	17/29 (57%)
Chemotherapy + 2° surgery	5/11 (45%)
TOTAL	42/63 (66%)
16 patients died of disease	
5 patients died of toxicity	

Data from Hammond, C. B., Weed, J. C., Jr., and Currie, J. L.: The role of operation in the current therapy of gestational trophoblastic disease, Am. J. Obstet. Gynecol. **136:**844, 1980.

Table 7-15. Recurrences in gestational trophoblastic neoplasia

Disease	Recurrences
Nonmetastatic	3/139 (2.1%)
Good prognosis metastatic	3/55 (5.4%)
Poor prognosis metastatic	13/63 (21%)

Data from Hammond, C. B., Weed, J. C., Jr., and Currie, J. L.: The role of operation in the current therapy of gestational trophoblastic disease, Am. J. Obstet. Gynecol. **136:**844, 1980.

Table 7-16. Results of treatment (Duke University)

Disease	Remission
Nonmetastatic	139/139 (100%)
Good prognosis metastatic	55/55 (100%)
Poor prognosis metastatic	42/63 (66%)
TOTAL	236/257 (92%)

Modified from Hammond, C. B., Weed, J. C., Jr., and Currie, J. L.: The role of operation in the current therapy of gestational trophoblastic disease, Am. J. Obstet. Gynecol. **136:**844, 1980.

Although the prognosis for poor prognosis GTN is considerably less than for non-metastatic and good prognosis metastatic disease, it has shown marked improvement over the years. As previously noted, of the first seven patients treated with single-agent chemotherapy, only one survived. During the 10 years from 1968 through 1978, 73% of the patients were placed into remission; however, during the last 3 years, 17 of 19 (90%) have gone into remission. This has been accomplished not only with the new chemotherapeutic regimens but also with the aggressive multiple-modality approach and conscientious support of these patients during their critical illness. Deaths from toxicity have also decreased considerably during this time.

Of the 63 patients with poor prognosis metastatic GTN, only 19 were able to preserve their reproductive capacity. Only four of these patients have had subsequent pregnancy, resulting in one spontaneous abortion and four normal deliveries.

Recurrence

Recurrence for all categories of GTN is presented in Table 7-15. In those patients with advanced initial disease, there is a greater chance of developing recurrence, as one would expect. Particularly in good and poor prognosis metastatic GTN, subsequent chemotherapy past the first normal titer is given as a precautionary measure in the hope of decreasing the chance of recurrence. It is of utmost importance that, once a patient is placed into remission, the follow-up protocol be adhered to strictly. With an aggressive multiple-modality approach developed through extensive experience, 100% of patients with nonmetastatic and good prognosis metastatic trophoblastic disease have been placed into remission. Only two thirds of the patients with poor prognosis metastatic disease have been placed into remission; however, this number has increased over the years, with 90% of those treated during the past 3 years in remission (Table 7-16). The fact that GTN is potentially curable in essentially 100% of the cases must be attributed to the patience and expertise as well as the ingenuity of those physicians who have developed and continually evaluate methods for making this the most curable of all gynecologic malignancies.

BIBLIOGRAPHY

Bagshawe, K. D.: Choriocarcinoma; the clinical biology of the trophoblast and its tumours, London, 1969, Edward Arnold (Publishers) Ltd.

Bagshawe, K. D.: Treatment of trophoblastic tumors; Ann. Acad. Med. **5:**273, 1976.

Bagshawe, K. D., and Wilde, C. E.: Infusion therapy for pelvic trophoblastic tumors, J. Obstet. Gynaecol. Br. Comm. **71:**565, 1964.

Brace, K. C.: The role of irradiation in the treatment of metastatic trophoblastic disease, Radiology **91:**539, 1968.

Brewer, J. I., Gerbie, A. B., Dolkart, R. E., and others: Chemotherapy in trophoblastic disease, Am. J. Obstet. Gynecol. **90:**566, 1964.

Brewer, J. I., Halpern, B., and Torok. E. E.: Gestational trophoblastic disease; selected clinical aspects and chorionic gonadotropin test methods. In Hickey, R. G., editor: Current problems in cancer, Chicago, 1979, Year Book Medical Publishers, Inc.

Brewer, J. I., Rinehart, J. J., and Dunbar, R.: Choriocarcinoma, Am. J. Obstet. Gynecol. **81:**574, 1961.

Curry, S. L., Hammond, C. B., Tyrey, L., and others: Hydatidiform mole; diagnosis, management, and long-term follow-up of 347 patients, Obstet. Gynecol. **45:**1, 1975.

Delfs, E.: Quantitative chorionic gonadotropin; prognostic value in hydatidiform mole and chorioepithelioma, Obstet. Gynecol. **9:**1, 1957.

Einhorn, L. H., and Donohue, J. H.: CIS-diammine-dichoplatinum, vinblastine and bleomycin; combination chemotherapy in disseminated testicular cancer, Ann. Intern. Med. **87**:293, 1967.

Goldstein, D. P.: Five year's experience with the prevention of trophoblastic tumors by the prophylactic use of chemotherapy in patients with molar pregnancy, Clin. Obstet. Gynecol. **13**:945, 1970.

Goldstein, D. P., and Reid, D.: Recent developments in management of molar pregnancy, Clin. Obstet. Gynecol. **10**:313, 1967.

Goldstein, D. P., Saracco, P., Osathanondh, R., and others: Methotrexate with citrovorum factor rescue for gestational trophoblastic neoplasms, Obstet. Gynecol. **53**:93, 1978.

Greene, R. R.: Chorioadenoma destruens, Ann. N.Y. Acad. Sci. **80**:143, 1959.

Hammond, C. B., Borchert, L. G., Tyrey, L., and others: Treatment of metastatic trophoblastic disease; good and poor prognosis, Am. J. Obstet. Gynecol. **115**:4, 1973.

Hammond, C. B., Hertz, R., Ross, G. T., and others: Primary chemotherapy for non-metastatic gestational trophoblastic neoplasms, Tex. Rep. Biol. Med. **24**:326, 1966.

Hammond, C. B., Hertz, R., Ross, G. T., and others: Diagnostic problems of choriocarcinoma and related trophoblastic neoplasms, Obstet. Gynecol. **29**:224, 1967.

Hammond, C. B., and Lewis, J. L., Jr.: Gestational trophoblastic neoplasms. In Schirra, J., editor: Davis' gynecology and obstetrics, vol. 1., Hagerstown, Md., 1977, Harper & Row, Publishers, Inc.

Hammond, C. B., and Parker, R. T.: Diagnosis and treatment of trophoblastic disease, Obstet. Gynecol. **35**:132, 1970.

Hammond, C. B., Weed, J. C., Jr., and Currie, J. L.: The role of operation in the current therapy of gestational trophoblastic disease, Am. J. Obstet. Gynecol. **136**:844, 1980.

Hertig, A. T.: Human trophoblast, Springfield, Ill., 1968, Charles C Thomas, Publisher.

Hertig, A. T., and Mansell, H.: Tumors of the female sex organs. I. Hydatidiform mole and choriocarcinoma. In Atlas of tumor pathology, Washington, D.C., 1956, Armed Forces Institute of Pathology.

Hertig, A. T., and Sheldon, W. H.: Hydatidiform mole—a pathological clinical correlation of 200 cases, Am. J. Obstet. Gynecol. **53**:1, 1947.

Hertz, R., Lewis, J. L., Jr., and Lipsett, M. B.: Five year's experience with chemotherapy of metastatic choriocarcinoma and related trophoblastic tumors in women, Am. J. Obstet. Gynecol. **82**:631, 1961.

Holland, J. F., Hreshchyshyn, M. M., and Glidewell, O.: Controlled clinical trials of methotrexate in treatment and prophylaxis of trophoblastic neoplasia. In Abstracts, 10th International Cancer Congress, May 1970, Houston, 1970, Medical Arts Publishers.

Hon, E. H.: A manual of pregnancy testing, Boston, 1961, Little, Brown & Co.

Lewis, J., Jr.: Chemotherapy for metastatic gestational trophoblastic neoplasms, Clin. Obstet. Gynecol. **10**:330, 1967.

Lewis, J., Jr., Gore, H., Hertig, A. T. and Goss, D. A.: Treatment of trophoblastic neoplasms; with rationale for the use of adjunctive chemotherapy at the time of indicated operation, Am. J. Obstet. Gynecol. **96**:710, 1966.

Lewis, J. L., Jr., Ketcham, A. S., and Hertz, R.: Surgical intervention during chemotherapy for gestational trophoblastic neoplasms, Cancer **19**:1517, 1966.

Li, M., Hertz, R., and Spencer, D. B.: Effects of methotrexate therapy upon choriocarcinoma and chorioadenoma, Proc. Soc. Exp. Biol. Med. **93**:361, 1956.

Maroulis, G. B., Hammond, C. B., Johnsrude, I. S., and others: Arteriography and infusional chemotherapy in localized trophoblastic disease, Obstet. Gynecol. **45**:397, 1975.

Miller, J. M., Jr., Surwit, E. A., and Hammond, C. B.: Choriocarcinoma following term pregnancy, Obstet. Gynecol. **53**:207, 1979.

Ober, W. B., and Fass, R. O.: The early history of choriocarcinoma, J. Hist. Med. Allied Sci. **16**:1, 1961.

Odell, W. B., Hertz, R., Lipsett, M. B., and others: Endocrine aspects of trophoblastic neoplasms, Clin. Obstet. Gynecol. **10**:290, 1967.

Park, W. W.: Choriocarcinoma; a study of its pathology, Philadelphia, 1971, F. A. Davis Co.

Ross, G. T., Goldstein, D. D., Hertz, R., and others: Sequential use of methotrexate and actinomycin D in the treatment of metastatic choriocarcinoma and related trophoblastic diseases in women, Am. J. Obstet. Gynecol. **93**:223, 1965.

Ross, G. T., Hammond, C. B., Hertz, R., and others: Chemotherapy of metastatic and non-metastatic gestational trophoblastic neoplasms, Tex. Rep. Biol. Med. **24**:326, 1966.

Vaitukaitis, J. B., Braunstein, G. D., and Ross, G. T.: A radioimmunoassay which specifically measures human chorionic gonadotrophin in the presence of human luteinizing hormone, Am. J. Obstet. Gynecol. **113**:751, 1972. ➡

CHAPTER EIGHT

Invasive cancer of the vulva

Invasive squamous cell carcinoma
Paget's disease
Melanoma
Sarcoma
Bartholin's gland carcinoma
Basal cell carcinoma

Historically, cancer of the vulva has accounted for 3% to 5% of all female genital malignancies. During recent years, it appears that this incidence has been increasing. Green reported that in his experience, carcinoma of the vulva amounted to 5% of all the patients with gynecologic malignancies seen from 1927 through 1961, but in the next 12 years it increased to 8%. He believes that this increase in incidence was due to the continued rise in the average age of the female population in recent years, causing an increase in the number of eligible to develop the disease. Vulvar cancer, with the exception of the rare sarcomas, appears most frequently in women in their mid-sixties, and in some series almost half will be 70 years of age or older. On the other hand, vulvar cancers can appear in young patients, and Rutledge and associates at the M. D. Anderson Hospital and Tumor Institute noted that about 15% of all vulvar cancers occur in women under the age of 40. Many of the associated features seen in patients with vulvar cancer, such as diabetes, obesity, hypertension, and arteriosclerosis, may just reflect the increased disease incidence as one gets older.

Over the years, the possible association of vulvar carcinoma and venereal or granulomatous lesions of the vulva has been noted. The incidence tends to be higher in the older literature and much lower in the most recent reports, probably reflecting to a certain degree a lower incidence of syphilis in the recent past. The association of condyloma acuminatum with vulvar carcinoma is well known, but no cause and effect relationship has been delineated.

HPV

185

Table 8-1. Incidence of vulvar neoplasms by histologic type*

Tumor type	Percent	
Epidermoid	86.2	
Melanoma	4.8	
Sarcoma	2.2	
Basal cell	1.4	
Bartholin's gland		
Squamous	0.4	
Adenocarcinoma	0.6	1.2
Adenocarcinoma	0.6	
Undifferentiated	3.9	

Modified from Plentl, A. A., and Friedman, E. A.: Lymphatic system of the female genitalia, Philadelphia, 1971, W. B. Saunders Co.
*Based on 1,378 reported cases.

INVASIVE SQUAMOUS CELL CARCINOMA
Histology

The overwhelming majority of all vulvar cancer is squamous in origin. The vulva is covered with skin, and any malignancy that appears elsewhere on the skin can occur in this region. Table 8-1 depicts the incidence of vulvar neoplasia from several collected studies in the literature. Our discussion will be aimed mainly at squamous carcinoma because of its preponderance, but as a generalization, the other lesions can also be treated in like fashion except as will be noted.

Clinical profile

The development of squamous cell carcinoma of the vulva may be quite similar to the process that occurs on the cervix. However, no race or culture is spared, and gravidity and parity are not involved in the pathogenesis of this neoplasm. Actually, vulvar cancer is common in the poor and elderly in most parts of the world, and this has led to the hypothesis that inadequate personal hygiene and medical care are often contributing factors in this disease. In truth, the cause of cancer of the vulva is unknown, and there is little data to support the concept that these neoplasms often develop from vulvar dystrophies. The initial lesion would appear in many cases to arise from an area of intraepithelial neoplasia, which subsequently develops into a small nodule that may break down and ulcerate (Fig. 8-1). On other occasions small, warty or cauliflower-like growths will evolve, and these may be confused with condyloma acuminatum. Long-term pruritus or a lump or mass on the vulva is present in more than 50% of patients with invasive vulvar cancer. In most reported series of carcinoma of the vulva, there is (1) delay in treatment of the patient, who has symptoms for 2 to 16 months before seeking medical attention, and/or (2) medical treatment of vulvar lesions for up to 12 months or longer without biopsy for definitive diagnosis or referral. Fortunately, vulvar cancer is commonly indolent, extends slowly, and metastasizes fairly late. Hence, we have a great opportunity for prevent-

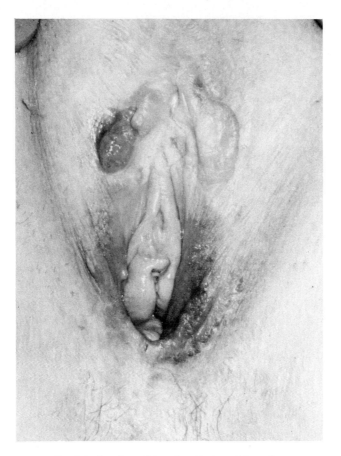

Fig. 8-1. Small, well-localized lesion of the vulva.

ing the serious advanced stages of this disease through education of both patients and physicians. Biopsy *must* be done on all suspicious lesions of the vulva, including lumps, ulcers, or pigmented areas, even in the patient not complaining of burning or itching.

Location and spread pattern

Primary disease can appear anywhere on the vulva, with approximately 70% arising primarily on the labia. Disease is more common on the labium majora; however, it may appear on the labium minora, clitoris, and perineum. The disease is usually localized and well demarcated, although occasionally it can be so extensive that the primary location cannot be determined (Fig. 8-2). Multifocal growth pattern in invasive squamous carcinoma of the vulva is uncommon, with the exception of the so-called kissing lesions that can occur as isolated lesions usually on the upper labia.

Fundamental to the understanding of therapy for invasive cancer of the vulva is proper knowledge of the lymphatic drainage of this organ. In general, the four his-

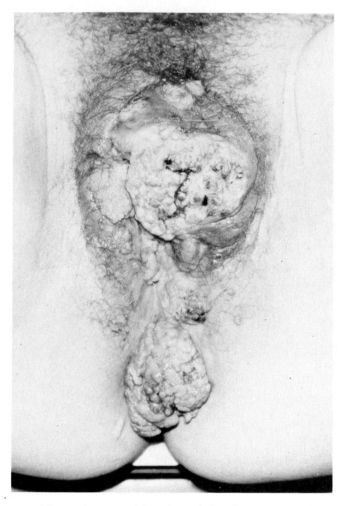

Fig. 8-2. Large, diffuse malignancy of the vulva including the perineum and perianal area.

tologic types of invasive cancer behave in a similar manner and use primarily the lymphatic mode for initial metastases.

Lymphatic drainage of the external genitalia begins with minute papillae, and these are connected in turn to a multilayered meshwork of fine vessels. These fine vessels extend over the entire labium minora, the prepuce of the clitoris, the forchette, and the vaginal mucosa up to the level of the hymenal ring. Drainage of these lymphatics extends toward the anterior portion of the labium minora, where they emerge into three or four collecting trunks whose course is toward the mons veneris bypassing the clitoris. Vessels from the prepuce anastomose with these lymphatics. In like manner, vessels from the labium majora proceed anteriorly to the upper part of the vulva and mons veneris, there joining the vessels of the prepuce and labium minora. These lymphatic vessels abruptly change direction, turning lat-

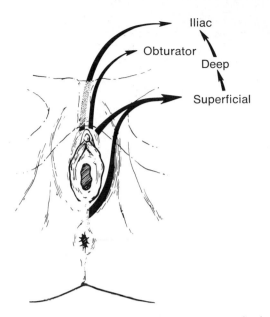

Fig. 8-3. Lymphatic spread of vulvar malignancy. See text for details.

erally, and terminate in ipsilateral or contralateral femoral nodes. Drainage is usually limited initially to the medial upper quadrant of the femoral node group. The nodes are located medial to the great saphenous vein above the cribriform fascia and in turn may drain secondarily through the cribriform fascia to the deep femoral group.

The superficial inguinal lymph glands, located immediately beneath the integument and Camper's fascia, are large and vary from eight to ten in number. All authors agree that the superficial inguinal lymph glands are the primary nodal group for the vulva and can serve as the sentinel lymph nodes of the vulva. The deep femoral nodes, which are located beneath the cribriform fascia, are the secondary nodal recipients and are involved before drainage into the deep pelvic nodes occurs. Cloquet's node is the last node of the deep femoral group and is located just beneath Poupart's ligament. The multilayered meshwork of lymphatics on the vulva itself is always limited to an area medial to the genitocrural fold (Fig. 8-3). Lymphatic drainage of the vulva is a very progressive systemic mechanism, and therapy can be planned depending on where in the lymphatic chain tumor is present.

Although lymphatics from the clitoris directly to the deep pelvic lymph nodes are described, their clinical significance appears to be minimal. It is unusual to find a case in which metastasis is present in the pelvic lymph nodes without metastatic disease in the inguinal lymph nodes, even when the clitoris is involved. Curry and associates noted 58 patients with clitoral involvement of 191 studied, and none had positive deep pelvic nodes without involvement of inguinal nodes also.

The incidence of positive inguinal and pelvic nodes varies considerably as noted in Table 8-2. Unfortunately most of these studies were unstaged, although, in gen-

Table 8-2. Incidence of positive nodes

Series	Number of cases	Positive groin and pelvic nodes (%)	Positive pelvic nodes (%)
Taussig (1938)	65	46.2	7.7
Cherry and Glucksman (1955)	95	44.2	—
Green and associates (1958)	238	58.8	—
Stening and Elliot (1959)	50	40.0	12.0
Way (1960)	143	42.0	16.1
Macafee (1962)	82	40.2	—
Collins and associates (1963)	71	31.0	8.5
Rutledge and associates (1970)	101	47.6	11.1
Fraukbeudal (1973)	55	22.0	—
Morley (1976)	374	37.0	—
Krupp and Bahm (1978)	195	21.0	4.6
Curry and associates (1980)	191	30.0	4.7

eral, the larger the tumor, the greater the propensity for inguinal and pelvic node metastases. Morley noted a 20.7% incidence of lymph node involvement if there was a T1 lesion (less that 2 cm in diameter). In T2 lesions (greater than 2 cm but limited to the vulva), the incidence of lymph node involvement more than doubled to 44.8%.

Staging

Historically, many staging systems have been applied to invasive cancer of the vulva. In 1971 the current FIGO staging system (Table 8-3), based on the TMN classification, was adopted for international use. This system of clinical staging is unfortunately contingent upon the ability of the clinician to assess node involvement by palpation. Yet even the most experienced observers often admit to a 25% to 40% error rate in such an evaluation. Survival does, however, mirror this classification.

Management

Since Way reported an improved survival rate in carcinoma of the vulva by using the en bloc dissection of radical vulvectomy plus inguinal and pelvic lymphadenectomy, this has become the mainstay of treatment in vulvar cancer. With this therapy, the corrected 5-year survival rate for stage I and II disease has been reported by many authors to be approximately 90%.

For many years, a deep pelvic lymphadenectomy was routinely performed along with the radical vulvectomy and inguinal lymphadenectomy irrespective of the size of the vulvar lesion or the presence or lack of disease in the inguinal lymph nodes. A growing number of surgeons now limit the initial procedure to radical vulvectomy and bilateral superifcial and deep inguinal lymphadenectomy and will not proceed

Table 8-3. FIGO staging (clinical) of invasive cancer of the vulva

Stage I	T1	N0	M0	All lesions confined to the vulva, with a
	T1	N1	M0	maximum diameter of 2 cm or less and
				no suspicious groin nodes.
Stage II	T2	N0	M0	All lesions confined to the vulva, with a
	T2	N1	M0	diameter greater than 2 cm and no
				suspicious groin nodes.
Stage III	T3	N0	M0	Lesions extending beyond the vulva but
	T3	N1	M0	without grossly positive groin nodes.
	T3	N2	M0	Lesions of any size confined to the vulva,
	T1	N2	M0	with suspicious groin nodes.
	T2	N2	M0	
Stage IV	T3	N3	M0	Lesions extending beyond the vulva, with
	T4	N3	M0	grossly positive nodes.
	T4	N0	M0	Lesions involving mucosa of rectum,
	T4	N1	M0	bladder, or urethra or involving bone.
	T4	N2	M0	
	T1	N3	M0	
	T2	N3	M0	
	M1A			All cases with distant or palpable deep
	M1B			pelvic metastases.

with pelvic lymphadenectomy unless metastasis is demonstrated in the inguinal node area. If the presence of tumor is documented in the inguinal nodes, a pelvic lymphadenectomy is performed on the involved side. This philosophy is a result of the observation that the deep pelvic nodes are essentially never involved with metastatic disease when the more superficial inguinal nodes are uninvolved. A recent study by Curry and associates of the M. D. Anderson Hospital data noted that in 191 patients, only nine (4.7%) had positive deep pelvic nodes, and all nine patients also had metastatic disease in the groin nodes. There is a definitive increase in morbidity from pelvic node dissection in conjunction with inguinal node dissection; thus, there is a valid reluctance to perform pelvic lymphadenectomy unless it is necessary. In some patients, the surgeons will elect to treat the pelvic nodes with radiation therapy rather than extend the operative procedure and incur the additional morbidity. The pelvic nodes will be positive approximately 25% of the time when the inguinal nodes have documented metastatic disease. In turn, approximately 20% of the patients with positive pelvic nodes will survive 5 years or more. Thus, if all patients with positive inguinal nodes underwent pelvic lymphadenectomy, the procedure would result in approximately a 5% salvage rate for that group of patients. It is this type of statistical reasoning that has encouraged many individuals to use radiation therapy when the deep pelvic nodes are at risk, especially in the elderly or medically infirm patient.

Combined radiation therapy and surgery, as well as radiation alone and local surgery alone, have been applied to this disease. No adequate prospective studies comparing various therapies or combinations of such are available for analysis. The older literature notes superior results with radical vulvectomy and lymphadenectomy as compared with radiation therapy alone or surgery plus radiation therapy. It was also noted that those patients who had vulvectomy alone did worse than if lymphadenectomy was also included.

Daly and Million have advocated radical vulvectomy combined with elective node irradiation for stage I and II squamous cell carcinoma of the vulva. In a small number of patients, they found that this treatment combination was well tolerated with no node failures, no irradiation complications, no delay in healing of the surgical site, and an average hospitalization of 13 days. The dose to the inguinal nodes was calculated between 5,000 and 5,500 rads, and the midplane pelvic dose was between 4,500 and 5,000 rads. Although this is an interesting approach, the small number of patients treated to date does not prove that elective node irradiation will eliminate subclinical node disease from vulvar carcinoma. Since the incidence of inguinal node involvement in stage I and II disease is in the neighborhood of 20% to 40%, it will take a reasonably large series of patients followed for a significant time to establish the validity of Daly and Million's hypothesis.

Boronow has also emphasized the possible role of irradiation therapy in vulvar vaginal cancers. His report dealt mostly with advanced disease involving vaginal mucous membrane, necessitating an exenterative type of procedure if a primary surgical approach were used. As an alternative, he recommends surgical extirpation of the lymph nodes with a combination of external and interstitial radiation for control of the central lesion. In a small, highly individualized series, this approach appeared promising. Radiotherapy has not hitherto been widely used for vulvar cancer because of the technical difficulties associated with directing external beam to this area and the very sensitive moist vulvar skin and mucous membrane, which tolerate irradiation poorly. Low anterior and posterior fields must be used, resulting in intense exposure of the vulvar skin as the axis of the x-ray beam runs parallel (and often within) the skin and mucous membrane. Vulvitis results, and interruption of therapy is often necessary because of patient discomfort. Similarly, radiation therapy to enlarged, obviously positive inguinal nodes becomes technically difficult, and removal of at least the enlarged nodes with subsequent x-ray therapy to the area has been our preference. Preoperative doses of 4,500 to 5,000 rads to either groin or vulvar areas produces a hazardous situation for any subsequent surgical approach.

Alternate approach to early vulvar cancer (microinvasive)

In 1974 Wharton and associates described an entity that they called microinvasive carcinoma of the vulva. These lesions were 2 cm or less in diameter and invaded the stroma to a depth of 5 mm or less. In 25 such patients, none had positive lymph nodes, developed recurrence, or died as a result of vulvar cancer. These results implied that microinvasive carcinoma of the vulva is a definable stage in that this group may be treated by conservative surgery. As a result of this article, several patients with stage I lesions and limited stromal invasion were treated by radical vulvectomy only. Several of these patients subsequently developed recurrent or metastatic carcinoma and died of their disease. In 1975, Parker and associates at Duke University presented their evaluation of patients with early invasive epidermoid carcinoma of the vulva. They felt that the term "microinvasive" was not applicable to vulvar neoplasia. Sixty of their patients had a stage I (T1) lesion of 2 cm or less, with 58 of these patients having stromal invasion 5 mm or less in depth. Three of the 58 patients (5%) had pelvic node metastases; two of these three showed invasion of vascular channels, and the third patient showed cellular anaplasia. The Duke study concluded that if a strict histologic evaluation was performed on the excised vulvar lesion and invasion of 5 mm or less was noted along with an absence of vascular or lymphatic channel invasion and no anaplasia, then an operational approach less radical than radical vulvectomy, inguinal dissection, and/or pelvic lymphadenectomy could be used for selected patients. This would reduce the morbidity while achieving comparable survival data.

There continues to be a lack of unanimity concerning what is the proper surgical approach to the patient with an early invasive carcinoma of the vulva. Reports illustrating metastatic disease in inguinal lymph nodes have conflicted with other reports suggesting radical vulvectomy only. The morbidity produced by radical vulvectomy, both to body image and sexual function, makes this issue worthy of serious consideration. As a result, DiSaia, Creasman, and Rich proposed an alternate approach to this early disease that attempts to preserve vulvar tissue without sacrificing curability when possible metastatic disease exists. This approach utilizes the superficial inguinal nodes as sentinel nodes in the treatment planning when the central lesion is 1 cm or less in diameter and focal invasion is limited to 5 mm or less in depth (see the description of metastatic lymph node spread pattern earlier in this chapter).

The patient is prepared for radical vulvectomy with a bilateral inguinal lymphadenectomy should the operative findings warrant a maximal surgical effort. An 8 cm incision is made parallel to the inguinal ligament two fingerbreadths (4 cm) beneath the inguinal ligament and two fingerbreadths (4 cm) lateral to the pubic tubercle (Fig. 8-4). This allows access to the superficial inguinal lymph nodes of both the upper oblique and inferior vertical set. The incision is carried down through Camper's fascia, and at this point skin flaps are bluntly and sharply dissected both superiorly and inferiorly, allowing access to the fat pad containing the superficial nodes. The sentinel nodes are located in the fatty layer of tissue beneath Camper's fascia anterior to the cribriform plate and the fascia lata (Fig. 8-5). The dissection should be carried superiorly to the inguinal ligament and inferiorly to a point approximately 2 cm proximal to the opening of Hunter's canal. The dissection should be carried laterally to the sartorius muscle and medially to the adductor longus muscle fascia (Fig. 8-6). Blunt dissection with the handle of the scalpel facilitates identification of the cribriform fascia, which is most easily identified just below the inguinal ligament or in the area of the saphenous opening. The cribriform fascia becomes one with the fascia lata and thus is contiguous with the fascia on the surface

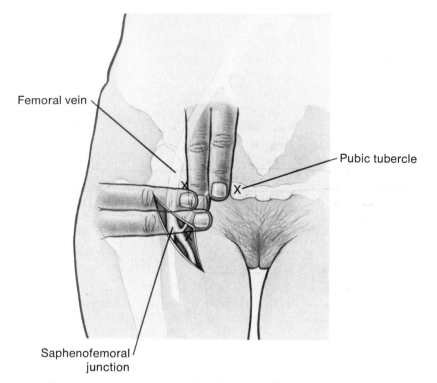

Femoral vein

Pubic tubercle

Saphenofemoral
junction

Fig. 8-4. An incision can be made as noted so that the superficial inguinal nodes can be removed easily.

of the adductor longus and sartorius muscles; this may facilitate its identification. The portion of the fascia covering the femoral triangle is perforated by the internal saphenous vein and by numerous blood and lymphatic vessels, hence the name cribriform fascia. If the dissection is carried out properly, the adventitia of the femoral vessels should not be clearly seen except through the vessel openings mentioned above.

The excised nodes are immediately sent for frozen section analysis, and the finding of positive nodes mandates a complete inguinal dissection including the deep femoral nodes as well as the pelvic nodes on the involved side. Absence of a report of metastatic disease is followed by simple closure of the incision with a subcuticular suture of polyglycolic acid (PGA) over two medium-size suction drainage tubes.

A wide local excision of the vulvar skin is then performed ensuring a margin of 3 cm of normal skin on all sides of the primary lesion. Adequate subcutaneous tissue should be taken, especially beneath the primary lesion. It has been our practice to submit both mucuous membrane and skin margins as separate specimens.

Hemostasis having been established, a decision must be made regarding primary closure of the defect versus intraposition of a split-thickness skin graft. When a split-thickness skin graft is employed, the graft is usually taken from the medial aspect of the right thigh at 0.018-inch thickness. With an air-driven dermatome, this can be

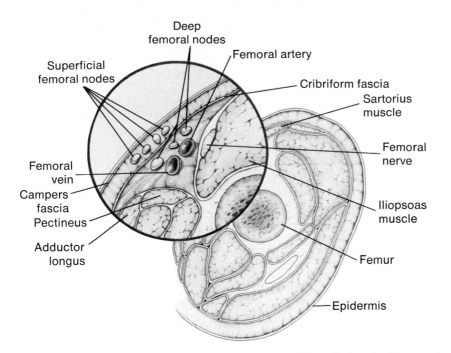

Fig. 8-5. Superficial nodes are located between Camper's fascia and the cribriform fascia as noted on the cross-section through the femoral triangle.

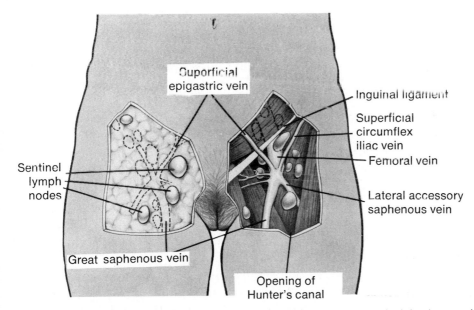

Fig. 8-6. The right side demonstrates the limit of the superficial node dissection. The left side notes the dissection after the cribriform fascia has been removed.

accomplished quite easily with minimal morbidity. The donor site is dressed with scarlet red gauze, and an occlusive pressure dressing is applied. The skin graft is then sutured to the defect using 4-0 PGA suture and a pressure dressing in a manner previously described by Rutledge and Sinclair.

In the event that metastatic disease is found in the inguinal nodes, a classical radical vulvectomy and inguinal lymphadenectomy must be performed. The approach outlined here attempts to gain optimum curability and preserve optimal cosmesis and sexual function. However, this plan has been carried out on a very limited number of patients and therefore must be considered investigational at this time.

Operative morbidity and mortality

In the early series of Way, the operative mortality approached 20%; however, in the last decade this has been reduced to 1% or 2%. Frequently, this procedure has been carried out in the ninth and tenth decades of life with surprising safety.

The complication encountered most frequently is wound breakdown, which occurs in well over 50% of patients in most series. This aspect of the morbidity is usually limited to skin loss at the margin of the groin incision. Removing lesser amounts of skin and decreasing the undermining of the skin flaps have reduced the incidence of wound breakdown. Suction drainage has also added to this decreasing morbidity. Careful debridement and vigorous care to keep the wounds clean and dry will almost always result in adequate healing.

Lymphedema of the lower extremities is another major problem, especially in patients who have had both inguinal and deep pelvic node dissection (Fig. 8-7). The incidence of this debilitating long-term complication can be reduced by routine use of custom-made elastic support hose during the first postoperative year while collateral pathways of lymph drainage are being developed. Rutledge has for many years advised that postlymphadenectomy patients also receive low-dose prophylactic antibiotic therapy (similar to that used to prevent subacute bacterial endocarditis) to prevent streptococcal lymphagitis in the lower extremities, which dramatically increases the incidence of lymphedema.

The development of a lymphocyst in the groin area is an infrequent occurrence, and it usually resolves spontaneously. The incidence can be lowered by careful ligation of all the lymph-bearing tissue during the groin dissection. Occasionally, intermittent aseptic aspiration of the fluid facilitates resolution of these collections.

Symptoms related to stress incontinence and the development of a cystocele or rectocele are sometimes reported by these patients. These conditions are secondary to the loss of the support of the lower end of the vagina and subsequent enlargement of the introitus. The findings may simply reflect the increased frequency of pelvic visceral prolapse among older women.

Removal of significant vulvar tissue, particularly the clitoris, can result in decreased sexual satisfaction. Loss of the subcutaneous tissue prevents mobility of the external genitalia, which can hinder sexual pleasure. Although this has been a detriment in some patients, others state that orgasm is still obtainable after vulvectomy.

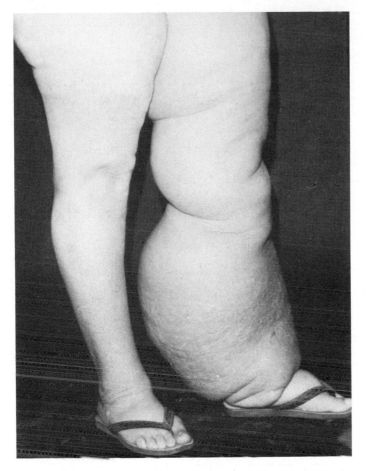

Fig. 8-7. Marked lymphedema of the left leg after inguinal and pelvic lymphadenectomy.

Survival results

Survival in cancer of the vulva is, as with all other malignancies, directly related to the extent of disease at the time that diagnosis and treatment are undertaken. Because this malignancy is initially diagnosed in the elderly woman, many of these individuals will succumb to intercurrent disease while tumor free. In stage I and II disease, the corrected 5-year survival rate should approach 90%. A 75% corrected 5-year survival rate for all stages of vulvar cancer is not unusual. If, however, the lymph nodes are negative irrespective of stage, over 90% of these patients will survive 5 years (corrected survival), whereas only a third will survive if the lymph nodes are positive (Table 8-4). Curry and associates noted that in those patients with three or less unilateral groin nodes involved with metastasis, the 5-year survival rate was still good (17/25, or 68%); however, if more than three nodes were involved, 0/5 patients survived. None of the patients with three or less unilateral involved nodes had deep pelvic node metastasis. Of the patients with more than four unilateral

Table 8-4. Survival rates for carcinoma of the vulva

Series	Status of nodes	Number of patients	Percent surviving	
			Positive	Negative
Way (1960)	Positive	45	42	
	Negative	36		77
Macafee (1962)	Positive	33	33	
	Negative	49		70
Collins and associates (1963)	Positive	19	21	
	Negative	32		69
Franklin and Rutledge (1971)	Positive	33	39	
	Negative	53		100
Morley (1976)	Positive	64	39	
	Negative	130		92
Krupp and Bahm (1978)	Positive	40	36	
	Negative	154		91
Green (1978)	Positive	46	33	
	Negative	61		87
Benedet and associates (1979)	Positive	34	53	
	Negative	86		81

Table 8-5. Survival rates for patients with positive pelvic nodes

Series	5-year survival rate (%)
Way (1957)	2/9 (22.2)
Green and associates (1958)	2/16 (12.5)
Way (1960)	3/8 (37.5)
Merrill and Ross (1961)	1/3 (33.3)
Collins and associates (1963)	1/6 (16.7)
Franklin and Rutledge (1971)	3/12 (25.0)
Morley (1976)	1/6 (16.7)
Curry and associates (1980)	2/9 (22.2)
TOTAL	15/69 (21.7)

nodes, 50% had deep pelvic node metastasis, and if bilateral groin nodes were involved, 26% had positive pelvic nodes. In those patients with positive pelvic nodes, the survival rate is poor. Collected series indicate that only one fifth of those patients with deep pelvic node metastasis survived 5 years (Table 8-5). The use of adjunctive radiation therapy in these patients is being evaluated, but no definitive statements can be made at this time concerning its effectiveness.

Recurrence

Recurrence may be local or distant, and over 80% will occur in the first 2 years after therapy, demanding close follow-up. Surprisingly, over half the recurrences are local and near the site of the primary lesion. This is more common in patients with large primary tumors and/or metastatic disease in the lymph nodes revealed at initial surgery. A study from M. D. Anderson Hospital would suggest that local recurrences are commonly seen even when the margins are declared clear on the original operative specimen. On the other hand, the high incidence of local recurrences demands careful attention to adequate margins in the removal of the primary lesion. In many instances, local recurrences can be successfully treated by local excision and/or interstitial radiation. Those patients with recurrent local disease in the lymph node area or distant disease are difficult to treat, and the salvage rate is poor.

PAGET'S DISEASE

Paget's disease of the vulva is a rare entity. Even among vulvar neoplasias it is an unusual finding. It occurs in women in the seventh decade of life but can be seen in the young patient, just as with squamous carcinoma of the vulva. Symptoms of pruritus and tenderness or the identification of a vulvar lesion are most frequently seen. These symptoms may be present for years before the patient seeks medical attention. The vulvar lesion may be localized to one labium or involve the entire vulvar epithelium. It is not unusual for the disease process to extend to the perirectal area, buttocks, inguinal area, or mons. Recently extension into the vagina itself has been reported.

Clinical and histologic features

On examination, the vulvar lesions are usually hyperemic, sharply demarcated, and thickened, with foci of excoriation and induration. Often the vulvar skin is thick and smooth, leading to the impression of leukoplakia. It is not unusual for the hyperemic areas associated with a superficial white coating to give the impression of "cake-icing effect." This finding is rather classic and, if present, is almost pathognomonic for Paget's disease (Fig. 8-8). On palpation, the vulvar changes appear to be superficial, and this maneuver is extremely important, for one must rule out an underlying adenocarcinoma, which is usually self-evident because of thickness or a masslike effect underneath the epithelial changes. It is unusual not to appreciate an underlying adenocarcinoma clinically; however, one must be diligent in taking adequate biopsies of the lesion, with regard not only to width but also to depth of tissue, for adequate histologic evaluation. It appears that there are probably two separate lesions: intraepithelial extramammary Paget's disease and Paget's disease associated with an underlying adenocarcinoma. Therapy for these two lesions is considerably different, and a definitive diagnosis is therefore imperative.

Typically, the histologic findings are that the epidermis is thickened, often acanthotic. Characteristic large cells with clear granular cytoplasm are found within the epidermis (Fig. 8-9). Often a single layer of squamous cells separates the Paget cells

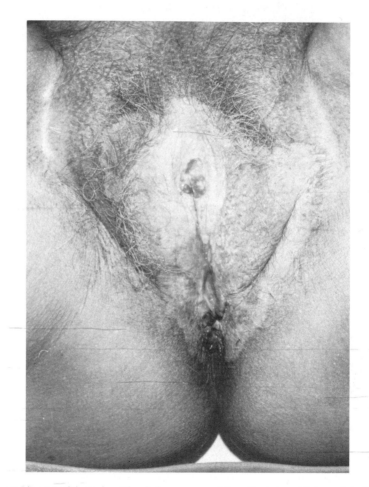

Fig. 8-8. Paget's disease of the vulva. The dark area around the clitoris is reddish, and the lighter area is white. Note the extent of disease perianally and onto the medial aspect of the left thigh.

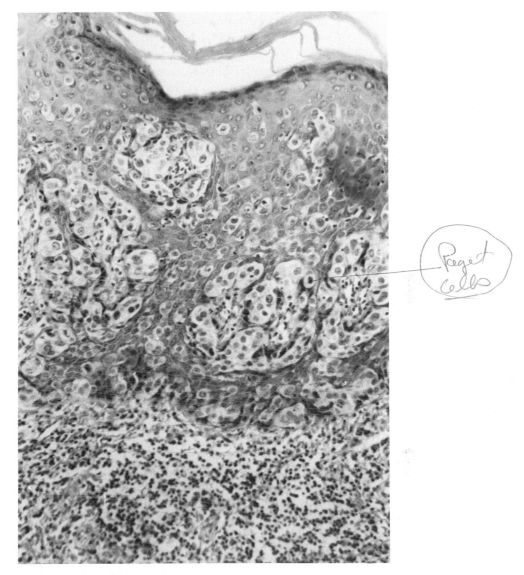

Fig. 8-9. Histologic picture of Paget's disease of the vulva. Large cells with clear cytoplasm are apparent in the epidermis. Note the heavy lymphocytic infiltration in the dermis.

from the epidermis, but neoplastic cells may be in immediate contact with the dermis. Intraepidermal formation of glands with true lumina may also be present. The hair follicles may also be involved with Paget cells. These cells contain intracytoplasmic mucin demonstrated by Mayer's mucicarmine or Alcian blue. A mixed inflammatory infiltrate of variable intensity composed usually of lymphocytes and plasma cells is present in the upper dermis. Misdiagnosis of carcinoma in situ or melanoma has been made; however, adequate tissue for evaluation and a proper clinical description would tend to eliminate this confusion. Sufficient tissue for histologic evaluation will readily identify an underlying adenocarcinoma.

Clinical course and management

If only the intraepithelial Paget's disease is present, the clinical course may be prolonged and indolent. In those patients who were originally diagnosed as having only intraepithelial Paget's disease, recurrence can occur but is seen as an intraepithelial lesion only without an underlying adenocarcinoma. From a review of our material as well as the literature, it is our opinion that when extramammary Paget's disease with an underlying adenocarcinoma is present, it is the result of simultaneous diagnoses. It appears that we are dealing with two separate disease entities and not a spectrum. Paget's disease with an underlying adenocarcinoma can be very aggressive, with metastasis to the regional lymph nodes as well as distant spread.

Since Paget's disease without an underlying adenocarcinoma appears to be a true intraepithelial neoplasia, it can be treated as such. Wide local excision to include the entire lesion is usually sufficient. Even with apparent wide margins, it is not unusual to find Paget's disease extending to the edge of the surgical margin. Histologically, one may find neoplastic cells present in normal-appearing skin for a variable, but often considerable, distance beyond the seemingly sharp margin of the clinically evident lesion. It is difficult to avoid cutting across intraepithelial tumor, and therefore intraoperative examination of the surgical margins by cryostat frozen sectioning is imperative. It is very common for recurrences to occur when the surgical margins contain neoplastic cells. These new lesions can be handled in the same manner as the primary disease, i.e., wide local excision. Since the lesion can be extensive in both the primary and recurrent stage, treatment should be given accordingly, and the use of a skin graft to cover the removed tissue may be warranted and should be used freely.

Patients in whom an underlying adenocarcinoma has been identified in association with Paget's disease of the vulva should be treated in the same manner as those individuals with other invasive malignancies of the vulva. This usually includes radical vulvectomy as well as inguinal lymphadenectomy. If the lymph nodes have no evidence of metastatic disease, the prognosis is quite good; however, if metastases are present in the lymph nodes, the prognosis is guarded. No statement concerning the role of chemotherapy in this disease entity can be made since the experience has been very limited and inconclusive.

MELANOMA

Melanoma of the vulva, although the second most common cancer occurring in this area, is still rare. This malignancy probably arises from lesions containing a junctional or compound nevus. As a result, it is suggested by some authorities that all pigmented nevi on the vulva should be prophylactically excised.

The clinical characteristics are as elsewhere on the body; melanomas are usually pigmented, raised, and may be ulcerated (Fig. 8-10). Melanomas are often misdiagnosed as undifferentiated squamous cell cancer, especially when they are histologically amelanotic. Electron microscopy can be very helpful when the diagnosis continues to be in doubt. The patient may have experienced pruritus, bleeding, or enlargement of a pigmented area. Most of the vulvar melanomas are located on the labium minora or clitoris. Prognosis is realted to the size of the lesion as well as the depth of invasion. The Clark classification, commonly used for melanomas elsewhere

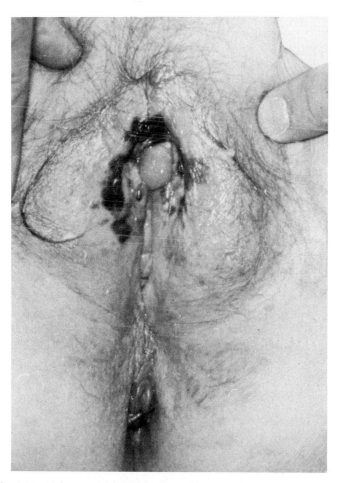

Fig. 8-10. Melanoma of the vulva. Typical pigmented neoplasm is present.

on the skin, has proved to be of prognostic benefit for the vulva also. Evidence exists that these lesions can metastasize to deep nodes in the absence of inguinal node involvement. Therapy should include a radical vulvectomy and inguinal and pelvic lymphadenectomy. If the disease is limited to the vulva, regardless of its extent, and the lymph nodes are negative, the survival rate is quite good. There are only scattered reports of survival in patients with positive nodes.

SARCOMA

Sarcoma of the vulva is rare, and even in large referral institutions the experience is quite limited. Symptoms and findings are the same as those noted with squamous carcinoma. DiSaia and associates in a review of 12 patients noted that this lesion occurred in a younger group of patients (mean age 38 years) than did other vulvar malignancies. The histologic grade of the sarcoma does appear to be the most important factor in prognosis. If a patient has an undifferentiated rhabdomyosarcoma, prognosis is quite poor, since these lesions tend to grow and metastasize very rapidly. However, a well-differentiated leiomyosarcoma will be slow growing and develop late recurrences. Therapy generally would be radical vulvectomy and bilateral inguinal lymphadenectomy except in the low-grade lesions, where nodal involvement is rare and wide local excision should be considered. Those patients undergoing wide local excision are at risk of local recurrence and should be observed closely.

BARTHOLIN'S GLAND CARCINOMA

Adenocarcinoma of Bartholin's gland is a rare lesion occurring only in about 1% of all vulvar malignancies. The peak incidence is in the mid-sixties, although it has been reported in a teenager. Because of its location, the tumor can be of considerable size before the patient is aware of symptoms. Dyspareunia may be one of the first symptoms, although the finding of a mass or ulcerative lesion may be the first indication to the patient of her disease process. An enlargement in the Bartholin gland area occurring in a postmenopausal woman should be considered a malignancy until proved otherwise. The lesion can have a tendency to spread in the ischiorectal fossa and can have a propensity for not only lymphatic spread to the inguinal nodes via the common lymphatic spread for vulvar cancer but also for posterior spread to the pelvic nodes directly. Almost half of all carcinomas said to be of Bartholin gland origin are squamous carcinomas. In most instances, strict histologic criteria have not been followed. Every attempt should be made to differentiate between a true Bartholin gland cancer and a squamous carcinoma of the vulva arising in proximity to the Bartholin gland. Prognosis is good if lymph node metastasis is not present.

Therapy includes radical vulvectomy with a large, wide, extensive dissection around the gland along with inguinal and pelvic lymphadenectomy. A considerable amount of vagina and, on occasion, part of the rectum may need to be removed in order to have adequate margins.

BASAL CELL CARCINOMA

Basal cell carcinoma is usually small, occurs on the labium majora, and may have a central ulceration. The stromal infiltration is usually circumscribed and orderly and, as elsewhere in the body, has a slow and indolent growth rate and rarely if ever involves the lymphatics. Local excision is quite adequate, with primary closure the usual rule. If a large lesion is present after local excision, a skin graft may be applied. Basal cell carcinoma must be differentiated pathologically from the so-called baso-squamous cell carcinoma, which must be treated as one would a squamous carcinoma of the vulva.

BIBLIOGRAPHY

Benedet, J. L., Turko, M., Fairey, R. N., and Boyes, D. A.: Squamous carcinoma of the vulva; results of treatment, 1938 to 1976, Am. J. Obstet. Gynecol. **134**:201, 1979.

Boronow, R. C.: Therapeutic alternative to primary exenteration for advanced vulvo-vaginal cancer, Gynecol. Oncol. **1**:233, 1973.

Boyce, C. R., and Mehran, A. H.: Management of vulvar malignancies, Am. J. Obstet. Gynecol. **119**:49, 1974.

Cabanas, R. M.: An approach to the treatment of penile carcinoma, Cancer **39**:456, 1977.

Curry, S. L., Wharton, J. T., and Rutledge, F.: Positive lymph nodes in vulvar squamous carcinoma, Gynecol. Oncol. **9**:63, 1980.

Daly, J. W., and Million, R. R.: Radical vulvectomy combined with elective node irradiation for T_xN_0 squamous carcinoma of the vulva, Cancer **34**:161, 1974.

DiPaola, G. R., Gomez-Rueda, N., and Arrighi, L.: Relevance of microinvasion in carcinoma of the vulva, J. Obstet. Gynecol. **45**:647, 1975.

DiSaia, P. J., Creasman, W. T., and Rich, W. M.: An alternate approach to early cancer of the vulva, Am. J. Obstet. Gynecol. **133**:825, 1979.

DiSaia, P. J., Rutledge, F. N., and Smith, J. P.: Sarcoma of the vulva, Obstet. Gynecol. **38**:180, 1971.

Forney, J. P., Morrow, C. P., Townsend, D. E., and DiSaia, P. J.: Management of carcinoma in situ of the vulva, Am. J. Obstet. Gynecol. **127**:8, 1977.

Franklin, E. W. III, and Rutledge, F. N.: Prognostic factors in epidermoid carcinoma of the vulva, Obstet. Gynecol. **37**:892, 1971.

Franklin, E. W. III, and Rutledge, F. N.: Epidemiology of epidermoid carcinoma of the vulva, Obstet. Gynecol. **39**:165, 1972.

Goss, C. M., editor: Gray's anatomy, ed. 29, Philadelphia, 1973, Lea & Febiger.

Green, T. H.: Carcinoma of the vulva, a reassessment, Obstet. Gynecol. **52**:462, 1978.

Helgason, N. M., Hass, A. C., and Latamette, H. G.: Radiation therapy in carcinoma of the vulva, Cancer **30**:997, 1972.

Hughes, R. P.: Early diagnosis and management of premalignant lesions and early invasive cancers of the vulva, South. Med. J. **64**:1490, 1971.

Jafari, K., and Cartnick, E. N.: Microinvasive squamous cell carcinoma of the vulva, Am. J. Obstet. Gynecol. **125**:274, 1976.

Japaze, H., Garcia-Bunel, R., and Woodruff, J. D.: Primary vulvar neoplasia, Obstet. Gynecol. **49**:404, 1977.

Kaufman, R. H., and Woodruff, J. D.: Historical background in developmental stages of the new nomenclature, J. Reprod. Med. **17**:133, 1976.

Krupp, P. J., and Bahm, J. W.: Lymph gland metastases in invasive squamous cell cancer of the vulva, Am. J. Obstet. Gynecol. **130**:943, 1978.

Kuppers, T.: Carcinoma of the vulva, Radiol. Clin. **44**:475, 1975.

Morley, G. W.: Infiltrative carcinoma of the vulva; results of surgical treatment, Am. J. Obstet. Gynecol. **124**:874, 1976.

Morris, J. M.: A formula for selective lymphadenectomy, its application in cancer of the vulva, Obstet. Gynecol. **50**:152, 1977.

Morrow, C. P., and Rutledge, F. N.: Melanoma of the vulva, Obstet. Gynecol. **39**:745, 1972.

Nakao, C. Y., and others: "Microinvasive" epidermoid carcinoma of the vulva with an unexpected natural history, Am. J. Obstet. Gynecol. **120**:1123, 1974.

Parker, R. T., Duncan, I., Rampone, J., and Creasman, W. T.: Operative management of early invasive epidermoid carcinoma of the vulva, Am. J. Obstet. Gynecol. **123**:349, 1975.

Piver, M. S., and Xymos, F. P.: Pelvic lymphadenectomy in women with carcinoma of the clitoris, Obstet. Gynecol. **49**:592, 1977.

Plentl, A. A., and Friedman, E. A.: Lymphatic system of the female genitalia, Philadelphia, 1971, W. B. Saunders Co.

Rutledge, F., and Sinclair, M.: Treatment of intraepithelial carcinoma of the vulva by skin excision and graft, Am. J. Obstet. Gynecol. **102:**806, 1968.

Rutledge, F., Smith, J. P., and Franklin, E. K.: Carcinoma of the vulva, Am. J. Obstet. Gynecol. **106:**1117, 1970.

Shingleton, H. M., Fowler, W. C., Palumbo, L.,

and others: Carcinoma of the vulva, influence of radical operation on cure rate, Obstet. Gynecol. **35:**1, 1970.

Way, S.: The surgery of vulvar carcinoma; an appraisal, Clin. Obstet. Gynecol. **5**(3):623, 1978.

Wharton, J. T., Gallager, S., and Rutledge, F. N.: Microinvasive carcinoma of the vulva, Am. J. Obstet. Gynecol. **118:**159, 1974.

Yazigi, R., Piver, M. S., and Tsukada, Y.: Microinvasive carcinoma of the vulva, Obstet. Gynecol. **123:**349, 1975.

CHAPTER NINE

Invasive cancer of the vagina and urethra

Squamous cancer of the vagina
Rare vaginal cancers
    Adenocarcinoma
    Sarcoma
    Malignant melanoma
Urethral cancer

SQUAMOUS CANCER OF THE VAGINA
Clinical profile

It is interesting that there is a greater frequency of malignant disease in the organs situated on either end of the vaginal canal than in the vagina itself. Indeed, one may say that primary cancer of the vagina is one of the rarest of the malignant processes in the human body (Table 9-1). The relative immunity of the vaginal tissues to malignant change is in sharp contrast to the uterine cervix. When primary cancer does occur in the vagina, it usually is in the upper half (Table 9-2), and it is generally epidermoid carcinoma. By convention, any malignant neoplasm involving both the cervix and vagina that is histologically compatible with origin in either organ is classified as cervical cancer. The age incidence of this disease is between 35 and 70 years. If the lesion arises in the upper portion of the vagina, extension occurs in much the same pattern as seen in cervical carcinoma; metastasis to obturator, iliac, and hypogastric lymph nodes is the usual spread pattern. If the lesion is low in the vagina, extension is similar to that observed in carcinoma of the vulva; inguinal nodes are involved early, with later extension to the deep pelvic nodes.

Secondary carcinoma of the vagina is seen much more frequently than primary disease. Extensions of cervical cancer to the vagina probably account for the greatest

Table 9-1. Incidence of vaginal cancer

Series	Number of genital malignancies	Percent vaginal cancer
Smith (1955)	8,199	1.5
Ries and Ludwig (1962)	14,785	2.1
Smith (1964)	6,050	1.8
Wolff and Douyon (1964)	4,665	1.8
Rutledge (1967)	5,715	1.2
Palumbo and associates (1969)	2,305	1.9
Daw (1971)	564	1.9

Table 9-2. Involvement of vagina

Series	Upper third	Middle third	Lower third
Livingstone (1950)	34	4	42
Bivens (1953)	22	3	14
Mobius (1956)	89	0	29
Arronet and associates (1960)	14	8	3
Whelton and Kottmeier (1962)	20	13	19
Blunt (1965)	13	15	10
Daw (1971)	24	14	13
TOTAL	216 (54%)	57 (14%)	130 (32%)

number of so-called vaginal cancers. In addition, true secondary lesions from more remote foci are not infrequently seen. Examples are cancers of the endometrium, ovary, urethra or bladder, and rectum and malignant trophoblastic disease. Primary lesions are usually in the histologic classification of squamous carcinoma. Melanoma, sarcoma, and recently adenocarcinoma have also been described as primary vaginal cancers. Most of the adenocarcinomas reported in the last decade have been secondary to intrauterine exposure to synthetic estrogen products.

The cause of squamous carcinoma of the vagina is unknown. The predominance of lesions in the upper third and on the posterior wall of the vagina (Fig. 9-1) has led to speculation concerning accumulation of irritating or macerating substances pooling in the posterior fornix and producing a chronic irritation leading to a malignant degeneration. Reports have been published concerning possible predisposing factors, such as use of a vaginal pessary, prolapse of the vaginal wall, syphilis, leukorrhea, and "leukoplakia," but none of these hypotheses has been validated.

The signs and symptoms of invasive vaginal cancer are very similar to those of cervical cancer. Vaginal discharge, often bloody, is the most frequent symptom in most series. Many patients with invasive lesions present with irregular or postmenopausal vaginal bleeding, and a gross lesion is obvious on speculum examination. Urinary symptoms are more common than with cervical cancer because neoplasms lower in the vagina are in close proximity to the vesicle neck with resulting compres-

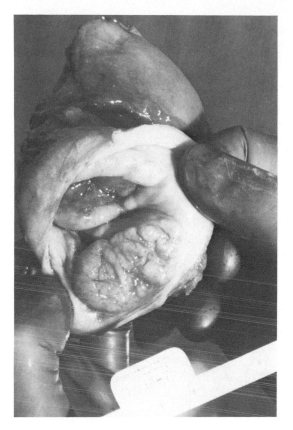

Fig. 9-1. Lesion of the posterior fornix in squamous cell carcinoma.

sion of the bladder at an earlier stage of the disease. As the lesion spreads locally it will often involve the paracolpium, bladder, rectum, and/or vulva. The elasticity of the posterior vaginal fornix allows lesions in this area to become quite large, especially in the sexually inactive elderly woman. The decreased distensibility of the anterior vaginal wall, creating bladder symptoms, would seem to favor these lesions in terms of early recognition and curability. However, the reverse is true, possibly because of early involvement of adjacent structures such as the bladder neck and urethra. The diagnosis of vaginal cancer is usually delayed. Several general explanations have been offered for this observation. Many patients are elderly, sexually inactive, and unlikely to have periodic vaginal examinations. In addition, the lesions are rare, and physicians often fail to consider the possibility until the patient has symptoms of advanced disease.

Lymphatic drainage of the vagina

The lymphatic vasculature of the vagina begins as an extremely fine capillary meshwork in the mucosa and submucosa (Fig. 9-2). In the deep layers of the sub-

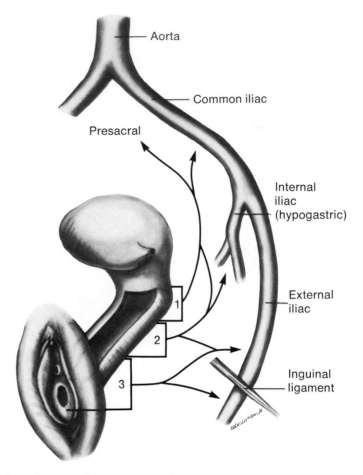

Fig. 9-2. Lymphatic drainage of the vagina: *(1)* channels from the lower third drain into femoral and external iliac nodes, *(2)* channels from the middle third drain into hypogastric nodes, *(3)* channels from the upper third drain into common iliac, presacral, and hypogastric nodes. (Modified from Plentl, A. A., and Friedman, E. A.: Lymphatic system of the female genitalia, Philadelphia, 1971, W. B. Saunders Co.)

mucosa and muscularis, there is a similar, parallel, but coarser network. Irregular anastomoses have been demonstrated between the two. Both systems drain into small trunks that combine at the lateral aspect of the vagina and form a number of collecting trunks. It is at this point that the efferent lymph drainage channels of the organ begin. The lymphatic trunks of the upper vagina drain into the most dorsal group of iliac nodes, usually represented by the common iliac and hypogastric nodes. The distal, or lower, vagina is drained by a lymphatic network that anastomoses with that of the vestibule to end in the regional lymph nodes of the femoral triangle. The lymphatic system of the vagina is complex, and the simple patterns suggested here are not necessarily always accurate. The course and destination of lymphatic channels from specific regions of the vagina are not entirely consistent, and there is a great deal of crossover. All lymph nodes in the pelvis may at one time or another serve as primary sites or regional drainage nodes for vaginal lymph and its contents.

Staging

Patients with invasive squamous cell carcinoma or other cancers of the vagina should be investigated for evidence of local or distant spread in a manner analogous to cervical cancer. All patients should have at least the following diagnostic studies in addition to a thorough history and physical examination: chest film, IVP, cystoscopy, and proctosigmoidoscopy. Optional, but often helpful, studies are lymphangiogram and barium enema. Barium enema is definitely indicated for patients suspected of having recent diverticulitis, because it may be important in planning radiation therapy for that individual. Staging according to FIGO is clinical and not surgical; a summary of the staging classification is as follows:

Stage I: Carcinoma is limited to the vaginal mucosa.
Stage II: Carcinoma has involved the subvaginal tissue but has not extended onto the pelvic wall.
Stage III: Carcinoma has extended onto the pelvic wall.
Stage IV: Carcinoma has extended beyond the true pelvis or has involved the mucosa of the bladder or rectum. Bullous edema or tumor bulge into the bladder or rectum is not acceptable evidence of invasion of these organs.

Management

Those cases of squamous carcinoma reported in the gynecologic literature have been treated primarily by radiotherapy. Treatment is tailored to the stage and extent of the disease. Large carcinomas of the vault or vaginal walls are treated initially with external irradiation. This shrinks the neoplasm so that local radiation therapy will be more effective. Cancers of the upper vagina in patients with an intact uterus are treated with techniques similar to those used for carcinoma of the cervix. External irradiation in a dose of 4,000 to 5,000 rads is given initially in bulky stage I and stage II cancers (Table 9-3). In some centers, upon completion of external therapy, vaginal ovoids plus an intrauterine tandem (Fletcher-Suit or similar applicators) are used to deliver a surface dose of 6,000 rads in 72 hours or 8,000 rads in 2 applications

Table 9-3. Radiotherapy of vaginal cancer

Stage	External irradiation	Vaginal therapy
Stage 0	Surgical excision preferred for localized disease	7,000 rads surface dose
Stage I		
1-2 cm lesion	Omit	Interstitial irradiation, 6,000-7,000 rads
Larger lesions	4,000-5,000 rads whole pelvis	Interstitial implant delivering 3,000-4,000 rads
Stage II	4,000-5,000 rads whole pelvis	Same as above
Stage III	5,000 rads whole pelvis optional (1,000-2,000 rads through reduced fields)	Interstitial implant, 2,000-3,000 rads (if tumor regression is optimal)
Stage IV (pelvis only)	Same as above	Same as above

of 48 hours each separated by 2 weeks, depending on the initial thickness and regression of the lesion. An interstitial implant is considered by others to be judicious instead of, or in combination with, the intracavitary technique described above. If the uterus has been previously removed, local therapy must be individualized, and one should consider the following: (1) ovoids, (2) transvaginal cone, and (3) an interstitial implant. Stage III and IV lesions anywhere in the vagina are treated initially with 5,000 rads external radiation over 5 to 6 weeks. The deep nodes must of course be included in the treatment fields, since large tumors have a high incidence of regional lymphatic metastasis. After receiving 5,000 rads, the patient should be reevaluated for an additional 1,000 to 2,000 rads external radiation to reduced fields. An interstitial implant in the residual disease is usually needed for these large neoplasms. A large-volume implant is often best delivered using a Syed/Neblet applicator (Fig. 9-3) and its accompanying perineal template (Fig. 9-4) to achieve a comprehensive isodose distribution (Fig. 9-5) to the paracolpium. Tumors involving the distal one third of the vagina frequently metastasize to the inguinal nodes, and these nodes are best treated by radical inguinal dissection. Postoperative radiation therapy can be delivered following inguinal lymphadenectomy. Small carcinomas of the vagina may be treated with interstitial radiation therapy alone; a single or double plane or even a volume implant may be necessary, depending on the location of the cancer. In most instances a minimum of 6,000 to 7,000 rads will be delivered to the neoplasm in 5 to 7 days.

In general, the treatment plan with regard to radiation therapy must consider the depth of invasion of the lesion. Lesions with appreciable invasion of the paracolpium must be treated with whole-pelvis irradiation followed by an interstitial implant in the tumor bed. As stated above, some have preferred intracavitary vaginal applicators to deliver the local radiation. However, interstitial therapy should be strongly considered for most patients, since surface applicators deliver a poor depth

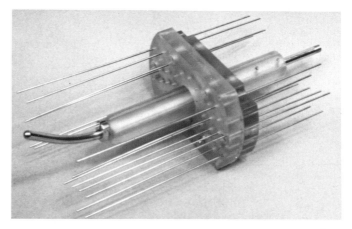

Fig. 9-3. Interstitial-intracavitary implant (Syed/Neblett applicator).

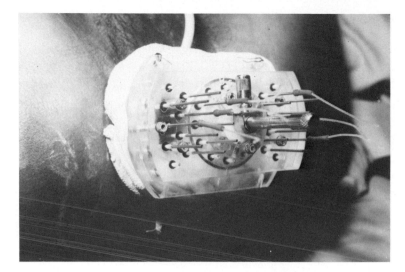

Fig. 9-4. Implant procedure completed.

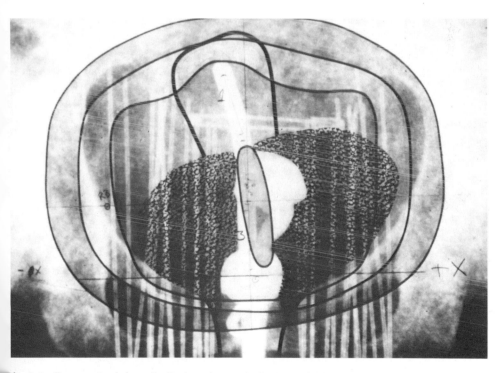

Fig. 9-5. Computerized dose distribution plot overlaid on x-ray localization film. There is extensive involvement of the parametria as well as the paracolpium.

dose to the submucosal tissue. An exception to the above recommendations may be valid in institutions where skilled personnel can give transvaginal external irradiation instead of interstitial irradiation to shallow residual lesions. Although one is often dealing with a radiosensitive neoplasm in a relatively radioresistant bed (the vagina), serious limitations may exist nonetheless. The proximity of relatively radiosensitive normal tissues, such as the bladder and rectum, provides a real challenge to the therapist, especially in the treatment of tumors located in the lower third of the vagina. Proper planning of radiation therapy and individualization of treatment plans are essential to minimize the more serious complications of acute and long-term radiation sequelae in these organs. The difficulty in applying radiation systems to vaginal cancer led some, such as Wertheim and Brunschwig, to advocate radical surgery as primary therapy. However, the complications associated with these radical procedures, especially in older patients, have become a serious limiting factor to the surgical approach. Our belief is that in most instances radical surgery should be reserved for radiation failures.

Survival results

Survival of patients with vaginal cancer has improved to a point where the pessimism detailed in the older literature can be abandoned. In a review of 104 patients, Smith (1955) found 6.8% survivors among 29 patients with cancer of the lower third of the vagina, 25.0% in 48 patients with middle-third tumors, and 37.0% in 27 patients with upper-third lesions. In 1958 Merrill and Bender reported a 29% survival rate in 14 patients with upper-third lesions and an 11% rate in 9 patients with distal-third involvement. A more encouraging study by Rutledge in 1967 reported 3- and 5-year survival rates of 42% and 44%, respectively, for patients treated primarily with radiotherapy. Comparable survival results were reported by Prempree and associates using radiotherapy for stage I (83%), stage II (63%), stage III (40%), and stage IV (0%) lesions at 5 years. Their absolute 5-year cure rate for all stages was 55.5%. A recent and still more encouraging report from the Rutledge service (M. D. Anderson Hospital) by Krepart and associates reveals considerable improvement, especially in early lesions (Table 9-4).

Table 9-4. Vaginal cancer

Stage	Number of patients	5-year (absolute) survival rate
I	25	65%
II	39	60%
III	28	35%
IV	22	39%
Overall	114	51%

Modified from Krepart, G., and others: Invasive squamous cell carcinoma of the vagina, Gynecol. Oncol., in press.

Recurrence

These neoplasms appear to behave like cervical or vulvar epidermoid cancer by first recurring locally. Over 80% of patients with recurrent disease have a pelvic recurrence noted clinically, and most recurrences occur within 2 years of primary therapy. Distant sites of involvement occur later and much less frequently. Recurrent or persistent vaginal cancer requires ultraradical surgery of an exenterative type, and very little has been written specifically on this subject. Recently, Krepart and associates reported a 51% overall recurrence rate in their series on vaginal cancers, and 40% of the patients with recurrent or persistent disease responded (apparent cures) when radical surgical procedures were carried out. Therefore, radiation therapy should be planned carefully, and the therapist should prepare for reevaluation of the patient during therapy for possible alterations in the treatment plan to give optimum results. Chemotherapy for recurrent squamous cell carcinoma of the vagina has in the past been relatively ineffectual, but cis-platinum appears to be an active agent when used in a manner similar to that for recurrent cervical cancer.

Special problems

Pride and Buchler suggested that vaginal carcinoma may occur more frequently in patients who had received pelvic irradiation 10 or more years before the appearance of the new lesion. The more frequent incidence of vaginal cancer with radiation therapy (5 or more years previously) than in those treated for cervical cancer with surgery was also noted by Murad and associates. The occurrance of abnormal vaginal cytologic findings following radiation is common, and many have ignored these dysplastic lesions as if they were a routine result of irradiation therapy. However, recently presented material from M. D. Anderson Hospital would suggest that 30% of these "dysplastic" or "intraepithelial" lesions will progress to invasive cancer if left untreated. In this report, 28 patients with dysplasia or carcinoma in situ of the vagina following previous pelvic radiation therapy were observed for progression, and nine developed invasive carcinoma. The median length of time from diagnosis of the intraepithelial lesion to invasion was 33.7 months. Therefore, treatment of these intraepithelial lesions by local excision or topical chemotherapy with 5-fluorouracil should be seriously considered.

Boronow has emphasized the possible role of radiation therapy in vulvovaginal cancers. His report dealt mostly with advanced disease involving a great deal of vaginal mucous membrane as well as the vulva, necessitating an exenterative type of procedure if a primary surgical approach were used. As an alternative he recommended surgical extirpation of the inguinal lymph nodes with a combination of external and interstitial irradiation for control of the central lesion. His results were encouraging.

When vaginal cancer occurs in a hysterectomized patient, the geometry is usually very unfavorable for local radiation therapy. In addition, the close proximity of the bladder base and urethra makes the risks of a urinary-vaginal fistula appreciable

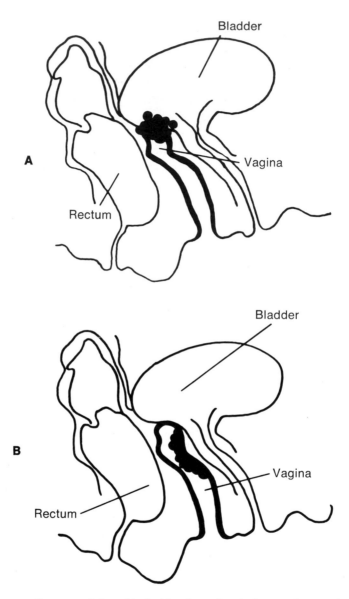

Fig. 9-6. Diagrammatic representation of typical locations of vaginal cancer in a previously hysterecto-mized patient illustrating the proximity of the bladder and urethra. **A,** Lesion at vaginal apex. **B,** Lesion at upper anterior vaginal wall. (Courtesy A. Robert Kagan, M.D., Los Angeles, California.)

(Fig. 9-6). Therapy must be individualized, and radical surgery should be held in reserve for failures. The radiotherapist must be flexible, using combinations of external radiation with transvaginal and/or interstitial and/or intracavitary therapy as necessary.

Barclay reported on 14 patients treated for intraepithelial or invasive cancer of the vagina subsequent to hysterectomy for severe dysplasia or carcinoma in situ of the cervix. He recommended partial or complete vaginectomy for in situ as well as early invasive disease. In all 14 of his patients the vaginal apex was involved. He found the bladder densely adherent to the cuff, and in two instances it was entered. When a total vaginectomy was necessary, a point was made to preserve at least 2 cm of vaginal mucosa proximal to the urethrovesical angle or to cover the denuded angle with a split-thickness skin graft. Postoperative radiation therapy was given to patients with early invasive disease following radical vaginectomy. The radical surgical approach allows removal of the medial parametrial and paravaginal tissues above the "ears" at the angles of the vagina on each side.

RARE VAGINAL CANCERS
Adenocarcinoma

Before 1965 adenocarcinoma arising in the vagina was one of the rarest gynecologic diseases. Rare case reports had been traceable to origins in paramesonephric epithelium, mesonephric remnants, and endometriosis. In 1971 Herbst and associates reported on eight cases of clear-cell adenocarcinoma of the vagina (see Chapter 2). This dramatic clustering of cases initiated an epidemiologic study that demonstrated an association of this malignancy with maternal ingestion of diethylstilbestrol (DES), a nonsteroidal estrogenic substance that in the previous 2 decades was sporadically used in the management of diabetic pregnancies, threatened abortion, habitual abortion, and other high-risk obstetric problems. The association of maternal ingestion of DES and subsequent development of clear-cell adenocarcinoma of the vagina in female offspring was confirmed in a national registry established by Herbst and associates. In 1979 the world registry contained approximately 340 cases of clear-cell adenocarcinoma of the vagina. In the cases where a maternal history was obtainable, two out of three were positive for ingestion of medication such as DES or chemically related estrogens. The youngest patient was 7 years of age at the time of diagnosis and the oldest 29 years, with a peak frequency at 19.5 years for those patients with a history of DES exposure. The risk of development of these carcinomas in the DES-exposed female through the age of 24 years has been calculated at 0.14 to 1.4 per 1,000. At the time of the 1978 report from the registry, 243 of 341 (71%) were free of disease, with the longest interval from diagnosis to the most recent examination being 11.3 years. Sixty-eight patients had recurrent disease, and 58 had died at the time of the report.

The preferred therapy for clear-cell carcinoma of the vagina and cervix has not been established. Approximately 40% of the cases do occur in the cervix and the other 60% primarily in the upper half of the vagina. The incidence of lymph node metastasis is fairly high: approximately 18% in stage I and 30% or more in stage II. If the neoplasm is confined to the cervix and upper vagina, radical hysterectomy and upper vaginectomy with pelvic lymphadenectomy are the recommended therapy, with preservation of the ovaries. More advanced tumors and lesions involving the lower vagina are more suitable for irradiation, which should include treatment of the pelvic nodes and parametrial tissues. Survival statistics are comparable to those for the squamous counterparts occurring in the cervix and upper vagina.

Rare cases of primary adenocarcinoma of the vagina occur unrelated to intrauterine DES exposure and often in postmenopausal women. These have been recognized and reported more frequently in the last decade because of the DES disclosures. Therapy for these adenocarcinomas is presently analogous to that for their squamous counterpart.

Sarcoma

Spindle cell sarcomas of the vagina such as leiomyosarcoma and fibrosarcoma have been rarely reported. Tavassoli and Norris reported on 60 smooth muscle tumors of the vagina. Only five neoplasms recurred, and these were all greater than 3 cm with more than five mitotic figures per ten HPF. Local excision was the treatment of choice when the tumor was well differentiated and well circumscribed and the margins were not infiltrated. In general, these lesions behave in a manner quite similar to their corresponding cell types on the vulva in that the well-differentiated lesions have a much better prognosis than the pleomorphic types, which tend to have a very poor prognosis regardless of therapy. The vagina, like the vulva, has a rich lymphatic and vascular network, possibly contributing to the early dissemination of these neoplasms (especially the pleomorphic types). In general, hematogenous dissemination occurs surprisingly late in the course of the disease, so that the importance of local therapy is underlined. However, after local excision of a circumscribed lesion and local radiation therapy postoperatively, the value of pelvic radiation therapy is unclear. In most instances where it has been successfully applied, the lesions were well differentiated and well circumscribed, suggesting that surgery itself was curative.

Another unusual and tragic lesion that predominately afflicts children is sarcoma botryoides (Fig. 9-7). These lesions are usually multicentric and tend to arise in the anterior wall at the apex of the vagina.

Malignant melanoma

Malignant melanoma of the vagina is very rare and comprises less than 0.5% of all vaginal malignancies. Multiple therapies have been attempted over the past several decades, and surgery remains the treatment of choice. The surgical approach must be tailored to the location of the lesions. Neoplasms that involve the lower third of the vagina are usually treated in a manner similar to vulvar melanoma, with radical vulvectomy and inguinal as well as deep node dissection. Those neoplasms that involve the upper two thirds of the vagina require some form of exenteration for

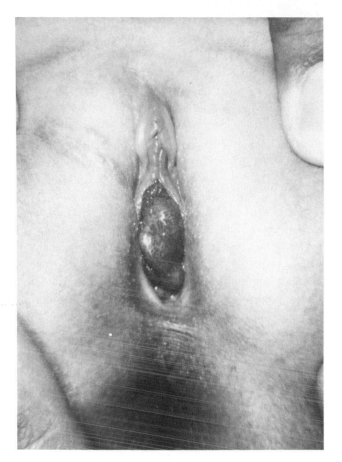

Fig. 9-7. Sarcoma botryoides (rhabdomyosarcoma) in a 10-month-old child.

optimum results. Radiation therapy has not proved to be effective, and the results of chemotherapy have been equally disappointing; thus, the radical surgical approach remains the primary therapy where applicable. Survival figures for this group of lesions are difficult to arrive at because of their infrequent occurrence. However, it would appear that the survival rate is quite poor if any nodes are found to be positive. The value of adjuvant chemotherapy in such instances has been disappointing to date. Patients who have disease involving the upper two thirds of the vagina and are treated by exenteration with negative nodes have roughly a 50% probability of surviving 5 years or more.

URETHRAL CANCER

The majority of urethral lesions are squamous growths originating from the mucosa and, less commonly, adenocarcinomas originating from the paraurethral ducts. Sarcomas and melanomas have been described rarely. Lesions of the distal third of the urethra present as elongated growths palpable through the anterior vaginal wall or as exophytic neoplasms obscuring the urethral orifice. Since they can be confused with a urethral carbuncle, urethral polyp, or mucosal ectropion, biopsy should be done to clarify the issue.

Unlike in vulvar cancer, the role of radiotherapy in this lesion is substantial. The proximal half of the urethra must be preserved to ensure urinary continence. This often leads to local failure when a surgical approach is chosen as the sole modality. Interstitial irradiation to the central lesion has thus gained wide acceptance for this site. Our recommendation has been to dissect the inguinal lymph nodes as both a diagnostic and a therapeutic procedure. Discovery of lymph node metastases should be followed by pelvic as well as local irradiation. Pelvic lymphadenectomy is usually omitted even with positive inguinal nodes, since whole-pelvis irradiation should follow as soon as the groin incisions have healed. In our experience, radiation therapy alone has been less successful in controlling groin metastases, leading to the difficult problem of a fungating necrotic lesion eroding through the skin of the groin in a previously irradiated area. No instances of local groin failure have resulted from removal of the inguinal node metastases with subsequent radiation therapy. Lesions of the distal urethra appear to have a better prognosis than those of the upper lumen. The poor results in carcinoma of the upper urethra appear to be due to early lymphatic dissemination to inaccessible pelvic and para-aortic nodes.

BIBLIOGRAPHY

Arronet, G. H., Latour, J. P. A., and Tremblay, P. C.: Primary carcinoma of the vagina, Am. J. Obstet. Gynecol. **79**:455, 1960.

Barclay, D. L.: Carcinoma of the vagina after hysterectomy for severe dysplasia or carcinoma in situ of the cervix, Gynecol. Oncol. **8**:1, 1979.

Bivens, M. D.: Primary carcinoma of the vagina; a report of forty-six cases, Am. J. Obstet. Gynecol. **65**:390, 1953.

Blunt, V. A. W.: Primary carcinoma of the vagina, Aust. N.Z. J. Obstet. Gynecol. **5**:29, 1965.

Boronow, R. C.: Therapeutic alternative to primary exenteration for advanced vulvovaginal cancer, Gynecol. Oncol. **1**:233, 1973.

Brown, A. R., Fletcher, G. H., and Rutledge, F. N.: Irradiation of in situ and invasive squamous cell carcinoma of the vagina, Cancer **28**:1278, 1971.

Chan, P. M.: Radiotherapeutic management of malignant tumor of the vagina, Am. J. Roentgenol. **89**:502, 1963.

Clement, P. B., and Benedet, J. L.: Adenocarcinoma in situ of the vagina, Cancer **43**:2479, 1979.

Daly, J. W., and Million, R. R.: Radical vulvectomy combined with elective node irradiation for T_xN_0 squamous carcinoma of the vulva, Cancer **34**:161, 1974.

Daw, E.: Primary carcinoma of the vagina, J. Obstet. Gynaecol. Br. Comm. **78**:853, 1971.

Dunn, L. J., and others: Primary carcinoma of vagina, Am. J. Obstet. Gynecol. **96**:1112, 1966.

Fagan, G. E., and Hertig, A. T.: Carcinoma of the female urethra, Obstet. Gynecol. **6**:1, 1955.

Flamant, F., and others: Embryonal rhabdomyosarcoma of the vagina in children—conservative treatment with curietherapy and chemotherapy, Cancer **15**:527, 1979.

Franklin, E. W. III, and Rutledge, F. N.: Prognostic factors in epidermoid carcinoma of the vulva, Cancer **30**:997, 1972.

Frick, H. C., and others: Primary carcinoma of the vagina, Am. J. Obstet. Gynecol. **101**:695, 1968.

Fricke, R. E., Van Herik, M., and Soule, E. H.: Treatment of rare lesions on the uterus and vagina, Radiology **63**:353, 1954.

Gray, L., and others: In situ and early invasive carcinoma of vagina, Obstet. Gynecol. **34**:226, 1969.

Greenwald, P., and others: Vaginal cancer after maternal treatment with synthetic estrogens, N. Engl. J. Med. **285**:390, 1971.

Helgason, N. M., Hass, A. C., and Latamette, H. B.: Radiation therapy in carcinoma of the vulva, Cancer **30**:997, 1972.

Herbst, A. L.: Current data from the clear cell adenocarcinoma registry. Presented at the Fifth Annual Meeting of the Society of Gynecologic Oncologists, Key Biscayne, Fla., January 9, 1974.

Herbst, A. L., editor: Intrauterine exposure to diethylstilbestrol in the human, Chicago, 1978, American College of Obstetricians and Gynecologists.

Herbst, A. L., Green, T. H., and Ulfelder, H.: Primary carcinoma of vagina, Am. J. Obstet. Gynecol. **106**:210, 1970.

Herbst, A. L., Ulfelder, H., and Roskunzer, D. C.: Adenocarcinoma of the vagina; association of maternal stilbestrol therapy with tumor appearance in young women, N. Engl. J. Med. **284**:878, 1971.

Herbst, A. L., and others: Clear cell adenocarcinoma of the genital tract in young females; registry report, N. Engl. J. Med. **287**:1259, 1972.

Huffman, J. W.: The gynecology of childhood and adolescence, Philadelphia, 1968, W. B. Saunders Co.

Ingemanson, C., and Alfredsson, J.: Recurrent fibromyoma of the vagina, Acta Obstet. Gynecol. Scand. **49**:271, 1970.

Japaze, H., Garcia-Bunuel, R., and Woodruff, J. D.: Primary vulvar neoplasia, Obstet. Gynecol. **49**:404, 1977.

Kaufman, R. H., and Gardner, H. L.: Tumors of the vulva and vagina; benign mesodermal tumors, Clin. Obstet. Gynecol. **8**:953, 1965.

Krepart, G., and others: Invasive squamous cell carcinoma of the vagina, Gynecol. Oncol., in press.

Krupp, P. J., and Bahm, J. W.: Lymph gland metastases in invasive squamous cell cancer of the vulva, Am. J. Obstet. Gynecol. **130**:943, 1978.

Kuppers, T.: Carcinoma of the vulva, Radiol. Clin. **44**:475, 1975.

Latourette, H. B.: End results of treatment of cancer of vagina, Ann. N.Y. Acad. Sci. **114**:1020, 1964.

Livingstone, R. G.: Primary carcinoma of the vagina, Springfield, Ill., Charles C Thomas, Publisher.

Mahesh Kumar, A. P., Wrenn, E. L., Jr., Fleming, I. D., and others: Combined therapy to prevent complete pelvic exenteration for rhabdomyosarcoma of the vagina or uterus, Cancer **37**:118, 1976.

Marcus, R., Jr., Million, R. R., and Daly, J. W.: Carcinoma of the vagina, Cancer **42**:2507, 1978.

Marley, G. W.: Infiltrative cancer of the vulva; results of surgical treatment, Am. J. Obstet. Gynecol. **87**:762, 1963.

Merrill, J. A., and Bender, W. T.: Primary carcinoma of the vagina, Obstet. Gynecol. **11**:3, 1958.

Mobius, W.: Uber das primare Scheidenkarzinom und seine Behandlung, Z. Geburtshilfe Gynak. **145**:253, 1956.

Murad, T. M., and others: The pathologic behavior of primary vaginal carcinoma and its relationship to cervical cancer, Cancer **35**:787, 1975.

Ortega, J. A.: A therapeutic approach to childhood pelvic rhabdomyosarcoma without pelvic exenteration, J. Pediatr. **94**:205, 1979.

Palmer, J. P., and Biback, S. M.: Primary cancer of the vagina, Am. J. Obstet. Gynecol. **67**:377, 1954.

Palumbo, L., and others: Primary carcinoma of the vagina, South. Med. J. **62**:1048, 1969.

Prempree, T., and others: Radiation management of primary carcinoma of the vagina, Cancer **40**(1):109, 1977.

Pride, G. L., and Buchler, D. A.: Carcinoma of vagina 10 or more years following pelvic irradiation therapy, Am. J. Obstet. Gynecol. **127**:513, 1977.

Pride, G. L., Schultz, A. E., Chuprevich, T. W., and Berchler, D. A.: Primary invasive squamous carcinoma of the vagina, Obstet. Gynecol. **53**(2):218, 1979.

Ries, J., and Ludwig, H.: Zur Therapie des primaren Karzinoms der Vagina, Strahlentherapie **118**:92, 1962.

Rutledge, F. N.: Cancer of vagina, Am. J. Obstet. Gynecol. **97**:635, 1967.

Rutledge, F. N., and Sullivan, M.: Sarcoma botryoides, Ann. N.Y. Acad. Sci. **142**:694, 1967.

Rywlin, A. M., Simmons, R. J., and Robinson, M. J.: Leiomyoma of vagina recurrent in pregnancy; a case with apparent hormone dependency, South. Med. J. **62**:1449, 1969.

Schram, M.: Leiomyosarcoma of the vagina; report of a case and review of the literature, Obstet. Gynecol. **12**:195, 1958.

Singh, B. P.: Primary carcinoma of vagina, Cancer **4**:1073, 1951.

Smith, F. R.: Primary carcinoma of vagina, Am. J. Obstet. Gynecol. **69**:525, 1955.

Smith, F. R.: Clinical management of cancer of the vagina, Ann. N.Y. Acad. Sci. **114**:1012, 1964.

Sogani, P. C., and Whitmore, W. F.: Solitary vaginal metastasis from unsuspected renal cell carcinoma, J. Urol. **121**(1):95, 1979.

Taggart, C. G., Cortro, J. R., and Rutledge, F. N.: Carcinoma of the female urethra, Am. J. Roentgenol. **114**:145, 1972.

Taussig, F. J.: Primary cancer of the vulva, vagina and female urethra, Surg. Gynecol. Obstet. **60**:477, 1935.

Tavassoli, F. A., and Norris, H. J.: Smooth muscle tumors of the vagina, Obstet. Gynecol. **53**:689, 1979.

Usherwood, M. McD.: Management of vaginal carcinoma after hysterectomy, Am. J. Obstet. Gynecol. **122**:352, 1975.

Wasserburger, K.: Zur Therapie des Karzinoms der weiblichen Hornrahre, Strahlentherapie **101:**485, 1956.

Way, S.: Primary carcinoma of the vagina, J. Obstet. Gynaecol. Br. Emp. **55:**739, 1948.

Wertheim, E.: Abdominal existirpierte Schiedenkarzinome, Abl. Gynak. **29:**1218, 1905.

Whelton, J. A., and Kottmeier, H. L.: Primary carcinoma of the vagina, Acta Obstet. Gynecol. Scand. **41:**22, 1962.

Whitehouse, W. L.: Primary carcinoma of vagina, J. Obstet. Gynaecol. Br. Comm. **69:**481, 1962.

Wolff, J. P., and Douyon, E.: Le cancer primitif du vagin, Gynecol. Obstet. (Paris) **63:**565, 1964.

CHAPTER TEN

The adnexal mass and early ovarian cancer

ADNEXAL MASS

Anatomically, the adnexa consists of the fallopian tube, round ligament, ovary, and those structures within the round ligament that were formed from embryologic rests. The differential diagnosis in management of the adnexal mass is complex because of the scope of the disorders that it encompasses and the numerous therapies that may be appropriate. It is the risk of malignancy (Table 10-1) that propels the system, as well as the fundamental concepts that early diagnosis and treatment in cancer are related to lessened mortality and morbidity. An adnexal mass often involves ovarian substance because of the propensity of the ovary for neoplasia. Fewer neoplasms occur in the fallopian tube, although that structure may commonly be involved in an inflammatory process that presents as an adnexal mass.

Table 10-1. Differential diagnosis of adnexal mass

Organ	Cystic	Solid

Ovary	Functional cyst
	Neoplastic cyst
	  Benign
	  Malignant
	Endometriosis
		Neoplasm
		  Benign
		  Malignant

Fallopian tube	Tubo-ovarian abscess Hydrosalpinx Parovarian cyst	Tubo-ovarian abscess Ectopic pregnancy Neoplasm

Uterus	Intrauterine pregnancy
	  in a bicornate uterus
		Pedunculated or
		  interligamentous myoma

Bowel	Sigmoid or cecum
	  distended with gas
	  and/or feces
		Diverticulitis
		Ileitis
		Appendicitis
		Colonic cancer

Miscellaneous	Distended bladder
	Pelvic kidney
	Urachal cyst
		Abdominal wall hematoma
		  or abscess
		Retroperitoneal
		  neoplasm

The differential diagnosis of an adnexal mass varies considerably with the age of the patient. In the premenarchal and postmenopausal woman, an adnexal mass should be considered highly abnormal and must be immediately investigated. In premenarchal patients, most neoplasms are germ cell in origin and require immediate surgical exploration. Postoperative treatment is usually required; in these young patients the kind of therapy depends on the stage of disease and the tumor type. Stromal, germ cell, and epithelial tumors are all seen in postmenopausal women; they should be considered malignant until proved otherwise. Any enlargement of the ovary is abnormal in this older age group. Many clinicians believe that any palpable ovary in a postmenopausal patient connotes malignancy and requires further study and likely laparotomy.

In the menstruating patient (reproductive age period), the differential diagnosis is quite varied; both benign and malignant tumors of multiple organs can occur. Occasionally, extragenital lesions, which are often quite large and cystic, are found on pelvic examination; exploratory laparotomy is indicated because of the size alone. These extragenital lesions may include peritoneal cysts, omental cysts, retroperitoneal lesions, and diseases of the gastrointestinal tract (cecum, appendix, sigmoid, and even small bowel, any of which may fall into the pelvis and become adherent). If one suspects gastrointestinal origin of the mass, appropriate radiographic studies will usually help in the definitive diagnosis.

The adnexal mass is usually secondary to disease of one of the genital organs in the menstruating patient. Detection of pelvic abnormalities is more frequent in women of reproductive age because these patients have relatively frequent periodic screening for cancer detection and contraceptive counseling. Although most pelvic masses occur in this age range, fortunately the majority are histologically benign.

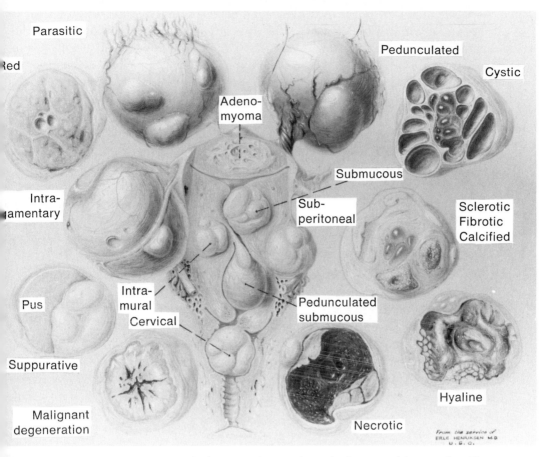

Parasitic

Red

Pedunculated

Cystic

Adeno-myoma

Intra-ligamentary

Submucous

Sub-peritoneal

Sclerotic
Fibrotic
Calcified

Pus

Intra-mural

Cervical

Pedunculated
submucous

Suppurative

Hyaline

Malignant
degeneration

Necrotic

From the service of
ERLE HENRIKSEN M.D.
U. S. C.

Fig. 10-1. Myomas can present in multiple sizes and states of growth, disease, and degeneration. (Courtesy Erle Henriksen, M.D., Los Angeles, California.)

Differential diagnosis

Adnexal mass of gynecologic origin. This category includes disorders of the uterus, fallopian tubes, ovaries, and their adjacent structures. The process that creates the mass may be congenital, functional, neoplastic, or inflammatory.

Uterine masses. Pregnancy should always be kept in mind as a cause of uterine enlargement. Most physicians are familiar with the unreliability of a menstrual history, and any patient in the reproductive age period with a pelvic mass should have pregnancy ruled out. This can be done by any of a variety of pregnancy tests or detection of fetal heart tones using some of the more sophisticated devices.

Myomas of the uterus are the most common uterine neoplasm (Fig. 10-1). They are usually discrete, relatively round tumors that are quite firm to palpation and may be single or multiple. Myomas may be located within the myometrium (intramural), just beneath the endometrial lining (submucous), or on the surface of the uterus (serous). Not infrequently a myoma may be found in the broad ligament attached to the lower uterine segment by a rather thin pedicle. This will often confuse the examiner and lead him to believe that the mass originates in the ovary or tube. In the United States, myomas are found in at least 10% of white women and 30% to 40% of black women over the age of 35. In the postmenopausal age group, it is said that the incidence increases to 30% in white women and 50% in black women. Fortunately these neoplasms usually shrink in size after menopause, especially in patients not receiving high doses of exogenous estrogen stimulation. It would appear that most of these benign neoplasms are somewhat estrogen dependent. Degeneration, infarction, and infection can occur in these lesions, and all of these complications are associated with impressive amounts of lower abdominal pain.

Other conditions that can cause enlargement of the uterus are adenomyosis and endometrial carcinoma. Endometrial carcinoma can enlarge the uterus up to four times that of normal size. The diagnosis of endometrial carcinoma is of course made by D&C of the endometrial cavity or some other appropriate endometrial sampling.

Ovarian masses

FUNCTIONAL CYSTS. Among the most frequently found masses involving the adnexa are the nonneoplastic cysts that are related to the process of ovulation and are sometimes referred to as functional cysts. They are by far the most common clinically detectable enlargements of the ovary occurring during the reproductive years. They are of great significance primarily because they cannot be readily distinguished from true neoplasms on clinical grounds alone. Among the nonneoplastic cysts and hyperplasias of the ovary are: (1) functional cysts, both follicular and corpus luteum types, (2) theca-lutein cysts, (3) pregnancy luteoma, (4) sclerocystic ovaries, and (5) endometriotic cysts.

If ovulation does not occur, a clear fluid-filled follicular cyst (Fig. 10-2) lined by granulosa cells may result and can reach sizes of up to 10 cm in diameter. These cysts usually resolve spontaneously within a few days to 2 weeks but can persist longer. When ovulation occurs, a corpus luteum is formed that may become abnormally enlarged through internal hemorrhage or cyst formation. Such cysts are often associated with variable delays in the onset of menses and confusion regarding the possibility of an ectopic pregnancy. Pregnancy testing has greatly facilitated this differential diagnosis. Theca-lutein cysts result from overstimulation of the ovary by human chorionic gonadotrophin (hCG) and are characterized by extensive luteinization of the stroma surrounding the follicle when studied histologically. Although theca-lutein cysts are uncommon in a normal pregnancy, they are often associated with hydatidiform moles and choriocarcinoma. Gross examination of the ovary containing theca-lutein cysts shows a structure almost completely replaced by lobulated thin-wall cysts that vary in size and are smooth and yellowish.

Corpus luteum, follicular, and theca-lutein cysts are benign and represent an exaggerated physiologic response of the ovary. In most instances they involute over a period of time, but they do present a problem requiring a differential diagnosis.

OVARIAN NEOPLASMS. Although it is not unrealistic to consider every ovarian neoplasm or ovarian mass potentially malignant, in truth only 20% of all ovarian

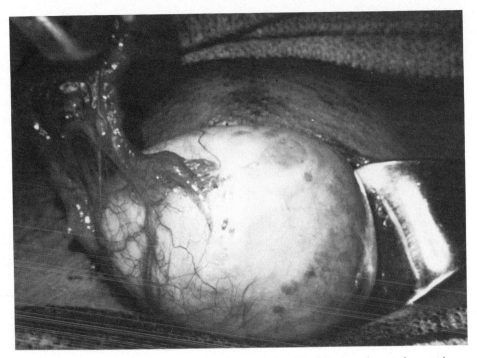

Fig. 10-2. Follicular cyst (8 cm). Fimbrial adhesions from the fallopian tube are also noted.

neoplasms are pathologically malignant. Only occasionally is it possible to differentiate benign from malignant tumors on the basis of history and physical examination. In most instances the diagnosis can only be made following gross and microscopic examination of the mass. The ovary is composed of tissue derived from coelomic epithelium, germ cells, and mesenchyme, and clinically, ovarian neoplasms may be divided into solid and cystic types.

By far the most common benign cystic tumors of the ovary are serous and mucinous cystadenomas and cystic teratomas (dermoids). Cystadenomas may vary from 5 to 20 cm in size and are thin-walled, ovoid, and unilocular. The fluid contained within the neoplasms is usually yellow tinged and thin to viscous in quality. Benign cystic teratomas are usually no greater than 10 cm and can be identified grossly by the presence of sebaceous material or hair noted on section of the neoplasm.

Malignant cystic neoplasms are usually of the serous or mucinous cystadenocarcinoma variety. In the absence of definite solid areas it may be difficult to distinguish these lesions from their benign counterparts. Papillary surface excrescences, areas of necrosis, and internal papillations are very suggestive of malignancy. However, in the absence of obvious implants elsewhere in the peritoneal cavity, histologic review of the material is necessary to establish the diagnosis.

Benign solid tumors of the ovary are usually of connective tissue origin (fibromas, thecomas, and Brenner tumors). They vary in size from very small nodules found on the surface of the ovary to very large neoplasms weighing several thousand grams.

On physical examination, these neoplasms are usually quite firm, slightly irregular in contour, and mobile. Meigs' syndrome is a very uncommon clinical entity in which a benign ovarian fibroma is seen with ascites and hydrothorax.

The malignant solid neoplasms of the ovary are most commonly adenocarcinomas arising in the ovary or metastatic from other sites. The very firm masses noted on pelvic examination often appear to be associated with the undifferentiated adenocarcinomas and a very poor prognosis. This clinical impression should be tempered by the knowledge that inflammatory processes (e.g., chronic pelvic inflammatory disease) can present as the firmest of palpable masses. In addition, elevated serum levels of several estrogens and androgens have been found in patients with solid ovarian neoplasms; fortunately, these neoplasms (arrhenoblastoma, gynandroblastoma, and hilus-cell tumor) are either benign or of low malignant potential.

Most neoplasms of the ovary are asymptomatic unless they have been subject to rupture or torsion. Widespread intraperitoneal dissemination can occur in ovarian carcinoma and be totally asymptomatic until ascites causes a presenting symptom of abdominal distention. On the other hand, any adnexal enlargement may cause menstrual abnormalities and a sensation of pelvic pressure from distortion of the bladder and rectum.

ENDOMETRIOSIS. Endometriosis is a condition in which implants of normal-appearing endometrial glands and stroma are found outside their normal location in the uterine cavity. The most common sites for the occurrence of endometriosis are the ovaries, supporting ligaments of the uterus, and peritoneum of the cul-de-sac and bladder. Endometriosis is most common in women 35 to 45 years of age and is more common in white and nulliparous women. When the ovary is involved, that structure may become enlarged and cystic as a collection of dark, chocolate-colored fluid accumulates within an ovarian cyst. These cysts rarely exceed a diameter of 12 cm but often are indistinguishable from ovarian neoplasms. Nodularity of the uterosacral ligaments and other structures within the cul-de-sac may be helpful in the differential diagnosis. Pelvic pain is by far the most common symptom of endometriosis. Although physical activity and sexual intercourse usually increase the discomfort, the amount of endometriosis present does not seem to correlate with the intensity of the symptoms. At times, pain produced from small peritoneal implants appears to be incapacitating.

Tubal masses. Neoplasms arising from the fallopian tube are quite rare. More commonly, adnexal masses secondary to tubal disease are inflammatory in nature or represent an ectopic pregnancy. Distinction between tubal and ovarian masses on the basis of examination alone is often quite difficult.

In the acute phase of salpingitis, the fallopian tube is distended by grossly purulent material. This infection may be secondary to gonorrhea or other organisms, including anaerobes. As the salpingitis process proceeds, the adjacent ovary may become involved, creating a so-called tubo-ovarian abscess. Although this acute process may resolve, the patient is often subject to reinfection. As a result of repeated chronic infectious processes, the tubal ostia may become closed or firmly adherent to the adjacent ovary, and the fallopian tube will be filled with a clear fluid. As the structure distends it creates a mass that can easily be mistaken for an ovarian cyst. Although the symptoms of acute pelvic inflammatory disease are quite distinct, with pelvic pain, fever, increased vaginal discharge, and abnormal uterine bleeding, those of chronic pelvic infection may be quite subtle. Even the traditional elevation of the erythrocyte sedimentation rate and/or leukocyte level may be absent in up to 30% of patients with chronic pelvic inflammatory disease and an adnexal mass.

A cystic mass in the adnexal region may be neither ovarian nor tubal in origin but caused instead by remnants of embryologic structures. The parovarium is located within the portion of the broad ligament containing the fallopian tube and consists of vestigial remnants of the wolffian duct. Parovarian cysts are found as distal remnants of the wolffian duct system (Fig. 10-3). They are characteristically located between the fallopian tube and the ovary and, when large, are often found with the fallopian tube stretched over the top of the cyst. These parovarian cysts are most commonly unilocular and filled with clear yellow fluid.

Approximately 98% of ectopic pregnancies are tubal. Unfortunately, a pelvic mass can be found on examination in less than half of the cases of tubal pregnancy, and urinary pregnancy tests may be negative. Rupture usually occurs when the distended fallopian tube reaches a diameter of 4 cm. Tubal pregnancy may be difficult

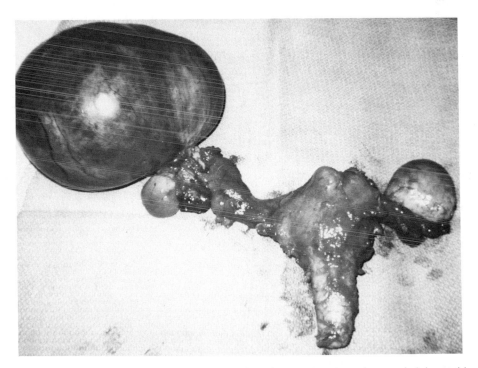

Fig. 10-3. Large fluid-filled parovarian cyst next to the right ovary (specimen from total abdominal hysterectomy and bilateral salpingo-oophorectomy).

to distinguish from pelvic inflammatory disease, torsion of the adnexa, or bleeding corpus luteum cysts, since all produce pain and/or abnormal bleeding. Culdocentesis may be quite helpful in ruling out a hemoperitoneum or pelvic inflammatory disease.

Carcinoma of the fallopian tube is very rare and accounts for less than 0.5% of all female genital tract malignancies. Indeed, most of these neoplasms are discovered by serendipity, with a preoperative diagnosis of ovarian neoplasm being most common. Grossly, the fallopian tube is usually enlarged, smooth walled, and sausage shaped.

Pelvic masses of nongynecologic origin

Bowel. By far the most common entity of the gastrointestinal tract presenting as an adnexal mass is fecal material in the sigmoid colon and/or cecum, which may on pelvic examination present as a soft, mobile, tubular mass. Patients suspected of this should be reexamined after appropriate cleansing enemas.

Inflammatory disorders of the large and small intestine can also be detected on pelvic examination. Symptoms of diarrhea, nausea and vomiting, anorexia, or passage of blood or mucus per rectum should suggest these gastrointestinal disorders. Patients with diverticulitis, even with abscess formation, are sometimes remarkable with regard to the minor degree of symptoms that they present with. Careful questioning in order to detect subtle changes in gastrointestinal symptoms is often very rewarding. Appendiceal abscesses may be formed as a result of rupture of the appendix and present as a pelvic mass. They are, unfortunately, variable in location, although they are generally found on the right side of the pelvis and are usually fixed in location, firm, and tender to palpation. Diverticulitis is a more common disorder with increasing age. Although it is most commonly located in the sigmoid colon, the mass may be midline or right-sided. Occasionally, inflammation of the ileum (regional ileitis) may present as a right adnexal mass as the loops of thickened and inflamed ileum become fixed in the pelvis.

Gastrointestinal malignancy is suggested by the presence of blood in the stool, anemia, and alterations in bowel habits. Neoplasms of the large intestine are particularly common with increasing age, and 80% occur on the left side within the reach of the palpating finger or sigmoidoscope. On the other hand, carcinoma of the cecum often presents as a right adnexal mass, and on examination induration and irregularity are often found in the involved area. Appropriate roentgenographic studies are very helpful in establishing these diagnoses (Table 10-2).

Table 10-2. Diagnostic evaluation of the patient with an adnexal mass

Complete physical examination
Sounding of uterus (after ruling out pregnancy)
IVP
Barium enema
Pelvic ultrasound (optional to rule out pregnancy)
Laparoscopy, laparotomy

Miscellaneous. Pelvic examination should always be performed under optimum circumstances, and this includes emptying the bladder. Many patients have been admitted to university hospitals with a 10-cm midline mass thought to be an ovarian neoplasm that disappeared with catheterization of the bladder. Whenever possible the rectum and rectosigmoid should also be empty when a pelvic examination is carried out. This avoids the problem of fecal material misdiagnosed as an adnexal mass.

Retroperitoneal disorders may also be evident on pelvic examination. Retroperitoneal sarcomas, lymphomas, and teratomas of the sacrococcygeal areas are commonly felt on rectovaginal examination.

Management

Pelvic examination remains the best method of identifying an ovarian mass in its earliest stages. The size, shape, contour, and general location within the pelvis help the physician arrive at the most likely diagnosis. Benign tumors are usually smooth walled, cystic, mobile, unilateral, and less than 8 cm (7 cm is the exact diameter of a new tennis ball). Malignant tumors are usually solid or semisolid, bilateral, irregular, fixed, and associated with nodules in the cul-de-sac. Ascites is usually found with malignant neoplasms.

Certain studies must precede surgical exploration. Roentgenologic examination of the abdomen may reveal the outline of a pelvic mass, and a finding of "teeth" indicates a benign teratoma. However, all calcifications are not "teeth," and psammoma bodies in serous adenocarcinoma of the ovary are commonly found radiopaque entities also noted on roentgenologic examination. Intravenous pyelography is useful in the management of a pelvic mass, because ureteral displacement and distortion of the bladder contour may be used to judge the size of the mass. In addition, kidney position and function can also be evaluated. Ureteral obstruction or displacement should be noted before laparotomy, particularly when retroperitoneal dissection is anticipated to remove tumor bulk.

Specific diagnostic assays (e.g., tumor markers) for ovarian cancer are rare. Some germ cell neoplasms produce hCG or alpha-fetoprotein (AFP), but the majority of ovarian neoplasms are not presently associated with a reliable tumor marker.

Contrast studies of the gastrointestinal tract should be used liberally, especially when there is any suspicion that the mass is gastrointestinal in origin. Barium enema should be seriously considered in most patients with an adnexal mass (Fig. 10-4). Ultrasonography has not been as diagnostically helpful as expected except to exclude intrauterine or extrauterine pregnancy. Although ultrasound can be helpful in detecting solid-fluid interfaces and distinguishing between solid and cystic masses, these determinations do not help in the eventual management of the patient and therefore seem redundant when a distinct mass has been palpated. Occasionally, ultrasound can be helpful in confirming the suspicion of an adnexal mass in an obese or uncooperative patient. Its routine use is discouraged.

Diagnostic laparoscopy may be quite helpful in distinguishing the presence of a uterine myoma versus an ovarian neoplasm. Laparoscopy is helpful in any situation

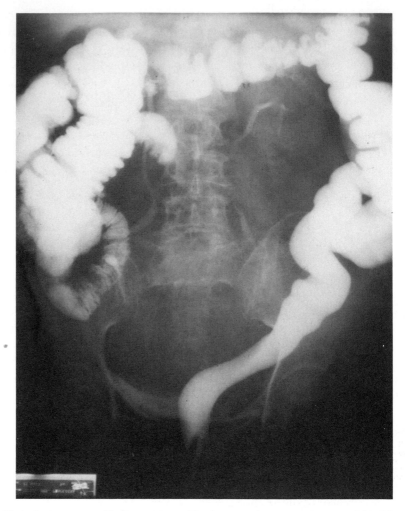

Fig. 10-4. Barium enema film in a patient with a large mucinous cystadenoma of the right ovary.

where the source of a pelvic mass is uncertain, and the source will determine whether treatment is surgical or nonsurgical. This is especially true with smaller masses (7 cm or less) occurring in patients of reproductive age, in whom expectant therapy should be seriously considered.

The decision as to which patient needs surgical exploration can best be determined by the characteristics of the adnexal mass. Any mass that is greater than 7 to 8 cm in diameter should usually be subjected to laparotomy and surgical exploration. Ninety-five percent of ovarian cysts less than 5 cm in diameter are nonneoplastic. In addition, functional cysts are seldom larger than 7 cm in diameter and are usually unilateral and freely mobile. During the reproductive years, an adnexal mass as described above can be presumed to be a functional or hyperplastic change of the ovary rather than a true neoplasm. The transitory existence of functional cysts is of prime importance in distinguishing them from true neoplasms. Tradition and clinical experience have taught us that functional cysts usually persist for only a few days to a few weeks, and reexamination during a later phase of the menstrual cycle has been a reliable procedure in confirming this diagnosis. Many gynecologists prescribe oral contraceptives to accelerate the involution of the functional cyst on the presumption that these cysts are gonadotrophin dependent. The theory is that the inhibitory effect of the contraceptive steroids on the release of pituitary gonadotrophins should shorten the life span of these cysts, hastening their identification as functional or nonneoplastic lesions. Failure of the enlargement to regress during the period of observation (4 to 6 weeks) mandates operative intervention. A very careful study by Spanos was conducted on 286 patients presenting with an adnexal cyst. Combination-type oral contraceptives were prescribed, and the women were reexamined in 6 weeks. In 72% of the women, the mass disappeared during the observation period. Of the 81 patients whose mass persisted, none were found to have a functional cyst at laparotomy. The fact that five of the removed tumors were malignant underscores the importance of avoiding unnecessary delay in the operative investigation of these patients.

In the premenarchal or postmenopausal period, any ovarian enlargement should result in surgical intervention.

BENIGN OVARIAN TUMORS (Table 10-3)

The differentiation between benign and malignant ovarian enlargements is often the exclusive decision of the pathologist, but a short discussion of these lesions is pertinent even in a textbook of oncology. Although functional ovarian cysts are usually asymptomatic, they can on occasion be accompanied by a minor degree of lower abdominal discomfort, pelvic pain, or dyspareunia. In addition, rupture of one of these fluid-filled structures can result in additional peritoneal irritation and possibly an accompanying hemoperitoneum; however, this is rarely of a serious nature. More intense lower abdominal discomfort will result when these ovarian tumors undergo torsion or infarction. Similar to functional cysts of the ovary, benign ovarian neoplasms do not produce any symptoms that readily differentiate them from malignant tumors or a variety of other pelvic diseases. Although these tumors are more prone to twist, resulting in infarction, malignant neoplasms may have the same fate. Indeed, one of the most unfortunate features of benign ovarian neoplasms is that they are *indistinguishable clinically from their malignant counterpart*. Although it is not known whether malignant ovarian tumors arise de novo or develop from benign tumors, there is strong inferential evidence that at least some benign tumors will become malignant. All too often, the first symptom of cancer in an ovarian tumor is increasing abdominal distention, although benign ovarian neoplasms may present as increasing abdominal girth, and indeed the "giant tumors" of the ovary are often benign mucinous cystadenomas. True functional cysts of the ovary will remit in a 4- to 6-week follow-up period of observation. *All persistent adnexal enlargements must be considered malignant until proved otherwise.*

Table 10-3. Benign ovarian tumors

I. Nonneoplastic tumors
   A. Germinal inclusion cyst
   B. Follicle cyst
   C. Corpus luteum cyst
   D. Pregnancy luteoma
   E. Theca-lutein cysts
   F. Sclerocystic ovaries
II. Neoplastic tumors derived from coelomic epithelium
   A. Cystic tumors
      1. Serous cystoma
      2. Endometrioma
      3. Mucinous cystoma
      4. Mixed forms
   B. Tumors with stromal overgrowth
      1. Fibroma, adenofibroma
      2. Brenner tumor
III. Tumors derived from germ cells
   A. Dermoid (benign cystic teratoma)

Serous cystadenoma

Serous cystadenomas are more common than the mucinous type of tumor and as a rule do not attain the very large size that is characteristic of their mucinous counterpart. Grossly, the characteristic feature is the presence of papillary projections on the surface of the tumor, which at times are so numerous as to produce a cauliflower pattern. Although most of the inner wall of the cyst may be smooth, it may also contain a large number of these papillae. Microscopically, the epithelium is usually of the low columnar type, and at times cilia are present. Particularly characteristic of this type of cyst is the frequent finding of small calcerous granules, the so-called psammoma bodies, which are an end product of degenertion of the papillary implants. Aure and associates have suggested that these psammoma bodies are indicative of a functional immunologic response. Associated fibrosis may lead to the so-called cystadenofibroma, which represents a similar lesion found in the breast.

Mucinous cystadenoma

Mucinous cystadenomas (Fig. 10-5) may attain a huge size, and several have been reported weighing 100 to 200 pounds. Grossly, they present as round or ovoid masses with a smooth capsule that is usually translucent, bluish-whitish gray. The interior is divided into a number of discrete septa or locules containing generally a clear, viscid fluid. Papillae are rarely noted. However, miscroscopically the lining epithelium is of a rather tall, pale-staining secretory type with nuclei at the basal pole; goblet cells are common. The cells will be found to be rich in mucin if suitable stains are obtained. It is believed that this type of cyst usually arises from simple metaplasia of the germinal epithelium. It may arise occasionally from a teratoma in which all of the other elements have been blotted out and rarely from a Brenner tumor in which there has been mucinous transformation of the epithelium.

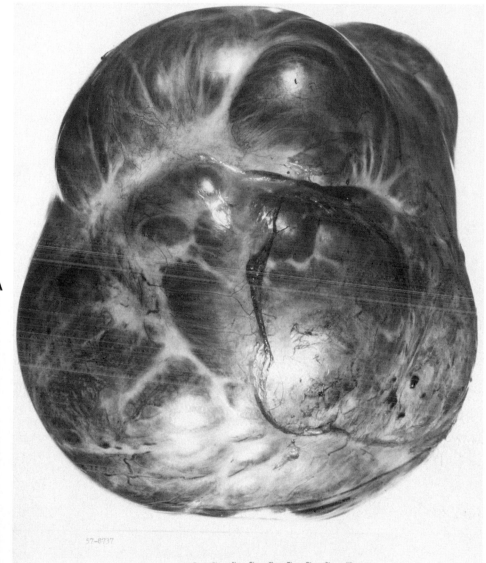

Fig. 10-5. Mucinous cystadenoma. **A,** Gross appearance.

Continued.

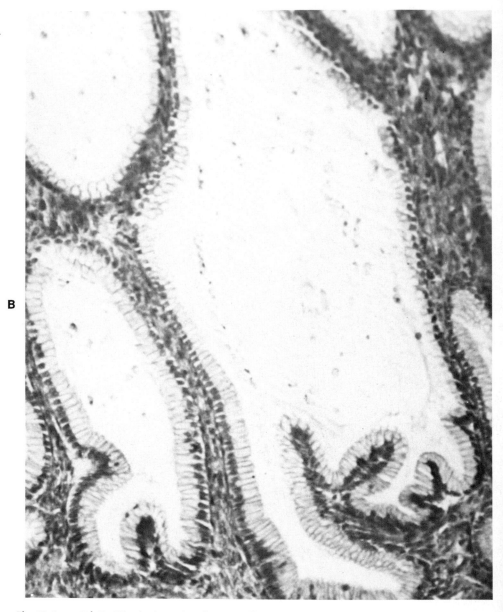

B

Fig. 10-5, cont'd. B, Histologic section showing tall epithelial lining with pale-staining nuclei at the basal pole.

Brenner tumor

Brenner tumor (Fig. 10-6) is a rather uncommon type of ovarian neoplasm and grossly is identical to a fibroma. Microscopically, one finds a markedly hyperplastic fibromatous matrix interspersed with nests of epithelioid cells. The epithelioid cells under high magnification show a "coffee bean" pattern due to the longitudinal grooving of the nuclei. The cell nests show a frequent tendency to central cystic degeneration, producing a superficial resemblance to a follicle. Although it was originally believed that Brenner tumors arise from simple Walthard rests, it has been conclusively demonstrated that Brenner tumors can arise from diverse sources, including the surface epithelium, rete ovarii, and ovarian stroma itself. It was originally stressed that Brenner tumors were uniformly benign, but in the last several decades there have been scattered reports of a number of malignant Brenner tumors. Brenner tumors are generally thought to be endocrinologically inert, but in recent years a number of cases have been associated with postmenopausal endometrial hyperplasia, and a frequent estrogen effect has been attributed to this neoplasm. Even more recently, a characteristic Brenner has been associated with virilism.

Dermoid cyst (benign cystic teratoma)

Dermoid cysts are rarely large, often bilateral (15% to 25%), and disproportionately frequent in the younger individual. Grossly, there is a rather thick, opaque, whitish wall, and on opening the cyst one frequently finds hair, bone, and cartilage as well as a large amount of greasy fluid, which rapidly becomes sebaceous on cooling. Microscopically one may find all types of mature ectoderm, mesoderm, and such endodermal elements as gastrointestinal mucosa. Stratified squamous epithelium, hair follicles, sebaceous and pseudoriferous glands, cartilage, neural and respiratory elements, and indeed all elements normally seen in fetal life may be present. Malignant degeneration can occur in these benign cystic teratomas and is usually of a squamous type; it has been reported in 1% to 3% of these tumors. These neoplasms are thought to arise from an early ovum that has been stimulated by some type of parthenogenetic stimulus.

Fibroma

Fibromas (Fig. 10-7) are not at all uncommon and sometimes present as a very small nodule on the ovarian cortex. In other instances they can be extremely large, filling the entire pelvis and lower abdomen. The tumors are characterized by their firmness and resemblance to myomas, which they are frequently misdiagnosed as. On the cut surface there is a homogeneous grayish-white and firm appearance, although areas of cystic degeneration are common in larger tumors. Microscopically one finds stellate or spindle-shaped cells arranged in fusiform fashion. The cells are uniformly well differentiated, with nothing to suggest malignancy. Hyalinization is frequent, particularly in the larger tumors, and if fat stains are done, admixtures of theca cells may be obtained. Meigs' syndrome is characterized by ascites, hydrothorax, and an ovarian tumor that was originally believed to be specifically a fibroma;

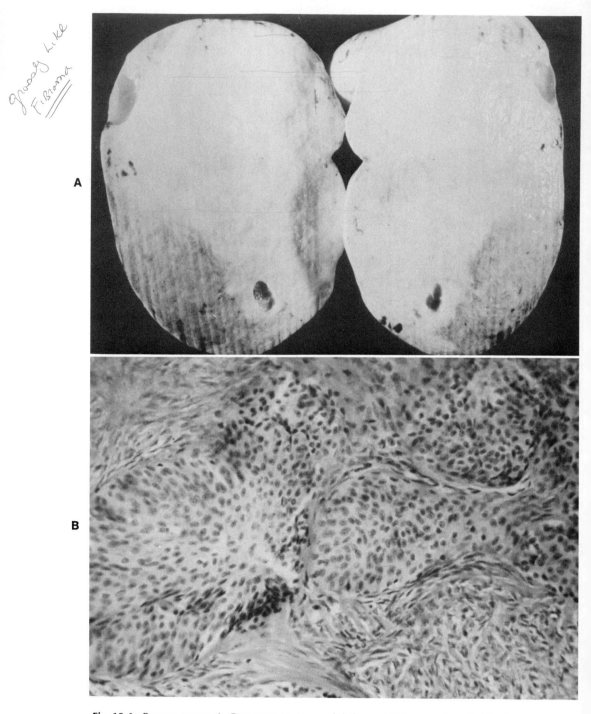

Fig. 10-6. Brenner tumor. **A,** Gross appearance—solid, firm, whitish cut surface. **B,** Histologic section—hyperplastic fibromatous matrix interspersed with nests of epithelioid cells.

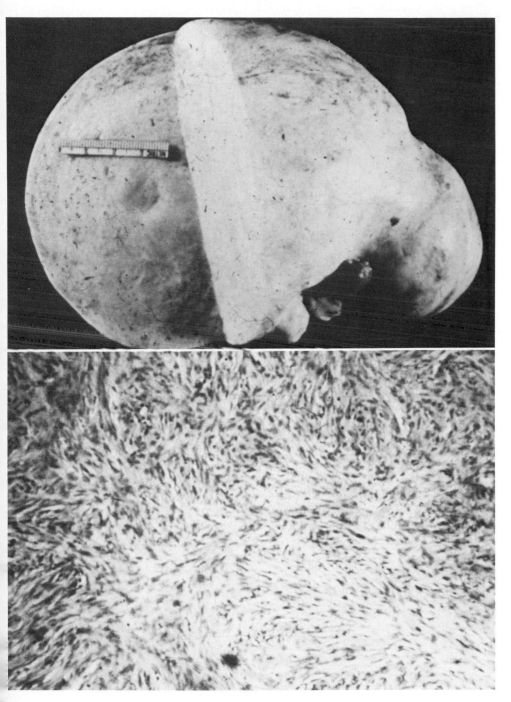

Fig. 10-7. Ovarian fibroma. **A,** Gross appearance—white, firm cut surface. **B,** Histologic section—whorls of the fibromatous matrix.

however, many other types of ovarian tumors are now known to be associated with this syndrome, such as Brenner tumors and Krukenberg tumors. The cause of Meigs' syndrome is not completely understood, but it would seem that the hydrothorax occurs via certain lymphatics through the diaphragm. Following removal of the ovarian neoplasm there is a prompt resolution of both abdominal and chest fluid.

PALPABLE POSTMENOPAUSAL OVARY (Fig. 10-8)

During the postmenopausal years, when the ovary becomes reduced in size and quiescent after cessation of menses, the presence of a palpable ovary must alert the physician to the possibility of an underlying malignancy. Physiologic enlargement and functional cysts should not be present in a postmenopausal ovary. The postmenopausal gonad atrophies to a size of 1.5 × 1 × ½ cm on the average, and at that size it should not be palpable on pelvic examination. The possibility of malignancy must therefore be carefully assessed when an ovary is palpable in a postmenopausal woman. Procrastination in this subset of patients can be fatal, and diagnostic laparotomy is indicated.

When laparotomy is performed, the approach should be with the assumption that the patient may have an early ovarian carcinoma. Cytologic washings and careful exploration of the abdomen should be carried out as in any patient being staged for ovarian cancer. A vertical abdominal incision is strongly recommended, which would allow careful assessment of the subdiaphragmatic surfaces. In our experience, only 10% of patients with a palpable postmenopausal ovary who are subjected to oophorectomy are found to have a malignant ovarian neoplasm. By far the most common findings are benign ovarian lesions such as fibroma and Brenner tumor.

Postmenopausal palpable ovary syndrome
The PMPO syndrome

Normal ovary
Premenopause
3.5 × 2 × 1.5 cm

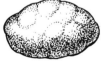

Early menopause
(1-2 years)
2 × 1.5 × 0.5 cm

Late menopause
(2-5 years)
1.5 × 0.75 × 0.5 cm

Fig. 10-8. Comparison of ovary size during progressive periods of a woman's life. (From Barber, H. R. K., and Graber, E. A.: The PMPO syndrome [postmenopausal palpable ovary syndrome], Obstet. Gynecol. Surv. **28:**357, 1973. © 1973 The Williams & Wilkins Co., Baltimore.)

BORDERLINE MALIGNANT EPITHELIAL OVARIAN NEOPLASMS

In the last decade, clear evidence has been presented for a group of epithelial ovarian tumors that have histologic and biologic features occupying a position between those of clearly benign and frankly malignant ovarian neoplasms. These borderline malignancies, which account for approximately 15% of all epithelial ovarian cancers, were often referred to as proliferative cystadenomas. A 10-year survival rate of approximately 95% has been obtained in these borderline neoplasms. However, symptomatic recurrence and death may occur as many as 20 years after therapy in a few patients, and these neoplasms are correctly labeled as being of low malignant potential.

Borderline serous epithelial tumors (Fig. 10-9) definitely occupy an intermediate position between the benign serous cystadenomas and the frankly malignant serous cystadenocarcinomas, in both their histologic features and prognostic aspects. Grossly, the borderline serous tumors are similar to the previously described benign serous cystadenomas with papillary projections, but the borderline tumors possibly show an increased incidence of bilaterality. In addition, the papillary component is usually more abundant in the borderline lesions than in the perfectly benign serous cystadenoma.

The histologic criteria characterizing the borderline tumors can be summarized as follows: stratification of the epithelial lining of the papillae, formation of microscopic papillary projections or tufts arising from the epithelial lining of the papillae, epithelial pleomorphism, atypicality, and mitotic activity. According to Janovski and Paramananthon, at least two of the above features must be present in order for the tumor to qualify as borderline. Although the borderline serous epithelial tumors of the ovary are well established and were accepted by FIGO in 1964, they remain a controversial issue. Although there is no doubt that there exists a group of low-grade malignant tumors among the serous cystadenocarcinomas of the ovary, it is doubtful whether qualifying terms such as "borderline" and the like are always appropriate. Unfortunately, terms like "borderline" may create a false sense of security among some physicians. These patients should be followed as closely as any patient with ovarian cancer.

In 1973 Hart and Norris reported a series of borderline mucinous tumors confined to one or both ovaries at the time of diagnosis, with a corrected 10-year actuarial survival rate of 96%. Whereas the origin of the serous tumors from germinal epithelium is generally accepted, the histogenesis of mucinous tumors is more problematic. Grossly, these neoplasms do not differ significantly from their benign counterpart. They are multilocular, cystic, frequently voluminous masses with a smooth outer surface. The interlining is also similar to that of benign mucinous cystadenomas and is generally smooth, although papillary structures and solid thickening of the capsule have been observed in about 25% to 50% of lesions reported. Microscopically, in contrast to the benign mucinous cystadenoma, the epithelial lining of the borderline tumor is characterized by stratification of two to three layers. Whereas in the benign tumors the cells show no atypism or pleomorphism, the

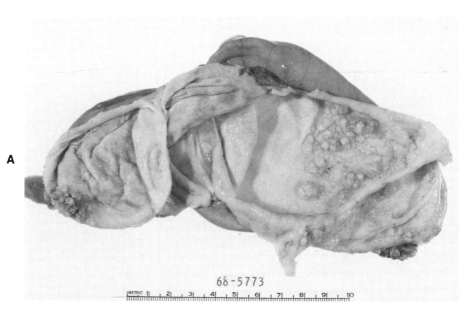

68-5773

Fig. 10-9.   Borderline serous carcinoma. **A,** Gross appearance.

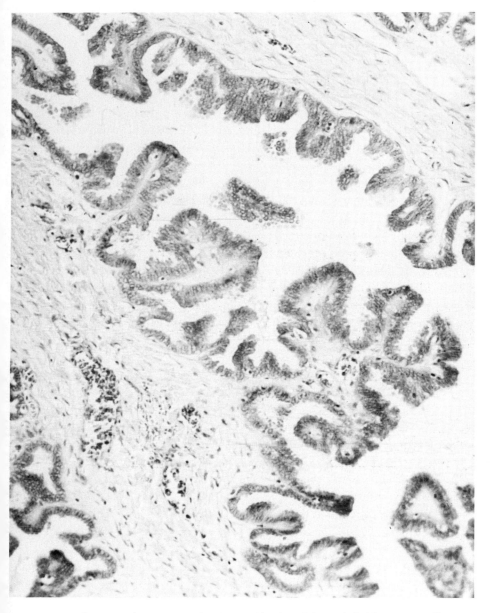

Fig. 10-9, cont'd. B, Histologic section showing stratification of the epithelial lining in papillary projections.

epithelium of the borderline lesions does demonstrate atypism, with irregular, hyperchromatic nuclei and enlarged nuclei. Mitotic figures are also encountered.

※ Treatment of borderline lesions should strive to completely extirpate the tumor. If unilateral, a salpingo-oophorectomy is appropriate, provided a thorough examination, including biopsy, of the contralateral ovary reveals no neoplasm there. If there is bilateral involvement, especially when papillary projections are found on the external surface of the tumor, or if peritoneal spread is noted, a more radical surgical approach such as total abdominal hysterectomy with bilateral salpingo-oophorectomy is advocated. Such extirpation of all the internal genitalia is curative in most patients with localized borderline tumors. Careful exploration of the entire abdominal cavity must be carried out at the time of exploratory laparotomy. Recurrences, peritoneal seeding, and death have been reported in patients who have been treated as if this were a benign lesion.

handwritten in margin: Some Room For Conservative Therapy

Appropriate treatment for stage I borderline neoplasms of the ovary, other than surgical resection, remains uncertain. Kolstad and associates randomized patients with stage I borderline lesions into two groups, one treated by pelvic radiotherapy and the other by pelvic radiotherapy and intraperitoneal radioactive colloidal gold. The actuarial survival rates were 92.5% and 87.2%, respectively, with several patients dying of complications of the gold therapy. In these instances, therapy seemingly resulted in a significant lowering of survival compared with three other series. Use of intraperitoneal chromic phosphate alone without pelvic radiotherapy is usually associated with fewer intra-abdominal complications and may be more appropriate therapy.

PROPER IDENTIFICATION OF AN EARLY LESION

The combined 5-year survival rates for stage I and II epithelial cancer of the ovary are variously quoted from 50% to 70% and from 40% to 50%, respectively. These survival rates are disappointing in view of the presumptive removal of all tumor at the time of surgery.

To date there have been several prospective studies evaluating metastasis to the diaphragm in women with presumed stage I and II ovarian carcinoma (Table 10-4). In each instance, the surgeon performing the initial procedure was of the opinion that the lesion was confined to the ovary and/or pelvis. The incidence of such unsuspected metastases was 15.7% in the collective series (11.3% for stage I and 23.0% for stage II).

Knapp and Friedman, Delgado and associates, and Musumeci and associates evaluated prospectively aortic node metastasis in patients with stage I and II ovarian carcinoma. Collectively they found that 10.3% of stage I and 10.0% of stage II patients had aortic node disease. Knapp and Friedman found that the omentum was a site of microscopic metastasis in 4.7% of the patients with stage I and II ovarian epithelial cancer. Keettel and associates were among the first to report that in the absence of clinical ascites, a significant number of patients with localized ovarian cancer have free-floating intraperitoneal cancer cells, demonstrated by cytologic

Table 10-4. Incidence of subclinical metastases in stage I and II ovarian carcinoma

Series	Diaphragm (%)	Aortic nodes (%)	Malignant cytologic washings (%)
Knapp and Friedman	—	12.5	—
Rosenoff and associates	43.7	—	—
Delgado and associates	0.0	20.0	—
Spinelli and associates	23.0	—	—
Musumeci and associates	—	7.0	—
Keettel and associates	—	—	36.0
Creasman and associates	—	—	10.0
Morton and associates	—	—	50.0
Piver and associates	3.2	0.0	25.8
TOTAL	15.7	10.3	29.8
Stage I	11.3	10.3	32.9
Stage II	23.0	10.0	12.5

Modified from Piver, M. S., Barlow, J. J., and Lele, S. B.: Incidence of subclinical metastasis in stage I and II ovarian carcinoma, Obstet. Gynecol. **52**:100, 1978.

washings. In their report, 36% of the stage I patients had malignant cells in the cytologic washings. This report and three other studies were collated by Piver and associates for a total of 87 women with presumed stage I and II ovarian carcinoma. A total of 29.8% of these patients were found to have free-floating cancer cells in the pelvis or paracolonic spaces. Therefore, many of the failures in the stage I and II category were undoubtedly patients with occult dissemination not appreciated at the time of the initial surgical procedure. (For recommendations on the optimal surgical procedure at initial laparotomy, see the section on Diagnostic Techniques and Staging in Chapter 11.)

MANAGEMENT OF EARLY OVARIAN CANCER IN YOUNG WOMEN

Traditionally, operative treatment has been the mainstay of management in ovarian carcinoma. The technical aspects of the initial laparotomy have a greater bearing on outcome than many subsequent therapeutic decisions. Hysterectomy with bilateral salpingo-oophorectomy continues to be the most cogent therapy for ovarian carcinoma. The opposite ovary is removed because of the frequency of bilateral synchronous tumors and the possibility of occult metastases, which in the normal-appearing opposite ovary have varied from 12% to 43%, depending on the report. Since the uterine serosa and endometrium are often sites of occult metastasis and since the prevalence of synchronous endometrial carcinoma is relatively high, hysterectomy is also indicated. Occasionally, however, unilateral oophorectomy has been carried out in a young, childless woman whose unilateral tumor later turned out to be malignant. Not proceeding with further therapy is a calculated risk, the justification for which exists in statements made by many authoritative gynecologists, which are summarized below.

For the young, nulliparous woman with a stage IA tumor, the safety of more

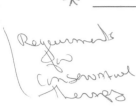

Table 10-5. Requirements for conservative management in epithelial ovarian cancer

1. Stage IA
2. Well differentiated
3. Young woman of low parity
4. Otherwise normal pelvis
5. Encapsulated and free of adhesions
6. No invasion of capsule, lymphatics, or mesovarium
7. Peritoneal washings negative
8. Bivalve of opposite ovary and omental biopsy negative
9. Close follow-up probable
10. Excision of residual ovary after completion of childbearing

Modified from DiSaia, P. J., Townsend, D. E., and Morrow, C. P.: The rationale for less than radical treatment for gynecologic malignancy in early reproductive years, Obstet. Gynecol. Surv. **29**:581, 1974.

conservative operations to preserve childbearing is uncertain. In reviewing 190 patients with stage IA ovarian carcinoma, Munnell found that of 144 patients whose reproductive organs were removed, 70% survived 5 years, whereas 61% of 46 patients treated by unilateral salpingo-oophorectomy survived 5 years. In patients with mucinous tumors, 78% with complete operation (23 patients) and 100% with conservative operation (8 patients) survived 5 years. Similarly, Parker and associates found no difference in the 5-year survival rate regardless of whether patients were treated by hysterectomy and bilateral salpingo-oophorectomy or by unilateral salpingo-oophorectomy alone. Julian and Woodruff evaluated 65 cases of low-grade papillary serous carcinoma of the ovary and found 100% of the 50 patients with unilateral adnexal removal and 90% of the 10 patients with complete operation alive at 5 years.

The requirements for conservative management of stage IA ovarian cancer are listed in Table 10-5. Unilateral salpingo-oophorectomy may be the definitive treatment of a young woman of low parity found to have a well-differentiated serous, mucinous, endometrioid, or mesonephric carcinoma of the ovary. The tumor must be unilateral, well encapsulated, free of adhesions, and not associated with ascites or evidence of extragonadal spread. Peritoneal washings for cytology should be taken from the pelvis and upper abdomen, and the opposite ovary should be bivalved for pathologic examination. The incidence of microscopic metastases in the opposite ovary has been calculated by Munnell and others to be approximately 12%. The periaortic and pelvic wall nodes must be carefully palpated and an adequate sample of the omentum taken for biopsy. In addition, the preserved pelvic organs should be reasonably normal, since there is little to be gained by retaining the opposite ovary in a patient who is not fertile. With the finding of carcinoma in any of these areas, conservative surgery must be abandoned. Dysgerminoma, granulosa cell tumor, and arrhenoblastoma may also be managed conservatively under these special circumstances. After the patient has completed her family, some consideration should be given to the removal of the other ovary because of the risk of eventually developing another ovarian malignancy.

Table 10-6. Dysgerminoma

	Cases	Treatment*	Recurrence rate	5-year survival rate
Radiumhemmet	22	CO + radiation therapy	18%	95%
AFIP	46	CO	22%	91%
AFIP	21	RO	10%	90%

*CO = unilateral oophorectomy, RO = total abdominal hysterectomy and bilateral salpingo-oophorectomy.

The key issue in patients treated conservatively for stage IA epithelial tumors of the ovary is the histology. Mucinous lesions fare better than serous lesions, the grade 1 and borderline lesions being the most easily treated conservatively. In a recent study of 33 women from the Mayo Clinic, ages 16 to 29, who had stage IA ovarian cancer, it was shown that unilateral salpingo-oophorectomy or just resection of the ovary was adequate to result in no recurrences in a period of follow-up from 3 to 10 years. These results are encouraging but are not the final answer, since many low-grade lesions are prone to late recurrence.

The management of dysgerminoma is frequently singled out as an example of conservative surgery. Table 10-6 shows the statistics in patients treated in various manners. The exquisite radiosensitivity of dysgerminoma allows us to be somewhat liberal in its management. Although the recurrence rate in this disease is approximately 20% in stage I, the overall survival rate approaches 95% because of the exceptional response to radical radiation therapy. Note that the incidence of recurrence is approximately the same despite the initial treatment. The treatment of recurrences results in approximately a 75% 5-year survival rate. However, the question that has not been answered is what the overall 5-year survival rate would be if all patients were treated with radical irradiation following conservative or radical surgery. Would we salvage the other 5%? It is difficult to answer this question, but we assume that not all of them would be salvaged since we are convinced that some of these patients who succumb to dysgerminoma have immature embryonal components that are not recognized.

SPILL OF TUMOR

The subject of tumor spill has been quite controversial in gynecologic oncology for some time. It is logical to assume that implantation and germination of cancer cells are conceivable and probable when a malignant cyst ruptures at the time of surgery. The question remains only to prove that this is so.

The early studies of Munnell did not support the theoretical possibility that rupture of a malignant ovarian tumor would enhance dissemination. He studied 99 patients with stage I and II ovarian cancer and had an overall 5-year survival rate of 71%. In his retrospective study, 27 of the patients had had spill at the time of surgery. Twenty-two (81%) of these patients survived 5 years. Of these 27 patients, postoperative irradiation was administered to 21, and there was a 66% 5-year survival rate

Table 10-7. Tumor-free survival in stage I ovarian cancer

Series	Neoplasm ruptured	Neoplasm unruptured
Purola and Nieminen (1968)	18/30 (60%)	83/100 (83%)
Williams and associates (1976)	3/7 (43%)	57/58 (98%)

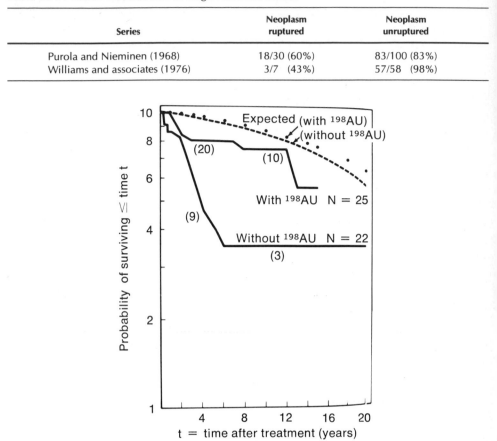

Fig. 10-10. Probability of survival in stage I epithelial ovarian cancer with rupture of the neoplasm at surgical removal, with and without intraperitoneal radioactive colloidal gold therapy. (From Decker, D. G., Webb, M. J., and Holbrook, M. A.: Am. J. Obstet. Gynecol. **115:**751, 1973.)

in this group of 21. Six of the patients did not receive x-ray therapy, and all six survived 5 years. It would appear from this very limited retrospective study that spill eruption does not endanger the patient's prognosis and that if this does occur postoperative irradiation is not necessarily indicated. It is obvious that the number of patients studied here is very small, and one would have to carefully study the histology in the six patients who did not receive x-ray therapy. One may find that these were highly differentiated lesions, maybe of borderline quality. There is, in addition, an obvious bias interjected here in that the patients with more malignant lesions probably received radiation therapy. There have been very few studies with enough patients to shed further light on this subject (Table 10-7). However, recently a report by Decker and associates of the Mayo Clinic involving some 223 stage I cases of ovarian epithelial cancer revealed that rupture during surgery did seem to lower the survival curve (Fig. 10-10). Another study by Grogan from Harvard analyzed 124 patients with ovarian cancer. Rupture of an ovarian tumor cyst during surgery occurred in 16 of 124 patients. For our purposes, however, only nine patients are worthy of consideration, since only these patients had stage I lesions. Six of these nine patients survived 5 years or more, one died of a massive myocardial infarction, and the other two succumbed to their malignancy. The six patients who survived had a well-differentiated grade 1 histologic pattern. Both of the patients who died of tumor presented with a poorly differentiated histologic picture. They had received radiation therapy following hysterectomy with bilateral salpingo-oophorectomy, but the radiation therapy was delivered in very moderate dosages of 2,500 to 3,000 rads on a 200-kv machine. This is far below optimum radiation therapy.

The issue is difficult to resolve because one is very prone to treat more vigorously patients who have spill at the time of surgery, and this may equalize the survival rates in the groups of patients. In the era when whole-abdomen irradiation with pelvic boost was the only therapy that could be offered these patients, some hesitation in instituting postoperative therapy appeared to be justified. However, we now have comparatively less toxic chemotherapeutic regimens that can be adequately used postoperatively. A reasonable and seemingly adequate recommendation in these instances is a year of chemotherapy administered in the form of melphalan (Alkeran) pulse therapy and then a "second-look" procedure to verify the absence of disease within the pelvic and abdominal cavity. Others have recommended the use of intraperitoneal colloidal isotopes such as P 32. No prospective study comparing these seemingly valid approaches has been reported to date. If rupture does occur, lavage of the peritoneal cavity with sterile water has been recommended to cause lysis of the cells, and this may be helpful.

BIBLIOGRAPHY

Abel, K. P.: Ovarian apoplexy, Lancet 1:136, 1964.

Abell, M. R.. The nature and classification of ovarian neoplasms, Can. Med. Assoc. J. 94:1102, 1966.

American Cancer Society: Cancer facts and figures, New York, 1978, The Society.

Arey, L. B.: Origin and form of Brenner tumor, Am. J. Obstet. Gynecol. 81:743, 1961.

Asadourian, L. A., and Taylor, H. B.: Dysgerminoma—an analysis of 105 cases, Obstet. Gynecol. 33:370, 1969.

Aure, J. C., Hoeg, K., and Kolstadt, P.: Psammoma bodies in serous carcinoma of the ovary, Am. J. Obstet. Gynecol. 109:113, 1971.

Aure, J. C., Hoeg, K., and Kolstadt, P.: Radioactive colloidal gold in the treatment of ovarian carcinoma, Acta Radiol. 10:399, 1971.

Bagley, C. M., Jr., Young, R. C., Canellos, G. P., and DeVita, V. T.: Treatment of ovarian carcinoma; possibilities for progress, N. Engl. J. Med. 287:856, 1971.

Barber, H. R. K., and Graber, E. A.: The PMPO syndrome (postmenopausal palpable ovary syndrome), Obstet. Gynecol. Surv. 28:357, 1973.

Barnes, P. H.: Oophorectomy in primary carcinoma confined to one ovary, Can. Med. Assoc. J. 79:416, 1958.

Beischer, N. A., and others: Ovarian tumors in pregnancy, Obstet. Gynecol. Surv. 27:429, 1972.

Bennington, J. L., Ferguson, B. R., and Haber, S. L.: Incidence and relative frequency of benign and malignant ovarian neoplasms, Obstet. Gynecol. 32:627, 1968.

Bergman, F.: Carcinoma of the ovary; a clinicopathological study of 86 autopsied cases with special reference to mode of spread, Acta Obstet. Gynecol. Scand. 45:211, 1966.

Berkowitz, R. L.: Massive ovarian enlargement in an obese patient, Obstet. Gynecol. 48:483, 1976.

Brody, S.: Clinical aspects of dysgerminoma of the ovary, Acta Radiol. 56:209, 1961.

Carlson, D. H., and Griscom, N. T.: Ovarian cysts

in the newborn, Am. J. Roentgenol. **116**:664, 1972.

Caspi, E., Schreyer, P., and Bukovsky, J.: Ovarian lutein cysts in pregnancy, Obstet. Gynecol. **42**:388, 1972.

Cianfrani, T.: Neoplasms in apparently normal ovaries, Am. J. Obstet. Gynecol. **41**:211, 1973.

Classification and staging of malignant tumours in the female pelvis, Acta Obstet. Gynecol. Scand. **50**:1, 1971.

Counseller, V. S., Hunt, W., and Haigler, F. H.: Carcinoma of the ovary following hysterectomy, Am. J. Obstet. Gynecol. **69**:538, 1955.

Creasman, W. T.: The adnexal mass; its diagnosis and management, Contemp. Ob/Gyn **9**:45, 1977.

Creasman, W. T., Fetter, B. F., Hammond, C. B., and Parker, R. T.: Germ cell malignancies of the ovary, Obstet. Gynecol. **53**:226, 1979.

Creasman, W. T., and Rutledge, F.: The prognostic value of peritoneal cytology in gynecologic malignant disease, Am. J. Obstet. Gynecol. **110**:773, 1971.

Creasman, W. T., Rutledge, F., and Smith, J. P.: Carcinoma of the ovary associated with pregnancy, Obstet. Gynecol. **38**:111, 1971.

Cutler, S. J., Myers, M. H., and Green, S. B.: Trends in survival rates of patients with cancer, N. Engl. J. Med. **293**:122, 1975.

De Bacalao, E. B., and Dominguez, I.: Unilateral gonadoblastoma in a pregnant woman, Am. J. Obstet. Gynecol. **105**:1279, 1969.

Decker, D. G., Mussey, E., Malkasian, G. D., and Johnson, C. E.: Adjuvant therapy for advanced ovarian malignancy, Am. J. Obstet. Gynecol. **97**:171, 1967.

Decker, D. G., Webb, M. J., and Holbrook, M. A.: Radiogold treatment of epithelial cancer of ovary; late results, Am. J. Obstet. Gynecol. **115**:751, 1973.

Delgado, G., Chun, B., Cogler, H., and others: Para-aortic lymphadenectomy in gynecologic malignancies confined to the pelvis, Obstet. Gynecol. **50**:418, 1977.

DiSaia, P. J., and others: Synopsis of gynecologic oncology, New York, 1975, John Wiley & Sons, Inc.

DiSaia, P. J., and others: Individualized treatment of ovarian cancers, Am. J. Obstet. Gynecol. **128**:619, 1977.

Dockerty, M. B., and Masson, J. C.: Ovarian fibromas; a clinical and pathological study of 283 cases, Am. J. Obstet. Gynecol. **47**:741, 1944.

Fathalla, M. F.: Factors in the causation and incidence of ovarian cancer, Obstet. Gynecol. Surv. **27**:751, 1972.

Fuller, M. E.: Oral contraceptive therapy for differentiating ovarian cysts, Postgrad. Med. **50**:143, 1971.

Gibbs, E.K.: Suggested prophylaxis for ovarian cancer, Am. J. Obstet. Gynecol. **111**:756, 1971.

Goldberg, B. B., Goodman, C. A., and Clearfield, H. R.: Evaluation of ascites by ultrasound, Radiology **96**:15, 1970.

Graham, J., Burstein, P., and Graham, R.: Prognostic significance of pleural effusion in ovarian cancer, Am. J. Obstet. Gynecol. **106**:312, 1970.

Graham, J. B., and Graham, R. M.: Ovarian cancer and asbestosis, Environ. Res. **1**:115, 1967.

Graham, J. B., Graham, R. M., and Schueller, E. F.: Preclinical detection of ovarian cancer, Cancer **17**:1414, 1964.

Grogan, R. H.: Accidental rupture of malignant ovarian cysts during surgical removal, Obstet. Gynecol. **30**:716, 1967.

Grogan, R. H.: Reappraisal of residual ovaries, Am. J. Obstet. Gynecol. **97**:124, 1967.

Hart, W. R., and Norris, H. J.: Borderline and malignant mucinous tumors of the ovary; histologic criteria and clinical behavior, Cancer **31**:1031, 1973.

Harvald, B., and Hauge, M.: Heredity of cancer elucidated by a study of unselected twins, J.A.M.A. **186**:749, 1963.

Henderson, W. J., Joslin, C. A. F., Turnbull, A. C., and Griffiths, K.: Talc and carcinoma of the ovary and cervix, J. Obstet. Gynecol. Br. Comm. **78**:6, 1971.

Hester, L. L., and White, L.: Radioactive colloidal chromic phosphate in the treatment of ovarian malignancies, Am. J. Obstet. Gynecol. **103**:911, 1969.

Itskovitz, J., Kerner, H., and Brandes, J. M.: Ovarian surface papillomatosis of borderline malignancy, J. Reprod. Med. **22**:144, 1979.

Janovski, N. A., and Paramananthon, T. L.: Ovarian tumors, Stuttgart, 1973, Georg Thieme Verlag K. G.

Jensen, R. D., and Norris, H. J.: Epithelial tumors of the ovary, Arch. Pathol. **94**:29, 1972.

Johnson, C. G.: Discussion of Randall, C. L., and Paloucek, F. P.: The frequency of oophorectomy at the time of hysterectomy, Am. J. Obstet. Gynecol. **100**:716, 1968.

Julian, C. G., and Woodruff, J. D.: The role of chemotherapy in the treatment of primary ovarian malignancy, Obstet. Gynecol. Surv. **24**:1307, 1969.

Julian, C. G., and Woodruff, J. D.: The biologic behavior of low-grade papillary serous carcinoma of the ovary, Obstet. Gynecol. **40**:860, 1973.

Kalstone, C. E., Jaffe, R. B., and Abell, M. R.: Massive edema of the ovary simulating fibroma, Obstet. Gynecol. 34:564, 1969.

Keettel, W. C., Fox, M. R., Longnecker, D. S., and Latourette, H. B.: Prophylactic use of radioactive gold in the treatment of primary ovarian cancer, Am. J. Obstet. Gynecol. 94:766, 1966.

Keettel, W. C., Pixley, E. E., and Buchsbaum, H. J.: Experience with peritoneal cytology in the management of gynecologic malignancies, Am. J. Obstet. Gynecol. 120:174, 1974.

Kistner, R. W.: Intraperitoneal rupture of benign cystic teratomas; review of the literature with a report of two cases, Obstet. Gynecol. Surv. 7:603, 1952.

Knapp, R. C., and Friedman, E. A.: Aortic lymph node metastases in early ovarian cancer, Am. J. Obstet. Gynecol. 119:1013, 1974.

Kolstad, P., and others: Individualized treatment of ovarian cancer, Am. J. Obstet. Gynecol. 128:619, 1977.

Kottmeier, H. L.: Clinical staging in ovarian carcinoma. In Gentil, F., and Junqueira, A. C., editors: Ovarian cancer, New York, 1968, Springer-Verlag New York, Inc.

Kottmeier, H. L.: Surgical management—conservative surgery. In Gentil, F., and Junqueira, A. C., editors: Ovarian cancer, New York, 1968, Springer-Verlag New York, Inc.

Kurman, R. J., and Craig, J. M.: Endometrioid carcinoma of the ovary, Cancer 29:1653, 1972.

Li, F. P., Rapoport, A. H., Fraumeni, J. F., and Jensen, R. D.: Familial ovarian carcinoma, J.A.M.A. 214:1559, 1970.

Malkasian, G. D., Jr., Dockerty, M. B., and Symmonds, R. E.: Benign cystic teratomas, Obstet. Gynecol. 29:719, 1967.

Malloy, J. J., Dockerty, M. B., Welch, J. S., and Hunt, A. B.: Papillary ovarian tumors. I. Benign tumors and serous and mucinous cystadenocarcinomas, Am. J. Obstet. Gynecol. 93:867, 1965.

Martin, C. B., Murata, Y., and Rabin, L. S.: Diagnostic ultrasound in obstetrics and gynecology; experience on a large clinical service, Obstet. Gynecol. 41:379, 1973.

McGowan, L., Davis, R. H., and Bunnag, B.: The biochemical diagnosis of ovarian cancer, Am. J. Obstet. Gynecol. 116:760, 1973.

McGowan, L., Stein, D. B., and Miller, W.: Cul-de-sac aspiration for diagnostic cytologic study, Am. J. Obstet. Gynecol. 96:413, 1966.

Meigs, J. V., and Cass, J. W.: Fibroma of the ovary with ascites and hydrothorax with a report of 7 cases, Am. J. Obstet. Gynecol. 33:249, 1937.

Moench, L. M.: A clinical study of 403 cases of adenocarcinoma of the ovary, Am. J. Obstet. Gynecol. 26:22, 1933.

Moore, D. W., and Langley, I. I.: Routine use of radiogold following operation for ovarian cancer, Am. J. Obstet. Gynecol. 98:624, 1967.

Morton, D. G., Moore, J. G., and Chang, N.: The clinical value of peritoneal lavage for cytologic evaluation, Am. J. Obstet. Gynecol. 81:1115, 1961.

Munnell, E. W.: The changing prognosis and treatment in cancer of the ovary; a report of 235 patients with primary ovarian carcinoma 1952-1961, Am. J. Obstet. Gynecol. 100:790, 1968.

Munnell, E. W.: Is conservative therapy ever justified in stage IA cancer of the ovary? Am. J. Obstet. Gynecol. 103:641, 1969.

Munnell, E. W.: Surgical treatment of ovarian carcinoma, Clin. Obstet. Gynecol. 12:980, 1969.

Munnell, E. W., and Taylor, H. C., Jr.: Ovarian carcinoma, Am. J. Obstet. Gynecol. 58:943, 1949.

Musumeci, R., Banfi, A., DePalo, G., and others: Lymphangiography in patients with ovarian epithelial cancer, Cancer 40:1444, 1977.

Neef, J. C. de, and Hollenbeck, Z. J. R.: The fate of ovaries preserved at the time of hysterectomy, Am. J. Obstet. Gynecol. 96:1088, 1966.

Nieminen, V., and Purola, E.: Stage and prognosis of ovarian cystadenocarcinomas, Acta Obstet. Gynecol. Scand. 49:49, 1970.

Norris, H. J., and Jensen, R. D.: Relative frequency of ovarian neoplasms in children and adolescents, Cancer 30:713, 1972.

Parker, R. T., Parker, C. H., and Wilbanks, G. D.: Cancer of the ovary; survival studies based upon operative therapy, chemotherapy, and radiotherapy, Am. J. Obstet. Gynecol. 108:878, 1970.

Parrish, H. M., Carr, C. A., Hall, D. G., and King, T. M.: Time interval from castration in premenopausal women to development of excessive coronary artherosclerosis, Am. J. Obstet. Gynecol. 90:155, 1967.

Peterson, W. F.: Solid histologically benign teratomas of the ovary, Am. J. Obstet. Gynecol. 72:1094, 1956.

Pezner, R. D.: Limited epithelial carcinoma of the ovary treated with curative intent by the intraperitoneal instillation of radiocolloids, Cancer 42:2563, 1978.

Piver, M. S.: Radioactive colloids in the treatment of stage IA ovarian cancer, Obstet. Gynecol. 40:42, 1972.

Piver, M. S., Barlow, J. J., and Lele, S. B.: Incidence of subclinical metastasis in stage I and II ovarian carcinoma, Obstet. Gynecol. 52:100, 1978.

Purola, E., and Nieminen, U.: Does rupture of cystic carcinoma during operation influence the prognosis? Ann. Chir. Gynaecol. Fenn. **57**:615, 1968.

Randall, C. L.: Background of statistical data on ovarian cancer. In Barber, H. R. K., and Graber, E. A., editors: Gynecologic oncology, Baltimore, 1970, The Williams & Wilkins Co.

Randall, C. L., Birtch, P. K., and Harkins, J. L.: Ovarian function after the menopause, Am. J. Obstet. Gynecol. **74**:719, 1957.

Randall, C. L., and Gerhardt, P. R.: The probability of the occurrence of the more common types of gynecologic malignancy, Am. J. Obstet. Gynecol. **68**:78, 1954.

Randall, C. L., and Hall, D. W.: Clinical considerations of benign ovarian cystomas, Am. J. Obstet. Gynecol. **62**:806, 1951.

Randall, C. L., Hall, D. W., and Armenia, C. S.: Pathology in the preserved ovary after unilateral oophorectomy, Am. J. Obstet. Gynecol. **84**:1233, 1962.

Randall, C. L., and Paloucek, F. P.: The frequency of oophorectomy at the time of hysterectomy, Am. J. Obstet. Gynecol. **100**:716, 1968.

Rosenoff, S. H., DeVita, V. T., Jr., Hubbard, S., and others: Peritoneoscopy in the staging and follow-up of ovarian cancer, Semin. Oncol. **2**:223, 1975.

Roth, L. M., and Sternberg, W. H.: Proliferating Brenner tumors, Cancer **27**:689, 1971.

Samanth, K. K., and Black, W. C.: Benign ovarian stromal tumors associated with free peritoneal fluid, Am. J. Obstet. Gynecol. **107**:538, 1970.

Smith, J. P., Rutledge, F. N., and Sutow, W. W.: Malignant gynecologic tumors in children; current approaches to treatment, Am. J. Obstet. Gynecol. **116**:261, 1973.

Spanos, W.: Preoperative hormonal therapy of cystic adnexal masses, Am. J. Obstet. Gynecol. **116**:551, 1973.

Spiert, H.: The role of ionizing radiations in the causation of ovarian tumors, Cancer **5**:478, 1952.

Spinelli, P., Luini, A., Pizzetti, P., and others: Laparoscopy in staging and restaging of 95 patients with ovarian carcinoma, Tumori **62**:493, 1976.

Stone, M. L., Weingold, A. B., and Lee, B. O.: Clinical applications of ultrasound in obstetrics and gynecology, Am. J. Obstet. Gynecol. **113**:1046, 1972.

Taylor, H. C., Jr.: Malignant and semimalignant tumors of the ovary, Surg. Gynecol. Obstet. **48**:204, 1929.

Terz, J. J., Barber, H. R. K., and Brunschwig, A.: Incidence of carcinoma in the retained ovary, Am. J. Surg. **113**:511, 1967.

Turner, J. C., Jr., Remine, W. H., and Dockerty, M. B.: Clinical pathologic study of 172 patients with primary carcinoma of the ovary, Surg. Gynecol. Obstet. **109**:198, 1959.

Walton, P. D., Jamieson, A. D., and Shingleton, H. M.: The expanding role of diagnostic ultrasound in obstetrics and gynecology, Surg. Gynecol. Obstet. **137**:753, 1973.

Webb, M. J., Decker, D. G., Mussey, E., and others: Factors influencing survival in Stage I ovarian cancer, Am. J. Obstet. Gynecol. **116**:222, 1973.

White, K. C.: Ovarian tumors in pregnancy, Am. J. Obstet. Gynecol. **116**:544, 1973.

Williams, T. J., and Dockerty, M. B.: Status of the contralateral ovary in encapsulated low grade malignant tumors of the ovary, Surgery **143**:763, 1976.

Williams, T. J., Symmonds, R. E., and Litwak, O.: Management of unilateral and encapsulated ovarian cancer in young women, Gynecol. Oncol. **1**:143, 1973.

Woodruff, J. D., and Julian, C. G.: Histologic grading and morphologic changes of significance in the treatment of semi-malignant and malignant ovarian tumors, Proc. Natl. Cancer Conf. **6**:346, 1970.

Wynder, E. L., Dodo, H., and Barber, H. R. K.: Epidemiology of cancer of the ovary, Cancer **23**:352, 1969.

Yoonessi, M., and Murray, R. A.: Brenner tumors of the ovary, Obstet. Gynecol. **54**:90, 1979.

Advanced epithelial ovarian cancer

Neoplasms of the ovary present an increasing challenge to the physician. They are the cause of more deaths than any other female genital cancer. There are about 18,000 new cases diagnosed each year, with about 11,000 deaths annually (Fig. 11-1). In the United States, a woman dies of ovarian cancer every 50 minutes. The gynecologic oncologist is frustrated by the paucity of knowledge of the etiologic factors in ovarian cancer and by the failure to achieve a significant reduction in mortality from these neoplasms over the past 5 decades.

253

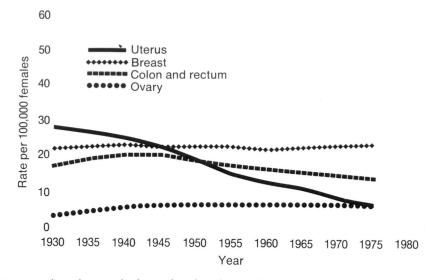

Fig. 11-1. Age-adjusted cancer death rates for selected sites in females, United States, 1930-1975. (From Cancer facts and figures, New York, 1979, American Cancer Society, Inc.)

CLASSIFICATION

The student of ovarian pathology is often confused by the prodigious variation in histologic structure and biologic behavior. Currently, the most popular and practical scheme of classification is based on the histogenesis of the ovary (Table 11-1). The early development of the ovary may be divided into four major stages. During the first stage, undifferentiated germ cells (primordial germ cells) become segregated and migrate from their sites of origin to settle in the genital ridges, which are bilateral thickenings of coelomic epithelium. The second stage occurs after arrival of the germ cells in the genital ridges and consists of proliferation of the coelomic epithelium and the underlying mesenchyme. During the third stage, the ovary becomes divided into a peripheral cortex and a central medulla. The fourth stage is characterized by the development of the cortex and the involution of the medulla. The histogenetic classification given in Table 11-1 categorizes ovarian neoplasms with regard to their derivation from coelomic epithelium, germ cells, and mesenchyme, respectively.

INCIDENCE, EPIDEMIOLOGY, AND ETIOLOGY (Fig. 11-2)

Approximately 23% of gynecologic cancers are of ovarian origin, but 47% of all deaths from cancer of the female genital tract are of this origin. Cancer of the ovaries is the fourth most frequent fatal cancer in women in the United States. It ranks high as a cause of female deaths in Canada, New Zealand, Israel, and countries of northern Europe. Approximately 12 out of every 1,000 women in the United States over the age of 40 will develop ovarian cancer (Table 11-2), but only two or three will be

Table 11-1. Histogenetic classification of ovarian neoplasms

I. Neoplasms derived from coelomic epithelium
    A. Serous tumor
    B. Mucinous tumor
    C. Endometrioid tumor
    D. Mesonephroid (clear-cell) tumor
    E. Brenner tumor
    F. Undifferentiated carcinoma
    G. Carcinosarcoma and mixed mesodermal tumor
II. Neoplasms derived from germ cells
    A. Teratoma
        1. Mature teratoma
            a. Solid adult teratoma
            b. Dermoid cyst
            c. Struma ovarii
            d. Malignant neoplasms secondarily arising from mature cystic teratoma *(1% usually sq)*
        2. Immature teratoma (partially differentiated teratoma)
    B. Dysgerminoma
    C. Embryonal carcinoma
    D. Endodermal sinus tumor
    E. Choriocarcinoma
    F. Gonadoblastoma
III. Neoplasms derived from specialized gonadal stroma
    A. Granulosa-theca cell tumors
        1. Granulosa tumor
        2. Thecoma
    B. Sertoli-Leydig tumors
        1   Arrhenoblastoma
        2. Sertoli tumor
    C. Gynandroblastoma
    D. Lipid cell tumors
IV. Neoplasms derived from nonspecific mesenchyme
    A. Fibroma, hemangioma, leiomyoma, lipoma, etc.
    B. Lymphoma
    C. Sarcoma
V. Neoplasms metastatic to the ovary
    A. Gastrointestinal tract (Krukenberg)
    B. Breast
    C. Endometrium
    D. Lymphoma

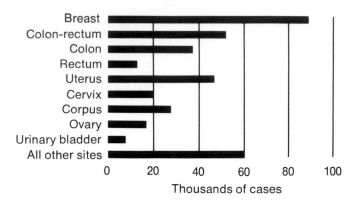

Fig. 11-2. Estimated incidence of cancer of leading sites in females, United States, 1975. (From Cancer facts and figures, New York, 1979, American Cancer Society, Inc.)

Table 11-2. Probability at birth of eventually developing cancer, United States, 1973

	White females	Black females
All sites	30.8	23.8
Breast	8.1	5.2
Cervix	1.5	3.0
Corpus	2.2	1.1
Other uterus	0.3	0.3
Ovary	1.5	0.9
Colon-rectum	5.2	3.6

Data from Biometry Branch, National Cancer Institute, 1973.

cured. The remainder will have repeated bouts of intestinal obstruction as the tumor spreads over the surface of the bowel, develop inanition and malnutrition, and literally starve to death.

Malignant neoplasms of the ovaries occur at all ages, including infancy and childhood. Throughout childhood and adolescence, U.S. death rates for neoplasms of the ovary are exceeded only by those for leukemia, lymphomas, and neoplasms of the central nervous system, kidney, connective tissue, and bone. Overall death rates for neoplasms of the ovary are higher in nonwhite Americans at ages under 39 years; after age 40, however, rates for white women are significantly higher. The major histologic types occur in distinctive age ranges (Table 11-3). Malignant germ cell tumors are most commonly seen in females under the age of 20, whereas epithelial cancers of the ovary are primarily seen in women over 50. The age-specific incidence for ovarian cancer shows a steady rise up to age 80 and drops off slightly in the older ages. The greatest number of cases is found in the age group 50 to 59 years. Studies of the Connecticut Tumor Registry would suggest that the age-adjusted rate for all ages has remained about the same over the last 30 years.

Several reports have described families in which girls and women of the same or

Table 11-3. Primary ovarian neoplasms related to age

Type	0-20 yr	20-50 yr	Over 50 yr
Coelomic epithelium	29%	71%	81%
Germ cell	59%	14%	6%
Specialized gonadal stroma	8%	5%	4%
Nonspecific mesenchyme	4%	10%	9%

Table 11-4. Age-standardized ovarian cancer death rates for various countries, 1970-71

Country	Death rate per 100,000 population
Denmark	12.9
Sweden	9.6
Norway	9.5
England and Wales	9.1
Scotland	8.5
Canada	7.3
United States	7.3
Ireland	5.8
Italy	3.3
Japan	2.1

From Cancer facts and figures, New York, 1979, American Cancer Society, Inc.

succeeding generations develop similar neoplasms of the ovaries. Most of these neoplasms were serous carcinomas, but other types were also observed. Cancers of the
breasts, colon, and other sites were also found more commonly in female members
of these afflicted families. Investigators at the National Cancer Institute have studied
four families in which women of two or three generations have developed papillary-
serous adenocarcinomas at ages past 35 years. The M. D. Anderson Hospital and
Tumor Institute is presently conducting a large study of the pedigree of patients with
ovarian cancer, and preliminary conclusions would suggest that there definitely are
family tendencies for this condition. In addition, the dysgenetic gonads of sex chromatin–negative individuals, most of whom are phenotypic females, are prone to develop a distinctive, ordinarily benign neoplasm called gonadoblastoma.

As with other prevalent epithelial cancers, epidemiologic evidence strongly suggests that environmental factors are a major etiologic determinant in cancer of the
human ovary. The highest rates are recorded in highly industrial countries (Table 11-
4), which suggests that physical or chemical products of industry are major causes of
epithelial neoplasms. A notable exception is highly industrialized Japan, where rates
for malignant neoplasms of the ovary have been among the lowest recorded in the
world. Interestingly, one observes a higher rate of ovarian cancer in Japanese im-
migrants in the United States and their offspring, eventually approaching that of

Anglo-Saxon whites by the second generation. This suggests strongly that the causative carcinogens are probably in the immediate environment, such as food, personal customs, and other influences that change gradually during the cultural transition. To date, there are no clues as to which possible dietary items or other environmental contacts might be specifically carcinogenic for the ovary.

No epidemiologic or experimental evidence exists to incriminate viruses in neoplasms of the human ovary. Attempts to isolate viruses from cultures of human ovarian cancer cells have been unsuccessful to date. Because of its gonadotropic properties, mumps virus is an obvious candidate among known viruses for oncogenic activity in the ovary. Case control studies have revealed a possible negative association with mumps parotitis, but these historic accounts were not supported by skin tests or serologic evidence of reactivity to mumps virus. Menczer and associates reported on 84 ovarian cancer patients and 84 controls with nonmalignant conditions matched by age and ethnic origin who were interviewed with regard to clinical mumps history and their sera tested for mumps complement-fixing antibodies. Ovarian cancer patients differed from the controls in the response to past mumps infection in two respects: (1) they appeared to be more likely to have developed subclinical mumps as evidenced by the lower rate of clinical mumps history in the presence of serologic evidence of similar infection rates among those with positive and those with negative clinical mumps history, and (2) they tended to have lower persistent mumps complement-fixing antibody titers. Menczer and associates interpreted these results as possibly indicating that an immunologic incompetence enables development of ovarian cancer possibly through a direct etiologic role of mumps virus. The evidence for mumps virus as an etiologic agent in ovarian cancer remains speculative.

Knowledge of the etiologic mechanisms involved in cancer of the ovary is limited to fragments of information. The multi-institution therapy programs offer an ideal population of women for case control studies. Each patient should be questioned for a history of preexisting gynecologic abnormalities, documented by clinical or laboratory data where possible, and for information about exposure to environmental carcinogens. Many programs of this nature are currently under way.

SIGNS, SYMPTOMS, AND ATTEMPTS AT EARLY DETECTION

Although diverse ovarian tumors generally manifest themselves in a similar manner, the diagnosis of early ovarian cancer is more a matter of chance than a triumph of the scientific method. As enlargement occurs (Fig. 11-3), there is progressive compression of the surrounding pelvic structures, producing vague abdominal discomfort, dyspepsia, urinary frequency, and "pelvic pressure" (Table 11-5). The insidious onset of ovarian cancer needs no elaboration. As the neoplasm reaches a diameter of 15 cm, it begins to rise out of the pelvis and may account for abdominal enlargement. It is time, however, to change the generally accepted notion that there are no early symptoms of ovarian cancer. Symptoms often include vague abdominal discomfort, dyspepsia, and other mild digestive disturbances, which may be present

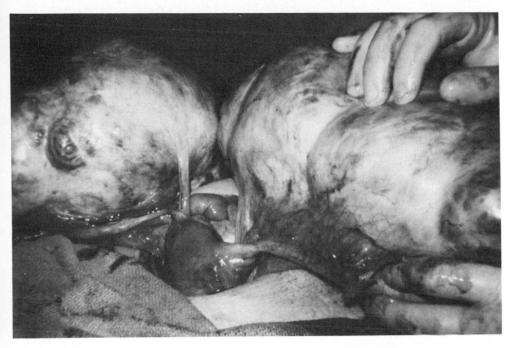

Fig. 11-3. Large bilateral ovarian neoplasms and low-grade mucinous adenocarcinoma.

Table 11-5. Most frequent presenting symptoms of ovarian cancer

Symptom	Relative frequency
Abdominal swelling	xxxx
Abdominal pain	xxx
Dyspepsia	xx
Urinary frequency	xx
Weight change	x

for several months before the diagnosis. Such complaints are usually not recognized as anything more than "middle-age indigestion." A high index of suspicion is warranted in all women between the ages of 40 and 69 who present with persistent gastrointestinal symptoms that cannot be diagnosed. Unfortunately, the majority of such nonspecific complaints are often functional in origin, causing the internist or family physician to overlook the possibility of ovarian cancer. Indeed, it is only when the patient presents with gross enlargement of the abdomen marking the occurrence of ascites and extension of the neoplastic process to the abdominal cavity (Fig. 11-4) that the patient receives appropriate diagnostic evaluation.

Methods for early diagnosis have been investigated in limited studies employing cul-de-sac aspiration for peritoneal cytology and frequent pelvic examinations. All of these endeavors have failed to show a significant impact on early diagnosis of this

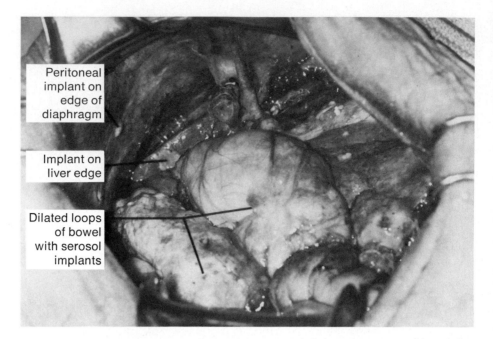

Fig. 11-4. Findings at laparotomy in a patient with stage III epithelial ovarian cancer and bowel obstruction. Note the wide distribution of surface implants.

Table 11-6. Surgical findings

	Benign	Malignant
1 Surface papilla	Rare	Very common
2 Intracystic papilla	Infrequent	Very common
3 Solid areas	Rare	Very common
4 Bilaterality	Rare	Common
5 Adhesions	Infrequent	Common
6 Ascites (100 ml)	Rare	Common
7 Necrosis	Rare	Common
8 Peritoneal implants	Rare	Common
9 Capsule intact	Common	Infrequent
10 Totally cystic	Common	Rare

disease. These ovarian neoplasms grow quickly and painlessly. Any ovarian enlargement should be an immediate indication for exploratory laparotomy. The diagnosis really rests with the pathologist. The size of the tumor does not indicate the severity of disease. Indeed, some of the largest neoplasms are benign histologically. In addition, many large adnexal masses may be of nonovarian etiology. Frequently encountered nonovarian causes of an apparent adnexal mass are diverticulitis, tubo-ovarian abscess, carcinoma of the cecum or sigmoid, pelvic kidney, and uterine or ligamentous myomas. At the time of surgery it may be difficult to discern the malignant potential of a particular ovarian neoplasm (Table 11-6). There is sufficient overlap of morphologic criteria to cause considerable confusion. Again the diagnosis rests with a histologic review of the specimen.

Immunologic diagnosis of subclinical ovarian cancer by means of identification of specific tumor-associated antigens in the serum awaits methodology for isolating these antigens in a purified form. The presence of such substances appears likely, but laboratory efforts at purification have been unsuccessful to date.

DIAGNOSTIC TECHNIQUES AND STAGING

Routine pelvic examinations will detect only one ovarian cancer in 10,000 asymptomatic women. However, pelvic examination remains the most reliable means of detecting early disease. Pain is usually a late complication and is seen with early disease only when associated with a complication such as torsion, rupture, or infection. Any ovary palpated in a patient 3 to 5 years or more after the menopause should raise a high index of suspicion for an early ovarian neoplasm. These patients should be considered for immediate laparoscopy and/or laparotomy.

Routine laboratory tests are not of great value in the diagnosis of ovarian tumors. The major value of laboratory tests is in ruling out other pelvic disorders (Table 11-7). Abdominal roentgenograms may reveal calcifications consistent with myomas or toothlike calcifications consistent with benign teratomas. Pyelogram and gastrointestinal series are often helpful in ruling out disease in adjacent pelvic structures. A barium enema is probably advisable with any pelvic mass, but the need for a gastrointestinal series can be individualized based on the patient's symptoms. A similar comment can be made for proctosigmoidoscopy, which is particularly valuable in patients who have lower intestinal symptoms. The outcome in ovarian cancer relies so heavily on early diagnosis that procrastination with numerous diagnostic procedures such as ultrasound is somewhat hazardous. Laparotomy is the ultimate test as to the nature of the disorder. Paracentesis for the purpose of obtaining a cell block and cytologic smear of the peritoneal fluid appears unnecessary and is, at times, dangerous. If one is dealing with a self-contained malignant cyst, such a procedure can result in a spill of malignant cells into the peritoneal cavity. In addition, whether or not the fluid reveals neoplastic cells, laparotomy is still necessary to either remove the large benign neoplasm or define the extent of the malignant process. In addition, up to 50% of ascitic fluid samples from patients with true ovarian malignancy will be negative for malignant cells on cell block analysis. Diagnostic paracentesis in a patient with ascites and a pelvic-abdominal mass is unnecessary and dangerous.

The staging of ovarian cancer is surgical (Table 11-8). A longitudinal midline incision is recommended to facilitate removal of the neoplasm and to permit adequate visualization of the entire abdominal cavity, including the undersurface of the diaphragm. Ovarian cancer is classically a serosal spreading disease, and thus all peritoneal surfaces must be carefully inspected, especially when disease is thought to be limited to the pelvis. Any peritoneal fluid encountered on opening of the peritoneal cavity should be aspirated and submitted for cytologic examination. In the absence

Table 11-7. Complete workup for ovarian cancer

> Careful history
> Physical examination
> Pelvic examination and Pap smear
> Proctosigmoidoscopy, where indicated
> CBC and urinalysis
> Blood chemistries
> Chest film
> IVP
> Barium enema
> Gastrointestinal series, where indicated

Table 11-8. FIGO stage-grouping for primary carcinoma of the ovary

Stage I	Growth limited to the ovaries.
	Stage IA: Growth limited to the ovary; no ascites.
	    1. No tumor on the external surface; capsule intact.
	    2. Tumor present on the external surface, or capsule(s) ruptured, or both
	Stage IB: Growth limited to both ovaries; no ascites.
	    1. No tumor on the external surface; capsule intact.
	    2. Tumor present on the external surface, or capsule(s) ruptured, or both.
	Stage IC: Tumor either stage IA or IB, but with ascites* present or with positive peritoneal washings.

Stage II	Growth involving one or both ovaries with pelvic extension. Stage IIA: Extension and/or metastases to the uterus and/or tubes. Stage IIB: Extension to other pelvic tissues. Stage IIC: Tumor either stage IIA or stage IIB, but with ascites* present or with positive peritoneal washings.
Stage III	Growth involving one or both ovaries, with intraperitoneal metastases outside the pelvis, or positive retroperitoneal nodes, or both. Tumor limited to the true pelvis with histologically proven malignant extension to small bowel or omentum.
Stage IV	Growth involving one or both ovaries with distant metastases. If pleural effusion is present, there must be positive cytology to allot a case to stage IV. Parenchymal liver metastasis equals stage IV.
Special category	Unexplored cases that are thought to be ovarian carcinoma.

From Manual for staging of cancer 1978, Chicago, 1978, American Joint Committee for Cancer Staging and End Results Reporting.
*Ascites is peritoneal effusion that, in the opinion of the surgeon, is pathologic, or clearly exceeds normal amounts, or both.

of peritoneal fluid, "four washings" should be taken by lavaging the peritoneal surfaces: the undersurface of the diaphragm as the first specimen (Fig. 11-5), lateral to the ascending and descending colon as the second and third specimens, and the pelvic peritoneal surfaces themselves as the fourth specimen. These specimens are obtained by lavaging these areas with 50 to 75 ml of saline solution and retrieving the fluid for cell block analysis. Care should be taken to visualize and palpate all

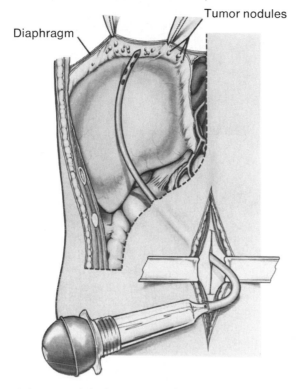

Diaphragm

Tumor nodules

Fig. 11-5. Technique of obtaining subdiaphragmatic cytologic washings at laparotomy. A saline lavage of the space between the diaphragm and the dome of the liver is easily accomplished, because the fluid pockets along the dura and is aspirated with the bulb syringe.

Table 11-9. Surgical therapy in ovarian cancer

1. Peritoneal cytology
2. Determination of extent of disease
   a. Pelvis
   b. Peritoneal surfaces
   c. Diaphragms
   d. Omentum
   e. Lymph nodes
3. Removal of all tumor possible (total abdominal hysterectomy and bilateral salpingo-oophorectomy) plus node sampling and partial omentectomy

Table 11-10. Aortic lymph node metastases in epithelial ovarian cancer

| Series | Stage I | | Stage II | | Stage III-IV | | Total |
	Positive lymphangiography	Positive biopsy	Positive lymphangiography	Positive biopsy	Positive lymphangiography	Positive biopsy	Positive lymphangiography
Hanks and Bagshaw (1969)	2/9	—	2/6	—	4/7	—	8/22
Parker and associates (1974)	3/13	—	2/29	—	12/27	—	17/69
Knapp and Friedman (1974)	—	5/26	—	—	—	—	—
Delgado and associates (1977)	1/5	—	1/5	—	—	3/5	2/10

Table 11-11. Relation of stage to prognosis

Stage		Number of patients	5-year survival rate
I		751	61
	A	528	65
	B	130	52
	C	80	52
II		401	40
	A	40	60
	B	205	38
III		539	5
IV		101	3

Reprinted by permission from Tobias, J. S., and Griffiths, C. T.: Management of ovarian carcinoma, New England Journal of Medicine **294**:818, 1976.

peritoneal surfaces, including the underside of the diaphragm, the surface of the liver, and the small and large bowel mesentery. Fiberoptic light sources are particularly helpful in properly visualizing the peritoneal surfaces of the upper abdomen through a vertical lower abdominal incision. The omentum should be carefully scrutinized and any suspicious areas removed by excision or biopsy. If the disease is apparently limited to the pelvis, it is judicious to remove the most dependent portion of the omentum or any portion of the omentum adherent to pelvic structures as a biopsy specimen. Often, microscopic disease will be present in the omentum but not obvious grossly. Recent data from one institution suggest that routine omentectomy may be of benefit in improving survival, but additional data are needed to confirm this observation. If the disease is limited to the pelvis, great care should be taken to avoid rupture of the neoplasm during its removal (Table 11-9). All roughened or suspicious surfaces in the peritoneal cavity should be removed as a biopsy specimen. This includes adhesions, which should be excised not incised, since often the adhesions contain microscopic disease. Several studies are under way to investigate the efficacy of "blind" peritoneal biopsies and routine retroperitoneal node dissections in the proper staging of early epithelial cancer of the ovary (Table 11-10). These studies are preliminary, and a firm recommendation must await their conclusion. At the present time, it has not been our practice to routinely perform biopsies on normal-appearing peritoneum or diaphragmatic surfaces. A high index of suspicion is always maintained for any abnormal-appearing surface, and biopsies are readily performed. Proper staging is the key to an accurate prognosis (Table 11-11). ✳

THERAPEUTIC OPTIONS FOR PRIMARY TREATMENT
Borderline malignant epithelial neoplasms

In the last decade, clear evidence has been presented for a group of epithelial ovarian tumors that have histologic and biologic features occupying a position between those of clearly benign and frankly malignant ovarian neoplasms. These bor-

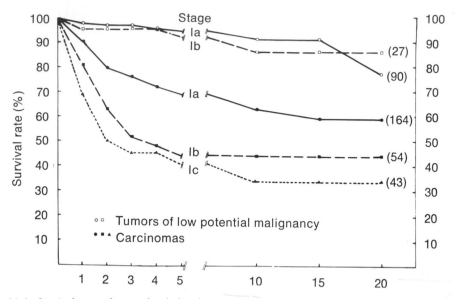

Fig. 11-6. Survival rates of stage I borderline lesions as compared with other grades of epithelial ovarian carcinoma. (From Aure, J. C., Hoeg, K., and Kolstad, P.: Obstet. Gynecol. **37**:1, 1971.)

15%

derline malignancies, which account for approximately 15% of all epithelial ovarian cancers, are often referred to as proliferative cystadenomas. A 10-year survival rate of approximately 95% has been obtained in these borderline neoplasms (Fig. 11-6). However, symptomatic recurrence and death may develop as many as 20 years after therapy in a few patients. These neoplasms can correctly be labeled as being of low malignant potential. On the basis of their almost benign behavior, many gynecologists have advocated conservative therapy, especially in patients who are desirous of further childbearing and have stage IA disease.

Malignant epithelial neoplasms

The most common epithelial cancers of the ovary are histologically categorized as serous, mucinous, endometrioid, and clear-cell (mesonephroid) types (Figs. 11-7 to 11-10). Although there has been some controversy in the past, it is now apparent that these different histologic varieties behave similarly stage for stage and grade for grade. Some types, such as the mucinous and endometrioid varieties, are more commonly found in lower stages, with more well-differentiated lesions accounting for the confusion in the earlier literature. Prognosis, survival, and therapy for these various forms of epithelial cancer are hereafter considered collectively.

Ovarian carcinoma initially grows locally, invading the capsule and mesovarium and then adjacent organs by contiguous growth and lymphatic spread. Once the malignancy has reached the external surface of the capsule, cells may exfoliate into the peritoneal cavity, where they are free to circulate and later implant. Local and regional lymphatic metastasis may occur that involves the uterus, fallopian tubes,

Text continued on p. 274.

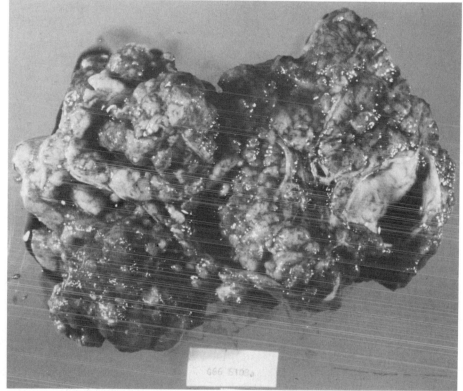

Fig. 11-7. Papillary serous adenocarcinoma of ovary. **A,** Gross appearance with soft, friable proliferating papillae.   *Continued.*

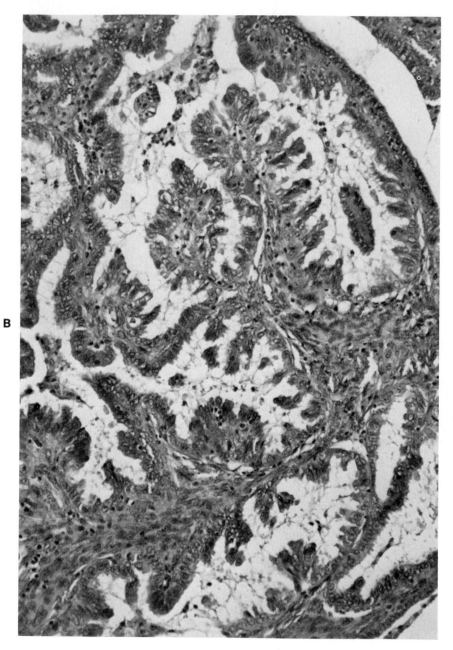

B

Fig. 11-7, cont'd. B, Histologic appearance with prominent fibrous stalks and non–mucin producing epithelial cells.

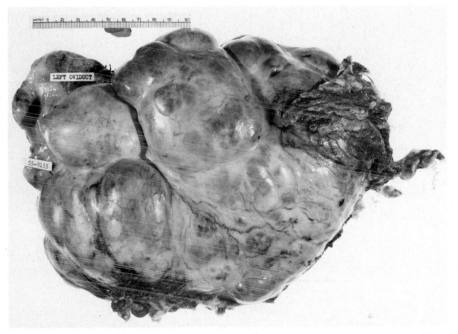

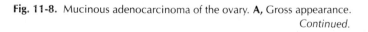

Fig. 11-8. Mucinous adenocarcinoma of the ovary. **A,** Gross appearance.
Continued.

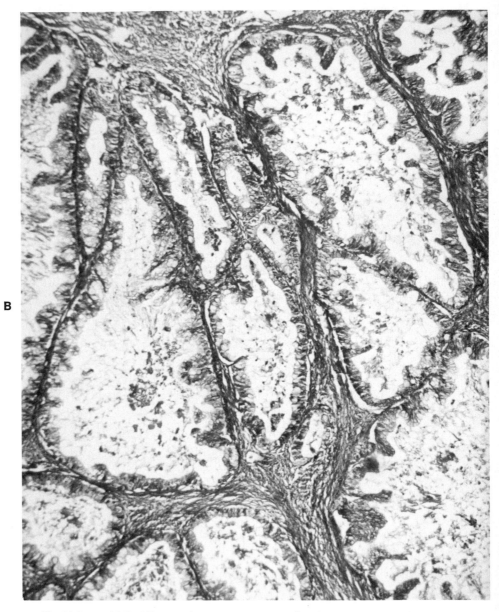

B

Fig. 11-8, cont'd. B, Microscopic appearance. Note tall, columnar, mucin-producing cells.

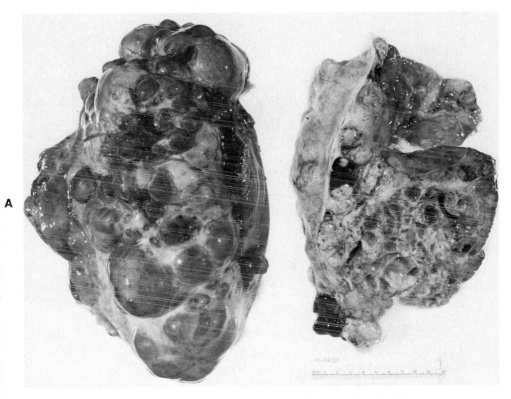

Fig. 11-9. Endometrioid adenocarcinoma of the ovary. **A,** Gross cystic and solid appearance.
Continued.

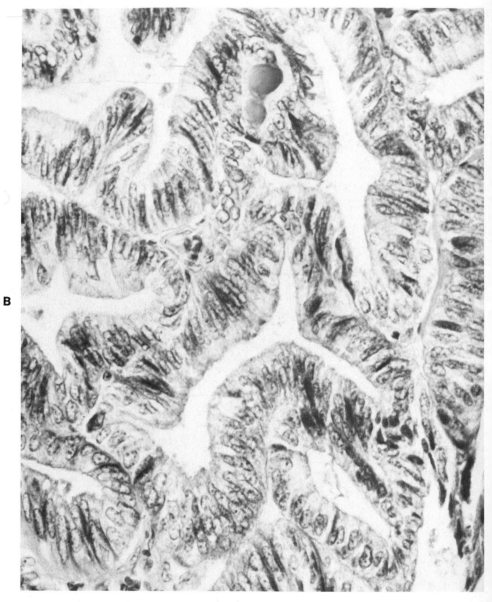

Fig. 11-9, cont'd. B, Histologic appearance with columnar and pseudostratified epithelial cells showing prominent elongated hyperchromatic nuclei.

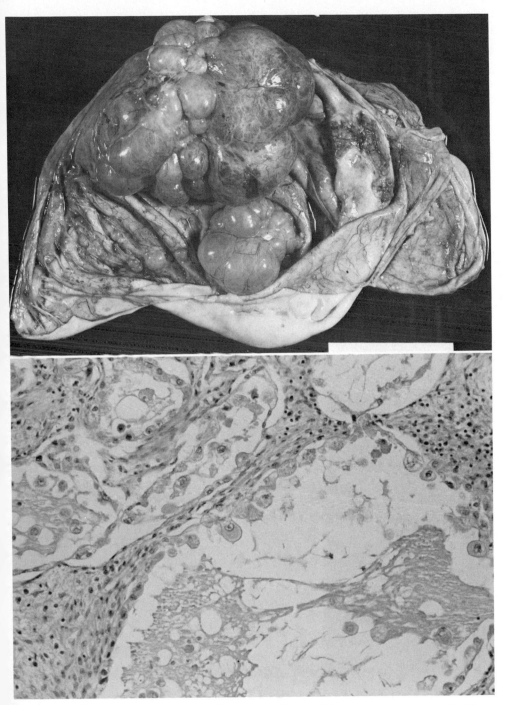

Fig. 11-10. Clear-cell adenocarcinoma of the ovary. **A,** Gross solid and cystic appearance. **B,** Microscopic view showing hobnail or peg cells.

and pelvic lymph nodes. Involvement of the para-aortic lymph nodes by way of the infundibulopelvic ligament is also common. Probably the most important variable influencing the prognosis in each case of ovarian cancer is the stage or extent of disease. A staging system has been devised that allows a comparison of treatment results among different institutions. Although staging does not mandate treatment, discussing treatment by stage is often helpful.

Survival depends on the stage of the lesion, the grade of differentiation of the lesion, the amount of residual tumor remaining following surgery, and the additional treatment following surgery. The 5-year survival figures from the FIGO report (Table 11-12) for the years 1958 to 1962 are: stage I, 61%; stage IB and IIA, 42%; stage IIB, 32%; stage III, 7%; and stage IV, 2.6%. The overall 5-year survival rate was 27%. There is improved survival stage for stage in those patients with well-differentiated lesions, in those with all or most of the tumor removed at surgery, and in those who received postoperative irradiation and/or chemotherapy.

Stage IA, IB, and IC. Total abdominal hysterectomy with bilateral salpingo-oophorectomy is undoubtedly the best therapy for stage I lesions (Table 11-13). At many institutions, omentectomy is also performed for stage I lesions, especially if adjunctive therapy is planned in the form of intraperitoneal instillation of radioactive phosphorus. In addition to being an organ that may harbor microscopic disease in patients with apparent stage I lesions, the omentum is an organ to which radioactive colloidal substances such as P 32 have a great affinity, and thus its removal theoreti-

Table 11-12. Survival rates (5-year) for epithelial ovarian cancer (1958-1962)

Stage IA	293/483 (61%)
Stage IB, IIA	124/295 (42%)
Stage IIB	141/446 (32%)
Stage III	57/824 (7%)
Stage IV	7/292 (2.6%)
Overall	622/2,320 (27%)

Modified from Kottmeier, H., and Kolstad, P., editors: Annual report on the results of treatment in carcinoma of the uterus, vagina, and ovary, vol. 15, Stockholm, 1973, FIGO (based on 2,320 reported cases).

Table 11-13. Stage I ovarian cancer (Mayo Clinic)

Extent grossly	Survival
Intracystic papillations	90%
Extracystic excrescences	68%
Ruptured cyst	56%
Adherent cyst	51%

Data from Webb, M. J., Decker, D. G., Mussey, E., and Williams, T. J.: Factors influencing survival in Stage I ovarian cancer, Am. J. Obstet. Gynecol. **116:**222, 1973.

cally allows a greater amount of radioactive substance to be available for distribution over the visceral and parietal peritoneal surfaces of the abdomen. The value of omentectomy in and of itself as a therapeutic modality for stage I disease is yet to be conclusively established. ·

Recent evidence suggests that pelvic and para-aortic nodes may be involved 10% to 20% of the time in stage I disease, and the value of lymphadenectomy as a diagnostic and therapeutic procedure is now under study. Creasman and associates reported four patients with ovarian cancer who, after chemotherapy or combined immunochemotherapy, were found to have retroperitoneal disease at the time of a second-look exploratory laparotomy, even though there was no evidence of intraabdominal residual cancer. Ovarian cancer can metastasize to both pelvic and para-aortic lymph nodes, and therefore these areas must be evaluated in order to assess appropriately the true extent of disease in patients with ovarian cancer.

Other institutions prefer chemotherapy with alkylating agents such as melphalan or chlorambucil as postoperative therapy. The drug is usually continued for a period of 12 to 18 months, after which time patients clinically free of disease are usually subjected to a second-look procedure. If no evidence of disease is found, therapy is discontinued. If residual disease is uncovered, appropriate radiotherapy or alternate chemotherapy may then be instituted. Not uncommonly, an isolated focus is judicious. In the management of low-grade (grade 1) lesions, the physician must weigh the possible benefits of adjuvant chemotherapy versus the risks suggested by some preliminary reports on the development of fatal acute leukemia in patients with ovarian cancer treated with alkylating agents and surviving 10 years or more. (See Carcinogenicity of Anticancer Drugs, p. 295.)

The most appropriate adjuvant therapy for patients with stage I lesions in whom total abdominal hysterectomy and bilateral salpingo-oophorectomy have been carried out is a subject of considerable controversy. Some have advocated no further therapy, whereas others have insisted on either a period of chemotherapy or intraperitoneal instillation of radioactive colloid. The only prospective study presently available that addresses this subject is found in some preliminary data of the Gynecologic Oncology Group (GOG) (Table 11-14). These data suggest that patients do

Table 11-14. Gynecologic Oncology Group protocol 1 (preliminary data): recurrences in terms of treatment of stage I epithelial ovarian cancer

Regimen*	Number of patients	Number of recurrences
1	29	5 (17.2%)
2	23	7 (30.4%)
3	34	2 (5.9%)

From Hreshchyshyn, M. H., Park, R. C., Blessing, J. A., and others: The role of adjunctive therapy in stage I ovarian cancer, Am. J. Obstet. Gynecol., in press.
*1, no further treatment; 2, 5,000 rads whole-pelvis irradiation; 3, melphalan, 0.2 mg/kg/day for 5 days every 4 weeks for 18 months.

better with adjuvant therapy, and chemotherapy appears to be the most appropriate modality. In the young woman with stage IA disease who is desirous of further childbearing, unilateral salpingo-oophorectomy may be associated with minimal increased risk of recurrence provided a careful staging procedure has been performed and due consideration has been given to grade and apparent self-containment of the neoplasm.

Stage IIA and IIB. In many institutions, the treatment of choice for stage IIA and IIB disease is total abdominal hysterectomy with bilateral salpingo-oophorectomy, omentectomy, and instillation of P 32. Other centers prefer abdominal plus pelvic irradiation as postoperative therapy. Still other institutions have had reasonable success with a combination of pelvic irradiation and systemic chemotherapy. A fourth, commonly used treatment plan is to follow surgery with 12 to 18 months of chemotherapy, usually with an alkylating agent, and to perform a second-look procedure if the patient is clinically free of disease at that time. As with stage I disease, the value of omentectomy remains inconclusive. Here, as in stage I disease, the variety of treatment plans is a reflection of retrospective studies that report acceptable survival rates following a number of therapy approaches. One issue appears to be clear: the entire abdomen should be considered at risk, and the treatment plan should include some form of therapy for all peritoneal surfaces. Even very large institutions have only a few cases of stage I or stage II disease, making prospective randomized studies difficult. Fortunately, these problems are currently being studied by cooperative groups, and some firm answers concerning optimum therapy may be forthcoming.

Stage III. In stage III, as with other stages, every effort should be made to remove the uterus with both adnexa. In addition, every effort should be made short of major bowel surgery to remove the bulk of the tumor, including large omental cakes. Retrospective studies have suggested strongly that the survival rate in patients with stage III disease relates to the residual tumor following surgery, such that those patients with minimal residual appear to have a better prognosis with adjunctive therapy. Adjunctive therapy in the form of abdominal plus pelvic irradiation is used in many centers but has found less and less favor in recent years. Unless the residual masses are no larger than 2 cm at any locus in the abdomen, irradiation is not likely to be effective. Thus, patients with bulky residual disease should be treated with chemotherapy (Table 11-15). Standard chemotherapy has been in the form of a single drug alkylating agent (melphalan, chlorambucil, thiotepa, or cyclophosphamide). The alkylating agent of choice in many institutions is melphalan (Alkeran), but comparable responses have been reported with the other agents in smaller series. The agent should be continued for at least 12 to 18 months or as long as clinical disease is apparent. Should the patient survive this period and have no clinical evidence of disease, a second-look procedure is usually recommended.

Recent evidence would suggest that even in the optimum group (patients with residua no greater than 2 cm in diameter at any site), the survival and response rate with single-agent chemotherapy is equivalent to that with abdominal and pelvic ir-

Table 11-15. Epithelial ovarian cancer

Size of largest tumor	Number of patients	Mean survival (months)
0	29	39
0-0.5	28	29
0.6-1.5	16	18
>1.5	29	11

From Griffiths, C. T.: Surgical resection of tumor bulk in the primary treatment of ovarian cancer, Natl. Cancer Inst. Monogr. **42:**101, 1975.

radiation. The morbidity of radiation therapy is, of course, much greater, and there-fore this finding may have considerable influence on future postoperative therapy for stage III disease. Initial prospective studies by several groups randomized pa-tients between single-agent chemotherapy and multiple-drug regimens, and most concluded (with regard to patient survival) that polychemotherapy had little advan-tage over single-agent regimens. This issue is quite important since the morbidity of polychemotherapy is considerably greater than that of the single drug alkylating agent regimen. Several recent and ongoing studies of still other drug combinations may significantly alter this preference for single-agent therapy (to be discussed later in this chapter).

Stage IV. The ideal management of stage IV disease is to remove as much cancer as possible and subject the patient to postoperative chemotherapy.

Maximal surgical effort on initial laparotomy

It has been axiomatic among many gynecologic oncologists that it is judicious to excise as much tumor tissue as possible when disseminated disease is encountered at the time of primary operation for ovarian cancer. Although it was known that significant palliation may be achieved by reduction of a heavy tumor burden, there had been little firm evidence that the usual "debulking" procedures directly improve survival until recent reports. Munnell reported a 28% 5-year survival rate among patients who had undergone a "maximal surgical effort" as compared with a 9% 5-year survival rate among patients who had had partial resection and a 3% 5-year survival rate among patients who had had biopsy only. In Munnell's 14 survivors, the "maximal surgical effort" consisted of hysterectomy, bilateral salpingo-oophorectomy, and omentectomy.

Aure and associates and Kottmeier demonstrated significant improvement in sur-vival among stage III patients only if all of the gross tumor had been removed (Fig. 11-11). Similar results were recently obtained by Griffiths, who used a multiple linear regression equation with survival as the dependent variable in order to control simultaneously for the multiple therapeutic and biologic factors that contribute to the ultimate outcome in the individual patient. The most important factors proved to be histologic grade of the tumor and size of the largest residual mass following primary surgery. The operation itself contributed nothing to survival unless it ef-

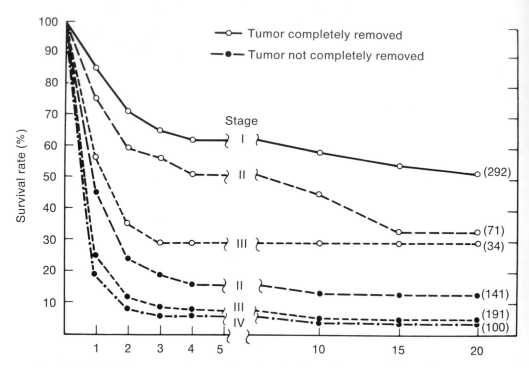

Fig. 11-11. Survival rates stage for stage in patients in whom all tumor was surgically removed versus those patients in whom all tumor was not completely removed. (From Aure, J. C., Hoeg, K., and Kolstad, P.: Obstet. Gynecol. **37:**1, 1971.)

fected the reduction in the size of the largest residual tumor mass below the limit of 1.6 cm.

The so-called debulking procedure has gained considerable attention in the management of ovarian cancer. The concept is simply to diminish the residual tumor burden to a point where adjuvant therapy will be optimally effective. All forms of adjuvant therapy are most effective when a minimal tumor burden exists. This is particularly true of ovarian carcinoma, which is one of the more sensitive solid tumors to chemotherapy. A careful and persistent surgeon can often remove large tumor masses that on first impression appear to be unresectable. Using the clear retroperitoneal spaces, one can usually identify the infundibulopelvic ligament and ureter and then isolate the vessels of the infundibulopelvic ligament and the blood supply of the ovary. Once these vessels have been ligated and transected, retrograde removal of large ovarian masses is easier and safer. The ureter is, of course, kept under direct vision throughout the dissection, and fear of traumatizing this pelvic structure is thereby minimized. A clear space also exists on the transverse colon whereby large omental cakes of ovarian carcinoma can be removed after the right and left gastroepiploic vessels have been ligated. Removal of large ovarian masses and omental involvement often reduces the tumor burden by 80% to 90%. The theoretical value of debulking procedures lies in the obvious reduction of cell num-

Table 11-16. Survival in terms of stage of epithelial ovarian cancer

	2-year	5-year
Stage I	80%	70%
Stage II	40%	25%
Stage III	18%	12%
Stage IV	5%	0%

bers and the advantage this affords to adjuvant therapy. This is especially relevant in bulky solid tumors such as ovarian cancer, where removal of large numbers of cells in the resting phase (G_0) can result in the propelling of the residual cells into the more vulnerable proliferating pool. Several careful retrospective studies have repeatedly demonstrated improved survival rate in patients who can be surgically brought to a status of minimal tumor burden. A recent report of the very large experience of the M. D. Anderson Hospital and Tumor Institute illustrated a significantly improved salvage rate in patients with stage II and stage III epithelial cancer of the ovary when initial surgery was followed by no gross residual tumor or no single residual tumor mass exceeding 1 cm in diameter. This report boasts of a 70% 2-year survival rate in stage III patients in whom no gross disease remained and a 50% survival rate when residual nodules were limited to 1 cm in diameter. This compares very favorably with the usually quoted overall survival rates (Table 11-16).

Role of radiation therapy

Radiation therapy techniques include intraperitoneal radioactive gold or chromium phosphate and external beam therapy to the abdomen and pelvis. Patients with epithelial carcinoma of the ovary selected to receive postoperative irradiation should receive treatment of the entire abdomen plus additional radiation to the pelvis. This broad treatment plan is based on an analysis of postirradiation recurrences of stage I and stage II disease that showed that most of the recurrences were outside the pelvis. There is no lid on the pelvis, and malignant cells are shed from the primary ovarian tumor and circulate throughout the entire abdominal cavity.

Two different radiation treatment techniques have been used for abdominal irradiation. Large portals may be employed, and a dose of 2,500 to 3,000 rads can be delivered over 4 to 5 weeks to the entire abdomen. The kidneys and possibly the right lobe of the liver are shielded with lead to limit the dose to 2,000 to 2,500 rads. Nausea and vomiting may be associated with this procedure, and therapy is frequently interrupted. In some centers the abdominal irradiation is delivered by the so-called moving strip technique. The abdomen, or the volume to be irradiated, is divided into contiguous segments or strips 2.5 cm wide. Both front and back are treated daily, and the treatment field is increased by one strip every 2 days until four strips (10 cm) have been treated. The 10-cm segment is moved up 2.5 cm every 2 days until the last strip is reached. The field is then reduced progressively one strip at a time, and on the last 2 days of treatment a single 2.5-cm strip is irradiated. Again the kidneys are shielded with lead, as is the upper portion of the liver, in an effort to reduce the dose to these organs. With this technique, each strip of the abdomen is irradiated from front and back for 8 days by the main beam and for 4 days by the penumbra (scatter), for a total of 12 days of irradiation. This treatment is usually delivered by a cobalt 60 machine, and a tumor dose of 2,600 to 2,800 rads, measured at the midline along a sagittal plane, can be delivered safely. It is calculated that this is biologically equivalent to approximately 4,000 rads given by the whole-abdomen technique. The fact that the dose is administered in a shorter time is the justification for this equivalent, and it is felt that since only a small portion of the abdominal cavity is irradiated at any one time, the treatment may be better tolerated. Nausea and vomiting are not uncommon when the upper abdomen is being treated, and diarrhea is frequent when the beam is low in the abdomen. Both the whole-abdomen and the moving strip techniques usually finish with a pelvic boost of approximately 2,000 to 3,000 rads.

As a better understanding of the effects of chemotherapeutic agents in ovarian cancer has been gained, the role of radiation therapy in this disease has diminished in prominence. The spread pattern of ovarian cancer and the normal tissue bed involved in the treatment of this neoplasm make effective radiation therapy difficult (Table 11-17). When the residual disease following laparotomy is bulky, radiation therapy is particularly ineffectual. The entire abdomen must be considered at risk, and therefore the volume that must be irradiated is very large, resulting in multiple limitations for the radiotherapist (Table 11-18).

As long as a decade ago, several institutions abandoned the use of irradiation as postoperative therapy in patients with bulky residual epithelial cancer of the ovary. However, these same institutions continued to test the applicability of irradiation in patients with minimal residual disease after surgery. Recently, a study was reported by Smith and associates from the M. D. Anderson Hospital that gave the results of a randomized prospective study of patients with minimal residual disease (no nodule greater than 2 cm) who were randomized between single drug alkylating agent chemotherapy and whole-abdomen irradiation (moving strip technique) with a pelvic boost. This study showed no advantage to the irradiation therapy and a significant

Table 11-17. Special problems in ovarian cancer

Limits of tumor spread often unknown
Variability of radiosensitivity
Total tumor burden usually very large
Free mobility of tumor cells within the abdominal cavity
Radiation dosage restricted by neighboring organs
Detection of early disease infrequent

Table 11-18. Dose restrictions

Tolerance of small intestine
Limited tolerance of kidneys
Bone marrow depression
Radiation enteritis due to large volume of intestine irradiated
Adhesive peritonitis

increase in morbidity. Based on this study, the role of radiation therapy in many institutions has become very limited for stage III and stage IV disease. The GOG tested the feasibility of using radiation therapy in conjunction with chemotherapy. A prospective randomized study using four arms and assessing radiation therapy alone, radiation therapy prior to chemotherapy (Alkeran), chemotherapy alone, and chemotherapy prior to radiation therapy was recently completed with no significant difference found in any of the four arms. It thus becomes difficult to justify the morbidity of extensive radiation therapy for this disease process.

The role of radiation therapy in localized disease also needs discussion. A recent prospective randomized study of stage I epithelial cancer of the ovary conducted by the GOG had the following results. Patients were randomized between three arms: (1) no further therapy, (2) Alkeran, and (3) pelvic radiation. Preliminary results would indicate that those patients who received Alkeran did the best, with no appreciable benefit being noted from the use of pelvic radiation. On the other hand, the role of pelvic radiation in stage II ovarian cancer has yet to be defined. Indeed, many institutions use pelvic radiation in conjunction with systemic chemotherapy as the customary treatment of stage II disease. Retrospective studies would suggest that pelvic radiation improves survival over and above the use of surgery alone (Table 11-19). The efficacy of pelvic radiation as compared with chemotherapy in stage II disease has yet to be tested in a prospective randomized study.

Radioisotopes

Radioisotopes have been widely used for the treatment of ovarian cancer. Both the pure beta emitter radioactive chromic phosphate (half-life of 14.2 days) and radioactive gold (10% gamma, half-life of 2.7 days) have been used. These isotopes emit radiation with an effective maximum penetration of 4 to 5 mm and therefore are only useful with minimal disease. Both agents are taken up by the serosal macrophages and transported to the retroperitoneal and mediastinal lymph nodes. The likelihood that the radioactive colloid will eradicate nodal metastases by selective lymphatic uptake is in considerable doubt, since studies suggest that malignant nodes do not take up the isotope but tumor-free nodes do. It has been estimated that 6,000 rads are delivered to the omentum and peritoneal surfaces and 7,000 rads

Table 11-19. Radiotherapy in FIGO stage II disease

Series	Number of patients		5-year survival rate (%)	
	Surgery alone	Surgery/ irradiation	Surgery alone	Surgery/ irradiation
Van Orden and associates	8	22	25	36.4
Barr and associates	27	91	33	48
Kent and McKay	32	36	28.2	52.8
Munnell	16	61	0	40
Clark and associates	6	51	16.7	31.4

to some retroperitoneal structures. If a free intraperitoneal distribution can be assured, chromic phosphate with a longer half-life and no gamma irradiation is the agent of choice. Decker and associates have demonstrated radioactive colloids to be advantageous in a selected group of patients with rupture of an ovarian tumor and surgery (80% 5-year survival rate versus 43% 5-year survival rate).

Radiotherapy with curative intent was used by Pezner to treat 104 patients with limited epithelial carcinoma of the ovary. All of these patients received intraperitoneal radioactive colloid therapy, optimally scheduled 3 to 6 weeks after laparotomy. The initial four patients received colloidal Au 198 (dose between 140 and 250 mCi). Subsequently, 94 patients received 15.0 mCi of P 32, and 6 patients received between 11.8 and 16.9 mCi of P 32. Pelvic radiotherapy was given to 56 out of 104 patients beginning approximately 6 weeks after intraperitoneal radioactive colloid therapy. The addition of pelvic radiotherapy did not appear to affect survival in limited disease stages and could not be shown to decrease the incidence of local recurrence in the pelvic region. The 5-year actuarial (no evidence of disease) survival rates, according to the FIGO staging classifications, were 95% for stage IA1, 82% for IA2, 73% for IB, 67% for IC, 67% for IIA, 67% for IIB without gross residual tumor, 25% for IIB with gross residual tumor, and 50% for III with minimal or no residual tumor. In the limited stages, the 5-year recurrence rate was 24% for patients treated with colloid alone and 31% for those treated with colloid plus pelvic radiotherapy. The incidence of small-bowel complication was related to the use of pelvic radiotherapy; these complications arose in 24% of the patients treated with colloid therapy and pelvic radiotherapy compared with only 2.2% of the patients treated with colloid therapy alone.

Experiments by Rosenshein and associates in the rhesus monkey suggest that adequate distribution of a radioactive colloidal substance instilled into the peritoneal cavity requires a volume of vehicle sufficiently large to slightly distend the peritoneal cavity. This function appears to be independent of multiple position changes. This may be particularly critical when it is desirable for therapeutic agents to reach the subdiaphragmatic area, where early microscopic metastasis from carcinoma of the ovary may exist. Myers and associates have shown the importance of position change and the value of Trendelenburg position for even distribution. Based on these observations, the following procedure for instillation of radioactive colloidal substances into the peritoneal cavity is suggested.

Technique. Radioactive colloidal chromic phosphate is either injected through a multiple perforated catheter (or catheters) that has been placed in the peritoneal cavity at surgery or inserted through a needle postoperatively. Proper placement of the catheter in the peritoneal cavity is confirmed by the instillation of 250 ml of normal saline solution. If there is free flow of saline, then technetium or Hypaque is instilled. After this, the patient is moved about to maximize distribution. Appropriate radiographs or fluoroscopy is obtained to confirm adequate distribution. Another 500 ml of saline is then instilled. Through a closed system similar to that shown in Fig. 11-12, 15 mCi of P 32 in 250 ml of saline is allowed to run into the abdomen at

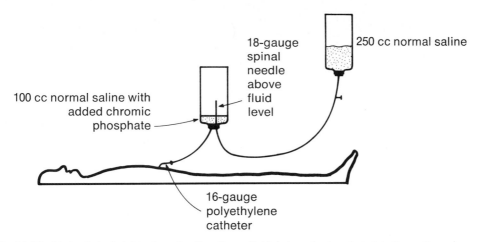

250 cc normal saline

18-gauge
spinal
needle
above
fluid
level

100 cc normal saline with
added chromic
phosphate

16-gauge
polyethylene
catheter

Fig. 11-12. Method of administration of radioactive colloidal chromic phosphate into the peritoneal cavity.

a rapid rate. Another 250 ml of saline is then run in from the upper bottle. The patient is instructed to change her position frequently so that a wide dispersion of the P 32 is obtained. The patient should be turned frequently into different positions to facilitate this distribution during the ensuing 90 to 120 minutes (Trendelenburg, 10 min; right side; left side; feet down; etc.).

Chemotherapy

Basic principles. The outcome of cancer chemotherapy is not fully predictable, but the chances of remission can be improved by judicious selection of patients, careful assessment of the tumor's growth pattern, and treatment of the neoplasm with the drug or drugs most likely to succeed.

Not all cancer patients can be treated with drugs. The suitability of a patient for chemotherapy depends on at least three critical criteria: (1) the nature of the neoplasm, (2) its extent of spread or stage, and (3) the patient's clinical condition. All cancers are not equally sensitive to drugs. Factors that determine a tumor's drug susceptibility include how the drug is distributed to the tumor, drug transport into the cell, whether a drug-sensitive biochemical pathway is present in the tumor cell, and the relative rates of intracellular activation and inactivation of the drug. In many instances, some of these factors are unknown for the drug and the tumor type. Investigational trials are currently going on with multiple agents in order to give us a better understanding of these parameters.

At present, only disseminated neoplasia is regularly treated with chemotherapy; surgery, radiotherapy, or both are the current treatment choice for localized disease. These concepts are rapidly changing, however, and the use of adjuvant chemotherapy soon after eradicative surgery is increasing, especially in the treatment of ovarian and uterine cancer. Treatment of a patient with metastatic disease should not mean waiting until the patient is cachetic or moribund. The patient should be treated as soon as she has symptoms attributable to the tumor, not only those as obvious as pain due to nerve route compression or dyspnea from lymphangitic pulmonary metastases but also anorexia and general weakness. Even asymptomatic patients who have diseases in which long remissions or cures can be achieved (such as choriocarcinoma or childhood acute leukemia) must be treated as early as possible. In most instances chemotherapy is palliative rather than curative; for this reason, side effects produced by these potent agents can only be justified by the more persistent removal of symptoms due to the tumor or by a reasonable expectation of improved survival even in the absence of symptoms. Chemotherapy in a severely debilitated patient is usually futile and often dangerous and thus should be avoided.

Chemotherapeutic agents are a crucial part of the physician's armamentarium in the ever broadening fight against cancer. With them he can ameliorate and, in a few instances, even cure diseases usually fatal in previous eras. Until recently, in most cases, chemotherapy has been reserved for relatively late stages of the disease, but its increasingly successful use, particularly in the treatment of hematologic malignancies, suggests that chemotherapy should be administered earlier. All physicians and surgeons must understand the nature and use of cancer chemotherapy so they can make rational decisions about when it may be indicated.

There are semiscientific rationales for modern treatment regimens. However, unfortunately, data on solid tumor response are still based on empirical observations. To understand the current literature on cell kinetics it is imperative to visualize cell cyling. All dividing cells follow a predictable pattern for replication called generation time. There are five basic phases as now described (Fig. 11-13). G_1 phase (G stands for gap and uncertainty as to purpose) lasts a variable amount of time but usually somewhere between 4 and 24 hours. If this phase is prolonged, we usually refer to the cell as being in the G_0, or resting, phase. The S phase is the phase of DNA synthesis and usually lasts between 6 and 8 hours. The G_2 phase is a premitotic phase lasting from 2 to 4 hours, and the M phase, when actual mitosis takes place, lasts between 1 and 4 hours. Tumors do not have faster generation times but have more cells in the active phases of replication than normal tissues. Normal tissues have a large number of cells in the G_0 phase.

Various chemotherapeutic agents appear to act at different phases of the cell cycle. Alkylating agents appear to act in all phases from G_0 to mitosis. They are termed cycle-nonspecific agents. Drugs such as hydoxyurea, doxorubicin (Adriamycin), and methotrexate appear to act primarily in the S phase. Bleomycin appears to act in the G_2 phase, and vincristine appears to act in the M phase. These drugs are termed cycle-specific agents because the chemotherapeutic drug acts only on cells that are in some phase of the cell generation cycle. Steroids, 5-fluorouracil, and cis-platinum have rather uniform activity around the cell generation cycle. In theory, if certain cancer therapeutic agents attack only cells that are dividing and more tumor cells are dividing than in normal tissues, then by properly spacing the chemotherapeutic agent and combining agents acting in different sites of the cell cycle, one

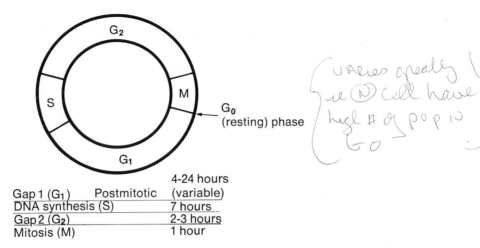

Gap 1 (G$_1$)	Postmitotic	4-24 hours (variable)
DNA synthesis (S)		7 hours
Gap 2 (G$_2$)		2-3 hours
Mitosis (M)		1 hour

Fig. 11-13. Cell generation time and sequence are similar for all mammalian cells.

should be able to kill tumor cells in far greater numbers than normal cells. Kinetic studies both in humans and animals suggest that tumors that have been cured by chemotherapy are those with a large fraction of cells in the proliferative phase (e.g., gestational choriocarcinoma and Burkitt's lymphoma). The extent of the disease rather than the total mass of tumor is the most important factor in considering curative radiation or surgery, but with chemotherapy the total mass is very important. Tumor volume reduction allows the remaining tumor cells to begin to divide actively (they are propelled from the G$_0$ phase into the more vulnerable cell generation cycle), thereby rendering them susceptible to chemotherapy. These chemotherapeutic agents, as with radiation therapy, kill by first-order kinetics, i.e., there is a reduction of the tumor population by a characteristic percentage regardless of the actual number of tumor cells initially present (Fig. 11-14). If the tumor burden is small, fewer cycles of chemotherapy may be necessary. One milligram of tumor usually consists of 10^6 cells. One cubic centimeter of tumor usually consists of 10^9 cells. Patient death usually occurs at 10^{12} cells.

Dynamics of chemotherapy. The time it takes a cell to complete one cycle of growth and division is its generation time. However, the time a tumor takes to double in size (doubling time) depends not only on generation time but also on cell death rate (Fig. 11-15). Thus, one cannot assume a long generation time simply because a tumor enlarges slowly. Slow tumor growth can result when a rapid generation time is combined with a high cell death rate. For similar reasons, a small tumor discovered on x-ray or physical examination is not necessarily an early tumor; only serial studies to judge its growth rate will help establish its age. Bulky tumors (diameters greater than 2 to 3 cm) enlarge more slowly than small ones because their cells, especially those of the inner core (farthest from the blood supply), have a long

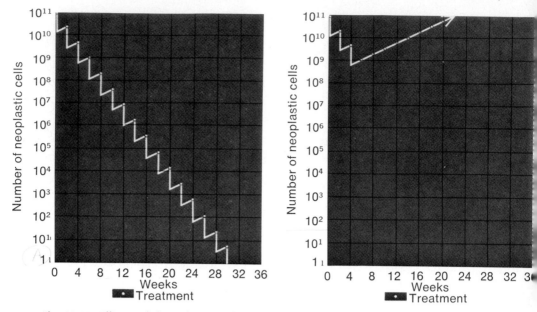

Fig. 11-14. Efficacy of chemotherapy related to tumor cell kinetics. (Figure by Miller, A., from Luce, J. K., and others: The systemic approach to cancer therapy, Hospital Practice, Vol. 2, No. 10. Reproduced with permission.)

generation time. Competition for nutrients and other less well defined competitive pressures reduce the activity of the whole mass.

Chemotherapy of cancer requires an edge, a physiologic mechanism that can be exploited to differentially kill cancer cells while sparing normal cells as much as possible. Tumor tissues have a more rapid growth rate compared with normal tissues, and this can be used against them. This is especially true because the growth of tumor cells is characteristically more synchronized than that of normal cells. This means that at any given time comparatively large numbers of cancer cells will be in the DNA synthesis phase (S phase) of the cell cycle, the only time during which cycle-dependent agents (those inhibiting DNA synthesis) can act. Thus, short-term high-dose chemotherapy with agents affecting DNA synthesis, such as methotrexate, is most effective in killing rapidly dividing tumor cells with relative sparing of normal bone marrow elements. Unfortunately, bone marrow cells and the epithelial cells that line the gastrointestinal tract as well as hair follicles have generation times comparable with those of tumors and are therefore vulnerable to compounds that inhibit DNA synthesis. However, compared with the more synchronously growing tumor cell population, only a small portion of the bone marrow cells are in their S phase at a given time, and this accounts for the selective toxicity of phase-dependent compounds. A course of therapy extending over a period of several days or even weeks may be required to kill a slow-growing tumor, in which only a few cells are in the stage of DNA synthesis at any one time. Agents that do not depend on DNA synthe-

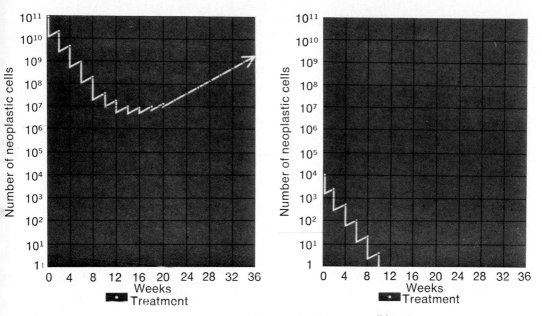

Fig. 11-14, cont'd. Efficacy of chemotherapy related to tumor cell kinetics.

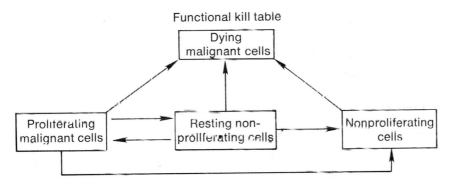

Functional kill table

Fig. 11-15. Dynamics of tumor growth showing the interrelationship of cell compartments contributing to the clinical presence of the tumor.

sis for their effects (cycle-nonspecific agents), such as alkylating agents, are most effective against bulky, slow-growing tumors. The cells remaining after treatment tend to divide more rapidly and are more susceptible to attack by cycle-specific agents. Thus, there is some flexibility in the interplay of chemotherapeutic agents.

The phenomenon of increased susceptibility of tumor cells during recovery from alkylating agents is the rationale for sequentially combining cycle-nonspecific and cycle-specific agents in many new regimens. If, in addition, drugs with different mechanisms of toxicity are combined, each drug can be given safely in the dose used when it is given alone. Each drug chosen for combination therapy should have antitumor activity when used alone.

Whenever possible, intermittent courses of chemotherapy are used to allow restoration of normal cells if they were reduced in number by treatment. In instances where an antidote to the chemotherapeutic agent is known, for example leucovorin (citrovorum factor–folinic acid) for methotrexate, this antidote can also be given to hasten normal cell recovery. Of course, the danger of revitalizing sublethally injured tumor cells also exists and must be evaluated with each new treatment regimen. Although careful studies are needed to compare each new combination with the single agents concerned, the trend in chemotherapy is unquestionably toward exploitation of drug combinations used simultaneously and sequentially.

Categories of drugs in current use (Table 11-20)

(A) *Cycle-nonspecific agents*

ALKYLATING AGENTS. Alkylating agents prevent cell division primarily by cross-linking strands of DNA. Because of continued synthesis of other cell constituents, such as RNA and protein, growth is unbalanced, and the cell dies. The activity of alkylating agents does not depend on DNA synthesis in the target cells. Cyclophosphamide, however, also inhibits DNA synthesis, which makes it distinctive among the alkylating agents in its mode and spectrum of activity. The alkylating agents currently in use in gynecologic oncology are:

1. Cyclophosphamide (Cytoxan)
2. Chlorambucil (Leukeran)
3. Melphalan (Alkeran)
4. Triethylenethiophosphoramide (thiotepa)

(B) *Cycle-specific agents*

① ANTIMETABOLITES. Antimetabolites act by inhibiting essential metabolic processes that are required for DNA and/or RNA synthesis. The currently used drugs in this category are:

(A) 5-Fluorouracil (5-FU)
(B) Methotrexate (MTX, Amethopterin)

② ANTIBIOTICS. A number of cytotoxic antibiotics have come into use for chemotherapy of certain neoplasms. Those used in gynecologic oncology are:

Dactinomycin (actinomycin D)
Bleomycin (Blenoxane)
Doxorubicin (Adriamycin)

③ PLANT ALKALOIDS. The two principal vinca alkaloids are very similar in structure, mode of action, and metabolism (mainly in the liver) but are very different in regard to dose, toxicity, and antitumor spectrum. They arrest cells in metaphase by

Text continued on p. 294.

Table 11-20. Chemotherapy agents used in treatment of gynecologic cancer

Drug	Dosage and route of administration	Acute side effects	Toxicity	Precautions*	Major indications
Alkylating agents					
Cyclophosphamide (Cytoxan)	500-1,500 mg/m² as a single dose IV or 60-120 mg/m²/day PO; dose decreased if severe leukopenia develops	Nausea and vomiting	Bone marrow depression, alopecia, cystitis	Maintain adequate fluid intake to avoid cystitis	Carcinoma of the cervix, ovary, endometrium, and fallopian tube
Chlorambucil (Leukeran)	0.1-0.2 mg/kg/day PO; dose decreased if severe bone marrow depression develops	Nausea, vomiting (with high doses)	Bone marrow depression	None	
Melphalan (Alkeran)	0.2 mg/kg/day PO for 4 days every 4-6 weeks	Nausea, vomiting (with high doses)	Bone marrow depression	None	
Triethylene-thiophosphoramide (thiotepa)	0.2 mg/kg/day IV for 5 days	None	Bone marrow depression	None	
Cycle-specific antimetabolites					
5-Fluorouracil (5-FU, fluorouracil)	12 mg/kg/day IV for 4 days; then alternate days at 6 mg/kg for 4 days or until toxicity; repeat course monthly or give weekly IV dose of 12-15 mg/kg; maximum dose 1 g for either regimen; often used as one drug in combination regimens at a dose of 500 mg/m² IV	Occasional nausea and vomiting	Bone marrow depression, diarrhea, stomatitis, alopecia	Decrease dose in patients with diminished liver, renal, or bone marrow function or after adrenalectomy	Carcinoma of the ovary and endometrium

*All alkylating agents and many other antineoplastic drugs should be used only if absolutely necessary in pregnant women, since they may be abortifacient or teratogenic.

Continued.

Table 11-20. Chemotherapy agents used in treatment of gynecologic cancer—cont'd

Drug	Dosage and route of administration	Acute side effects	Toxicity	Precautions*	Major indications
Cycle-specific antimetabolites—cont'd					
Methotrexate (MTX, Amethopterin)	Choriocarcinoma: 10-30 mg/day IV for 5 days Ovarian or cervical carcinoma: 200-2,000 mg/m² IV with concomitant and/or sequential systematic antidote leucovorin ("leucovorin rescue")	None	Bone marrow depression, megaloblastic anemia, diarrhea, stomatitis, vomiting; alopecia less common; occasional hepatic fibrosis, vasculitis, pulmonary fibrosis	Adequate renal function must be present, and urine output must be maintained	Choriocarcinoma, carcinoma of the ovary and cervix
Antibiotics					
Dactinomycin (actinomycin D, Cosmegen)	15 μg/kg/day IV or 0.5 mg/day for 5 days	Pain on local infiltration with skin necrosis; nausea and vomiting in many patients 2 hours after dose; occasional cramps and diarrhea	Bone marrow depression, stomatitis, diarrhea, erythema, hyperpigmentation with occasional desquamation in areas of previous irradiation	Administer through running IV infusion; use with care in liver disease and in presence of inadequate marrow function; prophylactic antiemetics are helpful	Embryonal rhabdomyosarcoma, choriocarcinoma, ovarian germ cell tumors
Mitomycin C (Mutamycin)	0.05 mg/kg/day IV for 6 days, then alternate days until 50-mg total dose	Nausea, vomiting, local inflammation and ulceration if extravasated	Neutropenia, thrombocytopenia, oral ulceration, nausea, vomiting, diarrhea	Administer through running IV infusion or inject with great care to prevent extravasation	Carcinoma of the cervix
Bleomycin (Blenoxane)	10-20 mg/m² IV or IM 1-2 times a week; start with 5 mg for first two doses in lymphoma	Fever, chills, nausea, vomiting; local pain and phlebitis less frequent	Skin: hyperpigmentation, thickening, nail changes, ulceration, rash, peeling, alopecia	Watch for hypersensitivity in lymphoma with first 1-2 doses; use with extreme cau-	Squamous cell carcinoma of the skin, vulva, and cervix; chorio-

Doxorubicin (Adriamycin)	60-100 mg/m² IV every 3 weeks	Nausea, vomiting, fever, local phlebitis, recrosis if extravasated, red urine (not blood)	Administer through running IV infusion; avoid giving to patients with significant heart disease, follow for ECG abnormalities and signs of heart failure	Adenocarcinoma of the endometrium, tube, ovary, and vagina; uterine sarcoma
		Bone marrow depression, alopecia, cardiac toxicity related to cumulative dose, stomatitis		
		monitis with dyspnea, rales, infiltrate can progress to fibrosis; more common in patients over 70 and with more than 400-mg total dose, but unpredictable	renal or pulmonary disease; start in hospital under observation, do not exceed total dose of 400 mg	
Plant alkaloids Vinblastine (Velban)	0.10-0.15 mg/kg week IV	Severe, prolonged inflammation if extravasated; occasional nausea, vomiting, headache, and paresthesias	Administer through running IV infusion or inject with great care to prevent extravasation; decrease dose in liver disease	Choriocarcinoma
		Bone marrow depression, particularly neutropenia; alopecia, muscle weakness, occasional mild peripheral neuropathy, mental depression 2-3 days after treatment, rarely stomatitis		

Continued.

Table 11-20. Chemotherapy agents used in treatment of gynecologic cancer—cont'd

Drug	Dosage and route of administration	Acute side effects	Toxicity	Precautions*	Major indications
Plant alkaloids—cont'd					
Vincristine (Oncovin)	0.4-1.4 mg/m² IV weekly in adults; 2 mg/m² weekly in children	Local inflammation if extravasated	Paresthesias, weakness, loss of reflexes, constipation; abdominal, chest, and jaw pain; hoarseness, foot-drop, mental depression; marrow toxicity generally mild, anemia and reticulocytopenia most prominent; alopecia	Administer through running IV infusion or inject with great care to prevent extravasation; decrease dose in liver disease; patients with underlying neurologic problems may be more susceptible to neurotoxicity; alopecia may be prevented by use of a scalp tourniquet for 5 minutes during and after administration	Uterine sarcoma, germ cell tumor of the ovary
Miscellaneous					
Hydroxyurea (Hydrea)	80 mg/kg PO every 3 days or 20-30 mg/kg/day	Anorexia and nausea	Bone marrow depression, megaloblastic anemia; stomatitis, diarrhea, and alope-	Decrease dose in patients with marrow and renal dysfunction	Carcinoma of the cervix (with radiotherapy)

chloroplatinum (cis-platinum)	3 weeks	ing, often severe	moderate myelo-suppression, neu-rotoxicity	to exceed 1 mg/min and only after 10-12 hours of hydration. Avoid nephrotoxic anti-bodies; watch renal function and discontinue if BUN exceeds 30 or creatinine ex-ceeds 2.0	ovary, endo-metrium, or cervix
Progestational agents				
Medroxyproges-terone acetate	400-800 mg/week IM or PO	None	Occasional liver function abnor-malities, occa-sional alopecia and hypersensitiv-ity reactions	Use with care in presence of liver dysfunction	Carcinoma of the endometrium
Hydroxyproges-terone caproate	1,000 mg IM twice weekly				
Megestrol acetate (Megace)	20-80 mg PO twice a day				

binding the microtubular protein used in the formation of the mitotic spindle. These drugs are:

Vinblastine (Velban)
Vincristine (Oncovin)

MISCELLANEOUS. A number of antineoplastic agents are available that do not clearly fit into any of the above categories. They are:

Dacarbazine (DTIC)
Nitrosoureas (carmustine or lomustine)
Hydroxyurea (Hydrea)
Cis-diamminedichloroplatinum (cis-platinum)

Supportive care. Since bone marrow depression can occur, facilities for supportive care should always be available. Platelet and erythrocyte transfusions and, where possible, leukocyte transfusions are often required until a patient's own normal bone marrow elements recover, a process that can take days or several weeks. The need for such support will increase with the widespread use of combination chemotherapy.

The supportive social workers, chaplains, and psychiatrists in a concentrated total care setting are of great value in enabling a patient to cope with the emotionally and financially shattering experience of having cancer. Although treatment of many patients must be conducted at large medical centers where new agents and multidisciplinary facilities are available, continuing collaboration between the medical center and the patient's primary physician is essential. Problems due to the disease or its treatment often arise when the patient has returned to her community. An informed local physician can rapidly evaluate these crises and take appropriate action.

Minimizing the most common side effects. Nausea and vomiting are common acute side effects of many antineoplastic drugs. Administration of the drug at night preceded by a sedative and phenothiazine, when possible, often minimizes these symptoms. Administration through an established intravenous line sometimes prevents drug extravasation and consequent pain and necrosis, which can occur with many of the agents. Phlebitis can often be prevented by administering the most irritating agents (such as actinomycin D and doxorubicin) through a running infusion. Continuation of the infusion will prevent dehydration.

Preliminary data reported by Rich and DiSaia suggest that short-term high-dose steroid therapy (methylprednisolone, 250 to 1,000 mg every 6 hours in 4 doses beginning 2 hours before administration of intravenous chemotherapy) can significantly reduce the nausea and vomiting caused by chemotherapy. One of the mechanisms of action proposed is associated with the inhibitory effect of steroids on prostaglandin synthesis, and other prostaglandin inhibitors may have a similar action.

Alopecia is a common consequence of therapy. The use of a scalp tourniquet during administration of such drugs as vincristine, actinomycin D, and doxorubicin

N + U

extravastn
Phlebit

Alopecia

has been reported to be helpful in preventing hair loss. These reports have not been confirmed widely.

Although many of the agents depress bone marrow elements at least transiently, it is important to emphasize that therapy should not be halted unless the depression is found to be prolonged. Infections due to neutropenia are uncommon until the absolute blood neutrophil count is less than 1,000/mm³, and therapy need not be interrupted until a falling blood count reaches 2,000 neutophils/mm³. Platelet counts in the range of 50,000 to 100,000/mm³ dictate cessation of therapy to avoid bleeding, which commonly occurs at levels less than 20,000/mm³. It is not necessary to increase the dose of an agent to amounts that cause leukopenia or thrombocytopenia to achieve a therapeutic result. Bone marrow depression is a toxic effect that limits the dose of a drug but is not a criterion of efficacy.

Calculation of dosage. Dosages of chemotherapeutic agents are usually discussed as mg per kg (of body weight) or mg per m² (of total body surface area). Dosage based on surface area is preferable to that based on weight, because surface area changes much less during the course of therapy, allowing a more consistent absolute amount of drug to be given throughout therapy. Dosages per unit are more comparable in adults and children (Figs. 11-16 and 11-17), and the variation in total dose between very obese and very thin people is minimized. Dosage in experimental animals expressed as mg per m² is more easily related to that in humans. In adults, mg per kg can be converted with reasonable accuracy to mg per m² by multiplying by 40.

Dose adjustments should be made for patients who are likely to have a compromised bone marrow reserve, i.e., those over 70 years of age, those who have received previous pelvic or abdominal irradiation, and those who have had previous chemotherapy. In these subsets of patients, consider beginning with a dose reduced by 35% to 50% and escalate up to full dose with subsequent courses if initial doses are well tolerated. In a similar manner, any moderate to severe toxicity encountered anywhere along the patient's course of therapy should be accompanied by a reduction in future doses. The adverse effects criteria table used by the GOG has been included in Appendix C.

Carcinogenicity of anticancer drugs. The carcinogenic potential of anticancer drugs must be kept in mind at all times. Clear evidence exists from several reports that the incidence of acute leukemia is increased in patients who have been treated with alkylating cystostatic agents for ovarian epithelial cancer. In 1976 Sotrel and associates reported two cases of advanced ovarian carcinoma treated with chlorambucil and terminating in acute leukemia. These patients were treated for 7 and 5 years, respectively, with continuous maintenance doses of chlorambucil. Recently other reviews of ovarian cancer patients surviving 3 years or more have pointed to similar increased incidences of acute leukemia in patients treated with melphalan pulse therapy. These well-tolerated chemotherapeutic agents that hitherto had been prescribed by gynecologists with little anxiety have emerged as potentially carcinogenic agents in and of themselves. Much of the data on the occurrence of acute leukemia in these patients treated with alkylating agents is clouded by detection

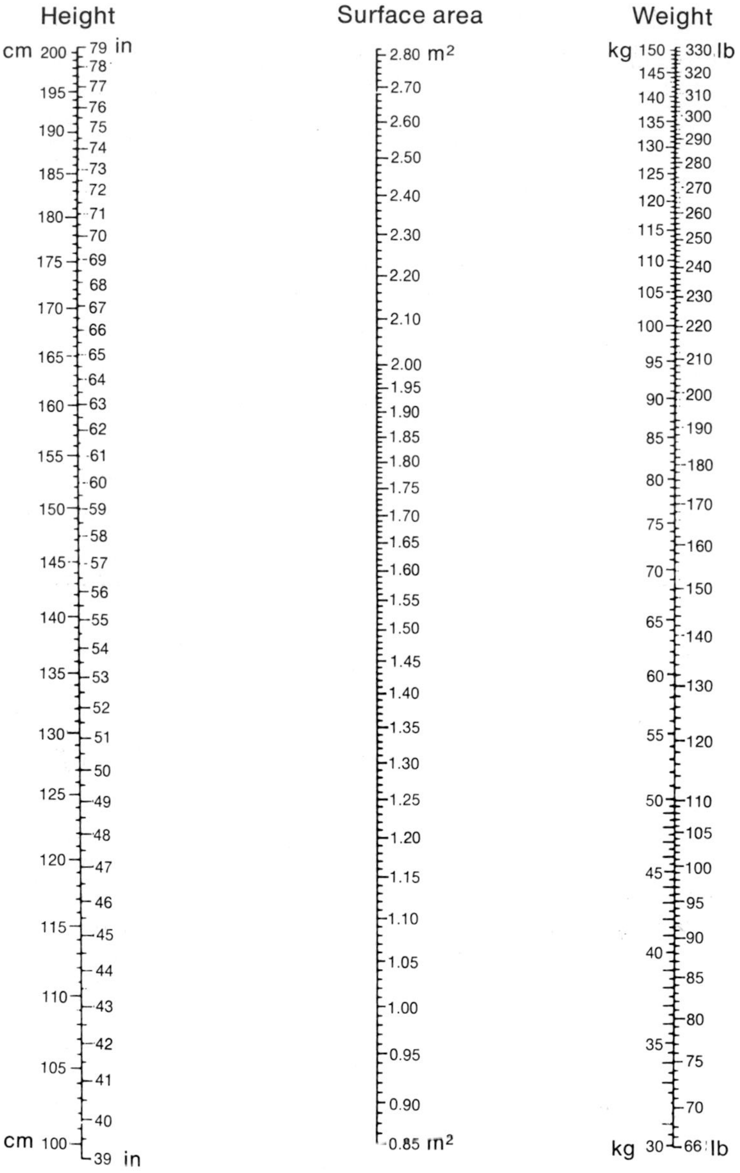

Fig. 11-16. Nomogram for calculating the body surface area of adults.

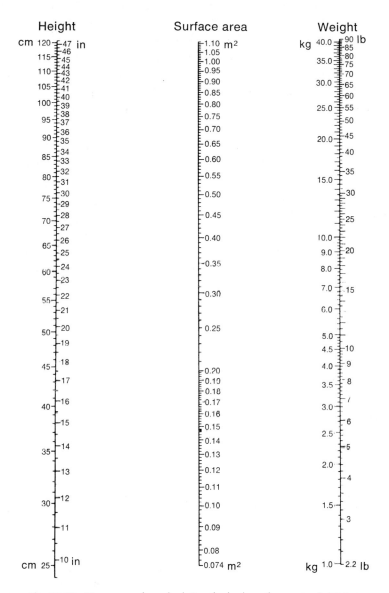

Fig. 11-17. Nomogram for calculating the body surface area of children.

bias. Obviously the patients who survive 3 years or more are a very small portion of the total group treated, since the disease claims the lives of most patients before 3 years. In addition, a significant number of the patients have received concomitant radiotherapy, and other patients have received additional chemotherapeutic agents. However, retrospective data would suggest strongly that alkylating agent therapy does result in a significant increase in the occurrence of acute leukemia in patients with ovarian cancer who survive following therapy.

This matter is of particular concern for the group of patients who are receiving adjuvant chemotherapy when the risk of recurrence is not great. An example of such a category would be individuals with stage I, grade 1 epithelial cancer of the ovary. In this category of patients and in similar groups where a reasonably high survival rate is anticipated, the risks of adjuvant therapy in the form of the traditional single drug alkylating agent must be weighed against the possible benefits. Since the benefits of adjuvant chemotherapy are uncear in this low-risk category, it would appear that therapy should be withheld until better evidence is available.

Nonalkylating agent chemotherapy. Since relatively high response rates have been traditional with alkylating agent chemotherapy (Table 11-21), there have been very few trials with other single agents in patients who have not previously received chemotherapy. Because previous drug therapy lessens the likelihood of response, response rates from nonalkylating agent chemotherapy, as often reported in the literature, may be falsely low (Table 11-22).

Table 11-21. Alkylating agent chemotherapy in stage III/IV ovarian cancer

Agent	Number of patients treated	Percent response
L-PAM (ALKERAN)	541	47
Cyclophosphamide (conventional dose)	335	43
Cyclophosphamide (intensive dose)	36	61
Chlorambucil	388	51
Triethylenethiophosphoramide (thiotepa)	337	48
Nitrosoureas	26	12

Reprinted by permission from Tobias, J. S., and Griffiths, C. T.: Management of ovarian carcinoma, New England Journal of Medicine **294:**818, 1976.

Table 11-22. Nonalkylating single agent chemotherapy in stage III/IV ovarian cancer

Agent	Average percent response
Hexamethylmelamine	42
Doxorubicin	36
Methotrexate	30
Cis-platinum	35
5-Fluorouracil	20

Hexamethylmelamine has recently been shown to be a very active agent in epithelial ovarian cancer. Wilson and associates reported five responses in 12 patients with ovarian cancer. Wampler confirmed these findings: three responses were seen in seven patients, and one was a complete response in a patient who had relapsed on chlorambucil and 5-fluorouracil. The most extensive experience with hexamethylmelamine (HXM) alone has been that of the M. D. Anderson Hospital, reported by Stanhope and associates, where a total of 22 previously untreated patients with stage III and IV epithelial cancer of the ovary were treated; seven complete and three partial responses were obtained, for an overall response rate of 45%. A study by the GOG for stage III and IV and recurrent epithelial cancer of the ovary with randomization prospectively between (1) melphalan, cyclophosphamide, and Adriamycin and (2) hexamethylmelamine and melphalan has shown in preliminary data a 32% complete response rate and a 22% partial response rate for patients receiving the latter regimen. Hexamethylmelamine is a very encouraging agent for further studies of combination chemotherapy in advanced epithelial ovarian cancer in spite of its moderately severe toxicity consisting primarily of gastrointestinal toxicity, myelosuppresion, and/or neurotoxicity with parkinsonian symptoms and abnormalities of gait.

In a report by Johnson and associates, hexamethylmelamine, 8 mg/kg/day for 14 days, was given to 21 patients with stage III/IV epithelial ovarian cancer resistant to alkylating agents. There were no complete remissions. Four patients had partial remission. The authors concluded that hexamethylmelamine is effective for the treatment of ovarian cancer and not invariably cross-resistant with conventional alkylating agents. Bonomi and associates reported four responders (one complete response and three partial responses) in 16 patients receiving hexamethylmelamine after failing to respond to alkylating agents. These four responses and others reported in the literature by Young and Chabner support the hypothesis that hexamethylmelamine may be suitable for combination therapy. Caution should be used in the administration of this agent in patients who have already had extensive chemotherapy because severe bone marrow suppression may occur.

Doxorubicin (Adriamycin) also has a broad spectrum of antineoplastic activity with great promise in epithelial cancer of the ovary. A review by Blum and Carter suggested that this drug had an 18% response rate in a collective group of patients with ovarian cancer, but in all of the series reviewed, the great majority of patients had failed on other chemotherapy. Second line chemotherapy in epithelial cancer of the ovary is notoriously ineffective. De Palo and associates carried out a prospective randomized study done primarily on previously untreated patients with stage III and IV ovarian cancer. Thirty-five patients were treated either with Adriamycin (75 mg/m² every 3 weeks) or L-PAM (6 mg/m²/day for 5 days every 4 to 5 weeks), and treatment was continued until relapse. Tumor regression occurred in eight of 13 patients treated with Adriamycin and in four of ten patients treated with L-PAM. After treatment failure, crossover was performed; Adriamycin produced regression in two out of two patients, and L-PAM was effective in one out of four.

Hubbard and associates reported the results of single agent Adriamycin therapy in 18 patients with stage III or IV ovarian carcinoma of epithelial origin who had developed recurrent disease or disease progression during or after systemic chemotherapy and/or local radiotherapy. Initial chemotherapy consisted of a single alkylating agent in 6 patients and intensive combination chemotherapy in 12 patients. These 18 patients received a total of 44 doses of single agent Adriamycin therapy. There were no responses of clinical benefit. One patient with a large abdominal mass obtained a 40% decrease in tumor size that lasted 2 months. The authors stressed the need for using Adriamycin in combination or as initial chemotherapy.

Bolis reported on the use of Adriamycin for the treatment of 38 women with stage III and IV ovarian carcinoma who had previously been treated with surgery and cyclophosphamide. Twelve patients had relapsed after response to cyclophosphamide, and 26 patients did not respond initially. Three of the 38 patients responded to Adriamycin therapy, and these three patients were in the group of 12 who had an initial response to cyclophosphamide. None of the 26 patients who failed to respond to cyclophosphamide subsequently responded to Adriamycin.

Of the antimetabolites, 5-fluorouracil has shown low but consistent efficacy in several trials. A review of these trials reveals 18 objective responses in 92 evaluable patients, for a response rate of 29%. In the opinion of most, 5-fluorouracil should not be considered as primary therapy; however, since it has some activity, can be administered orally, and has acceptable toxicity, it should be considered as a second line agent or as a possible member of combination therapy.

Methotrexate, the most widely used of the antifolate drugs, has been used only sporadically as a single agent in ovarian cancer. Sullivan and associates reported four responses in 16 patients, but this response rate has not be confirmed. Recently, interest in methotrexate has been stimulated by the observation that high doses of methotrexate followed by citrovorum factor "rescue" may have a higher therapeutic potential for several tumors. A recent report by Barlow and Piver in a randomized study of 55 patients with advanced stage epithelial ovarian cancer with progressive disease after prior chemotherapy evaluated the efficacy of high-dose methotrexate with citrovorum factor "rescue." All of the patients studied had had prior chemotherapy when treated with methotrexate-citrovorum factor rescue plus cyclophosphamide with and without pretreatment with vincristine. Vincristine did not enhance the efficacy of methotrexate-citrovorum factor rescue plus cyclophosphamide in terms of response rate. Objective responses of from 3 to 12 months were observed in 30% of the evaluable cases. The incidence of serious toxicity was acceptable in this group of patients who had had extensive prior chemotherapy.

Combination chemotherapy. The relatively low rates of response seen with most agents other than alkylating agents have stimulated investigators to search for combination schedules. Smith and associates reported one of the largest series to date, which consisted of 97 patients with stages II through IV epithelial cancer of the ovary, all of whom had residual masses of at least 2 cm and/or ascites following initial laparotomy. Patients were randomized into two groups, receiving either L-PAM or a combination of cyclophosphamide, 5-fluorouracil, and actinomycin D (ActFUCy). Fifty patients received a single agent, and 47 received a combination, and a stratification for stage of disease was carefully carried out. Despite a larger number of clinically complete responses in the combination group (30% compared with 20%), the survival times for the two groups were essentially the same (L-PAM, 51.5% at 1 year and 17% at 2 years; ActFUCy 40.6% at 1 year and 17% at 2 years). The toxicity was very much greater with the combination therapy.

Methotrexate has also been used in combination with other drugs. Greenspan reported on a series where methotrexate was given with thiotepa on an intermittent schedule, and a response rate of 63% was seen in 96 patients. Toxicity in this series of patients was considered, and there were three drug-related deaths. Brodovsky and associates reported on a series where L-PAM was compared with a combination of cyclophosphamide, methotrexate, and 5-fluorouracil. In both groups, response rates were unusually low; five out of 27 patients responsed to L-PAM, and eight out of 25 responded to the combination. There were no complete responses in the entire series. The addition of hexamethylmelamine to the three-drug combination appears to increase this response rate. Young and associates reported on 80 patients with advanced (FIGO stage III and IV) untreated epithelial ovarian cancer who were randomized to receive melphalan (PAM) (0.2 mg/kg/day orally for 5 days every 4 to 6 weeks) or combination chemotherapy (HEXA-CAF: 5-fluorouracil [600 mg/m²] and methotrexate [40 mg/m²] intravenously on days 1 and 8 plus cyclophosphamide and hexamethylmelamine [150 mg orally daily for 14 days]). Thirty-seven of 39 patients receiving PAM and 40 of 41 patients receiving HEXA-CAF were on therapy longer than 6 months at the time of the report and were evaluable for response. The two groups were similar in stage, age, histologic type, initial surgery, and residual disease. Approximately 80% of each group had residual disease greater than 2 cm after surgery. For the patients receiving PAM, the complete response rate was 16%, partial response rate 38% and no response 46%. For the patients receiving HEXA-CAF, the complete response rate was 33%, partial response rate 43%, and no response 25%. The difference between the 33% complete response rate with HEXA-CAF and the 16% complete response rate with PAM is statistically significant ($P = .02$). The overall response rate was 76% with HEXA-CAF versus 54% with PAM. In summary, HEXA-CAF showed a higher percentage of complete responses (33% versus 16%) and longer overall survival (29 months versus 17 months).

Many combinations using Adriamycin have also been reported. Barlow and associates used Adriamycin with bleomycin in six patients, but only one showed a response (partial). More recent reports using Adriamycin with cyclophosphamide have been more encouraging. Griffiths and associates reported on 24 patients who were treated on a 3-week schedule with Adriamycin, 40 mg/m², and cyclophosphamide, 500 mg/m². Eighteen patients were evaluable, and in this group of 18 the response rate was 50%, with five complete responses and four partial responses. The median duration of response was more than 8 months, and four of the five complete responders were doing well at the time of the report.

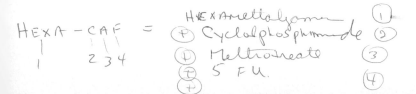

Table 11-23. Gynecologic Oncology Group (preliminary data): response in terms of treatment (for measurable disease patients)

Response	Treatment*			Total
	A	B	C	
Complete response	10 (16.7%)	19 (36.6%)	19 (31.7%)	= 48
Partial response	12 (20.0%)	9 (17.3%)	13 (21.7%)	= 34
No change	21 (35.0%)	13 (25.0%)	12 (20.0%)	= 46
Increasing disease	17 (28.3%)	11 (21.1%)	16 (26.6%)	= 44
TOTAL	60 (100.0%)	52 (100.0%)	60 (100.0%)	= 172

From Omura, G. A., Blessing, J. A., Buchsbaum, H. J., and Lathrop, J.: Randomized trial of melphalan vs. melphalan plus hexamethylmelamine vs. adriamycin plus cyclophosphamide in advanced ovarian adenocarcinoma, Proc. Am. Assoc. Cancer Res. **20**:358, 1979.
*A: melphalan, 7 mg/m² orally for 5 days every 4 weeks; B: cyclophosphamide, 500 mg/m² IV, plus Adriamycin, 50 mg/m² IV, every 3 weeks; C: melphalan, 7 mg/m² orally for 5 days, plus hexamethylmelamine, 150 mg/m² daily for 14 days, every 4 weeks.

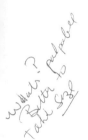

In a later report, Parker and associates reported on 41 evaluable women with stage III/IV ovarian cancer who received Adriamycin (45 to 100 mg/m²) and cyclophosphamide (500 to 2,000 mg/m²) every 3 weeks for five to ten cycles after surgery. The response rates were: complete response, 46%; partial response, 40%; no response, 15%. In this report they concluded that the absence of pretreatment palpable tumors was the major determinant of drug response but that further observation was required to demonstrate enhanced survival in this favorable group. Their results indicated that Adriamycin/cyclophosphamide can induce a complete response in 90% of stage III patients in whom the tumor has been resected below the level of palpability.

The GOG study quoted above (Table 11-23) showed a 36.6% complete response rate and a 17.3% partial response rate using Adriamycin at a dose of 50 mg/m² and cyclophosphamide at a dose of 500 mg/m² (repeated every 3 weeks as tolerated).

Turbow and associates reported on patients with stage III and IV epithelial carcinoma of the ovary and with recurrent ovarian carcinoma after previous radiation for stage I and II disease who were randomized between melphalan (0.2 mg/kg/day for 5 days) and Adriamycin (50 mg/m² intravenously on day 1) plus cyclophosphamide (250 mg/m² by mouth for 4 days). Both treatment programs were repeated every 4 weeks. Twenty-five patients were randomized: 11 patients to Adriamycin-cyclophosphamide and 14 patients to melphalan. The Adriamycin-cyclophosphamide combination had a significantly higher response rate. Eight of the 11 patients responded to Adriamycin-cyclophosphamide (two partial responses and six complete responses judged by clinical evaluation only). There were four responses in the 14 patients treated with melphalan (one complete response and three partial responses).

Cis-diamminedichloroplatinum (DDP), a heavy metal coordination compound with unique antitumor properties, is the first of this type of compound to undergo extensive clinical testing. Along with Adriamycin and hexamethylmelamine, it has shown itself to be a very active agent in epithelial cancer of the ovary. The response duration is often short. In 1976 Vogl and associates introduced the combination of DDP and Adriamycin. One of the five patients in their report responded to this therapy. Bruckner and associates reported a 70% overall response rate (28% complete response and 41% partial response) in 43 women who had not received prior chemotherapy; a 40% overall response rate was observed in another 60 previously treated patients. Less dramatic but similar results were obtained by Briscoe and associates, who reported on 24 women treated with DDP, 60 mg/m², and Adriamycin, 60 mg/m², every 3 to 4 weeks and recorded ten responses (four complete responses and six partial responses). An 80% response rate was recently reported by Ehrlich and associates. Their combination consisted of Adriamycin (50 mg/m²), DDP (50 mg/m²), and Cytoxan (750 mg/m²). The combination was repeated every 4 weeks. The patients treated were individuals with previously untreated advanced (stage III and IV) epithelial adenocarcinoma of the ovary.

There have been scattered reports of responses to progestin therapy alone in ovarian cancer. Every serious report in the literature suffers from small numbers of patients and poor evaluation of those patients. There have been many anecdotal reports of benefit from combining alkylating agents with progestin therapy for epithelial cancer of the ovary. No prospective randomized trial has been done to date. The use of progestins often creates an anabolic-like effect (increased appetite, etc.) in the patient and undoubtedly creates a subjective response. Whether it potentiates or improves the response to the chemotherapeutic agent is yet to be proved.

Immunochemotherapy. In the last few years there has been considerable interest in combining chemotherapy with immunotherapy for better results in patients with epithelial cancer of the ovary. Although these investigations are highly preliminary, some results have been published.

Recently, Creasman and associates reported a series of patients treated with Alkeran plus C-Parvum immunotherapy. The immunomodulating agent chosen for this study was a gram-positive bacterium, *Corynebacterium parvum*. This agent has been shown to increase nonspecific tumor resistance, to potentiate specific tumor rejections, to effect bone marrow proliferation, and to have additive antitumor effects when combined with alkylating agents. The pilot study done by Creasman and associates on 48 previously untreated stage III epithelial ovarian cancer patients showed a definite suggestion of improved response with the combination of chemotherapy and immunotherapy. The response rate in the group given Alkeran alone was 55%, whereas the response rate in the combination group was 65%. Further analysis of the material revealed that 44% of the patients in the Alkeran group had minimal residua at the commencement of therapy, whereas only 23% of the patients in the combination group had this favorable clinical finding. The author concluded that this was a promising combination, and a prospective randomized study comparing similar treatment groups is now being conducted by the GOG (Table 11-24). The results of that study are preliminary, and no significant difference has been found to date.

Table 11-24. Gynecologic Oncology Group protocol 25

Procedure: Exploratory laparotomy, plus total abdominal hysterectomy and bilateral salpingo-oophorectomy, plus omentectomy with debulking of tumor

Regimen A	Regimen B
Melphalan alone, 7 mg/m²/day orally for 5 days; repeat every 4 weeks	Melphalan alone, 7 mg/m²/day orally for 5 days; repeat every 4 weeks *plus* C-Parvum, 4 mg/m²/day IV on the 7th day following chemotherapy

From Creasman, W. T., Gall, S. A., Blessing, J. A., and others: Chemoimmunotherapy in the management of primary stage III ovarian cancer; a Gynecologic Oncology Group study, Cancer Treat. Rep. **63:**319, 1979.

Table 11-25. Chemoimmunotherapy

	A-C	A-C + BCG
Responses (CR + PR)	36%	53% (*P* <.05)
Alive at 36 months	46%	61% (*P* <.04)
Median survival time (months)	13.1	23.5

From Alberts, D. S., Moon, T. E., Stephens, R. A., and others: Randomized study of chemoimmunotherapy for advanced ovarian carcinoma; a preliminary report of a Southwest Oncology Group study, Cancer Treat. Rep. **63:**325, 1979.

Alberts and associates used a combination of Adriamycin and cyclophosphamide, with or without bacillus Calmette-Guerin (BCG), in 109 patients with stage III and IV or recurrent ovarian carcinoma who had not previously received chemotherapy. The effects of treatment were evaluable in 109 patients who had received two or more courses (Table 11-25). At the time of the report, five of the patients receiving A-C-BCG showed complete tumor regression. Partial remissions were noted in 22 of 56 patients receiving Adriamycin-cyclophosphamide alone and in 23 of 53 patients receiving A-C-BCG. The authors concluded that nonspecific immunostimulation therapy combined with chemotherapy could improve the results in advanced epithelial cancer of the ovary.

FOLLOW-UP TECHNIQUES AND TREATMENT OF RECURRENCES

As stated earlier, ovarian cancer is fast growing and insidious in that it is late to cause symptoms, and thus follow-up examinations are imperative to detect early recurrence. Even then, implants many centimeters in diameter can be hidden in the many crevices of the abdominal cavity and escape physical detection. There is a reasonable limit to the use of such sophisticated techniques as computerized axial tomography in the surveillance of a patient who has had ovarian cancer. The key to the proper assessment of the extent of disease is liberal use of surgical procedures (laparoscopy and laparotomy) to assay the contents of the abdominal and pelvic cavities.

Table 11-26. Ovarian cancer: stage vs. second-look findings

Stage	Number with no evidence of disease	Number with persistent carcinoma	Percent with no evidence of disease
I	18	9	66.7
II	14	17	45.2
III	17	88	16.2
IV	9	14	39.1

Data from Wharton, J. T., and others, M. D. Anderson Hospital.

"Second-look" operation

The so-called second-look operation was first defined by Owen Wangenstein in the late 1940s with reference to exploratory laparotomy procedures in colon cancer patients from whom he had previously removed all gross tumor but in whom there was a high risk of recurrence. At varying intervals, usually 6 months initially, he would explore these patients in the hope of detecting early recurrence at a time when secondary resection still offered a chance of cure. Since then, the term "second-look" has been used to describe many procedures. With reference to ovarian cancer, it appears that a second-look procedure may have three main indications: (1) to restage a patient who presents with probably localized disease who has not had a proper staging procedure as defined above; (2) to evaluate the effect of chemotherapy in patients receiving both standard and investigational regimens; in this regard, some centers have instituted serial laparoscopic examinations in order to assess the extent of regression or progression of bulk disease several months after commencement of chemotherapy, with the option to offer other therapy should a poor response be noted; and (3) to evaluate patients who are clinically free of disease after receiving what is considered a sufficient course of chemotherapy (10 to 18 months) and are then eligible for assessment as to possible "cure" and discontinuation of therapy (Table 11-26). This last indication has been the most widely used and has resulted in small numbers of patients with even advanced disease who are free of detectable malignant cells at the second procedure. The most difficult second-look procedure is that in which no evidence of disease apparently exists, since very extensive and thorough surgery must be performed to establish lack of disease.

These second-look procedures are often begun with a laparoscopic examination to rule out widespread disease. Should this lesser procedure reveal diffuse miliary studding (which was not clinically detectable), a laparotomy is not necessary. It is obvious that these patients need to continue receiving therapy of some sort and are not candidates for a second attempt at surgical resection. On the other hand, at the present state of knowledge, a negative laparoscopic examination is not sufficient evidence for classifying the patient as without evidence of disease, and a laparotomy must be carried out. At the time of laparotomy a detailed exploration of the abdominal cavity must be conducted in a manner quite similar to the initial staging procedures previously described. Should focal residual disease be encountered it should be surgically resected and the area marked with metal clips for regional radiation therapy. Careful inspection of the entire abdominal cavity, including the undersurface of the diaphragm, the root of the mesentery, and all parietal and visceral peritoneal surfaces, must be tediously carried out with liberal use of biopsy for suspicious areas.

Creasman and associates reported four patients with ovarian cancer who, after chemotherapy or combined immunochemotherapy, were found to have retroperitoneal disease at the time of second-look exploratory laparotomy, even though there was no evidence of intra-abdominal residual cancer. Ovarian cancer can metastasize to both pelvic and periaortic lymph nodes, and therefore these areas must be evaluated in order to assess appropriately the true extent of disease in patients with ovarian cancer.

Smith and associates recently reported on 103 patients with advanced ovarian cancer who underwent a second-look operation following chemotherapy. They concluded that patients should have ten or more courses of chemotherapy before a second-look operation. Those patients with no evidence of disease at second-look laparotomy are eligible for discontinuation of all therapy. Patients who continued chemotherapy after the second-look operation did better than those who were treated with radiation after surgery in this series. They also found that only those patients with clinical remission of disease benefited from a second-look procedure. They proposed the following reasons for a second-look operation: (1) the patient may have received sufficient drug and is clinically free of disease, (2) the patient has had ten or more courses of chemotherapy, (3) the tumor has had almost complete clinical remission and is possibly resectable, (4) the patient has had maximum benefit from one type of chemotherapy and it is advantageous to change to a different chemotherapy, and (5) the suspected tumor mass watched during chemotherapy, which had served as a guide to treatment, is now suspected to be other than a neoplastic mass.

With the religious use of an extensive second-look operation (Table 11-27), one can expect a very low subsequent recurrence rate should the results be negative. In the hands of most physicians, less than 10% of these patients will subsequently appear with evidence of recurrent disease. Thus, these procedures can significantly influence the physician's ability to give an accurate prognosis to the patient and allow the patient to approach the future with reasonable expectations. In the absence of

Table 11-27. Steps taken in second-look laparotomy

1. Midline incision
2. Cytologic washings from several areas of the abdomen and pelvis
3. Inspection of the omentum
4. Visualization of all peritoneal surfaces, including the undersurface of the diaphragm, serosa, and mesentery of the bowel
5. Submission of all *excised* adhesions for histologic review
6. Careful inspection of all pelvic organs and pelvic peritoneum
7. Retroperitoneal inspection of pelvic and para-aortic nodes

reliable tumor markers in epithelial cancer of the ovary, these second-look operations have great value.

Second line chemotherapy

In all forms of ovarian cancer, second line chemotherapy has to date been very
disappointing. When effective drug combinations are initially used and fail, there is
virtually no chance of inducing a significant response with a second drug or combination of drugs. A partial response and control of malignant effusions can be achieved
on occasion, but these are usually short-lived. However, most gynecologic oncologists attempt to treat these drug failure patients using a reasonable second line regimen usually consisting of active chemotherapeutic agents that have not been used
in the first treatment plan (Table 11-28). It is hoped that as new agents evolve, a
more effective second echelon of drugs will be available for use. Although second
line surgery is not generally advocated, every experienced gynecologic oncologist
has a group of patients who have responded well to a second surgical attack on local
or regional recurrent disease that initially had not responded to chemotherapy. This
is especially relevant to the patient who, at the time of second-look operation following chemotherapy, has what appears to be localized persistent disease.

Malignant effusions

Fortunately, malignant effusions are nowhere near the problem that they were a
decade ago. Chemotherapeutic regimens control malignant effusions in a full 90% of
the cases. The patient who presents with a distended abdomen and probable ascites
is the initial problem. There is a tendency to perform paracentesis for diagnostic
purposes when the situation is somewhat doubtful. We would like to make a plea for
not performing paracentesis in patients who are highly suspect of ovarian malignancy, for the following reasons:
1. Cytologic examination of fluid may be negative in the presence of malignancy,
   and laparotomy is still indicated.
2. Even when cytologic examination of the fluid is positive, it seldom provides
   a sufficient clue to the origin of the primary tumor, and laparotomy is indicated.
3. If the patient has a large fluid-filled cyst (Fig. 11-18) rather than ascites, rup-

Table 11-28. Agents used in epithelial ovarian cancer

Active agents	Inactive agents	Not known
Alkylating agents	BCNU	Procarbazine
Hexamethylmelamine	Vincristine	Mithramycin
Doxorubicin	6-MP	Bleomycin
Cis-platinum	Actinomycin D	Dacarbazine (DTIC)
5-Fluorouracil		Mitomycin C
Methotrexate		Hydroxyurea

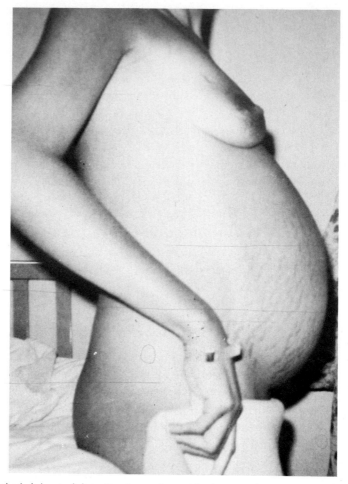

Fig. 11-18. Marked abdominal distention in a patient with a large grade 2 mucinous adenocarcinoma of the ovary.

ture of the cyst and seeding into the peritoneal cavity may occur, often long before laparotomy (Fig. 11-19).

4. Paracentesis may be associated with complications other than seeding, such as rupture of an intra-abdominal viscus, bleeding, infection, and severe depletion of electrolytes and proteins. We would therefore recommend that these patients be investigated short of paracentesis and that the disease be defined at laparotomy, when the situation can be controlled with more ease.

Our comments are to discourage paracentesis as a diagnostic tool, but in instances where intra-abdominal pressure causes respiratory embarrassment or severe pain, the procedure should be performed as therapy. Often, improved gastrointestinal function and relief of nausea and vomiting as well as constipation may be seen following therapeutic paracentesis.

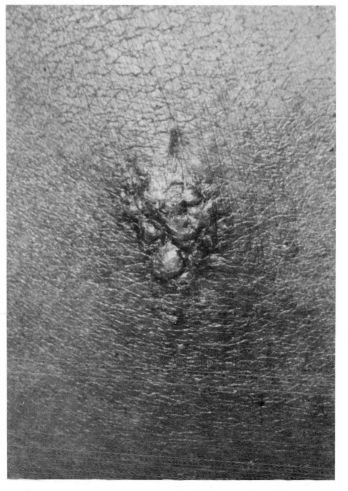

Fig. 11 19. Skin implant in the patient seen in Fig. 11-18. This was found at the site of the abdominal paracentesis performed 4 weeks earlier and represented the only disease identified outside of a large self-contained neoplasm.

It is a long-standing practice to instill antineoplastic agents into the peritoneal cavity at the time of exploratory laparotomy if unresectable tumor is found. It has been shown by multiple animal studies and other testing in humans that this topical use or intraperitoneal instillation of chemotherapeutic agents is effective primarily by absorption from the peritoneal cavity into the systemic circulation. Since this is the case, it would follow that a much more scientific and controlled situation can be achieved by direct systemic use of the drug. Other agents, such as quinacrine (Atabrine) and nitrogen mustard, have an effect on effusions by producing an adhesive serositis that will partially obliterate the peritoneal or pleural cavity, making the accumulation of ascites more difficult. However, these agents also create a situation in which further surgical intervention is almost impossible. When ascites reaccumulates following surgery, it is almost always a problem associated with unresectable carcinoma, and these patients usually can be controlled with systemic chemotherapy of one form or the other. Should one drug fail, other combinations should be tried and are sometimes successful. Unfortunately, there are some patients whose ascites cannot be completely controlled by systemic chemotherapy, and often these patients can be kept comfortable by periodic paracentesis. This can be done on an outpatient basis at intervals determined by the patient's symptoms. The site of paracentesis is usually at the lateral border of the rectus muscle and at the level of the umbilicus. The midline is avoided since tumor or adhesions are often present and complications can result. It is advisable to infiltrate the abdominal wall with a small amount of local anesthetic and then, using the same syringe and needle explore for a clear spot in the peritoneal cavity. A larger trocar can then be inserted over the exact area of exploration, and in this way one can avoid the complication of inserting a trocar into an adherent segment of bowel. Measurements of weight and abdominal girth are recorded before and after paracentesis, and the volume of fluid is also noted. Sometimes fluid will continue to leak out of the trocar sites, and attaching a urostomy bag to the area will provide some comfort for the patient. Irradiation techniques are usually not recommended in the management of ascites because systemic chemotherapy is so effective. Instillation of P 32 or Au 198 is often difficult because of the need to obtain a uniform distribution of the radioactive substance. In addition, one is usually dealing with a situation where large individual tumor masses are present, and even the gamma emission of radioactive gold is effective for only 2 to 4 mm. There are situations where a diffuse miliary spread of disease is suspected and ascites is only partially controlled with chemotherapy. In these instances radioactive chromium phosphate (a beta emitter) may be very beneficial and provide minimum chance of severe injury to the bowel.

Pleural effusion is another problem in the management of ovarian cancer. Approximately one third of the patients with ascites will have a pleural effusion. This usually responds to systemic chemotherapy along with the ascites. Pleural effusion in the absence of ascites usually indicates involvement of the pleura with disease. The same techniques that have been outlined for the management of ascites can be used. Nitrogen mustard or quinacrine (Atabrine) injected into the pleural cavity is associated with a high success rate. Obliteration of the pleural cavity prevents the accumulation of fluid in that space. A dose of 10 or 15 mg of nitrogen mustard creates enough pleural reaction to cause obliteration of the potential space, resulting in relief of this troublesome symptom for patients who are not responding optimally to systemic chemotherapy. Another method recently employed with some success is the instillation of bleomycin (60 to 120 mg) into the pleural cavity after thoracentesis. This drug can be used with systemic chemotherapy because of its minimal myelosuppressive effect.

The cause of malignant effusions is not known. The most common explanations are: (1) an irritant effect of the tumor on normal serous membranes, (2) lymphatic obstruction, and (3) venous obstruction. Graham studied ascites circulating in patients with peritoneal carcinomatosis. He noted a large increase in the production of fluid by *noncancer* bearing peritoneal surfaces that was most marked from the omentum and small-bowel surfaces. He also noted a significant elevation of portal pressure in the presence of ovarian cancer with ascites as compared with normal patients and patients with ovarian cancer without ascites.

The surgical approach to recurrent malignant effusions has been somewhat limited. In the case of pleural effusion, decortication of the lung and pleurectomy have been used with varying results. Instillation of nitrogen mustard and similar caustic compounds has essentially replaced these procedures. Other agents have been used to create pleuritis, including hypertonic glucose and talc. Again, they have variable success rates, depending on the investigator. A surgical procedure for uncontrollable ascites called ileoentectropy was promoted by Brunschwig at Memorial Hospital. Some of the patients with ascites due to ovarian cancer had control of their effusion by this method, but it has not proved to be a practical approach.

CURRENT AREAS OF RESEARCH

Most of the advances that have been made in the treatment of cancer of the ovary in the last 10 years have used the multimodality approach. A combination of modalities used in a logical and flexible manner can achieve notable successes on an individual basis. This combined with improved chemotherapeutic agents and the possible addition of immunotherapy as a new modality will hopefully result in improved outcome for this devastating group of malignancies.

By far the greatest advance on the horizon is in the area of early detection by immunodiagnostic techniques. Several crude experimental procedures have strongly suggested the presence of commonly shared tumor-associated antigens in epithelial cancers of the ovary. Unfortunately, isolation of these antigens has been more difficult than initially conceived and is essential to the creation of a clinically useful immunodiagnostic tool. Given that there are commonly shared tumor-associated antigens in epithelial cancer of the ovary and that a small amount of this antigen or an antibody to it are detectable in the sera of patients with subclinical disease, all the ingredients for a dramatic improvement in the battle against this disease are at hand.

Widder and associates have reported on magnetically responsive microspheres for targeting of antitumor agents. The technique described by these investigators offers considerable promise for targeting of antineoplastic agents to restricted anatomic sites and specific target areas. They reported on magnetically responsive small albumin microspheres (biodegradable) that could be injected intra-arterially and localized at specific target sites by application of appropriately directed magnetic fields. Magnetite (Fe_3O_4) was used as the magnetically responsive material, and this was incorporated into the albumin matrix. Adriamycin was used as the prototype drug, was encapsulated, and was found to distribute with the carrier. In preliminary studies the released drug appeared to retain its biologic activity. Innovative approaches such as this may afford an opportunity to overcome the problems of adequate drug concentration in tumor tissue and systemic toxicity (e.g., cardiac toxicity with Adriamycin) seen with conventional intravenous use.

REHABILITATION

The nature of ovarian cancer is such that the major vital organs such as the lung, heart, liver, and kidneys remain unaffected. The disease itself and its therapy appear to attack the gastrointestinal tract primarily. Indeed, the terminal event for most patients who succumb to this disease is electrolyte imbalance due to prolonged gastrointestinal obstruction, malnutrition, and significant protein and electrolyte loss from repeated paracentesis and thoracentesis. It is necessary to support these patients with various forms of alimentation during therapy in order to sustain the host sufficiently to tolerate the somewhat vigorous therapy often prescribed. Intermittent episodes of partial small- and large-bowel obstruction are common, and they must be treated conservatively initially and surgically ultimately if the patient is to continue the fight. The issue as to whether a patient with a high-grade small-bowel obstruction from ovarian cancer carcinomatosis should be explored for a possible bypass procedure to reestablish the continuity of the alimentary tract is a subject that has been long debated. Management of these patients is extremely difficult because of the intactness of their vital organs and their alert mental status. Although most of these patients will not survive 6 months from the time of the bowel obstruction, surgical intervention should be considered in light of the difficulty that all individuals have observing the slow process of death by starvation. Any procedure that can result in the patient returning to her home and family seems to be worthy of consideration even in these hopeless cases. If nothing else, the performance of a gastrostomy to avoid the uncomfortable nasogastric intubation or persistent agony of constant vomiting is in itself humane and allows more easy return of the patient to a home setting, where the gastrostomy can be used to decompress the patient as the need arises.

In general, the most discouraging aspect in the management of ovarian cancer patients is the apathy of many physicians. In all truth these diseases are discouraging, but an offensive attitude is both medically sound and reassuring to the patient. Significant numbers of patients referred as "unresectable" have been debulked and responded nicely to postoperative therapy. Still other patients have survived after receiving a complicated combination of multiple surgical and adjuvant therapies. A positive approach to the disease restores hope in the patient with this devastating illness and is justified on that basis alone.

CONCLUSIONS ON MANAGEMENT

Although adenocarcinoma of the ovary remains one of the most sensitive solid tumors to chemotherapeutic regimens, the mortality from this disease remains high. There appears, however, to be great promise with newer developments in the management of this disease. The following general principles should be kept in mind:

1. An optimal surgical procedure should be carried out whenever possible. This is defined as the removal of all bulk tumor with the intent to leave minimal residual (no individual mass greater than 1 to 2 cm in diameter). It is not possible to advocate any one operation for all patients, and the clinician must make a judgment at the time of surgery. Unquestionably, patients with small

residual tumor volumes have a better prognosis with any postoperative therapy. Even when optimal debulking is not possible, bilateral salpingo-oophorectomy, total abdominal hysterectomy, and omentectomy may afford significant palliations for the patient. Resection of a portion of the bowel should be considered only when such a resection will result in removal of all gross tumor. A careful exploration of the entire abdomen including the diaphragmatic surfaces must be carried out by a methodical surgeon to ensure proper staging of the disease.

2. The conventional view of radiation therapy as the most important postoperative modality for gynecologic cancer must be discarded with respect to adenocarcinoma of the ovary. In advanced (stage III and IV) disease, there is little evidence that radiation therapy has significant value over chemotherapy. A major limiting factor with radiotherapy in advanced disease is the hepatic and renal toxicity that follows adequate doses of whole-abdomen radiation. Shielding of these vital organs will lead to undertreatment, especially in commonly involved areas such as the undersurface of the diaphragm. The place of radiotherapy appears at present to be limited to earlier disease, and here too there is considerable doubt. Too few valid studies comparing radiotherapy with chemotherapy for stage I and II disease are at hand.

3. A large number of reports in the literature have confirmed that chemotherapy with alkylating agents can produce responses in 30% to 60% of patients with advanced disease. Experience with other solid tumors has suggested strongly that an improved complete response rate with any particular chemotherapeutic regimen correlates well with eventual improved survival rate. Recently several nonalkylating agent chemotherapeutic drugs have been identified with considerable activity in ovarian cancer, e.g., hexamethylmelamine, doxorubicin, and cis-platinum. Several reports have confirmed significant improvement in complete response rates when a combination of drugs containing two or more of these active agents was used. It is hoped that, as in other solid tumors, these preliminary reports of improved complete response rates will eventuate in later reports of improved overall survival rates.

4. Prognosis depends very much on stage, but other factors are also quite pertinent. Undifferentiated lesions have a worse prognosis regardless of stage. Those patients with bulk residual disease following laparotomy are much less likely to respond to subsequent therapy.

5. Chemotherapy appears to be the most effective method of controlling ascites. First line chemotherapy will be effective in 90% of patients with ascitic fluid for varying periods.

6. The use of intraperitoneal colloidal isotopes such as P 32 has great theoretical value for patients with microscopic residual disease following laparotomy. However, distribution of the drug within the peritoneal cavity in a patient postoperatively may buffer the theoretical advantages. No good prospective randomized study comparing intraperitoneal colloidal isotopes with other modalities such as chemotherapy has yet been reported.

BIBLIOGRAPHY

Alberts, D. S., Hilgers, R. D., Moon, T. E., and others: Combination chemotherapy for alkylator-resistant ovarian carcinoma; a preliminary report of a Southwest Oncology Group trial, Cancer Treat. Rep. **63**:301, 1979.

Alberts, D. S., Moon, T. E., Stephens, R. A., and others: Randomized study of chemoimmunotherapy for advanced ovarian carcinoma; a preliminary report of a Southwest Oncology Group study, Cancer Treat. Rep. **63**:325, 1979.

Allan, M. S., and Hertig, A. T.: Carcinoma of the ovary, Am. J. Obstet. Gynecol. **58**:640, 1949.

Annegers, J. F., Strom, H., Decker, D. G., and others: Ovarian cancer—incidence and case control study, Cancer **43**:723, 1979.

Ansfield, F. J., Schroeder, J. M., and Curreri, A. R.: Five years' clinical experience with 5-fluorouracil, J.A.M.A. **181**:295, 1962.

Aure, J. C., Hoeg, K., and Kolstad, P.: Clinical and histologic studies of ovarian carcinoma; long-term follow-up of 990 cases, Obstet. Gynecol. **37**:1, 1971.

Aure, J. C., Hoeg, K., and Kolstad, P.: Psammoma bodies in serous carcinoma of the ovary; a prognostic study, Am. J. Obstet. Gynecol. **109**:113, 1971.

Azoury, R. S., and Woodruff, J. D.: Primary ovarian sarcomas; report of 43 cases from the Emil Novak Ovarian Tumor Registry, Obstet. Gynecol. **37**:920, 1971.

Bagley, C. M., Jr., Young, R. C., Canellos, G. P., and DeVita, V. T.: Treatment of ovarian carcinoma; possibilities for progress, N. Engl. J. Med. **287**:856, 1972.

Baillie, A. H., Ferguson, M. M., and Hart, D. M.: Histochemical evidence of steroid metabolism in the human genital ridge, J. Clin. Endocrinol. **26**:738, 1966.

Bales, G., and others: Adriamycin in ovarian cancer patients resistant to cyclophosphamide, Eur. J. Cancer **14**:1401, 1978.

Barclay, D. L., Leverich, E. B., and Kemmerly, J. R.: Hyperreactio luteinalis; postpartum persistence, Am. J. Obstet. Gynecol. **105**:642, 1969.

Barlow, J. J., and Dillard, P. H.: Serum protein-bound fucose in patients with gynecologic cancers, Obstet. Gynecol. **39**:727, 1972.

Barlow, J. J., and Piver, M. S.: Second-line efficacy of intermediate high-dose methotrexate with citrovorum factor rescue plus cyclophosphamide in ovarian cancer, Gynecol. Oncol. **7**:233, 1979.

Barlow, J. J., Piver, M. S., Chuang, J. T., and others: Adriamycin and bleomycin, alone and in combination in gynecologic cancers, Cancer **32**:735, 1973.

Barr, W., Cowell, M. A. C., and Chatfield, W. R.: The management of ovarian cancer; a review of 420 cases, Scott. Med. J. **15**:250, 1970.

Beck, R. D., and Boyes, D. A.: Treatment of 126 cases of advanced ovarian carcinoma with cyclophosphamide, Can. Med. Assoc. J. **98**:539, 1968.

Bergman, F.: Carcinoma of the ovary; a clinicopathological study of 86 autopsied cases with special reference to mode of spread, Acta Obstet. Gynecol. Scand. **45**:211, 1966.

Blum, R. H., and Carter, S. K.: Adriamycin—a new anticancer drug with significant clinical activity, Ann. Intern. Med. **80**:249, 1974.

Blum, R. H., Livingston, R. B., and Carter, S. K.: Hexamethylmelamine—a new drug with activity in solid tumors, Eur. J. Cancer **9**:195, 1973.

Bolis, G., D'Incalci, M., Gramellini, F., and Mangioni, C.: Adriamycin in ovarian cancer patients resistant to cyclophosphamide, Eur. J. Cancer **14**:1401, 1978.

Bonomi, P. D., Miadineo, J., Morrin, B., and others: Phase II trial of hexamethylmelamine in ovarian carcinoma resistant to alkylating agents, Cancer Treat. Rep. **63**:137, 1979.

Brady, L., Blessing, J., Homesley, H., and Leives, G. C.: Radiotherapy, chemotherapy, and combined therapy in Stage III epithelial ovarian cancer, Proc. Am. Assoc. Cancer Res. **20**:218, 1979.

Brennan, M. J., and Vaitkevicius, V. K.: 5-Fluorouracil in clinical cancer; experience with 155 patients, Cancer Chemother. Rep. **6**:8, 1960.

Briggs, M. H., Caldwell, A. D. S., and Pitchford, A. G.: The treatment of cancer by progestogens, Hosp. Med. Lond. **2**:63, 1967.

Briscoe, K. E., Pasmantier, M. W., Ohnuma, T., and Kennedy, B. J.: Cis-dichlorodiammineplatinum (II) and adriamycin treatment of advanced ovarian cancer, Cancer Treat. Rep. **62**:2027, 1978.

Brodovsky, H. S., Pocock, S. J., Sears, M., and others: A comparison of melphalan with 5-fluorouracil, Cytoxan and methotrexate in patients with ovarian cancer, Proc. Am. Soc. Clin. Oncol. **15**:165, 1974.

Bruckner, H. W., Cohen, C. J., Gusberg, S. B., and others: Chemotherapy of ovarian cancer with adriamycin (ADM) and cis-platinum (DDP), Proc. Am. Assoc. Cancer Res. **17**:287, 1976.

Bruckner, H. W., Cohen, C. J., Wallach, R. C., and others: Prospective controlled randomized trial comparing combination chemotherapy of advanced ovarian carcinoma with adriamycin and cis-platinum +/− cyclophosphamide and hexamethylmelamine, Proc. Am. Assoc. Cancer Res. **20**:414, 1979.

Bruckner, H. W., Pagano, M., Falkson, G., and

others: Controlled prospective trial of combination chemotherapy with cyclophosphamide, adriamycin, and 5-fluorouracil for the treatment of advanced ovarian cancer; a preliminary report, Cancer Treat. Rep. **63**:297, 1979.

Bruckner, H. W., Wallach, R. C., Kabakow, B., and others: Cis-platinum (DDP) for combination chemotherapy of ovarian carcinoma; improved response rate and survival, Proc. Am. Assoc. Cancer Res. **19**:373, 1978.

Buckner, C. D., Rudolph, R. H., Fefer, A., and others: High dose cyclophosphamide therapy for malignant disease; toxicity, tumor response and the effects of stored autologous marrow, Cancer **29**:357, 1972.

Buka, N. J, and MacFarlane, K. T.: Malignant tumors of the ovary, Am. J. Obstet. Gynecol. **90**:383, 1964.

Burns, B. C., Jr., Rutledge, F. N., Smith, J. P., and Delclos, L.: Management of ovarian carcinoma; surgery, irradiation and chemotherapy, Am. J. Obstet. Gynecol. **98**:374, 1967.

Carcinoma of the ovary; panel discussion. In Carcinoma of the uterine cervix, endometrium and ovary, The University of Texas M. D. Anderson Hospital and Tumor Institute. Fifth Clinical Conference on Cancer, 1960, Chicago, 1962, Year Book Medical Publishers, Inc.

Cariker, M., and Dockerty, M.: Mucinous cystadenomas and mucinous cystadenocarcinomas of the ovary; a clinical and pathological study of 335 cases, Cancer **7**:302, 1954.

Chung, A., and Birnbaum, S. J.: Ovarian cancer associated with pregnancy, Obstet. Gynecol. **41**:211, 1973.

Clark, D. G. C., Hilaris, B., Roussis, C., and others: The role of radiation therapy in the treatment of cancer of the ovary; results of 614 patients, Prog. Clin. Cancer **5**:227, 1973.

Corbett, T. H., Griswold, D. P., Mayo, J. G., and others: Cyclophosphamide-Adriamycin combination chemotherapy in transplantable murine tumors, Cancer Res. **35**:1568, 1975.

Creasman, W. T., Abu-Ghazaleh, S., and Schmidt, H. J.: Retroperitoneal metastatic spread of ovarian cancer, Gynecol. Oncol. **6**:447, 1978.

Creasman, W. T., Gall, S. A., Blessing, J. A., and others: Chemoimmunotherapy in the management of primary stage III ovarian cancer; a Gynecologic Oncology Group study, Cancer Treat. Rep. **63**:319, 1979.

Cruikshank, D. P., and Buchsbaum, H. J.: Effects of rapid paracentesis; cardiovascular dynamics and body fluid composition, J.A.M.A. **225**:1361, 1973.

Czernobilsky, B., and LaBarre, G. C.: Carcinoma and mixed mesodermal tumor of the ovary; a clinicopathologic analysis of 9 cases, Obstet. Gynecol. **31**:21, 1968.

Czernobilsky, B., Silverman, B. B., and Enterline, H. T.: Clear-cell carcinoma of the ovary; a clinicopathologic analysis of pure and mixed forms and comparison with endometrioid carcinoma, Cancer **25**:762, 1970.

Decker, D. G., Malkasian, G. D., Jr., Mussey, E., and Johnson, C. E.: Cyclophosphamide; evaluation in recurrent and progressive ovarian cancer, Am. J. Obstet. Gynecol. **97**:656, 1967.

Decker, D. G., Mussey, E., Malkasian, G. D., and Johnson, C. E.: Adjuvant therapy for advanced ovarian malignancy, Am. J. Obstet. Gynecol. **97**:171, 1967.

Decker, D. G., Webb, M. J., and Holbrook, M. A.: Radiogold treatment of epithelial cancer of the ovary; late results, Am. J. Obstet. Gynecol. **115**:751, 1973.

Dehner, L. P., Norris, H. J., and Taylor, H. B.: Carcinosarcomas and mixed mesodermal tumors of the ovary, Cancer **27**:207, 1971.

Delclos, L., and Fletcher, G. H.: Postoperative irradiation for ovarian carcinoma with the cobalt 60 moving strip technique, Clin. Obstet. Gynecol. **12**:993, 1969.

Delclos, L., and Quinlan, E. J.: Malignant tumors of the ovary managed with postoperative megavoltage irradiation, Radiology **93**:659, 1969.

Delclos, L., and Smith, J. P.: Tumors of the ovary. In Fletcher, G., editor: Textbook of radiotherapy, Philadelphia, 1973, Lea & Febiger.

Delgado, G., Chun, B., Caglar, H., and Bepko, F.: Paraaortic lymphadenectomy in gynecologic malignancies confined to the pelvis, Obstet. Gynecol. **50**:418, 1977.

Dembo, A. J., Bush, R. S., Beale, F. A., and others: The Princess Margaret Hospital study of ovarian cancer; stages I, II and asymptomatic III presentations, Cancer Treat. Rep. **63**:249, 1979.

De Palo, G., De Lena, M., Bajetta, E., and others: Controlled study with L-phenylalanine mustard versus Adriamycin in stage IV ovarian cancer. In Proceedings of the Eleventh International Cancer Congress, Florence, 1974.

De Palo, G. M., De Lena, M., and Bonadonna, G.: Adriamycin versus adriamycin plus melphalan in advanced ovarian carcinoma, Cancer Treat. Rep. **61**:355, 1977.

Donald, I.: On launching a new diagnostic science, Am. J. Obstet. Gynecol. **103**:609, 1969.

Dunnihoo, D. R., Grieme, D. L., and Woolf, R. B.: Hilar-cell tumors of the ovary; report of two new cases and review of the world literature, Obstet. Gynecol. **27**:703, 1966.

Edmonson, J. H., Fleming, T. R., Decker, D. G., and others: Different chemotherapeutic sensitivities and host factors affecting prognosis in advanced ovarian carcinoma versus minimal residual disease, Cancer Treat. Rep. **63:**241, 1979.

Ehrlich, C. E., and others: Combination of ovarian carcinoma with cis-dichlorodiammineplatinum (DDP), adriamycin (ADR) and Cytoxan (CTX), Proc. Am. Assoc. Cancer Res. **19:**379, 1978.

Ehrlich, C. E., Einhorn, L., Williams, S. D., and Morgan, J.: Chemotherapy for stage III-IV epithelial ovarian cancer with cis-dichlorodiammineplatinum (II), adriamycin, and cyclophosphamide; a preliminary report, Cancer Treat. Rep. **63:**281, 1979.

Einhorn, L. H., and Williams, S. D.: The role of cis-platinum in solid-tumor therapy, N. Engl. J. Med. **300:**289, 1979.

Fenn, M. E., and Abell, M. R.: Carcinosarcoma of the ovary, Am. J. Obstet. Gynecol. **110:**1066, 1971.

Frei, E.: Selected considerations regarding chemotherapy as adjuvant in cancer treatment; a commentary, Cancer Chemother. Rep. **50:**1, 1966.

Frei, E., Jaffe, N., Tattersall, M. H. N., and others: New approaches to cancer chemotherapy with methotrexate, N. Engl. J. Med. **292:**846, 1975.

Frick, H. C. II, Tretter, P., Tretter, W., and others: Disseminated carcinoma of the ovary treated by L-phenylalanine mustard, Cancer **21:**508, 1968.

Geisler, H. E., Minor, J. R., and Eastlund, M. E.: Treatment of advanced ovarian carcinoma with high dose, intravenous cyclophosphamide, Gynecol. Oncol. **4:**43, 1976.

Gentil, F., and Junqueira, A. C., editors: Ovarian cancer, New York, 1968, Springer-Verlag New York, Inc.

Godfrey, T. E., King, A., and Rentschler, R.: 1, 3-bis(2-chloroethyl)-1-nitrosourea; effects on advanced ovarian carcinoma, Am. J. Obstet. Gynecol. **115:**576, 1973.

Graham, J. B., Graham, R. M., and Schueller, E. F.: Preclinical detection of ovarian cancer, Cancer **17:**1414, 1964.

Gray, L. A., and Barnes, M. L.: Endometrioid carcinoma of the ovary, Obstet. Gynecol. **29:**694, 1967.

Greenspan, E. M.: Thio-tepa and methotrexate chemotherapy of advanced ovarian carcinoma, J. Mt. Sinai Hosp. **32:**52, 1968.

Griffiths, C. T.: Surgical resection of tumor bulk in the primary treatment of ovarian cancer, Natl. Cancer Inst. Monogr. **42:**101, 1975.

Griffiths, C. T., and Fuller, A. F.: Intensive surgical and chemotherapeutic management of advanced ovarian cancer, Surg. Clin. North Am. **58:**1978.

Griffiths, C. T., Grogan, R. H., and Hall, T. C.: Advanced cancer; primary treatment with surgery, radiotherapy and chemotherapy, Cancer **29:**1, 1972.

Griffiths, C. T., Parker, L. M., and Fuller, A. F.: Role of cytoreductive surgical treatment in the management of advanced ovarian cancer, Cancer Treat. Rep. **63:**235, 1979.

Halpin, T. F., and McCann, T. O.: Dynamics of body fluids following the rapid removal of large volumes of ascites, Am. J. Obstet. Gynecol. **110:**103, 1971.

Hanks, G. E., and Bagshaw, M. A.: Megavoltage radiation therapy and lymphangiography in ovarian cancer, Radiology **93:**649, 1969.

Harris, C. C.: The carcinogenicity of anticancer drugs; a hazard to man, Cancer **37:**1014, 1976.

Hester, L. L., Sr., and White, L.: Radioactive colloidal chromic phosphate in the treatment of ovarian malignancies, Am. J. Obstet. Gynecol. **103:**911, 1969.

Hirabayashi, K., and Graham, J.: Genesis of ascites in ovarian cancer, Am. J. Obstet. Gynecol. **106:**492, 1970.

Hoogstraten, B., Gottlieb, J. A., Caoili, E., and others: CCNU (1-(2-chloroethyl)-3-cyclohexyl-1-nitrosourea) in the treatment of cancer; phase II study, Cancer **32:**38, 1973.

Hubbard, S. M., Barkes, P., and Young, R. C.: Adriamycin therapy for advanced ovarian carcinoma recurrent after chemotherapy, Cancer Treat. Rep. **62:**1375, 1978.

Hudson, C. N., and Dendy, P. P.: Aspects of treatment of more advanced cases of ovarian cancer, Proc. R. Soc. Med. **67:**798, 1974.

Johansson, H.: Clinical aspects of metastatic ovarian cancer of extragenital origin, Acta Obstet. Gynecol. Scand. **39:**681, 1960.

Johnson, B. L., Fisher, R. I., Bender, R. A., and others: Hexamethylmelamine in alkylating agent-resistant ovarian carcinoma, Cancer **42:**2157, 1978.

Johnson, C. E., Decker, D. G., Van Herik, M., and others: Advanced ovarian cancer; therapy with radiation and cyclophosphamide in a random series, Am. J. Roentgenol. **114:**136, 1972.

Jolles, B.: Progesterone in the treatment of advanced malignant tumors of breast, ovary and uterus, Br. J. Cancer **16:**209, 1962.

Jorgensen, E. O., Malkasian, G. D., Webb, M. J., and others: Pilot study evaluating 1, 2-bis(2-chloroethyl)-1-nitrosourea in the treatment of advanced ovarian carcinoma, Am. J. Obstet. Gynecol. **116:**769, 1973.

Julian, C. G., and Woodruff, J. D.: The role of chemotherapy in the treatment of primary ovarian malignancy, Obstet. Gynecol. Surv. **24:**1307, 1969.

Kane, R., Harvey, H., Andrews, T., and others: Phase II trial of cyclophosphamide, hexamethylmelamine, adriamycin, and cis-dichlorodiammineplatinum (II) combination chemotherapy in advanced ovarian carcinoma, Cancer Treat. Rep. **63:**307, 1979.

Kaslow, R. A., Wisch, N., and Glass, J. L.: Acute leukemia following cytotoxic chemotherapy, J.A.M.A. **219:**75, 1972.

Kennedy, B. J., and Theologides, A.: The role of 5-fluorouracil in malignant disease, Ann. Intern. Med. **55:**719, 1961.

Kent, S. W., and McKay, D. G.: Primary cancer of the ovary, Am. J. Obstet. Gynecol. **80:**430, 1960.

Kerr, H. D., and Elkins, H. B.: Carcinoma of the ovary, Am. J. Roentgenol. **66:**184, 1951.

Klaassen, D. J., Boyes, D. A., Gerulath, A., and others: Preliminary report of a clinical trial of the treatment of patients with advanced stage III and IV ovarian cancer with melphalan, 5-fluorouracil, and methotrexate in combination and sequentially; a study of the clinical trials group of the National Cancer Institute of Canada, Cancer Treat. Rep. **63:**280, 1979.

Knapp, R. C., and Friedman, E. A.: Aortic lymph node metastases in early ovarian cancer, Am. J. Obstet. Gynecol. **119:**1013, 1974.

Kottmeier, H. L.: The classification and treatment of ovarian tumors, Acta Obstet. Gynecol. Scand. **31:**313, 1952.

Kottmeier, H. L.: Carcinoma of the female genitalia, Baltimore, 1953, The Williams & Wilkins Co.

Kottmeier, H. L.: Problems relating to classification and stage-grouping of malignant tumors in the female pelvis. In Cancer of the uterus and ovary, The University of Texas M. D. Anderson Hospital and Tumor Institute. Eleventh Annual Clinical Conference on Cancer, Chicago, 1966, Year Book Medical Publishers, Inc.

Kottmeier, H. L.: Treatment of ovarian cancer with thio tepa, Clin. Obstet. Gynecol. **11:**428, 1968.

Kottmeier, H. L.: Cancer of the uterus and ovary, Chicago, 1969, Year Book Medical Publishers, Inc.

Kottmeier, H. L.: Ovarian cancer with special regard to radiotherapy, Am. J. Roentgenol. **111:**417, 1971.

Kurman, R. J., and Craig, J. M.: Endometrioid and clear cell carcinoma of the ovary, Cancer **29:**1653, 1972.

Latour, J. P. A., and Davis, B. A.: A critical assessment of the value of x-ray therapy in primary ovarian carcinoma, Am. J. Obstet. Gynecol. **74:**968, 1957.

Levi, M. M.: Antigenicity of ovarian and cervical malignancies with a view toward possible immunodiagnosis, Am. J. Obstet. Gynecol. **109:**689, 1971.

Levi, M. M., Parshley, M. S., and Mandl, I.: Antigenicity of papillary serous cystadenocarcinoma tissue culture cells, Am. J. Obstet. Gynecol. **101:**433, 1968.

Lokich, J. J., and Skarin, A. T.: Five-drug combination chemotherapy for disseminated adenocarcinoma, Cancer Chemother. Rep. **56:**761, 1972.

Long, M. E., and Taylor, H. C., Jr.: Endometrioid carcinoma of the ovary, Am. J. Obstet. Gynecol. **90:**936, 1964.

Long, R. T. L., Johnson, R. E., and Sala, J. M.: Variation in survival among patients with carcinoma of the ovary, Cancer **20:**1195, 1967.

Lurain, J. R., and Piver, M. S.: Familial ovarian cancer, Gynecol. Oncol. **8:**185, 1979.

Malkasian, G. D., Jr., Decker, D. G., Mussey, E., and Johnson, C. E.: Observations on gynecologic malignancy treated with 5-fluorouracil, Am. J. Obstet. Gynecol. **100:**1012, 1968.

Mangioni, C., Bolis, G., Molteni, P., and Belloni, C.: Indications, advantages and limits of laparoscopy in ovarian cancer, Gynecol. Oncol. **7:**47, 1979.

Masterson, J. G., and Nelson, J. H., Jr.: The role of chemotherapy in the treatment of gynecologic malignancy, Am. J. Obstet. Gynecol. **93:**11102, 1965.

McGown, L., Parent, L., Lednar, W., and Norris, H. J.: The woman at risk for developing ovarian cancer, Gynecol. Oncol. **7:**315, 1979.

Menczer, J., Modan, M., and others: Possible role of mumps virus in the etiology of ovarian cancer, Cancer **43:**1375, 1979.

Moore, G. E., Bross, I. D. G., Ausman, R., and others: Effects of chlorambucil in 374 patients with advanced cancer, Cancer Chemother. Rep. **52:**661, 1968.

Morris, J. M., and Scully, R. E.: Endocrine pathology of the ovary, St. Louis, 1958, The C. V. Mosby Co.

Munnell, E. W.: Is conservative therapy ever justified in stage I (Ia) cancer of the ovary? Am. J. Obstet. Gynecol. **103:**641, 1969.

Myers, M. A.: Peritoneography; normal and pathologic anatomy, Am. J. Roentgenol. **117:**353, 1973.

Myers, R. A., Belinson, J., Yates, J. W., and Krakoff, I.: Combination chemotherapy of ovarian carcinoma, Proc. Am. Assoc. Cancer Res. **20:**405, 1979.

Neijt, J. P., van Lindert, A. C., Vendrik, C. P., and others: Hexa-CAF combination chemotherapy and other multiple-drug regimens in advanced ovarian carcinoma; present and future, Neth. J. Med. **22:**(2):38, 1979.

Nieminen, V., and Purola, E.: Stage and prognosis of ovarian cystadenocarcinomas, Acta Obstet. Gynecol. Scan. **49:**49, 1970.

Norris, C. C., and Murphy, D. P.: Malignant ovarian neoplasms; with a report of the end results in a series of 93 cases, Am. J. Obstet. Gynecol. **23:**833, 1933.

Norris, H. J., and Robinowitz, M.: Ovarian adenocarcinoma of mesonephric type, Cancer **28:**1074, 1971.

Nye, E. B.: Ovarian carcinoma; improvement in survival time after chemotherapy, J. Obstet. Gynaecol. Br. Comm. **79:**550, 1972.

O'Bryan, R. M., Luce, J. K., Talley, R. W., and others: Phase 2 evaluation of Adriamycin in human neoplasia, Cancer **32:**1, 1973.

Omura, G. A., Blessing, J. A., Buchsbaum, H. J., and Lathrop, J.: Randomized trial of melphalan vs. melphalan plus hexamethylmelamine vs. adriamycin plus cyclophosphamide in advanced ovarian adenocarcinoma, Proc. Am. Assoc. Cancer Res. **20:**358, 1979.

Ozols, R. F., Garvin, A. J., Costa, J., and others: Histologic grade in advanced ovarian cancer, Cancer Treat. Rep. **63:**255, 1979.

Ozols, R. F., Locker, G. Y., Doroshow, J. H., and others: Chemotherapy for murine ovarian cancer; a rationale for ip therapy with adriamycin, Cancer Treat. Rep. **63:**269, 1979.

Parker, L. M., Griffiths, C. T., and others: Adriamycin/cyclophosphamide and surgical treatment of advanced ovarian cancer, Proc. Am. Assoc. Cancer Res. **19:**399, 1978.

Parker, L. M., Griffiths, C. T., Yankee, R. A., and others: High-dose methotrexate with leucovorin rescue in ovarian cancer; a phase II study, Cancer Treat. Rep. **63:**275, 1979.

Parker, L. M., Kokich, J. J., Griffiths, C. T., and others: Adriamycin-cyclophosphamide therapy in ovarian cancer, Proc. Am. Soc. Clin. Oncol. **16:**263, 1975.

Parker, R., and others: The role of lymphography in patients with ovarian cancer, Cancer **34:**100, 1974.

Parker, R. T., Parker, C. H., and Wilbanks, C. D.: Cancer of the ovary, Am. J. Obstet. Gynecol. **108:**878, 1970.

Perez, C. A., and Bradfield, J. S.: Radiation therapy in the treatment of carcinoma of the ovary, Cancer **29:**1027, 1972.

Pezner, R. D.: Limited epithelial carcinoma of the ovary treated with curative intent by the intraperitoneal instillation of radioactive colloids, Cancer **42:**2563, 1978.

Pitman, S. W., Parker, L. M., Tattersall, M. H. N., and others: Clinical trial of high dose methotrexate-citrovorum factor; toxicologic and therapeutic observations, Cancer Chemother. Rep. **6:**43, 1975.

Piver, M. S., Barlow, J. J., and Bhattacharya, M.: Treatment and immunodiagnosis of advanced ovarian adenocarcinoma; a preliminary report, Cancer Treat. Rep. **63:**265, 1979.

Piver, M. S., Barlow, J. J., and Lele, S. B.: Incidence of subclinical metastasis in stage I and II ovarian carcinoma, Obstet. Gynecol. **52:**100, 1978.

Piver, M. S., Barlow, J. J., Lele, S. B., and others: Cis-dichlorodiammineplatinum (II) as third line chemotherapy in advanced ovarian adenocarcinoma, Cancer Treat. Rep. **62:**559, 1978.

Piver, M. S., Barlow, J. J., Yazigi, R., and Blumenson, L. E.: Melphalan chemotherapy in advanced ovarian carcinoma, Obstet. Gynecol. **51:**352, 1978.

Purola, E.: Serous papillary ovarian tumors; a study of 233 cases with special reference to the histological type of tumor and its influence in prognosis, Acta Obstet. Gynecol. Scand. **42:**7, 1963.

Purola, E., and Nieminen, U.: Does rupture of cystic carcinoma during operation influence the prognosis? Am. Clin. Gynecol. Fenn. **57:**615, 1968.

Rozencweig, M., von Hoff, D. D., Slavik, M., and others: Cis-diamminedichloroplatinum (II); a new anticancer drug, Ann. Intern. Med. **86:**803, 1977.

Rosenshein, N., and others: The effect of volume on the distribution of substances instilled into the peritoneal cavity, Gynecol. Oncol. **6:**106, 1978.

Rosenshein, N., Leichner, P., and Vogelsang, G.: Radiocolloids in the treatment of ovarian cancer, Obstet. Gynecol. Surv. **34:**708, 1979.

Rubin, P.: A critical analysis of current therapy of carcinoma of the ovary; introduction to symposium, Am. J. Roentgenol. **88:**833, 1962.

Sall, S., and Stone, M. L.: The treatment of ovarian cancer, Prog. Clin. Cancer **5:**249, 1973.

Sampson, J. A.: Endometrial carcinoma of ovary arising in endometrial tissue in that organ, Arch. Surg. **10:**1, 1925.

Schueller, E. F., and Korol, P. M.: Prognosis in

endometrial carcinoma of the ovary, Obstet. Gynecol. **27**:850, 1966.

Scully, R. E.: Recent progress in ovarian cancer, Hum. Pathol. **1**:73, 1970.

Scully, R. E., and Barlow, J. F.: "Mesonephroma" of the ovary; tumor of Mullerian nature related to the endometrioid carcinoma, Cancer **20**:1405, 1967.

Shanks, H. G. I.: Pseudomyxoma peritonei, J. Obstet. Gynaecol. Br. Comm. **68**:212, 1961.

Smith, J. P., Delgado, G., and Rutledge, F.: Second-look operation in ovarian carcinoma, Cancer **38**:1438, 1976.

Smith, J. P., and Rutledge, F.: Chemotherapy in the treatment of cancer of the ovary, Am. J. Obstet. Gynecol. **107**:691, 1970.

Smith, J. P., Rutledge, F., and Sutow, W. W.: Malignant gynecologic tumors in children; current approaches to treatment, Am. J. Obstet. Gynecol. **116**:261, 1973.

Smith, J. P., Rutledge, F., and Wharton, J. T.: Chemotherapy of ovarian cancer; new approaches to treatment, Cancer **30**:1565, 1972.

Smith, J. P., and others: Results of chemotherapy as an adjunct through surgery in patients with localized ovarian cancer, Semin. Oncol. **2**:277, 1975.

Sotrel, G., Jafari, K., Lash, A. F., and others: Acute leukemia in advanced ovarian carcinoma after treatment with alkylating agents, Obstet. Gynecol. **47**:67S, 1976.

Stanhope, R. C., Smith, J. P., and others: Second trial drugs in ovarian cancer, Gynecol. Oncol. **5**:52, 1977.

Stone, M. L., Weingold, A. B., Sall, S., and others: Factors affecting survival of patients with ovarian carcinoma, Surg. Gynecol. Obstet. **116**:351, 1963.

Sullivan, R. A., Miller, E., Zurek, W. Z., and others: Reevaluation of methotrexate as an anticancer drug, Surg. Gynecol. Obstet. **125**:319, 1967.

Tepper, E., Sanfilippo, L. J., Gray, J., and others: Second look surgery after radiation therapy for advanced stages of carcinoma of the ovary, Am. J. Roentgenol. **112**:755, 1971.

Tobias, J. S., and Griffiths, C. T.: Management of ovarian carcinoma, N. Engl. J. Med. **294**:818, 1976.

Tobias, J. S., Parker, L. M., Tattersall, M. H. N., and others: Adriamycin-cyclophosphamide and Adriamycin-melphalan in advanced L1210 leukemia, Br. J. Cancer, in press.

Turbow, M. M., and others: Chemotherapy of ovarian carcinoma; randomization between melphalan and adriamycin-cyclophosphamide, Proc. Am. Assoc. Cancer Res. **19**:394, 1978.

Van Orden, D. E., MacAllister, W. B., Zerne, S. R. M., and others: Ovarian carcinoma; the problems of staging and grading, Am. J. Obstet. Gynecol. **94**:195, 1966.

Varga, A., and Henriksen, E.: Effect of 17-alpha-hydroxyprogesterone 17-N-caproate on various pelvic malignancies, Obstet. Gynecol. **23**:51, 1964.

Vider, M., Deland, F. H., and Maruyama, Y.: Loculation as a contraindication to intracavitary 32P–chromic phosphate therapy, letter, J. Nucl. Med. **17**:150, 1976.

Vogl, S. E., Berenzweig, M., Kaplan, B. H., and others: The CHAD and HAD regimens in advanced ovarian cancer; combination chemotherapy including cyclophosphamide, hexamethylmelamine, adriamycin, and cis-dichlorodiammineplatinum (II), Cancer Treat. Rep. **63**:311, 1979.

Vogl, S. E., Greenwald, E., and Kaplan, B. H.: The CHAD regimen (cyclophosphamide, hexamethylmelamine, adriamycin and diamminedichloroplatinum) in advanced ovarian cancer, Proc. Am. Assoc. Cancer Res. **20**:384, 1979.

Vogl, S., Ohnuma, T., Perloff, M., and others: Combination chemotherapy with Adriamycin and cis-diamminedichloroplatinum in patients with advanced neoplastic diseases, Cancer **38**:21, 1976.

Vogler, W. R., and Jacobs, J.: Toxic and therapeutic effects of methotrexate-folinic acid (leucovorin) in advanced cancer and leukemia, Cancer **28**:894, 1971.

Wallach, R. C., Kabakow, B., Blinick, G., and Antopol, W.: Thio-tepa chemotherapy for ovarian carcinoma; influence of remission and toxicity on survival, Obstet. Gynecol. **35**:278, 1970.

Wampler, G. L., Mellette, S. J., and Kuperminc, M.: Hexamethylmelamine in the treatment of advanced cancer, Cancer Chemother. Rep. **56**:505, 1972.

Ward, H. W. C.: Progestogen therapy for ovarian carcinoma, J. Obstet. Gynaecol. Br. Comm. **79**:555, 1972.

Weeth, J. B.: Large dose progestin palliation; valuable in solid tumor patients, Proc. Am. Soc. Clin. Oncol. **15**:165, 1974.

Wharton, J. T., Rutledge, F., Smith, J. P., and others: Hexamethylmelamine; an evaluation of its role in the treatment of ovarian cancer, Am. J. Obstet. Gynecol. **133**:833, 1979.

Widder, K. J., Senyei, A. E., and Ranney, D. F.: Magnetically responsive microspheres and other carriers for the biophysical targeting of anti-tumor agents, Adv. Pharmacol. Chemother. **16**:213, 1979.

Williams, T. J., Symmonds, R. E., and Litwak, O.: Management of unilateral and encapsulated ovarian cancer in young women, Gynecol. Oncol. **1**:143, 1973.

Wilson, W. L., Bisel, H. F., Cole, D., and others: Prolonged low dosage administration of hexamethylmelamine, Cancer **25**:568, 1970.

Wilson, W. L., Schroeder, J. N., Bisel, H. F., and others: Phase II study of hexamethylmalamine, Cancer **23**:132, 1969.

Wiltshaw, E., and Carr, B.: Cis-platinum (II) diamminedichloride; clinical experience of the Royal Marsden Hospital and Institute of Cancer Research, London. In Connors, T. A., and Roberts, J. J., editors: Platinum coordination complexes in cancer chemotherapy; recent results in cancer research, New York, 1974, Springer-Verlag New York, Inc.

Wiltshaw, E., and Kroner, T.: Phase II study of cis-dichlorodiammineplatinum (II) (NSC-119875) in advanced adenocarcinoma of the ovary, Cancer Treat. Rep. **60**:55, 1976.

Woodruff, J. D., Bie, L. S., and Sherman, R. J.: Mucinous tumors of the ovary, Obstet. Gynecol. **16**:699, 1960.

Woodruff, J. D., and Novak, E. R.: Papillary serous tumors of the ovary, Am. J. Obstet. Gynecol. **67**:1112, 1954.

Woodruff, J. D., and others: Mucinous cystadenocarcinoma of the ovary, Obstet. Gynecol. **51**:483, 1978.

Yesair, D. W., Momitt, S., Tobias, J. S., and others: Importance of schedule in Adriamycin/cyclophosphamide combination chemotherapy, Eur. J. Cancer **14**:141, 1978.

Young, R. C.: Ovarian carcinoma; an optimistic epilogue, Cancer Treat. Rep. **63**:333, 1979.

Young, R. C., Canellos, G. P., Chabner, B. A., and others: Chemotherapy of advanced ovarian carcinoma; a prospective randomized comparison of L-phenylalanine mustard and high dose cyclophosphamide, Gynecol. Oncol. **1**:489, 1974.

Young, R. C., Chabner, B. A., Hubbard, S. P., and others: Advanced ovarian adenocarcinoma; a prospective clinical trial of melphalan (L-PAM) versus combination chemotherapy, N. Engl. J. Med. **299**:1261, 1978.

Young, R. C., and Fisher, R. I.: The staging and treatment of epithelial ovarian cancer, Can. Med. Assoc. J. **119**:249, 1978.

Young, R. C., Hubbard, S. P., and De Vita, V. T.: The chemotherapy of ovarian carcinoma, Cancer Treat. Rev. **1**:99, 1974.

Young, R. C., Wharton, J. T., Decker, D. G., and others: Staging laparotomy in early ovarian cancer, Proc. Am. Assoc. Cancer Res. **20**:399, 1979.

Young, R. C., and others: Advanced ovarian adenocarcinoma; melphalan (PAM) versus combination chemotherapy (HEXA-CAF), Proc. Am. Assoc. Cancer Res. **19**:393, 1978.

CHAPTER TWELVE

Germ cell, stromal, and other ovarian tumors

GERM CELL TUMORS
Classification

This group of ovarian neoplasms is composed of a number of histologically differ-ent tumor types and embraces all the neoplasms considered to be ultimately derived from the primitive germ cells of the embryonic gonad (Fig. 12-1). This concept of

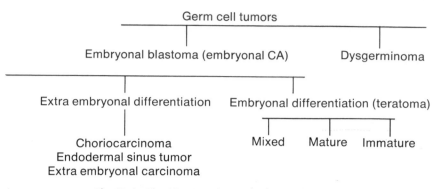

Fig. 12-1. Classification of germ cell tumors of the ovary.

germ cell tumors as a specific group of gonadal neoplasms has evolved in the last 4 decades and has become generally accepted. This concept is based primarily on the common histogenesis of these neoplasms, on the relatively frequent presence of histologically different tumor elements within the same tumor mass, on the presence of histologically similar neoplasms in extragonadal locations along the line of migration of the primitive germ cells from the wall of yolk sac to the gonadal ridge, and on the remarkable homology between the various tumor types in the male and the female. In no other group of gonadal neoplasms has this homology been better illustrated. An example of this is the striking similarity between the testicular seminoma and its ovarian counterpart, the dysgerminoma. These were the first neoplasms to become accepted as originating from germ cells. A number of classifications of germ cell neoplasms of the ovary have been proposed over the past few decades. Table 12-1 is a modification of a classification originally described by Teilum and is very similar to that proposed by the World Health Organization, which divides the germ cell tumors into a number of groups and also includes neoplasms composed of germ cells and "sex" stroma derivatives.

Clinical profile

Germ cell tumors represent a relatively small proportion (about 20%) of all ovarian tumors (Table 12-2) but are becoming increasingly important in the clinical practice of obstetrics and gynecology. Most of these neoplasms occur in young women, and extirpation of the disease involves decisions concerning childbearing and probabilities of recurrence. Recent developments in chemotherapy have dramatically changed the prognosis for many of the patients who develop the more aggressive types of germ cell tumors. Knowing the classification of these lesions and how the pathologist arrives at the diagnosis, as well as the clinical significance of that diagnosis, has great practical value for the practicing obstetrician/gynecologist. Most of these lesions are found in the second and third decades of life and are frequently diagnosed by finding a palpable abdominal mass, often associated with pain (Fig. 12-2). Except for the benign cystic teratoma, ovarian germ cell tumors are usually rap-

Table 12-1. Classification of germ cell neoplasms of the ovary

I. Germ cell tumors
   A. Dysgerminoma
   B. Endodermal sinus tumor
   C. Embryonal carcinoma
   D. Polyembryoma
   E. Choriocarcinoma
   F. Teratoma
      1. Immature (solid, cystic, or both)
      2. Mature
         a. Solid
         b. Cystic
            (1) Mature cystic teratoma (dermoid cyst)
            (2) Mature cystic teratoma (dermoid cyst) with malignant
                transformation
      3. Monodermal or highly specialized
         a. Struma ovarii
         b. Carcinoid
         c. Struma ovarii and carcinoid
         d. Others
   G. Mixed forms (tumors composed of types A through F in any
      possible combination)
II. Tumors composed of germ cells and sex cord stroma derivative
   A. Gonadoblastoma
   B. Mixed germ cell- sex cord stroma tumor

Table 12-2. Relative frequency of ovarian neoplasms

Type	Percent
Celomic epithelium	50-70
Germ cell	15-20
Specialized gonadal stroma	5-10
Nonspecific mesenchyme	5-10
Metastatic tumor	5-10

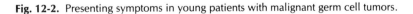

Frequency
Acute abdominal pain
Chronic abdominal pain
Asymptomatic mass
Abnormal vaginal bleeding
Abdominal distention

Fig. 12-2. Presenting symptoms in young patients with malignant germ cell tumors.

idly enlarging abdominal masses that often cause considerable abdominal pain. At times the pain is exacerbated by rupture or torsion of the neoplasm. One of the classic presenting signs of a dysgerminoma is hemoperitoneum from rupture of the capsule of the lesion as it rapidly enlarges.

Dysgerminoma

Dysgerminoma is composed of germ cells that have not differentiated to form embryonic or extraembryonic structures (Fig. 12-3). Its stroma is almost always infiltrated with lymphocytes and often contains granulomas similar to those of sarcoid. Grossly, the tumor may be firm or fleshy and cream colored or pale tan; both its external and section surfaces may be lobulated. A small proportion of dysgerminomas arise in sexually abnormal individuals, particularly those with pure or mixed gonadal dysgenesis or testicular feminization. In such cases the dysgerminoma often develops in a previously existing gonadoblastoma.

The symptoms of dysgerminoma are not distinctive, and they are similar to those observed in patients with other solid ovarian neoplasms. The duration of symptoms is usually short, and despite this the tumor is often large, indicating a rapid growth of the tumor. The most common presenting symptoms are abdominal enlargement and the presence of a mass in the lower abdomen. In a number of cases the tumor

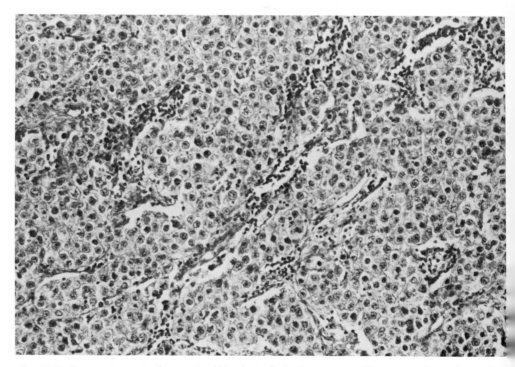

Fig. 12-3. Dysgerminoma is characterized histologically by the presence of large, round, ovoid or polygonal cells with stroma infiltrated by lymphocytes.

has been found incidentally at cesarean section or as a cause of dystocia in labor. Dysgerminoma is one of the two most common ovarian neoplasms observed in pregnancy, the other being serous cystadenoma. The relatively common finding of dysgerminoma in pregnant patients is nonspecific and relates to the age of the patient rather than the pregnant state. Dysgerminoma may also be discovered incidentally in patients investigated for primary amenorrhea, and in those cases it is not infrequently associated with gonadal dysgenesis and a gonadoblastoma. Occasionally, menstrual and endocrine abnormalities may be the presenting symptoms, but this tends to be more common in patients with dysgerminoma combined with other neoplastic germ cell elements, especially choriocarcinoma.

Dysgerminomas are notable by their predilection for lymphatic spread and their acute sensivity to irradiation. In patients under the age of 35 years with a tumor that has spread beyond the ovary or in patients with testicular feminization, the ideal treatment is removal of all internal genitalia. In the young woman with a unilateral encapsulated dysgerminoma who is desirous of future childbearing, conservative management is indicated (see Chapter 10). In those patients in whom unilateral salpingo-oophorectomy is performed, careful inspection of the other ovary and exploration to rule out disseminated disease are mandatory. These patients should then be followed closely for 2 to 3 years with periodic examinations including liberal use of lymphangiography and "second-look" procedures for possible recurrences. Approximately 90% of recurrences will occur in the first 2 years after initial therapy. Fortunately, 75% of recurrences can be successfully eradicated with radiotherapy, and it is this knowledge that permits the conservative management of patients as outlined in Chapter 10. The overall 5-year survival rate has been quoted between 70% and 95%.

Often lesions that consist primarily of dysgerminoma elements will contain small areas of more malignant histology (e.g., embryonal carcinoma or endodermal sinus tumor). When the dysgerminoma is not pure and these more malignant components are present, the prognosis and therapy are determined by the poorly differentiated elements and the dysgerminoma is disregarded.

Endodermal sinus tumor

The endodermal sinus tumor is the second most frequent form of malignant germ cell tumor of the ovary, accounting for 22% of germ cell lesions in one large series. Three fourths of the patients present with a combination of abdominal pain and abdominal or pelvic mass; the median age of the patients is 19 years. Alpha-fetoprotein (AFP) levels are often elevated in this group of tumors. The endodermal sinus tumor is characterized by extremely rapid growth and extensive intra-abdominal spread; nearly half the patients present with symptoms of 1 week's duration or less. Schiller called these neoplasms "mesonephroma," but most pathologists now consider them a variety of germ cell tumor unrelated to the mesonephros. They were thought to originate from germ cells that differentiate into extraembryonal yolk sac, because the tumor structure is very similar to that in the endodermal sinuses of the rat yolk sac. The tumors consist of scattered tubules or spaces lined by single layers of flattened cuboidal cells, loose reticular stroma, numerous scattered PAS-positive globules, and, within some spaces or clefts, a characteristic invaginated papillary structure with a central blood vessel (Schiller-Duval body) (Fig. 12-4).

The prognosis for patients with endodermal sinus tumor of the ovary has been unfavorable, with most patients dying of the disease within 12 to 18 months of diagnosis. Up until recently there had only been a few known 5-year survivors. The majority of these patients had tumors confined to the ovary, and in a number of cases the tumor was composed of endodermal sinus tumors admixed with other neoplastic germ cell elements, frequently dysgerminoma. The clinical course in most patients

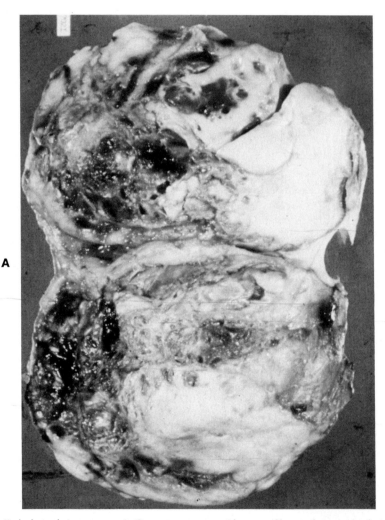

Fig. 12-4. Endodermal sinus tumor. **A,** Gross appearance with areas of hemorrhage and gelatinous necrosis.

with tumors composed of endodermal sinus tumor associated with dysgerminoma or other neoplastic germ cell elements does not differ greatly from that in patients with pure endodermal sinus tumor.

The treatment of patients with endodermal sinus tumor of the ovary has, in the past, been frustrating. The tumor is not sensitive to radiation therapy, although there may be an initial response. Optimum surgical extirpation of the disease has been advocated, but this alone is unsuccessful in producing a significant number of cures. In recent years there have been optimistic reports of sustained remissions in some patients treated by surgery and chemotherapy using a combination of actinomycin D, 5-fluorouracil, and cyclophosphamide (ActFUCy) or actinomycin D, vincristine, and cyclophosphamide (VAC). Forney and associates and Smith and associates reported long-term survivors in patients with advanced disease treated with these vigorous chemotherapeutic regimens. Creasman and associates have had comparable results using a combination of methotrexate, actinomycin D, and chlorambucil (MAC), and in addition, they have suggested that the VAC or MAC regimen is effective when administered for a period of no more than 6 months. This series needs confirmation but is particularly interesting in view of the growing philosophy advo-

(handwritten margin notes: "1° prognosis based on worse element", "not radios.")

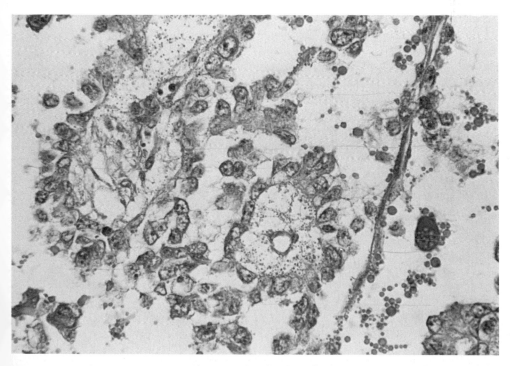

Fig. 12-4, cont'd. B, Microscopic appearance with isolated papillary projections containing single blood vessels and having a peripheral lining of neoplastic cells (Schiller-Duval body).

cating unilateral salpingo-oophorectomy only for these patients who desire preservation of childbearing capacity.

Most centers are recommending that all these patients receive intensive chemotherapy for periods of 6 to 18 months. Cis-platinum appears to be an active agent in this disease and will probably be included in future combination chemotherapy, as is the case with similar neoplasms of the testes. The most promising combination was suggested by Einhorn and Donohue and consists of vinblastine, bleomycin and cis-platinum. Trials are currently under way to define the minimum number of months of chemotherapy that produces optimum curability for these devastating lesions. Preliminary results are very encouraging, and its success, at least in some cases, may lead to the reassessment of the value of radical surgery and loss of childbearing ability in patients in whom the lesion is confined to one ovary.

From a practical point of view, serum AFP determination is considered to be a useful diagnostic tool in patients with endodermal sinus tumor. It can be of value in monitoring the results of therapy and in detecting metastasis and recurrences following therapy. Recent reports suggest that recurrences may occur in the retroperitoneal nodes in the absence of recognizable intraperitoneal disease.

Embryonal carcinoma

Embryonal carcinoma is one of the most malignant cancers arising in the ovary. The neoplasm, only recently described, closely resembles the embryonal carcinoma of the adult testes, where it is relatively common. However, it represents only 4% of the malignant ovarian germ cell tumors. Its rarity in the ovary and its confusion with choriocarcinoma and endodermal sinus tumors in the past account for its late identification as a distinct entity. It usually presents as an abdominal mass or pelvic mass, occurring at a mean age of 15 years. More than half the patients have hormonal abnormalities, including precocious puberty, irregular uterine bleeding, amenor-

Table 12-3. Comparison of embryonal carcinoma with endodermal sinus tumor

	Endodermal sinus tumor (71 cases)	Embryonal carcinoma (15 cases)
Median age	19 years	15 years
Prepubertal status	23%	47%
Precocious puberty	0	43%
Positive pregnancy test	None (0/15)	All (9/9)
Vaginal bleeding	1%	33%
Amenorrhea	0	7%
Hirsutism	0	7%
Survival, stage I patients	16%	50%
Human chorionic gonadotrophin	Negative (0/15)	Positive (10/10)
Alpha-fetoprotein	Positive (15/15)	Positive (7/10)

From Kurman, R. J., and Norris, H. J.: Endodermal sinus tumor of the ovary; a clinical and pathological analysis of 71 cases, Cancer **38:**2404, 1976.

rhea, or hirsutism. The tumors consist of large primitive cells with occasional papillary or glandlike formations. The cells have eosinophilic cytoplasm with distinct borders and round nuclei with prominent nucleoli. Numerous mitotic figures, many atypical, are seen, and scattered throughout the tumor are multinucleated giant cells that resemble syncytial cells.

These tumors contain human chorionic gonadotrophin (hCG), syncytiotrophoblastlike cells, and AFP in the large primitive cells. This tumor most likely arises from primordial germ cells, but it develops before there is much further differentiation toward either embryonic or extraembryonic tissue. In a review of 15 patients, Kurman and Norris had an actuarial survival rate of 39% for the whole group; for those with stage I tumors, it was 50% (Table 12-3). This is significantly better than with the endodermal sinus tumor. Optimal therapy, though not yet established, is probably similar to that for endodermal sinus tumor. Progress can be monitored by following hCG and AFP levels.

Polyembryoma

Polyembryoma is a very rare ovarian germ cell neoplasm composed of numerous embryoid bodies resembling morphologically normal embryos. Similar homologous neoplasms occur more frequently in the human testes. To date only seven cases of ovarian polyembryoma have been reported in the literature. In most instances the polyembryoma has been associated with other neoplastic germ cell elements, mainly immature teratoma.

Polyembryoma is a highly malignant germ cell neoplasm, and in the majority of cases it has been associated with invasion of adjacent structures and organs and extensive metastases that are mainly confined to the abdominal cavity. The tumor is not sensitive to radiotherapy, and its response to chemotherapy is unknown.

Choriocarcinoma

Choriocarcinoma, a very rare, highly malignant tumor that may be associated with sexual precocity, can arise in one of three ways: (1) as a primary gestational choriocarcinoma associated with ovarian pregnancy, (2) as a metastatic choriocarcinoma from a primary gestational choriocarcinoma arising in other parts of the genital tract, mainly the uterus, and (3) as a germ cell tumor differentiating in the direction of trophoblastic structures and arising admixed with other neoplastic germ cell elements. Choriocarcinoma of the ovary may also be divided into two broad groups: gestational choriocarcinoma, encompassing the first two groups mentioned above, and nongestational choriocarcinoma, a germ cell tumor differentiating toward trophoblastic structures. Only nongestational choriocarcinoma of the ovary will be discussed here.

In the majority of cases the tumor is admixed with other neoplastic germ cell elements, and their presence is diagnostic of nongestational choriocarcinoma except for the remote possibility of the tumor being a gestational choriocarcinoma metastatic to an ovarian germ cell tumor. The tumor, in common with other malignant germ cell neoplasms, occurs in children and young adults. Its occurrence in children has been emphasized, and in some series 50% of cases occurred in children who had not yet reached puberty. This high incidence in children may result from the previous reluctance of investigators to make the diagnosis in adults.

These neoplasms secrete hCG. This is particularly noticeable in prepubertal children, who show evidence of isosexual precocious puberty with mammary development, growth of pubic and axillary hair, and uterine bleeding. Adult patients may present with signs of an ectopic pregnancy, because the nongestational choriocarcinoma, like its gestational counterpart, is associated with an increased production of hCG. Estimation of urinary or plasma hCG levels is a very useful diagnostic test in these cases. The prognosis of patients with choriocarcinoma is unfavorable, and the influence of modern chemotherapy regimens is unclear at this time. Unlike gestational choriocarcinoma, the treatment of which has been revolutionized by the discovery of its response to methotrexate and actinomycin D, nongestational choriocarcinoma is *not* exquisitely sensitive to these chemotherapeutic agents, although prolonged remissions have been achieved by Creasman and associates in four cases using the MAC combination chemotherapy. Some responses have been seen with combination chemotherapy using methotrexate as one of the drugs in the regimen. In most instances the other drugs used in the combinations have been actinomycin D and an alkylating agent.

Teratoma

Mature cystic teratoma. Accounting for over 95% of all ovarian teratomas, the dermoid cyst, or mature cystic teratoma, is one of the most common ovarian neoplasms. Teratomas themselves account for approximately 15% of all ovarian tumors. They are the most common ovarian tumors in women in the second and third decades of life. Fortunately, the overwhelming majority of benign cystic lesions contain mature tissue of ectodermal, mesodermal, and/or endodermal origin. The most common elements are ectodermal derivatives such as skin, hair follicles, and sebaceous or sweat glands, accounting for the characteristic histologic and gross appearance of teratomas (Fig. 12-5). These tumors are usually multicystic and contain visible hair intermixed with foul-smelling, sticky, keratinaceous and sebaceous debris. Occasionally, well-formed teeth are seen along with cartilage or bone. If the tumor is composed of only ectodermal derivatives of skin and skin appendages, it is a true dermoid cyst. A mix of other, usually mature tissues (gastrointestinal, respiratory) may be present.

The clinical manifestation of this slow-growing lesion is usually related to its size, compression, or torsion or to a chemical peritonitis secondary to intra-abdominal spillage of the cholesterol-laden debris. The latter event tends to occur more commonly when the tumor is large. Torsion is the most frequent complication, being observed in up to 16% of the cases in one large series, and it tends to be more common during pregnancy and the puerperium. Mature cystic teratomas are said to comprise from 22% to 40% of ovarian tumors in pregnancy, and from 0.8% to 12.8%

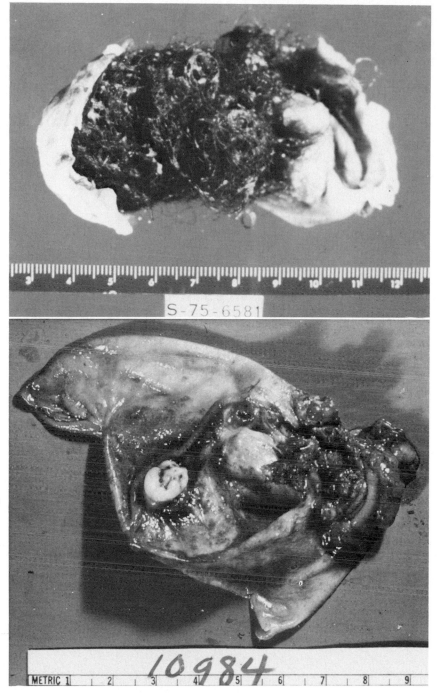

S-75-6581

10984

METRIC 1   2   3   4   5   6   7   8   9

Fig. 12-5. Benign cystic teratoma. **A** and **B**, Gross appearance.

Continued.

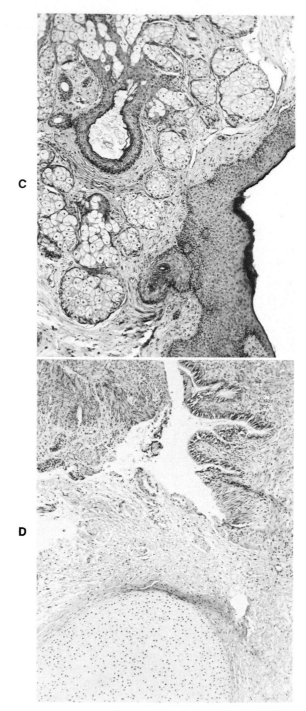

Fig. 12-5, cont'd. C, Microscopic view of ectodermal elements (skin and skin appendages). **D,** Microscopic view of another area with cartilage and respiratory epithelium.

of reported cases of mature cystic teratoma have occurred in pregnancy. In general, torsion is more common in children and younger patients. The patients usually present with severe acute abdominal pain, and the condition is considered an acute abdominal emergency. Rupture of a mature cystic teratoma is an uncommon complication, occurring in approximately 1% of cases, but it is much more common during pregnancy and may manifest itself during labor. The immediate result of rupture may be shock or hemorrhage, especially during pregnancy or labor, but the prognosis even in these cases is favorable. Rupture of the tumor into the peritoneal cavity may be followed by a chemical peritonitis caused by the spillage of the contents of the tumor. This may result in a marked granulomatous reaction and lead to the formation of dense adhesions throughout the peritoneal cavity. Infection is an uncommon complication of mature cystic teratoma and occurs in approximately 1% of cases. The infecting organism is usually a coliform, but *Salmonella* infection causing typhoid fever has also been reported. Removal of the neoplasm by oophorectomy or by ovarian cystectomy appears to be adequate therapy.

Mature solid teratoma. Mature solid teratoma is a very rare ovarian neoplasm and a very uncommon type of ovarian teratoma. The agents in it are similar to the agents in immature solid teratoma, which occurs mainly in children and young adults. The presence of immature elements immediately excludes the tumor from this group, and by definition only tumors composed entirely of mature tissues may be included. The tumor is usually unilateral and therefore adequately treated by unilateral oophorectomy. Although this neoplasm is considered benign, occasionally mature solid teratomas may be associated with peritoneal implants composed entirely of mature glial tissue, and in spite of the extensive involvement that may be present, the prognosis is excellent.

Immature teratoma. Immature teratomas are composed of tissue derived from the three germ layers—ectoderm, mesoderm, and endoderm—and, in contrast to the very much more common mature teratoma, they contain immature or embryonal structures. These tumors have had a variety of names: solid teratoma, malignant teratoma, teratoblastoma, teratocarcinoma, and embryonal teratoma. These names have arisen because immature teratomas have been incorrectly considered mixed germ cell tumors or secondary malignant tumors originating in mature benign teratomas. Mature tissues are frequently present and sometimes may predominate. Immature teratoma of the ovary is an uncommon tumor, comprising less than 1% of ovarian teratomas. In contrast to the mature cystic teratoma, which is encountered most frequently during the reproductive years but occurs at all ages, the immature teratoma has a very specific age incidence, occurring most commonly in the first 2 decades of life and being almost unknown after the menopause. Neural tissue is the most frequently found immature element and is usually represented by neuroepithelial tubules of varying degrees of differentiation, and according to Norris the quantity of immature neural tissue alone determines the grade. Neuroblastomatous elements, glial tissue, and immature cerebellar and cortical tissue may also be seen. These tumors are graded histologically on the basis of the amount and degree of cellular immaturity. The range is from grade 1 (mature teratoma containing only rare immature foci) through grade 3 (large portions of the tumor consist of embryonal tissue with atypicality and mitotic activity). Generally, older patients tend to have lower grade primary tumors than do younger patients. When the neoplasm is solid grossly and all elements are well differentiated histologically (solid mature teratoma), a grade 0 designation is given (Table 12-4).

Immature teratomas are virtually never bilateral, though occasionally a benign teratoma is found in the opposite ovary. These tumors commonly have multiple peritoneal implants at the time of initial surgery, and the prognosis is closely correlated with the histologic grade of the primary tumor and the implants. Norris and associates studied 58 patients with immature teratomas and reported an 82% survival rate for patients with grade 1 primary lesions, 63% for grade 2, and 30% for grade 3 (Table 12-5). Multiple sections of the primary lesion and wide sampling of the peritoneal implants are necessary to properly grade the tumor. In the majority of cases the implants are more well differentiated than the primary tumor. Both the primary lesion and the implants should be graded according to the most immature tissue present.

Since the lesion is rarely bilateral in its ovarian involvement, the present method of therapy consists of unilateral salpingo-oophorectomy with wide sampling of peritoneal implants. Total abdominal hysterectomy with bilateral salpingo-oophorectomy

Table 12-4. Immature teratoma—grading system

Grade	Criteria
0	All cells well differentiated
1	Cells well differentiated except in rare small foci of embryonal tissue
2	*Moderate* quantities of embryonal tissue present; cells are atypical and show mitotic activity
3	*Large* quantities of embryonal tissue present; cells are atypical and show mitotic activity

From Thurlbeck, W. M., and Scully, R. E.: Solid teratoma of the ovary; a clinicopathologic analysis of 9 cases, Cancer **13:**804, 1960.

Table 12-5. Immature (malignant) teratomas

Grade	n	Tumor deaths	Percent
1	22	4	(18)
2	24	9	(37)
3	10	7	(30)

From Norris, H. J., Zirkin, H. J., and Benson, W. L.: Immature (malignant) teratoma of the ovary; a clinical and pathologic study of 58 cases, Cancer **37:**2359, 1976.

does not seem to be indicated, since it does not influence the outcome for the patient. Radiotherapy has also been shown to be of little value. If the primary tumor is grade 1 and all peritoneal implants (if they exist) are grade 0, no further therapy is recommended. However, if the primary tumor is grade 2 or 3 or if implants or recurrences are grade 1, 2, or 3, triple-agent chemotherapy has recently been shown to be quite helpful. The VAC regimen has proved to be highly effective and is generally recommended at this time. Many have reported prolonged survival times in patients who have undergone such therapy. DiSaia and associates reported on three patients with disseminated disease treated with this chemotherapeutic regimen. At second-look laparotomy these three patients were free of immature elements but retained peritoneal implants containing exclusively mature elements. This was labeled chemotherapeutic retroconversion of immature teratoma of the ovary. All of these patients have had an uneventful follow-up, with the mature implants apparently remaining in a static state.

Experience with the treatment of 25 patients (mean age at diagnosis 19 years) with malignant teratoma of the ovary was reported by Curry and associates. Four patients received postoperative external radiation therapy to the pelvis and/or abdomen either alone or with a single chemotherapeutic agent, two were treated with postoperative single-agent chemotherapy, and two had no treatment other than surgical removal of the tumors. All of these eight patients died of their disease; the longest survival time was 40 months, and six of the eight patients survived less than 12 months after the initial treatment. Five patients received postoperative combination chemotherapy, either with a combination of methotrexate, actinomycin D, and cyclophosphamide or with a combination of actinomycin D, 5-fluorouracil, and cyclophosphamide. Two are surviving at 73 and 50 months after the initiation of chemotherapy. The combination of vincristine (1.5 mg/m^2), actinomycin D (0.5 mg), and cyclophosphamide (500 mg) was administered to 12 patients. The drugs were administered intravenously every week for 12 consecutive weeks, and then a 5-day intravenous course was given every 4 weeks for 2 years. At the time of their report, all of the ten patients who initially responded were surviving 16 to 28 months after the initiation of chemotherapy. Two of the 12 patients died at 3 and 26 months, respectively.

Monodermal or highly specialized teratomas

Struma ovarii. Another tumor thought to represent the one-sided development of benign teratoma is struma ovarii, which is composed totally or predominantly of thyroid parenchyma. This is an uncommon lesion and should not be confused with benign teratomas that contain small foci of thyroid tissue. Between 25% and 35% of patients with strumal tumors will have clinical hyperthyroidism. The gross and microscopic appearance of these lesions is similar to that of typical thyroid tissue, although the histologic pattern may resemble that in adenomatous thyroid. These ovarian tumors may undergo malignant transformation, but they are usually benign and easily treated by simple surgical resection.

Carcinoid tumors. Primary ovarian carcinoid tumors usually arise in association with gastrointestinal or respiratory epithelium present in mature cystic teratoma. They may also be observed within a solid teratoma or a mucinous tumor, or they may occur in an apparently pure form. Primary ovarian carcinoid tumors are uncommon. Approximately 50 cases have been reported. The age distribution of patients with ovarian carcinoid is similar to that of patients with mature cystic teratoma, although the average age may be somewhat higher in ovarian carcinoid. Many patients are postmenopausal.

One third of the reported cases have been associated with the typical carcinoid syndrome, in spite of the absence of metastasis. This is in contrast to intestinal carcinoids, which are associated with the syndrome only when there is metastatic spread to the liver. Excision of the tumor has been associated with the rapid remission of symptoms in all of the described cases and the disappearance of 5-hydroxyindoleacetic acid from the urine. The primary ovarian carcinoids are only occasionally associated with metastasis; metastasis was observed in only three out of 47 reported cases in one review. The prognosis after excision of the primary tumor is very favorable, and in the majority of cases a cure results.

Strumal carcinoid is an even rarer entity. It represents a close admixture of the previously discussed struma ovarii and carcinoid tumors and may actually represent medullary carcinoma arising in thyroid tissue. Most cases follow a benign course.

Gonadoblastoma

Gonadoblastoma is a rare ovarian lesion composed of germ cells resembling those of dysgerminoma and gonadal stromal cells resembling those of a granulosa or Sertoli tumor. Sex chromatin studies usually show a negative nuclear pattern (45XO) or a sex chromosome mosaicism (XO/XY). Patients who have a gonadoblastoma usually present with primary amenorrhea, virilization, or developmental abnormalities of the genitalia, and the discovery of gonadoblastoma is made in the course of investigation of these conditions. Another not infrequent presenting symptom is the presence of a gonadal tumor. The majority of patients with gonadoblastoma (80%) are phenotypic females, and the remainder are phenotypic males with cryptorchidism, hypospadias, and internal female secondary sex organs. Among the phenotypic females, 60% are virilized and the remainder are normal in appearance.

The prognosis of patients with gonadoblastoma is excellent provided the tumor and the contralateral gonad, which may be harboring a macroscopically undetectable gonadoblastoma, are excised. When gonadoblastoma is associated with or overgrown by dysgerminoma, the prognosis is still excellent. Metastases tend to occur later and more infrequently than in dysgerminoma arising de novo. Complete agreement has not been reached on whether the uterus should be excised together with the gonads. In the opinion of many, the uterus should be retained for psychologic reasons and exogenous estrogen therapy given for periodic bleeding.

TUMORS DERIVED FROM SPECIAL GONADAL STROMA
Classification

This category of ovarian tumors includes all those that contain granulosa cells, theca cells and luteinized derivatives, Sertoli cells, Leydig cells, and fibroblasts of gonadal stromal origin. Sex cord–stromal tumors as a group account for approximately 5% of all ovarian tumors, but functioning neoplastic groups of this variety comprise only 2%. Five to 10% of ovarian cancers belong in the sex cord–stromal group; most of these are granulosa cell tumors, which are a low grade of malignancy.

Granulosa-stromal cell tumors

Granulosa and theca cell tumors occur about as frequently in women in the reproductive age group as they do in women who are postmenopausal. Only about 5% of granulosa cell tumors occur before puberty (Table 12-6). Most granulosa and theca cells produce estrogen, but a few are androgenic. The exact proportion of these neoplasms that have function is really not known, because the endometrium is often not examined microscopically and appropriate laboratory tests are not done preoperatively. About 80% to 85% of granulosa cell and theca cell neoplasms are palpable on abdominal or pelvic examination, but occasionally an unsuspected tumor is found when a hysterectomy is done on a patient who has abnormal bleeding as a result of endometrial hyperplasia or endometrial carcinoma. A recent study by Evans and associates from the Mayo Clinic of 76 patients with granulosa cell tumor in whom endometrial tissue was available shows a high incidence of endometrial stimulation (Table 12-7).

Table 12-6. Granulosa cell tumors—age distribution of 118 cases

Age	Number
Child	3
12-40	27
41-50	28
51-60	32
61-79	28
	118

Data from Evans, A. J. III, Gaffey, T. A., Malkasian, G. D., Jr., and Annegers, J. T.: Clinicopathologic review of 118 granulosa and 82 theca cell tumors, Obstet. Gynecol. **55**(2):213, 1980.

Table 12-7. Granulosa cell tumor (76 patients)

Endometrial histology	Number	Percent
Proliferative endometrium	19	25
Atrophic endometrium	5	7
Hyperplastic endometrium	42	55
Adenocarcinoma	10	13

Data from Evans, A. J. III, Gaffey, T. A., Malkasian, G. D., Jr., and Annegers, J. T.: Clinicopathologic review of 118 granulosa and 82 theca cell tumors, Obstet. Gynecol. **55**(2):213, 1980.

Granulosa cell tumors vary greatly in gross appearance (Fig. 12-6). Sometimes they are solid tumors that feel soft or firm, depending on the relative amounts of neoplastic cells and fibrothecomatous stroma they contain, and are yellow or gray, depending on the amount of intracellular lipid in the lesion. More commonly, the granulosa cell tumor is predominantly cystic and, on external examination, may resemble mucinous cystadenoma or cystadenocarcinoma. However, when sectioned, this cyst is generally found to be filled with serous fluid or clotted blood. About 15% of patients who have granulosa cell tumors of the cystic variety are first examined for an acute or subacute abdomen associated with hemoperitoneum.

Thecomas are not quite as frequent as granulosa cell tumors but have a similar appearance. They are solid fibromatous lesions that show varying degrees of yellow or orange coloration. Whereas granulosa cell tumors are found to be bilateral in 2% to 5% of patients, thecomas are almost always confined to one ovary. On microscopic examination, most tumors in the granulosa-theca cell category are found to contain both cell types. If more than a very small component of granulosa cells is present, the term granulosa cell tumor, rather than granulosa-theca cell tumor, is generally applied. The designation theca cell tumor or thecoma should be reserved for neoplasms consisting entirely of theca cells that are benign.

Both
CellTypes

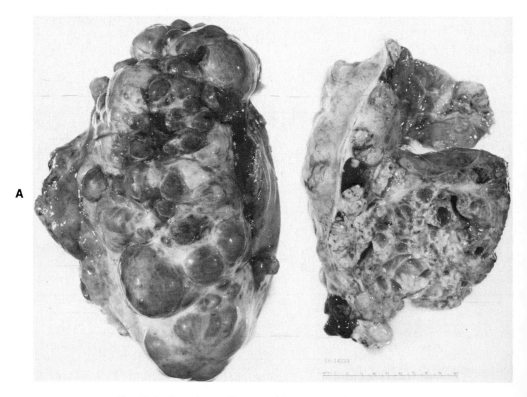

A

Fig. 12-6. Granulosa cell tumor of the ovary. **A,** Gross appearance.

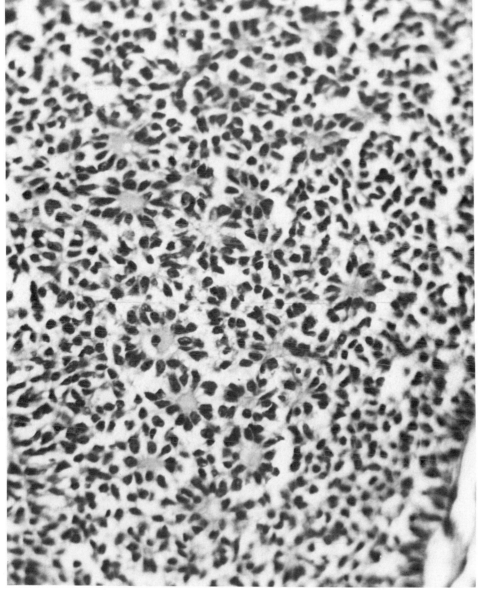

B

Fig. 12-6, cont'd. B, Microscopic appearance.

On the basis of their differentiation, granulosa cell tumors should be divided into two general categories: well differentiated and moderately differentiated. The former pattern may have various presentations, including microfollicular, macrofollicular, trabecular, solid-tubular, and watered-silk. Tumors in the moderately differentiated category have a diffuse pattern that has also been designated "sarcomatoid." Although attempts have been made by many authors, no distinct correlation between histologic structure and prognosis has yet been substantiated.

It is important that undifferentiated carcinomas, adenocarcinomas, and carcinoids, all of which may superficially resemble granulosa cell tumors, not be so misdiagnosed. Each of these tumors has a strikingly different prognosis. One characteristic feature is the appearance of the nuclei. Oval or angular, grooved nuclei are typical of granulosa cell tumors ("coffee bean appearance"). The Call-Exner bodies are also of diagnostic importance but unfortunately are not often sharply defined.

True granulosa tumors are low-grade malignancies, the great majority of which are confined to one ovary at the time of diagnosis. Only 5% to 10% of the stage I cases will subsequently recur, and they often appear more than 5 years after initial therapy. The prognosis for these patients is excellent, with long-term survival rates from 75% to 90% having been reported for all stages. These lesions are adequately managed during the reproductive years by removing the involved ovary and ipsilateral tube. The uterus and uninvolved adnexa should be removed in the perimenopausal and postmenopausal age groups, as is the practice with other benign or low malignant potential tumors. In a series from the Mayo Clinic, 92% of the patients had survived 5 to 10 years (76 patients, 82% of which had stage I lesions). The recurrence pattern in this same series (18.6% overall recurrence rate) revealed that 23% of the recurrences were more than 13 years after initial therapy. Most of the recurrences occurred in preserved genital tract structures. This is the kind of data that has prompted our recommendation that the preserved internal genitalia be removed in the perimenopausal patient in whom preservation may have been appropriate during the childbearing period.

Thecomas consist of neoplastic cells of ovarian stromal origin that have accumulated moderate to large amounts of lipid. Sometimes such tumors contain clusters of lutein cells, in which case the term luteinized thecoma is often used. Occasionally, tumors fall into a gray zone between thecomas and fibromas. Although the latter also arise from the ovarian stromal cell, they differentiate predominantly in the direction of collagen-producing fibroblasts. Tumors in the gray zone may be designated thecoma-fibroma. They are almost always unilateral and virtually never malignant. Several tumors have been reported as malignant thecomas in the literature, but at least some of these are better interpreted as fibrosarcomas or diffuse forms of granulosa cell tumors. In cases in which preservation of fertility is important, a thecoma may be treated adequately by unilateral oophorectomy. However, total hysterectomy with bilateral salpingo-oophorectomy is recommended in most postmenopausal and perimenopausal women.

Often, recurrent tumors have been effectively treated by means of reoperation, radiation therapy, chemotherapy, or a combination thereof. Although radiation therapy has been advocated for these tumors by many authors, careful search of the literature shows a paucity of evidence relating enhanced curability to the use of radiation therapy. There has never been a prospective study comparing one form of therapy with another for patients with advanced or recurrent disease. The question of adjuvant radiotherapy in the postmenopausal woman found to have granulosa cell tumor is often an issue. Our practice has been to recommend no further therapy in patients with stage I lesions. We have continued to use pelvic radiation in patients with stage II lesions. Stage III or recurrent granulosa cell tumor is probably best treated with systemic chemotherapy. Doxorubicin (Adriamycin) has proved to be an effective agent in this category of neoplasms; combination chemotherapy probably has a role (including doxorubicin), but sufficient evidence is wanting.

Sertoli-Leydig cell tumors

Sertoli-Leydig cell tumors contain Sertoli cells and/or Leydig cells in varying proportions and varying degrees of differentiation. Because less well differentiated neoplasms within this category may recapitulate the development of the testes, the terms androblastoma and arrhenoblastoma have been used as synonyms for Sertoli-Leydig cell tumors. However, their connotation of associated masculinization is misleading, because some of these tumors have no endocrine manifestation and others

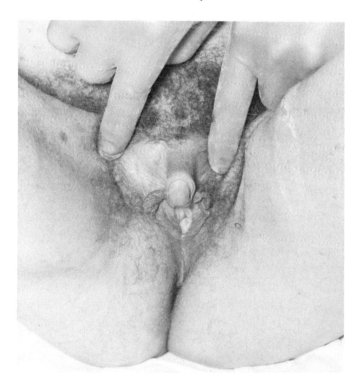

Fig. 12-7. Enlarged clitoris in a patient with a Sertoli-Leydig cell tumor (arrhenoblastoma).

may even be accompanied by an estrogenic syndrome. Nevertheless, the World Health Organization has selected androblastoma as an alternate term for Sertoli-Leydig cell tumor. These neoplasms account for less than 0.5% of all ovarian tumors but are among the most fascinating from both pathologic and clinical viewpoints. They occur in all age groups but are most often encountered in young women, who usually become virilized (Fig. 12-7). In some cases, the Sertoli cells may produce estrogenic hormones, as they do in feminizing canine testicular Sertoli cell tumors. In other instances, such tumors are found to be made up predominantly or exclusively of Leydig cells that either secrete estrogens directly or produce androgens that are converted to estrogens in extraovarian tissues. Thus, one can see the multifaceted clinical presentation of this fascinating neoplasm. Classically, there is progressive masculinization that is heralded by hirsutism, temporal balding, deepening of the voice, and enlargement of the clitoris.

Sertoli-Leydig cell tumors with heterologous elements may contain a variety of unusual cell types, but the degree of differentiation of the tumor is probably of greater importance than its content of unexpected tissue in determining its prognosis. The overall 5-year survival rate of patients with Sertoli-Leydig cell tumors has been reported to be in the range of slightly over 70% to slightly over 90%. Because these tumors occur predominantly in young women and are bilateral in fewer than 5% of the cases, conservative removal of the tumor and adjacent fallopian tube is justifiable if preservation of fertility is an important consideration and there is no evidence of extension beyond the involved ovary. Like granulosa cell tumors, they are considered to have low malignant potential.

Gynandroblastoma

Rarely, a gonadostromal tumor contains unequivocal granulosa cell elements combined with tubules and Leydig cells characteristic of an arrhenoblastoma. Designated as gynandroblastomas, these mixed tumors may be associated with either androgen or estrogen production, and they can be expected to behave as low-grade malignancies similar to the individual components.

Lipid cell neoplasms

Lipid cell neoplasms are a heterologous group of tumors that have in common a parenchyma composed of polygonal cells containing lipid. They include neoplasms that have been designated as either hilus cell tumors, Leydig tumors, adrenal rest tumors, stromal luteomas, or masculinovoblastomas. Leydig cell tumors are unilateral and are commonly found in the medulla or hilus region of the ovary. Tumors that have spread to contiguous organs or have a microscopic cellular pleomorphism with high mitotic activity should be considered malignant. Reinke's crystals, normally occurring in mature Leydig cells of the testes, are often found in these neoplasms, and their presence may be interpreted as signifying a benign lesion. Regardless of the presence or absence of Reinke's crystals, neoplasms smaller than 8 cm in diameter can be expected to act in a benign fashion.

TUMORS DERIVED FROM NONSPECIFIC MESENCHYME

Benign and malignant tumors, including fibromas, hemangiomas, leiomyomas, soft-tissue sarcomas, lymphomas, and rare neoplasms, may arise in the ovary from nonspecific supporting tissues that are common to most organs. The most common and most important tumors in this category are the fibroma and the lymphoma.

The mixed mesodermal sarcoma of the ovary (analogous to its uterine counterpart) has been more widely recognized in the last decade. It is an extremely rare neoplasm but one that is invariably fatal. A recent review by Hernandez and associates suggested that 50% of the patients present with stage III tumors, and the patients are most commonly diagnosed in the sixth decade of life. Various forms of combination chemotherapy, including a vigorous regimen with the VAC combination, have been advocated with mixed results.

METASTATIC TUMORS TO THE OVARY

Roughly 6% of ovarian cancers encountered by a surgeon exploring a pelvic or abdominal mass are metastases, most often either metastatic breast tumors or metastatic adenocarcinoma of large intestinal origin. Metastases from carcinomas of the breast are among the more common surgical specimens of the ovary, especially if one includes those found incidentally. They are almost always incidental findings in therapeutic oophorectomy and rarely form symptomatic masses that require surgical removal. The term Krukenberg tumor should be reserved for those metastases that contain significant numbers of signet-ring cells in a cellular stroma derived from the ovarian stroma. This restriction is important because tumors with those microscopic characteristics also have distinctive gross pathologic and clinical features. Almost all have metastasized from the stomach, but some have arisen in the breast, intestine, or other mucus gland–containing organs. Krukenberg tumor forms a solid, often uniform mass, the sectioned surface of which typically exhibits gelatinous necrosis and hemorrhage.

Metastatic adenocarcinomas of large intestinal origin have been more common than Krukenberg tumors in the past 2 decades with the gradual decline in the incidence of carcinoma of the stomach. These lesions are characterized microscopically by the presence of large acini similar to those of primary intestinal carcinomas. Grossly, they may form solid metastases but more often appear as large, partly cystic tumors with areas of hemorrhage and necrosis (Fig. 12-8). In such instances they are easily confused with cystic forms of primary ovarian cancers.

The ovary is a fairly frequent site of metastasis from certain primary carcinomas. Approximately 10% of ovarian tumors are not primary in origin. The most common metastasis is in the form of a carcinoma arising in the endometrium. There is no doubt that cancer of the endometrium metastasizes to the ovaries, but difficulty may be encountered in distinguishing metastasis of an endometrial cancer from a separate ovarian tumor. This is particularly true in the case of ovarian endometrioid carcinoma, which according to Scully is associated with a similar tumor in the endometrium in one third of cases.

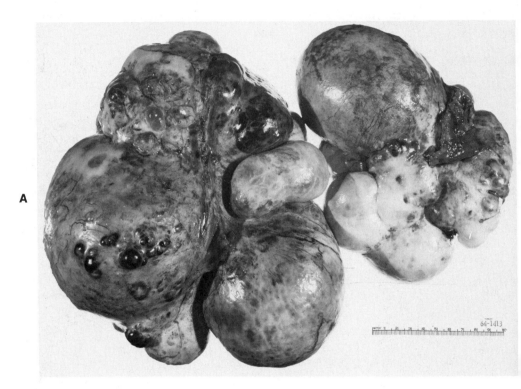

Fig. 12-8. Metastatic tumor to ovary from adenocarcinoma of the colon. **A,** Gross appearance.

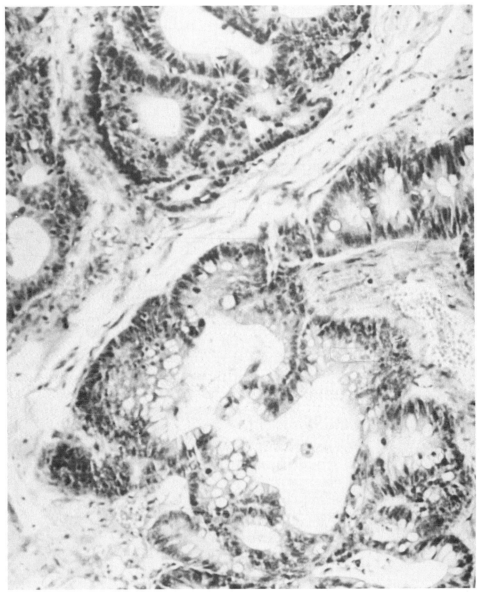

Fig. 12-8, cont'd. B, Histologic appearance. Note large acini similar to those of intestinal carcinoma.

There are four possible pathways of spread of tumors to the ovary: (1) direct continuity, (2) surface papillation, (3) lymphatic metastasis, and (4) hematogenous spread. Lymphatic metastasis is undoubtedly the most common pathway for spread to the ovary. The rich network of lymph nodes and lymphatic channels in the pelvis readily explains the metastatic pathway of tumors in the uterus and contralateral ovary. The rare finding of clusters of tumor cells limited to lymphatics in the medulla of the ovary in cases of breast carcinoma confirm that this is the pathway of spread to the ovary. As yet, no one has convincingly described the pathway of metastasis to the ovaries from cancer of the stomach. It is known that the lymphatic channels that drain the upper gastrointestinal tract ultimately link up with the lumbar chain of lymph nodes. Ovarian lymphatics drain into the lumbar glands. This could well be the route of spread to the ovaries in these cases.

There have been cases of metastatic ovarian carcinoma in which there was a clinical presentation consistent with hormonal activity. Both androgen and estrogen excretion have been described. Endometrial hyperplasia has been described in post-menopausal patients with metastatic ovarian carcinoma, presumably indicating estrogen activity within the metastatic lesion or its normal tissue capsule.

MALIGNANT OVARIAN TUMORS IN CHILDREN

Ovarian tumors, cysts, and torsion are more frequent indications for surgical intervention in infancy and childhood than is commonly realized. The symptoms they produce may be the same as those of appendicitis, and it is not always appreciated how often they mimic this condition. The proportion of all tumors of the abdomen in this age group that are ovarian in origin has not been reported. Pain is the most frequently reported symptom. A palpable abdominal mass is found in half of the patients with a neoplasm. Roughly 10% of the patients present with isosexual precocity, which includes patients who demonstrate precocious puberty as well as those with an early onset of sexual development. The initial signs are areolar pigmentation and breast development. Some patients have vaginal discharge or bleeding, and others have the appearance of pubic hair. These changes usually completely regress after surgical extirpation of the responsible endocrine-secreting tumor. Granulosa-theca cell tumors are by far the most common ovarian neoplasms found in these patients with isosexual precocity and adnexal enlargement.

Most ovarian cancers in children are of germ cell origin. Cangir and associates reported on 21 girls under the age of 16, with a median age of 13.5. Of the 21 patients, 8 had malignant teratomas, 6 had mixed germinal tumors, 6 had endodermal sinus tumors, and 1 had a stromal cell tumor (Sertoli-Leydig type). There were 8 stage I, 1 stage II, 7 stage III, and 5 stage IV patients.

Fortunately the most common germ cell neoplasm is the benign teratoma. A significant number of additional patients are found to have benign functional cysts of the ovary. All patients are treated in a manner similar to the adolescent or older patient in the early reproductive age period.

BIBLIOGRAPHY

Abell, M. R., and Holtz, F.: Ovarian neoplasms in childhood and adolescence. II. Tumors of non-germ cell origin, Am. J. Obstet. Gynecol. **93**:850, 1965.

Abell, M. R., Johnson, V. J., and Holtz, F.: Ovarian neoplasms in childhood and adolescence. I. Tumors of germ cell origin, Am. J. Obstet. Gynecol. **92**:1059, 1965.

Acosta, A., Kaplan, A. L., and Kaufman, R. H.: Gynecologic cancer in children, Am. J. Obstet. Gynecol. **112**:944, 1972.

Albites, V.: Solid teratoma of the ovary with malignant gliomatosis peritonei, Int. J. Gynaecol. Obstet. **12**:59, 1974.

Anderson, W. R., Levine, A. J., and MacMillan, D.: Granulosa-theca cell tumors; clinical and pathologic study, Am. J. Obstet. Gynecol. **110**:32, 1971.

Arias-Bernal, L., and Jones, H. W.: Chromosomes of a malignant ovarian teratoma, Am. J. Obstet. Gynecol. **100**:785, 1968.

Asadourian, L. A., and Taylor, H. B.: Dysgerminoma; an analysis of 105 cases, Obstet. Gynecol. **33**:370, 1969.

Ashley, D. J. B.: Origin of teratomas, Cancer **32**:390, 1973.

Azoury, R. S., and Woodruff, J. D.: Primary ovarian sarcomas; report of 43 cases from the Emil Novak Ovarian Tumor Registry, Obstet. Gynecol. **37**:920, 1971.

Barber, H. R. K., and Graber, E. A.: Gynecological tumors in childhood and adolescence, Obstet. Gynecol. Surv. **28**:357, 1973.

Blackwell, W. J., Dockerty, M. B., Masson, J. C., and Mussey, R. D.: Dermoid cysts of the ovary, their clinical and pathologic significance, Am. J. Obstet. Gynecol. **51**:151, 1946.

Boczkowski, K., Teter, J., and Sternadel, Z.: Sibship occurrence of XY gonadal dysgenesis with dysgerminoma, Am. J. Obstet. Gynecol. **113**:952, 1972.

Boivin, Y., and Richart, R. M.: Hilus cell tumors of the ovary; a review with a report of 3 new cases, Cancer **18**:231, 1965.

Braun, P. A., and Richart, R.M.: Functioning ovarian carcinoid tumors, Obstet. Gynecol. **24**:390, 1969.

Breen, J. L., and Neubecker, R. D.: Ovarian malignancy in children with special reference to the germ cell tumors, Ann. N.Y. Acad. Sci. **142**:208, 1962.

Breen, J. L., and Neubecker, R. D.: Malignant teratoma of the ovary; an analysis of 17 cases, Obstet. Gynecol. **21**:669, 1963.

Brody, S.: Clinical aspects of dysgerminoma of the ovary, Acta Radiol. **56**:209, 1961.

Cangir, A., Smith, J., and van Eys, J.: Improved prognosis in children with ovarian cancers following modified VAC (vincristine sulfate, dactinomycin, and cyclophosphamide) chemotherapy, Cancer **42**:1234, 1978.

Carlson, D. H., and Griscom, N. T.: Ovarian cysts in the newborn, Am. J. Roentgenol. **116**:664, 1972.

Chalvardjian, A., and Scully, R. E.: Sclerosing stromal tumors of the ovary, Cancer **31**:664, 1973.

Chan, L. K. C., and Prathap, K.: Virilization in pregnancy associated with an ovarian mucinous cystadenoma, Am. J. Obstet. Gynecol. **108**:946, 1970.

Chatterjee, K., and Heather, J. C.: Carcinoid heart disease from primary ovarian carcinoid tumors; a case report and a review of the literature, Am. J. Med. **45**:643, 1968.

Chung, A., and Birnbaum, S. J.: Ovarian cancer associated with pregnancy, Obstet. Gynecol. **41**:211, 1973.

Climie, A. R. W., and Heath, L. P.: Malignant degeneration of benign cystic teratomas of the ovary, Cancer **22**:824, 1968.

Creasman, W. T., Fetter, B. F., Hammond, C. B., and Parker, R. T.: Germ cell malignancies of the ovary, Obstet. Gynecol. **53**:226, 1979.

Creasman, W. T., Rutledge, F. N., and Smith, J. P.: Carcinoma of the ovary associated with pregnancy, Obstet. Gynecol. **38**:111, 1971.

Curry, S. L., Smith, J. P., and Gallagher, H. S.: Malignant teratoma of the ovary; prognostic factors and treatment, Am. J. Obstet. Gynecol. **131**:845, 1978.

Dehner, L. P., Norris, H. J., and Taylor, H. B.: Carcinosarcomas and mixed mesodermal tumors of the ovary, Cancer **27**:207, 1971.

Dinnerstein, A. J., and O'Leary, J. A.: Granulosa-theca cell tumors; a clinical review of 102 patients, Obstet. Gynecol. **31**:654, 1968.

Einhorn, L. H., and Donohue, J.: Cis-diammine-dichloroplatinum, vinblastine, and bleomycin combination chemotherapy in disseminated testicular cancer, Ann. Intern. Med. **87**:293, 1977.

Emig, O. R., Hertig, A. T., and Rowe, F. J.: Gynadroblastoma of the ovary; review and report of a case, Obstet. Gynecol. **13**:135, 1959.

Evans, A. J. III, Gaffey, T. A., Malkasian, G. D., Jr., and Annegers, J. T.: Clinicopathologic review of 118 granulosa and 82 theca cell tumors, Obstet. Gynecol. **55**(2): 213, 1980.

Favara, B. E., and Franciosi, R. A.: Ovarian teratoma and neuroglial implants on the peritoneum, Cancer **31**:678, 1973.

Felmus, L. B., and Pedowitz, P.: Clinical malignancy of endocrine tumors of the ovary and dysgerminoma, Obstet. Gynecol. **29**:344, 1967.

Ferenczy, A., Okagaki, T., and Richart, R. M.: Para-endocrine hypercalcemia in ovarian neoplasms; report of mesonephroma with hypercalcemia and review of literature, Cancer **27**:427, 1971.

Forney, J. P., DiSaia, P. J., and Morrow, C. P.: Endodermal sinus tumor; a report of two sustained remissions treated postoperatively with a combination of actinomycin D, 5-fluorouracil and cyclophosphamide, Obstet. Gynecol. **45**:186, 1975.

Fox, L. P., and Stamm, W. J.: Krukenberg tumor complicating pregnancy; report of a case with androgenic activity, Am. J. Obstet. Gynecol. **92**:702, 1965.

Freel, J. H., Cassir, J. F., Pierce, V. K., and others: Dysgerminoma of the ovary, Cancer **43**:798, 1979.

Genadry, R., Parmley, T., and Woodruff, J. D.: Case report—secondary malignancies in benign cystic teratomas, Gynecol. Oncol. **8**:246, 1979.

Gillibrand, P. N.: Granulosa-theca cell tumors of the ovary associated with pregnancy; case report and review of the literature, Am. J. Obstet. Gynecol. **94**:1108, 1966.

Goldstein, D. P., and Lamb, E. J.: Arrhenoblastoma in first cousins; report of 2 cases, Obstet. Gynecol. **35**:444, 1970.

Goldstein, D. P., and Piro, J. A.: Combination chemotherapy in the treatment of germ cell tumors containing choriocarcinoma, Surg. Gynecol. Obstet. **134**:61, 1972.

Goldston, W. R., Johnston, W. W., Fetter, B. F., and others: Clinicopathologic studies in feminizing tumors of the ovary, Am. J. Obstet. Gynecol. **112**:442, 1972.

Goldston, W. R., Wilbanks, G. D., and Campbell, J. A.: A granulosa cell tumor in tissue culture, Am. J. Obstet. Gynecol. **114**:652, 1972.

Gompel, C., and Silverberg, S. G.: Pathology in gynecology and obstetrics, Philadelphia, 1977, J. B. Lippincott Co.

Greenblatt, R. B., Mahesh, V. B., and Gambrell, R. D.: Arrhenoblastoma; three case reports, Obstet. Gynecol. **39**:567, 1972.

Greene, R. R.: Feminizing tumors of the ovary and carcinoma of the endometrium, Obstet. Gynecol. Annu. **10**:393, 1973.

Groeber, W. R.: Ovarian tumors during infancy and childhood, Am. J. Obstet. Gynecol. **86**:1027, 1963.

Gusberg, S. B., and Kardon, P.: Proliferative endometrial response to theca-granulosa cell tumors, Am. J. Obstet. Gynecol. **111**:633, 1971.

Hale, R. W.: Krukenberg tumor of the ovaries; a review of 81 records, Obstet. Gynecol. **22**:221, 1968.

Hart, W. R., and Burkons, D. M.: Germ cell neoplasms arising in gonadoblastomas, Cancer **43**:669, 1979.

Hay, D. M., and Stewart, D. B.: Primary ovarian choriocarcinoma, J. Obstet. Gynaecol. Br. Comm. **76**:941, 1969.

Hernandez, W., DiSaia, P., Morrow, C., and Townsend, D.: Mixed mesodermal sarcoma of the ovary, Obstet. Gynecol. **49**:59, 1977.

Huntington, R. W., and Bullock, W. K.: Yolk sac tumors of the ovary, Cancer **25**:1357, 1970.

Joshi, V. V.: Primary Krukenberg tumor of ovary; review of literature and case report, Cancer **22**:1199, 1968.

Judd, H. L., Benirschke, K., DeVane, G., and others: Maternal virilization developing during a twin pregnancy; demonstration of excess ovarian androgen production associated with theca-lutein cysts, N. Engl. J. Med. **288**:118, 1973.

Kase, N.: Steroid synthesis in abnormal ovaries. II. Granulosa cell tumor, Am. J. Obstet. Gynecol. **90**:1262, 1964.

Kase, N., and Conrad, S.: Steroid synthesis in abnormal ovaries. I. Arrhenoblastoma, Am. J. Obstet. Gynecol. **90**:1251, 1964.

Kelley, R. R., and Scully, R. E.: Cancer developing in dermoid cysts of the ovary, Cancer **14**:989, 1961.

Kempers, R. D., Dockerty, M. B., Hoffman, D. L., and others: Struma ovarii-ascitic, hyperthyroid and asymptomatic syndromes, Ann. Intern. Med. **72**:883, 1970.

Koller, O., and Gjonnaess, H.: Dysgerminoma of the ovary; a clinical report of 20 cases, Acta Obstet. Gynecol. Scand. **43**:268, 1964.

Kosloske, A. M., Favara, B. E., Hays, T., and others: Management of immature teratoma of the ovary in children by conservative resection and chemotherapy, J. Pediatr. Surg. **11**:839, 1976.

Krumerman, M. S., and Chung, A.: Squamous carcinoma arising in benign cystic teratoma of the ovary, Cancer **29**:1237, 1977.

Kurman, R. J., and Norris, H. J.: Endodermal sinus tumor of the ovary; a clinical and pathological analysis of 71 cases, Cancer **38**:2404, 1976.

Kurman, R. J., and Norris, H. J.: Malignant mixed germ cell tumors of the ovary; a clinical and pathological analysis of 30 cases, Obstet. Gynecol. **48**:579, 1976.

Kurman, R. J., and Norris, H. J.: Malignant germ cell tumors of the ovary, Hum. Pathol. **8**:551, 1977.

Luisi, A.: Metastatic ovarian tumors. In Gentil, F., and Junqueira, A. C., editors: Ovarian cancer, New York, 1968, Springer-Verlag New York, Inc.

Lyon, F. A., Sinykin, M. B., and McKelvey, J. L.: Granulosa-cell tumors of the ovary; review of 23 cases, Obstet. Gynecol. **21**:67, 1963.

Malkasian, G. D., Jr., Dockerty, M. B., and Symmonds, R. E.: Benign cystic teratomas, Obstet. Gynecol. **29**:719, 1967.

Malkasian, G. D., Jr., and Symmonds, R. E.: Treatment of the unilateral encapsulated ovarian dysgerminoma, Am. J. Obstet. Gynecol. **90**:379, 1964.

Marshall, J. R.: Ovarian enlargements in the first year of life; review of 45 cases, Ann. Surg. **161**:372, 1965.

Moore, J. G., Schifrin, B. S., and Erez, S.: Ovarian tumors in infancy, childhood and adolescence, Am. J. Obstet. Gynecol. **99**:913, 1967.

Neubecker, R. D., and Breen, J. L.: Embryonal carcinoma of the ovary, Cancer **15**:546, 1962.

Neubecker, R. D., and Breen, J. L.: Gynandroblastoma; a report of five cases, with a discussion of the histogenesis and classification of ovarian tumors, Am. J. Clin. Pathol. **38**:60, 1962.

Nogales, F. F., Jr., Favara, B. E., Major, F. J., and others: Immature teratoma of the ovary with a neural component ("solid" teratoma); a clinicopathologic study of 20 cases, Hum. Pathol. **7**:625, 1976.

Nogales-Fernandez, F., Silverberg, S. G., Bloustein, P. A., and others: Yolk sac carcinoma (endodermal sinus tumor); ultrastructure and histogenesis of gonadal and extragonadal tumors in comparison with normal human yolk sac, Cancer **39**:1462, 1977.

Norris, H. J., and Jensen, R. D.: Relative frequency of ovarian neoplasms in children and adolescents, Cancer **39**:713, 1972.

Norris, H. J., and Taylor, H. B.: Prognosis of granulosa-theca tumors of the ovary, Cancer **21**:255, 1968.

Norris, H. J., and Taylor, H. B.: Virilization associated with cystic granulosa tumors, Obstet. Gynecol. **34**:629, 1969.

Norris, H. J., Zirkin, H. J., and Benson, W. L.: Immature (malignant) teratoma of the ovary; a clinical and pathologic study of 58 cases, Cancer **37**:2359, 1976.

Novak, E. R., Kutchmeshgi, J., Mupas, R. S., and Woodruff, J. D.: Feminizing gonadal stromal tumors; analysis of the granulosa-theca cell tumors of the Ovarian Tumor Registry, Obstet. Gynecol. **38**:701, 1971.

Novak, E. R., and Long, J. H.: Arrhenoblastoma of the ovary; a review of the ovarian tumor registry, Am. J. Obstet. Gynecol. **92**:1082, 1965.

Novak, E. R., and Mattingly, R. F.: Hilus cell tumor of the ovary, Obstet. Gynecol. **15**:425, 1960.

O'Hern, T. M., and Neubecker, R. D.: Arrhenoblastoma, Obstet. Gynecol. **19**:758, 1962.

Pedowitz, P., and O'Brien, F. B.: Arrhenoblastoma of the ovary; review of the literature and report of 2 cases, Obstet. Gynecol. **16**:62, 1960.

Peterson, W. F.: Malignant degeneration of benign cystic teratomas of the ovary; a collective review of the literature, Obstet. Gynecol. Surv. **12**:793, 1957.

Peterson, W. F., Prevost, E. C., Edmunds, F. T., and others: Benign cystic teratomas of the ovary; a clinico-statistical study of 1,007 cases with a review of the literature, Am. J. Obstet. Gynecol. **70**:568, 1955.

Qizilbach, A. H., Trebilcock, R. G., Patterson, M. C., and others: Functioning primary carcinoid tumor of the ovary, Am. J. Clin. Pathol. **62**:629, 1974.

Robboy, S. J., Norris, H. J., and Scully, R. E.: Insular carcinoid primary in the ovary, Cancer **36**:404, 1975.

Robboy, S. J., and Scully, R. E.: Ovarian teratoma with glial implants on the peritoneum; an analysis of 12 cases, Hum. Pathol. **1**:643, 1970.

Robboy, S. J., Scully, R. E., and Norris, H. J.: Carcinoid metastatic to the ovary; a clinicopathologic analysis of 35 cases, Cancer **33**:798, 1974.

Robboy, S. J., Scully, R. E., and Norris, H. J.: Primary trabecular carcinoid of the ovary, Obstet. Gynecol. **49**:202, 1977.

Rosenshein, N. B., Grumbine, F. C., Woodruff, J. D., and Ettinger, D. S.: Pregnancy following chemotherapy for an ovarian immature embryonal teratoma, Gynecol. Oncol. **8**:234, 1979.

Roth, L. M., and Panganiban, W. G.: Gonadal and extragonadal yolk sac carcinomas; a clinicopathologic study of 14 cases, Cancer **37**:812, 1976.

Santesson, L., and Marrubini, G.: Clinical and pathological survey of ovarian embryonal carcinomas, including so-called "mesonephromas" (Schiller) or "mesoblastomas" (Teilum), treated at the Radiumhemmet, Acta Obstet. Gynecol. Scand. **36**:399, 1957.

Schellhas, H. F., Trujillo, J. M., Rutledge, F. N., and Cork, A.: Germ cell tumors associated with XY gonadal dysgenesis, Am. J. Obstet. Gynecol. **109**:1197, 1971.

Schuster, M., Mendoza-Divino, E., and Joselson,

H.: Carcinoid tumor metastasizing to the ovaries, Obstet. Gynecol. **36:**515, 1970.

Scully, R. E.: Gonadoblastoma; a gonadal tumor related to the dysgerminoma (seminoma) and capable of sex hormone production, Cancer **6:**455, 1953.

Scully, R. E.: Gonadoblastoma; a review of 74 cases, Cancer **25:**1340, 1970.

Scully, R. E.: Ovarian tumors of germ cell origin. In Sturgis, S. H., and Taymor, M. L., editors: Progress in gynecology, ed. 5, New York, 1970, Grune & Stratton, Inc.

Scully, R. E.: Recent progress in ovarian cancer, Hum. Pathol. **1:**73, 1970.

Scully, R. E.: Ovarian tumors; a review, Am. J. Pathol. **87:**686, 1977.

Simmons, R. L., and Sciarra, J. J.: Treatment of late recurrent granulosa cell tumors of the ovary, Surg, Gynecol. Obstet. **124:**65, 1967.

Sjostedt, S., and Wahlen, T.: Prognosis of granulosa cell tumors, Acta Obstet. Gynecol. Scand. **40** (Suppl. 6):1, 1961.

Slayton, R. E., Hreshchyshyn, M. M., Silverberg, S. C., and others: Treatment of malignant ovarian germ cell tumors; response to vincristine, dactinomycin, and cyclophosphamide (preliminary report), Cancer **42:**390, 1978.

Smith, J. P., Rutledge, F., and Sutow, W. W.: Malignant gynecologic tumors in children; current approaches to treatment, Am. J. Obstet. Gynecol. **116:**261, 1973.

Spadoni, L. R., Lindberg, M. C., Mottet, N. K., and Herrman, W. L.: Virilization coexisting with Krukenberg tumor during pregnancy, Am. J. Obstet. Gynecol. **92:**981, 1965.

Stenwig, J. T., Hazekamp, J., and Beecham, J.: Granulosa cell tumors of the ovary; a clinicopathological study of 118 cases with long term follow-up, Gynecol. Oncol. **7:**136, 1979.

Talerman, A., Haije, W. G., and Baggerman, L.: Serum alpha fetoprotein (AFP) in the diagnosis and management of endodermal sinus (yolk sac) tumor and mixed germ cell tumor of the ovary, Cancer **41:**272, 1978.

Teilum, G.: Classification of testicular and ovarian androblastoma and Sertoli cell tumors, Cancer **11:**769, 1958.

Teilum, G.: Endodermal sinus tumors of the ovary and testes; comparative morphogenesis of the so-called mesonephroma ovarii (Schiller) and extraembryonic (yolk sac allantoic) structure of the rat placenta, Cancer **12:**1029, 1959.

Teilum, G.: Classification of endodermal sinus tumor (mesoblastoma vitellinum) and so-called "embryonal carcinoma" of the ovary, Acta Pathol. Microbiol. Scand. **64:**407, 1965.

Teilum, G.: Tumors of germinal origin. In Gentil, F., and Junqueira, A. C., editors: Ovarian cancer, New York, 1968, Springer-Verlag New York, Inc.

Teter, J.: Prognosis, malignancy, and curability of the germ-cell tumor occurring in dysgenetic gonads, Am. J. Obstet. Gynecol. **108:**894, 1970.

Thurlbeck, W. M., and Scully, R. E.: Solid teratoma of the ovary; a clinicopathologic analysis of 9 cases, Cancer **13:**804, 1960.

Turner, H. B., Douglas, W. M., and Gladding, T. C.: Choriocarcinoma of the ovary, Obstet. Gynecol. **24:**918, 1964.

Ungerleider, R. S., Donaldson, S. S., Warnke, R. A., and Wilbur, J. R.: Endodermal sinus tumor; the Stanford experience and the first reported case arising in the vulva, Cancer **41:**1627, 1978.

Wider, J. A., Marshall, J. R., Bardin, C. W., and others: Sustained remissions after chemotherapy for primary ovarian cancers containing choriocarcinoma, N. Engl. J. Med. **280:**1439, 1969.

Wisniewski, M., and Deppisch, L. M.: Solid teratomas of the ovary, Cancer **32:**440, 1973.

Woodruff, J. D., Murthy, Y. S., Bhaskar, T. N., and others: Metastatic ovarian tumors, Am. J. Obstet. Gynecol. **107:**202, 1970.

Woodruff, J. D., Noli Castillo, R. D., and Novak, E. R.: Lymphoma of the ovary; a study of 35 cases from the Ovarian Tumor Registry of the American Gynecological Society, Am. J. Obstet. Gynecol. **85:**912, 1963.

Woodruff, J. D., and Novak, E. R.: The Krukenberg tumor; a study of 48 cases from the Ovarian Tumor Registry, Obstet. Gynecol. **15:**351, 1960.

Woodruff, J. D., Protos, P., and Peterson, W. F.: Ovarian teratomas, Am. J. Obstet. Gynecol. **102:**702, 1968.

Woodruff, J. D., Rauh, J. T., and Markley, R. L.: Ovarian struma, Obstet. Gynecol. **27:**194, 1966.

CHAPTER THIRTEEN

Carcinoma of the fallopian tube

Signs and symptoms
Diagnosis
Therapy
Prognosis
Sarcomas

Adenocarcinoma of the fallopian tube is one of the rarest malignancies of the female genital tract. Its frequency in relationship to all gynecologic cancers is usually considered to be in the range of 1% or less. Approximately 950 cases of fallopian tube carcinoma have been reported, mostly in small series and, in many instances, single case reports. Therefore, the experience of any one physician (even at a large cancer referral institution) is rather limited. As a result, it is not at all surprising that the diagnosis is infrequently made preoperatively. In many instances, this lesion presents as an unexpected operative finding, and cases have been reported in individuals who were undergoing tubal sterilization. There does appear to be an associated increase of tubal infections with this malignancy, and in many instances, pelvic inflammatory disease is the preoperative diagnosis.

RARE
1%

usually found at Surgery

SIGNS AND SYMPTOMS

Most patients with this malignancy will present with symptoms such as vaginal bleeding or discharge, lower abdominal pain, abdominal distention, and pressure. In many instances, these are vague and nonspecific. Vaginal bleeding is the most common symptom of tubal carcinoma and is present in over 50% of the patients. Since this lesion occurs most frequently in the postmenopausal patient, postmenopausal bleeding is common, and as a result, carcinoma of the endometrium is the first consideration in the differential diagnosis. One must seriously consider the diagnosis of fallopian tube carcinoma when the D&C is negative and symptoms persist. Vaginal bleeding is caused by blood that has accumulated from the lesion in the

Discharge
Bleeding ✱ → Most common
Pain
Swelling

351

TRIAD ① PAIN
② Bleeding
③ LEUKORRHEA

fallopian tube, subsequently passes into the uterine cavity, and finally exits into the vagina. Pain is a very frequent symptom in tubal carcinoma, is usually colicky in nature, and often accompanies the vaginal bleeding. The pain is caused by distention of the tubal wall and stimulation of peristaltic activity. This pain, in many instances, is relieved with the passage of blood or watery discharge. Vaginal discharge, which is usually clear, is a common finding in tubal carcinoma.

Pain combined with a profuse, watery vaginal discharge is referred to as hydrops tubae profluens. Although the triad of pain, menorrhagia, and leukorrhea is considered pathognomonic for tubal carcinoma, it occurs infrequently. Pain with bloody vaginal discharge is a more frequent finding. If a patient is examined during the time that hydrops tubae profluens is present, a palpable pelvic mass is a frequent finding. The mass can actually decrease in size during the examination as the watery discharge continues. With the cessation of watery discharge and decrease in pelvic mass, the pain also decreases. Hydrops tubae profluens is caused by the effusion produced by the tumor that accumulates within the tube and causes the distention, which in turn produces the colicky pain. The same symptoms are present when bleeding occurs into the tubal lumen. Ascites is infrequent in this tumor but can occur. A pelvic mass is palpable in about 60% of the cases. The mass is usually

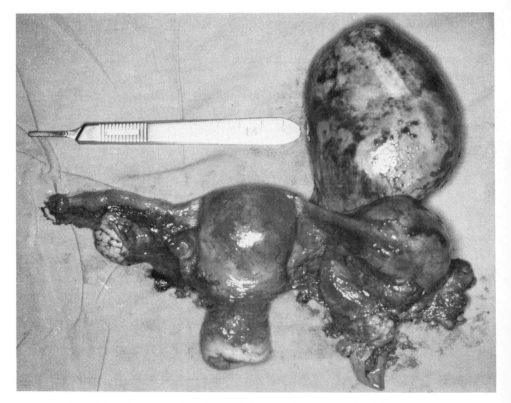

Fig. 13-1. A left large adnexal mass. Enlargement of left fallopian tube is apparent.

adnexal in location, and in most instances it is interpreted as a pedunculated fibroid or ovarian neoplasm (Fig. 13-1).

Malignant cells in cervical cytologic preparations have been said to be present in as many as 60% of patients with tubal carcinoma, although that is probably a very optimistic statistic. Certainly, in those patients with hydrops tubae profluens, the chances of obtaining malignant cells should be relatively high.

DIAGNOSIS

As previously noted, the diagnosis of this malignancy preoperatively is unusual if not rare. X-ray films of the pelvis may depict a mass that can be confirmed with ultrasound or CAT scan. However, these are usually not any more specific than the pelvic examination. Hysterosalpingography has been reported by some investigators to show diagnostically helpful abnormalities in the tube; however, many are hesitant to use this technique because of potential spread of malignant cells into the peritoneal cavity.

Histologic diagnosis may be difficult. The carcinoma should arise in the mucosa of the endosalpinx and have a papillary pattern with histologic characteristics of the endosalpinx. A transition between the benign and malignant tubal epithelium should be demonstrated. When the ovaries are involved, differentiation between a primary tubal or primary ovarian malignancy should be attempted. When ovarian cancer extends to the tube, serosal involvement is usually quite evident, and the mucosa of the endosalpinx may not be involved. In such situations, the correct diagnosis is apparent. Interestingly, in tubal carcinoma there is usually intraperitoneal involve- ment before the ovaries are affected. Because of the possibility of early intraperitoneal cytologic spread even with only mucosal involvement, the role of peritoneal cytology is extremely important in this disease entity. In patients with disease limited to the tube, the exact extent should be ascertained. If only the mucosa is involved, an "in situ" lesion is present, and the prognosis is quite good. Once the muscularis is invaded, the prognosis worsens, even with disease limited to the tube.

Intra-peritoneal Spread

THERAPY

In view of the fact that the diagnosis is rarely established preoperatively, one must be prepared to proceed with definitive therapy at the time of exploratory laparotomy for any adnexal mass or when this lesion is found coincidently with other disease. There is no staging classification for tubal carcinoma; however, many authors have suggested that the FIGO staging for ovarian cancer be used since the two organs are closely related anatomically and the spread pattern appears to be similar (see Table 11-8). Therapy guidelines should be essentially the same as for ovarian carcinoma, and a total abdominal hysterectomy with bilateral salpingo-oophorectomy is minimum therapy. Even with apparent early disease, this malignancy can be bilateral. Peritoneal cytologic specimens should be obtained on opening of the peritoneal cavity not only from the pelvis but also from the lateral paracolonic gutters and supradiaphragmatic areas. A partial omentectomy should be performed as well. Any disease outside the areas already extirpated should be removed if technically

No staging

Hyst BSO

Table 13-1. Suggested management for adenocarcinoma of the fallopian tube

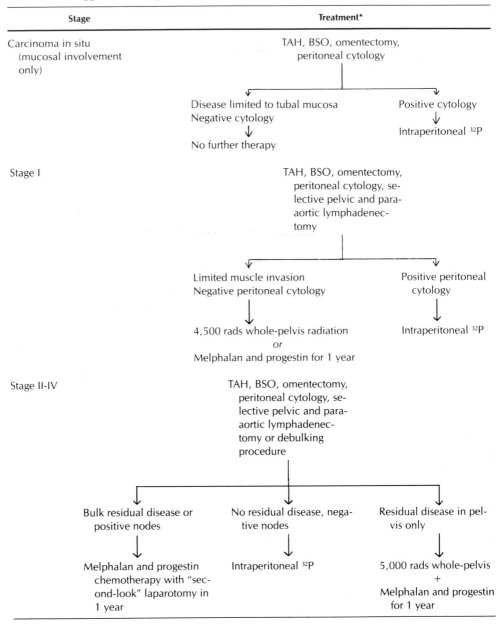

Stage	Treatment*

*TAH, total abdominal hysterectomy; BSO, bilateral salpingo-oophorectomy.

feasible. Debulking as described in ovarian carcinoma would also be applicable to this malignancy. It is believed that the lymphatic spread of this malignancy is mainly to the para-aortic lymph nodes, and this area should be examined, particularly in early stage disease. It has been established that lymphatic metastasis can also occur to the pelvic lymph nodes in both early ovarian and uterine cancer, and therefore these areas should also be carefully evaluated.

Postoperative therapy is needed as in ovarian carcinoma. In those instances in which disease is limited to the tube and ovary or uterus but no gross residual is left behind, radioactive chromic phosphate has been used and would appear to be efficacious. Radiation therapy after surgery has probably been used in more patients than any other subsequent therapy; again the results mimick those of ovarian carcinoma in that if disease is limited to the pelvis radiation therapy may be helpful, but once it is outside of those confines the entire intraperitoneal cavity must be treated (Table 13-1).

The role of chemotherapy has not been well studied; on an empirical basis, alkylating agents have been used since they have been the primary treatment for ovarian carcinoma. Progestin has been added in many circumstances because the endosalpinx is anatomically, embryologically, and histologically similar to the uterine endometrium. Boronow has reported a patient who had metastatic fallopian tube carcinoma that responded to a combination of an alkylating agent and progestin and had a negative "second-look" laparotomy. Since doxorubicin and cis-platinum are effective chemotherapeutic agents in both ovarian and endometrial carcinomas, it would appear worthwhile to use these drugs in tubal carcinoma, particularly with large residual disease. Data concerning the effectiveness of these two drugs, however, are not available.

PROGNOSIS

Since this disease is rare and the treatment varies, prognosis may be prejudiced. Sedlis noted that the 5-year survival rate for all cases of tubal carcinoma was 38% regardless of stage. Other authors have noted 5-year survival rates as high as 88% in stage I fallopian tube carcinoma, with diminishing survival rates as the stage increases. In fact, prognosis mimicks ovarian carcinoma when stage is used as a discriminating factor. Improved survival rates can be accomplished only when patients seek prompt medical care once symptoms have developed and when the physician has a high index of suspicion so that proper evaluation and therapy can be performed expeditiously.

SARCOMAS

Sarcomas are extremely rare. They have been reported in adolescents as well as in the elderly. Prognosis is very guarded. Treatment should be surgery initially, as in adenocarcinoma of the tube. Adjunctive chemotherapy with doxorubicin would appear to be treatment of choice after surgery. Presently, a patient is being treated with doxorubicin and is currently doing well on this regimen.

BIBLIOGRAPHY

Benedet, J. L., White, G. W., Fairey, R. N., and Boyes, D. A.: Adenocarcinoma of the fallopian tube, Obstet. Gynecol. **50:**654, 1977.

Boronow, R. C.: Chemotherapy for disseminated tubal cancer, Obstet. Gynecol. **42:**62, 1973.

Boutselis, J., and Thompson, J.: Clinical aspects of primary carcinoma of the fallopian tube, Am. J. Obstet. and Gynecol. **111:**98, 1971.

Dodson, M. G., Ford, J. H., and Averette, H. E.: Clinical aspects of fallopian tube carcinoma, Obstet. Gynecol. **36:**935, 1970.

Erey, S., Kaplan, A. L., and Wall, T. A.: Clinical staging of carcinoma of the uterine tube, Obstet. Gynecol. **30:**547, 1967.

Henderson, S. R., Harper, R. C., Salazar, O. M., and Rudolph, J. H.: Primary carcinoma of the fallopian tube; difficulties of diagnosis and treatment, Gynecol. Oncol. **5:**168, 1977.

Jones, O. V.: Primary carcinoma of the uterine tube, Obstet. Gynecol. **26:**122, 1965.

Kawase, N., Hirasawa, T., Akashi, E., and Hashimato, M.: Primary carcinoma of the fallopian tube, Acta Obstet. Gynaecol. Jap. **22**(1):20, 1975.

Kinzel, G. E.: Primary carcinoma of the fallopian tube, Am. J. Obstet. Gynecol. **125:**816, 1976.

Momtazee, S., and Kempson, R. L.: Primary adenocarcinoma of the fallopian tube, Obstet. Gynecol. **32:**649, 1968.

Phelps, H. M., and Chapman, K. E.: Role of radiation therapy in treatment of primary carcinoma of the uterine tube, Obstet. Gynecol. **43:**669, 1974.

Schiller, H. M., and Silverberg, S. G.: Staging and prognosis in primary carcinoma of the fallopian tube, Cancer **28:**389, 1971.

Sedlis, A.: Carcinoma of the fallopian tube, Surg. Clin. North Am. **58:**121, 1978.

CHAPTER FOURTEEN

The gynecologist and breast disease

Despite governmental denials, the obstetrician/gynecologist functions as the primary care physician for women, especially during the reproductive and perimenopausal years. Therefore, the diagnosis of breast cancer in its most curable forms lies within this speciality for large number of women. Breast cancer is the most common neoplasm in women. One out of every 13 women, or about 7%, will develop breast cancer during her lifetime. In 1978 there were nearly 95,000 new cases in the United States alone. Breast cancer is also the leading cause of cancer death in women, as well as the leading cause of death from all causes in women 40 to 44 years old. Every 15 minutes a woman dies of this disease. Nearly 35,000 deaths in the United States during 1978 can be attributed to breast cancer. These startling statistics clearly call for an immediate attack against this dread disease. Obviously, the most direct approach would be to find its cause and eradicate its inception. Unfortunately, the cause of breast cancer seems to be multifactorial, due to a constellation of risk factors rather than a single factor. Among the most important causes of breast cancer are: genetic predisposition, loss of the host's immunologic defense mechanism, and vi-

357

ruses as well as other carcinogens. Hormones, especially estrogens, were once considered to be primary carcinogenic agents but are now believed to act more as powerful promoters in carcinogenesis. Therefore, despite all the research aimed at finding the cause of breast cancer, this avenue does not seem to hold promise for the near future.

Next to finding the cause of breast cancer, the most important aspect in combatting the disease is diagnosis at an early stage when the prognosis for cure with appropriate therapy is excellent. By instructing the patient in the art of monthly breast examination, by performing careful periodic breast examinations in the office, and by judiciously using diagnostic aids, especially in those patients with increased risk for the disease, the physician has a golden opportunity to detect breast cancer at an early and highly curable stage.

BENIGN CONDITIONS OF THE BREAST

Most women discover their own breast tumors by chance or by periodic self-examination. Two thirds of the tumors found by all methods during a woman's reproductive years are benign and represent cystic changes, dysplasia, fibroadenomas, and papillomas. However, 50% of the palpable masses in perimenopausal women and the majority of lesions in postmenopausal patients are malignant.

Cystic breast changes and mammary dysplasia are common, often symptomatic, and require considerable judgment on the part of the physician in choosing the appropriate therapy. The incidence of these benign changes peaks in women 30 to 50 years of age and may be the result of estrogen stimulation in the absence of cyclic corpus luteum formation and the cyclic production of progesterone. Continued estrogen stimulation may be a factor in the development of the so-called macrocyst. The fact that breast tenderness often occurs premenstrually suggests that progesterone may also play a role in the development and symptoms of cystic alterations in the breast tissue. However, the proportional effect of each of these hormones on the cause of benign breast conditions is unclear and needs further clarification.

A more thorough understanding of the embryologic and prepubertal development of the breast will aid in the study of benign breast lesions. The mammary glands are highly specialized skin derivatives of ectodermal origin. The epithelial ridge that will develop into breast tissue undergoes a series of proliferations to form the lactiferous ducts. Primitive breast tissue is under the gonadal control of fetal androgen production, which causes a suppression of breast growth during the period of gestation, when the tissue is under the simultaneous influence of increasing levels of growth-promoting estrogen and progesterone. Following birth, breast tissue remains dormant until adolescence, when estrogen produces a proliferation of ductal epithelium and progesterone produces rapid growth of the acini. However, breast growth and development are not totally dependent on estrogen and progesterone levels. Insulin, cortisol, thyroxine, growth hormone, and prolactin are also required for complete functional development. Minor deficiencies in any one of these hormones can be compensated for by an excess of prolactin, the interesting hormone found in mammals that suckle their young.

During pregnancy, increasing amounts of estrogen, progesterone, and human placental lactogen produce active growth of functional breast tissue. Serum prolactin rises from prepregnant levels of 10 ng/ml to term levels of 200 ng/ml. Amniotic fluid prolactin levels are more than 100 times greater than the levels seen in maternal or fetal blood early in pregnancy. It is not known whether the fetal pituitary gland or the trophoblast secretes the hormone into the amniotic fluid, but one hypothesis suggests that prolactin may help the embryo survive its aquatic environment much as it helps the teleost fish in its journey from salt to fresh water to spawn. Elevated levels of estradiol parallel those of prolactin and indicate that estriol may be responsible for increases in prolactin. Although estrogen may initiate prolactin secretion, high levels block its physiologic effects. Prolactin secretion is also controlled by the prolactin-inhibiting factor. A decrease of estrogen level following delivery and suppression of the prolactin-inhibiting factor by suckling increases prolactin levels. If breast-feeding does not occur, serum prolactin levels decrease to prepregnant levels in about 1 week. The final episode in nature's plan to provide the newborn with milk from its mother's breast is the contraction of the duct system by the release of oxytocin from the posterior pituitary and the delivery of milk to the nipples. After 3 to 4 months of breast-feeding, suckling appears to be the only stimulus required for lactation.

Diagnosis and management

There is considerable controversy as to whether the patient with benign cystic changes in the breast is at greater risk for the development of cancer. Some authorities believe that the risk of cancer is two to four times greater in the patient with cystic changes. These cystic changes produce lumpy, tender breasts, particularly during the premenstrual phase. In advanced stages, there may be discrete, tender, and turgid cystic masses within the breast. The following benign conditions are commonly found.

Fibrocystic disease. The lesions are commonly bilateral and multiple. They are characterized by dull, heavy pain, a sense of fullness, and tenderness. These symptoms increase premenstrually, as does lump size. In the case of a cyst, the patient will often report that there was a sudden appearance of a tender lump and that she or her doctor recently examined her breast and did not notice a lump. The lumps are cystic to palpation, tender, well delineated, slightly mobile, and clear on transillumination. Aspiration reveals a typical turbid, nonhemorrhagic, yellow, greenish, or brownish fluid (Fig. 14-1). Deeply imbedded cysts, a cluster of cysts, or dominant areas due to sclerosing adenosis or dense fibrous dysplasia can produce a mass that clinically mimics cancer.

Fibroadenoma. Another common benign lesion is the fibroadenoma, which appears predominantly in young women and occasionally in adolescents. It presents as

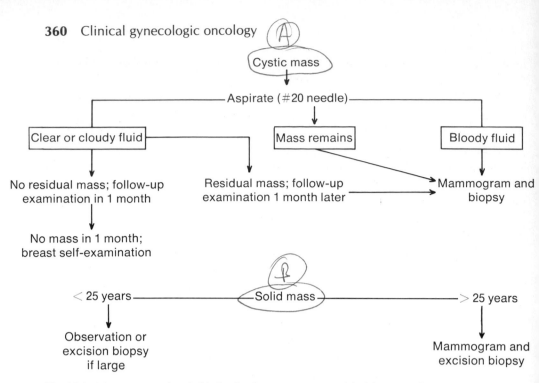

Fig. 14-1. Management of probable benign breast masses. (Modified from Marchant, D. J.: Female patient, vol. 4, no. 3, March 1979, P. W. Communications Inc.)

a firm, painless, mobile mass and may be very large, particularly in adolescents. Fibroadenomas are multiple and bilateral in about 14% to 25% of patients.

Intraductal papilloma. Intraductal papilloma presents as a serous, serosanguineous, or watery type of nipple discharge. In the absence of a mass, the most frequent cause of bloody nipple discharge is an intraductal papilloma. The discharge is usually spontaneous and from a single duct and is commonly unilateral. Most discharges are due to benign conditions and do not require surgical intervention. The color and consistency of the discharge is important, however, and cytologic examination of the nipple discharge and, occasionally, mammography are important diagnostic aids. Tranquilizers, particularly the phenothiazines, may cause bilateral nipple discharge, principally because they decrease the prolactin-inhibiting factor and thus elevate prolactin levels.

Ductal ectasia. Ductal ectasia is also commonly manifested by nipple discharge. However, this discharge is usually multicolored and sticky, bilateral, and from multiple ducts. Frequently a patient experiences a burning, itching, or dull drawing type of pain around the nipple and areola, and there are palpable tortuous tubular swellings under the areola. When the condition is more advanced, a mass can develop that may resemble a locally advanced stage III breast carcinoma.

• • •

A careful, methodical examination is essential to the detection of pathologic breast conditions. A complete breast examination requires a full 5 minutes of the physician's time and should include instruction to the patient in the technique of self-examination. The breasts are first inspected with the patient in the sitting or standing position. Contour, symmetry, and skin changes are observed. These changes may be exaggerated by asking the patient to place her hands on her hips and contract the pectoral muscles. Palpation is performed with the flat of the hand, and the axilla is palpated while the patient's arm is supported by the opposite hand. Regional lymph nodes are also sought in the supraclavicular area before the patient is asked to assume a supine position, where palpation is repeated. The areola and the nipples should also be carefully examined and palpated.

Most patients discover their own breast masses and then consult their physician. It is essential that an active diagnosis be made and proper treatment be initiated with minimal delay (Fig. 14-2). Definitive treatment of cystic alterations and mammary dysplasia depends on the age of the patient and the size and characteristics of the lesion. An obvious fibroadenoma may be observed safely in patients under 25, but large dominant masses should be removed, even if the mammogram is negative, because continued growth may cause local destruction of functioning breast tissue. Solid masses should also be excised by means of a circumareola incision. Obvious cystic masses can be aspirated and the fluid sent for cytologic analysis. Some authorities feel that cytologic examination of clear breast fluid is unnecessary, but it would seem that pathologic analysis of the fluid is prudent in all circumstances. The presence of serosanguineous or bloody fluid demands further tissue biopsy. Women over the age of 25 who have a dominant mass should have a mammogram as a baseline reading before any biopsy or aspiration is performed. Since breast cancer is exceedingly rare in patients under 25, a mammogram need not be done in this age group.

The gynecologist should recognize that there are three special groups of women who are at added risk for development of breast cancer (Table 14-1). First, those with a family history of breast cancer (grandmother, mother, aunt, or sister) develop at least twice as many breast cancers as do the control group. Second, those patients who have already had cancer in one breast develop more than five times as many cancers in the remaining breast as occur in the control group. Third, there are those patients with gross cystic disease in whom subsequent breast cancer (apparently unrelated to the cysts themselves) is reported to occur two to four times more frequently than in the control group. Women in each of these groups should have a breast examination every 3 to 6 months for the duration of their lives. Women between the ages of 40 to 44 and those over 60 have a higher risk, especially if they have not been pregnant or have not borne their first child before the age of 34. Whites are at higher risk as compared with blacks and Orientals. In addition, patients who experience early menarche and late menopause are apparently at higher risk.

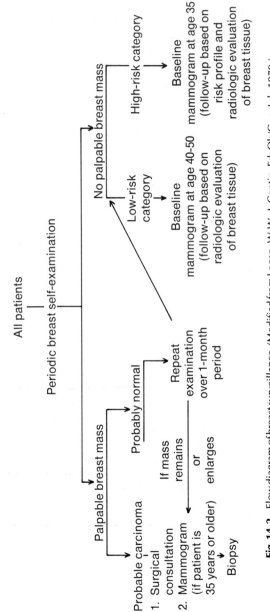

Fig. 14-2. Flow diagram of breast surveillance. (Modified from Logan, W. W.: J. Contin. Ed. Ob/Gyn, July 1979.)

Table 14-1. High-risk factors in breast cancer

1. Over 40 years of age
2. Family history: positive maternal
3. Obstetric history: late parity
4. Previous cancer in one breast
5. Other organ cancer, e.g., endometrium and ovary
6. Fibrocystic disease
7. Adverse hormonal milieu
8. Lower immunologic competence
9. Excess exposure of the breast to radiation
10. High dietary fat intake

Outpatient biopsy has become increasingly popular and inconveniences the patient minimally. A biopsy is not an office procedure and is best performed in a regular operating room setting with a standard team of assistants. Local anesthesia can be used, and in most instances a circumareolar incision is made. Meticulous hemostasis must be achieved during these biopsies in order to minimize postoperative complications. Biopsy and definitive diagnosis are becoming more popular even for lesions that appear to be malignant. Available data suggest that a 12-week delay in treatment does not adversely influence survival in breast cancer, so that the diagnostic and therapeutic procedures need not be combined in the same surgical procedure.

BREAST CANCERS
Early detection and diagnosis

More than 70% of all breast cancers are accidentally detected by the patient. Masses found by patients in this manner are likely to be sizeable, and methods are needed for detection of earlier disease. The signs and symptoms of breast cancer, such as localized skin edema, nipple retraction, localized erythema, swelling, skin retraction, changes in contour, ulceration, and enlargement of the axillary nodes, represent manifestations of locally advanced disease. Minimal breast cancer is occasionally found accidentally when an abnormality actually due to benign breast disease leads to the performance of a biopsy and minimal carcinoma is found accidentally in adjacent tissue by histologic examination. Such fortuitous events are obviously unusual and not the main method of diagnosis. In order to detect breast cancer before the development of signs of advanced disease, mass population screening is necessary. The modalities available for screening are physical examination, mammography, and thermography.

Physical examination of the breast in a screening center consists of rigidly systematic palpation and inspection, usually carried out by trained paramedical specialists. In one or two earlier attempts at breast cancer screening, physical examination alone was used and was found to be effective in increasing the frequency of node-negative breast cancer cases. More productive, however, is a combination of mammography and physical examination. The examination period also provides an opportunity for instruction of the patient in breast self-examination (BSE). She is shown how to conduct the examination and introduced to the variations that may be present in her own breast. A good instructor in BSE attempts to instill strong motivation in the woman to do a monthly assessment of her own breasts.

Mammographic examination usually consists of two views of each breast. In most of the breast detection demonstration project centers, xeroradiographic apparatus is used. Images are obtained by trained radiographic technicians and interpreted by radiologists who have special training and experience in this radiographic discipline.

Thermography as a means of breast cancer detection is unproved. Early studies gave hope that it might be useful in prescreening to identify a group of women most at risk. Experience in most centers, however, has been disappointing. The number of false-negative and false-positive results obtained by thermography has been unacceptably high, and at present the examination has been dropped from the screening routine in all but a few centers, where it is retained as a research tool.

Recently, technical improvements in ultrasonic imaging techniques have led to the suggestion that this modality might also be used in breast cancer detection. The proposal is attractive because ultrasonography exposes the breast to only trivial levels of energy, on the order of a few milliwatts per square centimeter. Although a considerable amount of preliminary work has been carried out that indicates that there are differences in the absorption of ultrasound by normal and neoplastic tissue, neither the practical aspects of application nor the specific diagnostic parameters have, as yet, been accurately defined. At present the procedure is experimental.

The experience gained through the Breast Cancer Detection Demonstration Project (BCDDP) (Table 14-2) has been helpful in drawing some conclusions. Analysis of their data suggests that screening for breast cancer does lead to earlier detection. Although the high yield encountered in that project may in part be due to self detection of the patient population, a significant number of the cancers detected were small. The women involved in the screening project were volunteers, and it had been hoped that they would be primarily asymptomatic; however, it appeared that there was a significant factor of self-detection because of individual concerns about breast disease. Up until 1977, approximately 1,200 carcinomas had been discovered by biopsy on the basis of an initial recommendation through the screening

Table 14-2. Breast cancers by modality of detection at first screening (BCDDP)*

Total cancer detected		734
Modality of detection known		683 (100%)
Mammography only	354 (51.8%)	
Mammography and physical examination	269 (39.4%)	
Physical examination only	60 (8.8%)	

Data from National Institutes of Health, Department of Health, Education, and Welfare, March 1977.
*BCDDP, Breast Cancer Detection Demonstration Project.

program. Many of these tumors were very small, and it can be concluded that at least part of the increase in survival was due to early recognition of tumors that under ordinary circumstances would have been undetectable until a later date. Mammography proved to be highly successful in early breast detection in this program. Physical examination is less likely to be effective in influencing end results but plays an important role in detection of cancers missed by radiographic examination. Until mammography can achieve total accuracy of diagnosis, physical examination must remain an integral part of the screening examination.

Since the BCDDP data are tainted by the absence of a control group of women, a high detection rate of early cancer in women under 50 years of age merits further evaluation. However, there are some risks associated with repeated mammography in patients in this age group. The report of Upton and his National Cancer Institute group, issued in February 1977, on the risks associated with mammography in mass screening for the detection of breast cancer noted that epidemiologic studies reveal an excess of breast cancer in three groups: American women treated with x-radiation of the breast for postpartum mastitis, American and Canadian women subjected to multiple fluoroscopic examinations of the chest during artificial pneumothorax treatment of pulmonary tuberculosis, and Japanese women surviving atomic bomb irradiation who were more than 10 years old at the time of the exposure. From these observations, it was possible for Upton and his group to estimate the carcinogenic risk to the breast associated with the far lower doses of mammography, if the dose-response relationship was assumed to remain linear, irrespective of dose, dose rate, and age at irradiation. Based on this assumption, along with the adjustment for the effects of age difference and susceptibility, the risk was assumed to be approximately 3.5 to 7.5 cases of breast cancer per million women of ages 35 or older at risk per year per rad to both breasts, from the tenth year after irradiation throughout the remainder of life. According to this model, a single mammographic examination performed with a technique that involves an average dose to the breast of less than 1 rad should be expected to increase a woman's subsequent risk of developing breast cancer by much less than 1% of the natural risk of 7% at the age of 35 and by a progressively smaller percentage with increasing age at examinations thereafter, i.e., from a risk of 7% (since one out of 13 American women develops breast cancer) to a risk of 7.07%. Whether the risk is greater in women affected by other high-risk factors remains to be determined. With newer technology and less exposure to the breast from high-quality mammograms we would expect that these estimates would be reduced.

Based on this type of reasoning, the following recommendations are made for the use of mammography:

1. Mammography should be performed at any age when clinical findings indicate a significant suspicion of cancer.
2. Mammography should not be performed in women under the age of 35 except when there is a specific strong clinical indication. The incidence of carcinoma in this age group is very low.

3. A baseline mammogram should be considered in women between 35 and 40 because a baseline study provides the groundwork for assessing subtle changes in subsequent mammograms that may indicate mammary cancer. Many authorities argue with this indication for mammography, preferring to await clinical indications.

4. Periodic mammography with low-level radiation may be performed in women between the ages of 35 and 49 only after the risk factors have been thoroughly evaluated. Patients who are at high risk or who are clinically suspect would of course be included in this category.

5. For women 50 years of age or older, the National Cancer Institute agrees that annual or other periodic mammography is statistically justified to screen asymptomatic women for breast cancer.

There is no single 100% effective method of diagnosing all breast carcinomas. The major value of mammography lies chiefly in the detection of nonpalpable, hitherto totally unsuspected lesions (for example, on a baseline mammogram in a woman who is at high risk or in the left breast of a woman who has had palpable mass or cyst in the right breast). Another valuable role lies in spurring on the surgeon to operate sooner, instead of observing a breast mass of borderline significance over a period of time, when the radiologic diagnosis is that of a definite malignancy. The undesirable situation in which a surgeon delays biopsy or the gynecologist delays referral of the patient to a surgeon based on a report of a "normal" mammogram should not occur if the decision to perform biopsy or to refer the patient is carried out despite the mammogram report. The gynecologist must remember that mammography is not the first step one takes in evaluating a breast mass; it is an additional step. When a heightened suspicion exists, the patient should be further evaluated regardless of the mammogram report (Table 14-3).

Breast cancer accounts for 26% of all nonskin cancers and 20% of all cancer deaths in women (Table 14-4). The incidence of breast cancer has increased steadily since 1930, but the mortality has remained between 35% and 50%. After an improvement in the 5-year survival rate from 53% for patients diagnosed between 1940 and 1949 to 60% during the next decade, further gains were modest. In children under 15 years of age, breast cancer is relatively rare and appears to follow a favorable course. Between 1% and 3% of all female mammary cancers occur in women under the age of 30 years, 5% in women below 35 years, and 10% to 15% in women less than 41 years. At age 45 the incidence curve approaches its first peak. More than 75% of breast cancers are detected by women themselves and are merely confirmed by the physician. Early diagnosis, which greatly improves the results of breast cancer treatment, would be possible if all women were taught to examine their own breasts; at present, regular self-examination is practiced by less than 20% of American women. Physical findings characteristic of malignant disease often occur relatively late. Moreover, in young women palpable masses are notoriously difficult to evaluate clinically and radiographically.

Table 14-3. Wolfe classification of mammogram results with recommendations

NI breast	Composed mainly of fat Low risk for cancer Self breast examination Yearly physical examination Rare mammography
PI breast	Prominent subareolar ducts Invading only a small portion of breast Low risk Recommendations same as NI
P2 breast	More prominent ductal pattern Considerable risk Yearly mammography
DY breast	Severe involvement with mammary dysplasia $+/-$ ductal pattern High risk Yearly mammography

From Wolfe, J. N.: Risk for breast cancer development determined by mammographic parenchymal patterns, Cancer **37**:5, 1976.

Table 14-4. Breast cancer incidence by age

Age	Incidence
20-30	3/100,000
50	150/100,000
80	450/100,000

Data from Cancer facts and figures 1978, New York, 1978, American Cancer Society, Inc.

Clinical staging of patients with suspected operable mammary cancer begins with measurement of the primary tumor in two or three diameters and with a description of its location and attachments. Palpation of regional lymph node areas should be thorough. Although about one fourth of the patients with enlarged axillary nodes (stage II) are without nodal metastasis, about 40% of those without palpable nodes (stage I) have nodal metastasis. The clinical staging, nevertheless, correlates well with 5- to 10-year survival rate and is the basis for selection of therapy in many cases. Biopsy should be done on enlarged supraclavicular nodes before mastectomy, and other signs of local spread of tumor outside the breasts (stage III) should be sought (see Table 15-5 for staging).

Primary treatment by modern modalities results in a 10-year survival rate of 55% for operable cases. Seventy percent of patients without axillary node involvement, but only 40% of operable cases with positive axillary nodes, survive 10 years. Size and histopathologic character of the neoplasms are correlated with curability. All patients with suspected progression of disease beyond clinical stage I, on the basis of the history and physical examination, require careful laboratory search for distant metastasis as well. The most useful tests are bone scans and x-ray films of bones with abnormal uptake on the scan, as well as films of the chest and contralateral breast.

Differences in the extent of the disease in the presence of asymptomatic but possibly detectable metastasis at the time of initial diagnosis may explain much of the variability in the results of therapy. Large clinical series indicate a frequency of stage IV disease of between 2% and 13% at the time of presentation. Without including the number of patients who were not scanned or x-rayed, Roberts and associates reported that 18% of new breast cancer patients with normal bone radiographs had scans with evidence of bone metastasis. Such a frequency of bone involvement in patients presenting with clinically localized and operable breast cancer appears extensive in view of the 17% total recurrence rate at all sites observed by others in the first 18 months after surgery in patients with operable breast cancer. With a trend toward lesser surgery and systemic adjuvant therapy, the importance of proper staging becomes crucial. One objective of adjuvant chemotherapy is eradication of minimal "microscopic" disease. If patients with detectable primary metastatic disease contaminate the true adjuvant population, results of such therapy may be obscured. Moreover, patients with primary metastatic disease should be considered for alternative therapeutic options, such as endocrine therapy before or in combination with chemotherapy.

Treatment

In recent years a change in attitude has created controversies concerning the extent of surgery for primary operable tumors, and at present there is no one best operation for breast cancer. Radical mastectomy has been the standard procedure ever since Halsted published his first series in 1894. There was universal acceptance of his concept of wide en bloc resection of the primary tumor together with the lymphatic pathway of spread to the axillary lymph nodes. This mode of treatment was dominant for about 50 years in spite of the fact that cure rates left much to be desired. Thereafter, dissatisfaction with the standard radical mastectomy began to gain momentum, and the trend toward lesser procedures has been widespread in the past decade. The surgical world is now in a dilemma, and the enlightened public is well aware of the controversies over the extent of surgery for the cure of primary operable breast cancer. There are proponents for essentially three types of treatment: standard radical mastectomy, modified radical mastectomy, and local excision plus radiation. Statistical data gathered on a worldwide basis from each of these groups indicate that all arrive at essentially similar survival figures.

There are a number of reasons for the gradual decline of use of the radical mastectomy. The cosmetic defect produced by loss of the pectoral muscles was unacceptable to many women, and the morbidity included a 30% incidence of chronic arm edema. It also became apparent that even increasing the extent of the surgery to include the internal mammary chain of nodes did not improve the salvage rates.

For primary operable lesions, the 10-year survival rate stayed at about 50%. Early critics indicated that the radical operation was not necessary if a small lesion was localized and uselessly destructive if there were metastases that ruled out cure. They also questioned the simplistic explanation of tumor spread from tumor site to regional nodes and then to distant sites. The concept of breast cancer as a systemic disease developed and led to the reevaluation of the role of axillary node dissection. Is it therapeutic or simply a diagnostic maneuver? Those who limit the extent of surgery to primary excision rely on radiation therapy to sterilize not only regional node areas but also multicentric foci that might remain in the involved breast. Increasing knowledge of chemotherapy and the kinetics of cancer kill and growth is having a major impact on ideas concerning the total management of primary operable breast cancer. There is good evidence that micrometastases can be handled by immune mechanisms and/or multiagent chemotherapy.

The trend toward lesser surgery really began when the concept of removing the breast and axillary contents and leaving the chest wall muscles intact was first introduced. It was demonstrated that simple mastectomy followed by radiation resulted in salvage rates equal to those of radical mastectomy. The trend was completed with recent reports advocating local excision and radiation. The present dilemma stems from the fact that absolute data on survival in randomized control series are almost impossible to obtain. There are many operative control studies going on at the present time, but increasing restrictions of an ethical and legal nature are making it difficult to gather significant data. In most studies, survival figures are compared with those of studies based on the Halsted radical mastectomy. It is significant that all lesser procedures reveal similar end results but none surpass those obtained with radical surgery. Accordingly, many proponents of Halsted's radical mastectomy will continue to use that operation until offered an alternative that will yield better 10-year salvage rates. A detailed discussion of the advantages and disadvantages of the alternatives for primary therapy in patients with potentially curable breast cancer is beyond the scope of this text. The reader is referred to the bibliography at the end of the chapter for more detailed information concerning this interesting and current controversy.

The treatment of locally advanced breast cancer (stages III and IV) is often palliative. Many of these patients have detectable distant metastasis at the time they seek medical treatment, and their prognosis is quite poor (10-year survival rate of 14%). For palliation, systemic endocrine therapy or chemotherapy is necessary. In addition, several groups have reported good results with aggressive preoperative radiotherapy, reducing the frequency of local recurrences after mastectomy. Removal of tumor bulk by mastectomy is usually recommended, but the value of postoperative radiotherapy is equivocal. Preoperative or postoperative radiotherapy does not appear to improve the 5- or 10-year survival rates, and radiation to regional lymph nodes may have detrimental immunosuppressive effects. Any local control achieved is usually not appreciated, with the appearance of distant metastasis.

The treatment of metastatic breast cancer includes a cooperative effort on the

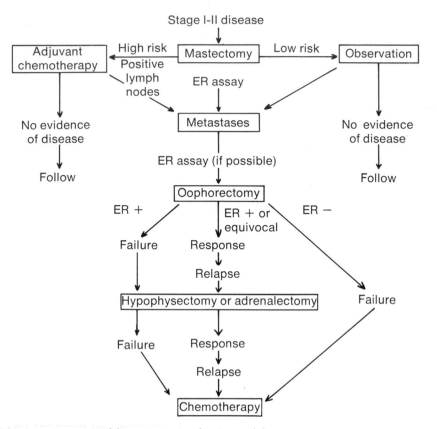

Fig. 14-3. Treatment of the premenopausal patient with breast cancer. (ER, estrogen receptor.)

part of surgeons. radiotherapists, endocrinologists, and medical oncologists to produce a systemic therapy supplemented by local measures to lesions in immediate need of palliation (Fig. 14-3).

Estrogen receptors are proteins found in hormonally dependent malignant and nonmalignant tissue. The amount of receptor present in the breast cancer specimen is predictive of the success or failure of endocrine therapy. The identification of the estrogen receptor protein in certain human mammary cancers and the subsequent explanation of the role of estrogen in tumor growth clarified a clinical relationship that had been observed for a century. In 1917, Beatson produced regression of mammary cancer by oophorectomy. Later, Huggins and Bergenstal demonstrated in 1952 that some mammary and prostatic cancers were not autonomous but were under the partial control of the endocrine system. Regressions of mammary cancer were continually obtained by removing the source of endogenous circulating hormones via oophorectomy, adrenalectomy, and hypophysectomy. Alternatively, breast cancer regressions were also achieved by administering large doses of estrogen, androgen, progesterone, and glucocorticoids. The choice of a particular endocrine therapy has been in large part empirical, guided by certain clinical features such as menopausal status, disease-free interval, site of dominant lesion, and response to previous therapy. Regardless of the method of endocrine therapy employed, objective regressions were obtained in no more than one third of breast cancer patients. As a result of basic investigations by Jensen and others of steroid hormone metabolism, there have developed a series of assays that can identify with considerable accuracy those breast cancers that are not autonomous and will respond to endocrine manipulation. Such a method of predicting a priori those cancers that will be responsive to changes in endocrine milieu greatly enhances the usefulness of hormonal therapy and allows the structuring of such treatments on a plausible biochemical basis.

Knowledge of the estrogen receptor content of either the primary or the recurrent mammary cancer must be viewed within the proper clinical perspective. This one determination is but a single piece in the mosaic of the subcellular biochemistry of breast cancer. To deprecate the clinical importance of this determination because some patients with significant estrogen receptor content will not respond to hormonal treatment (because of eventual escape from hormonal regulation or because of lack of understanding of the role of other steroid or protein hormone receptors) begs the question. Knowledge of the estrogen receptor content of either a primary or a metastatic tumor does allow the physician to predict the hormonal dependency of a tumor with enough accuracy to be rationally employed in the selection of appropriate palliative treatment.

Bilateral oophorectomy at the time of documented metastatic locally recurrent disease appears to be the most useful treatment for a premenopausal patient with an estrogen receptor–containing tumor. Castration is also indicated when the receptor status cannot be assessed, whereas patients with negative analyses should benefit more from chemotherapy. Responses are less frequent below the age of 35 and are rare if the disease-free interval is less than 24 months. Soft-tissue and bone lesions respond more frequently than do visceral and metastatic lesions and inoperable primary disease.

With the recent development of the transsphenoidal microsurgical approach to the pituitary, the mortality and morbidity of hypophysectomy can be reduced to very low levels. The time of hypophysectomy is of importance. Oophorectomy has generally been carried out in premenopausal patients when the recurrent disease was first recognized. If the patient seems to meet the criterion of a previous response to castration, hypophysectomy should be performed when disease progression is again identified.

The rationale that led to the consideration of adrenalectomy for the treatment of advanced metastatic cancer of the breast was also based on the concept of hormone dependence. Although there had been no evidence that the human adrenal cortex secretes estrogens, it is now well established that in postmenopausal women an adrenal androgen, androstenedione, is peripherally converted to estrogens. It has been demonstrated that women with breast cancer after menopause or oophorectomy still excrete significant amounts of estrogen hormones in the urine; these hormones are further reduced or become unmeasurable after adrenalectomy. Although a number of investigators have felt that hypophysectomy is superior to adrenalectomy, this assertion has been very difficult to prove statistically. One of the problems in answering this question is that it has been very difficult to compare one series with another because the criteria for operation and the definition of remission are likely to differ from one series to another. In one clinical trial where a randomization was carried out, the difference in response was 13% in favor of the hypophysectomy group. Investigations are under way using chemical adrenal blockers to achieve a nonsurgical adrenalectomy.

Chemotherapy

For decades the primary therapy for women with breast cancer has been surgery or radiation, or a combination of both. At present many women are being treated with steroid hormones and cytotoxic agents for advanced or metastatic breast cancer. However, these two classes of drugs have different modes of action and toxic effects. Both are most effective when these differences are taken into account and chemotherapy is employed selectively. The choice depends essentially on whether breast cancer in a given patient is a hormone-dependent neoplasm. It has been established that about half of all breast cancers are somewhat hormone dependent, and it is also evident that hormone dependence is associated with specific estrogen receptors, or cytoplasmic estrogen-binding proteins, in neoplastic cells. On this basis, one can first determine the presence or absence of estrogen receptors and proceed accordingly. Hormonal therapy is the treatment of choice in hormone-related breast cancer. Judicious use of cytotoxic agents is indicated if an assay proves receptor-negative or if initial hormone treatment is unsuccessful.

Several cytotoxic agents have commonly been used either singly or in combination for the treatment of advanced breast cancer. Agents that have been found to be active are the antimetabolites 5-fluorouracil and methotrexate, alkylating agents such as cyclophosphamide and melphalan, vincristine, and cytotoxic antibiotics such as doxorubicin and mitomycin C.

The use of multiple drug combinations in cancer chemotherapy was introduced more than a decade ago. Although superior clinical results with combination therapy have been reported, acceptance of the use of multiple drug therapy has been slow, mainly because of the fear of increased toxicity. Most combination programs were designed empirically, and it appears well proved that combination chemotherapy yields clinical results superior to those achieved with single-agent therapy. The various combinations that are commonly used in the treatment of breast cancer are cyclophosphamide and 5-fluorouracil (CF), cyclophosphamide, prednisone, and 5-fluorouracil (CPF), cyclophosphamide, methotrexate, and 5-fluorouracil (CMF), doxorubicin (Adriamycin) and cyclophosphamide (AC), and cyclophosphamide, methotrexate, 5-fluorouracil, vincristine, and prednisone (CMFVP).

Adjuvant chemotherapy. The rationale for adjuvant chemotherapy is based on the premise that minimal residual disease after primary resection of a carcinoma (which may account for subsequent development of metastasis) may be eliminated by early systemic therapy with cytotoxic chemotherapeutic drugs. The goal is an improvement in cure rate. An early study using thiotepa as adjuvant therapy after mastectomy had suggested a delay in recurrence in patients receiving this drug. This finding, however, was observed only in premenopausal patients. A more recent study using melphalan (L-PAM) as adjuvant therapy for an extended period (more than 1 year after mastectomy) again demonstrated a beneficial effect (delay of recurrence) in premenopausal women with high-risk cancer. Interestingly, the postmenopausal patients receiving postoperative melphalan treatment showed no significant increase in the recurrence-free period as compared with the control group, in which patients were not given adjuvant chemotherapy. A trial with drug combinations such as cyclophosphamide, methotrexate, and 5-fluorouracil as adjuvant therapy following mastectomy in women with high-risk breast cancer has yielded results similar to those seen in the study using melphalan. Again, an increase in the recurrent-free period was observed in the premenopausal but not the postmenopausal women. Clinical and laboratory studies have shown that cytotoxic alkylating agents and antimetabolites induce marked suppression of ovarian function and cessation of menstruation. It is conceivable that the beneficial effect of adjuvant chemotherapy in premenopausal patients is partially the result of a suppression of ovarian activity by these drugs. Some authors used cytotoxic chemotherapeutic agents as adjuvant therapy only in high risk breast cancer patients whose tumors were found to be negative for estrogen receptors. These same investigators recommend endocrine ablation as adjuvant therapy in high-risk patients whose tumors contain estrogen receptors.

BIBLIOGRAPHY

Atkins, H., Hayward, J. L., Klugman, D. J., and others: Treatment of early breast cancer; a report after ten years of a clinical trial, Br. Med. J. 2:423, 1972.

Barrett, A., DeSouza, I., Morgan, L., and others: A breast carcinoma dependent on human placental lactogen, letter, Lancet 1:1347, 1975.

Bonadonna, G., Brusamolino, E., Valagussa, P., and others: Combination chemotherapy as an adjuvant treatment in operable breast cancer, N. Engl. J. Med. 294:405, 1976.

Bonadonna, G., Rossi, A., Valagussa, P., and others: The CMF program for operable breast cancer with positive axillary nodes; updated analysis on the disease free interval, site of relapse and drug tolerance, Cancer 39:2904, 1977.

Bonadonna, G., and Valagussa, P.: Chemotherapy of breast cancer, N. Engl. J. Med. 294:1345, 1976.

Byrne, R.: Utilization of thermography as a risk indicator in the detection of breast cancer, Bull. N.Y. Acad. Med. 52:741, 1976.

Canellos, G. P., DeVita, V. T., Gold, G. L., and others: Combination chemotherapy for advanced breast cancer; response and effect on survival, Ann. Intern. Med. 84:389, 1976.

Carbone, P. P.: The role of chemotherapy in the treatment of cancer of the breast, Am. J. Clin. Pathol. 64:774, 1975.

Carter, A. C. Sedransk, N., Kelly, R., and others: Diethylstilbestrol; recommended dosages for different categories of breast cancer patients; report of the Cooperative Breast Cancer Group, J.A.M.A. 237:2079, 1977.

Chan, L., and O'Malley, B. W.: Mechanism of action of the sex steroid hormones, N. Engl. J. Med. 294:1322, 1372, 1430, 1976.

Constanza, M. E.: The problem of breast cancer prophylaxis, N. Engl. J. Med. 293:1095, 1975.

Cook, D. C., Dent, O., and Hewitt, D.: Breast cancer following multiple chest fluoroscopy; the Ontario experience, Can. Med. Assoc. J. 111:406, 1974.

Cutler, S. J.: Classification of extent of disease in breast cancer, Semin. Oncol. 1:91, 1974.

Ferguson, D. J., and Meier, P.: Results of the treatment of mammary cancer at the University of Chicago, 1960-1969, Surg. Clin. North Am. **56:**103, 1976.

Final Reports of the National Cancer Institute Ad Hoc Working Groups on Mammography Screening for Breast Cancer and A Summary Report of Their Joint Recommendations, National Institutes of Health, DHEW Publication No. (NH) 77-1400, Washington, D.C., 1977, Department of Health, Education, and Welfare.

Fisher, B., Carbone, P., Economous, S. G., and others: *l*-Phenylalanine mustard (L-PAM) in the management of primary breast cancer; a report of early findings, N. Engl. J. Med. **292:**117, 1975.

Fisher, E. R., Gregorio, R. M., and Fisher, B.: The pathology of invasive breast cancer; a syllabus derived from findings of the National Surgical Adjuvant Breast Project (Protocol No. 4), Cancer **36:**1, 1975.

Gilbertsen, V. A.: The earlier detection of breast cancer, Semin. Oncol. **1:**87, 1975.

Gogas, J., and Skalkeas, G.: Prognosis of mammary carcinoma in young women, Surgery **78:**339, 1975.

Gorten, R. J.: Nuclear medicine procedures in obstetrics and gynecology, Radiol. Clin. North Am. **12:**147, 1974.

Haagensen, C. D.: The choice of treatment for operable carcinoma of the breast, Surgery **76:**685, 1974.

Haberman, J. D., and others: Thermography; a primary consideration in noninvasive testing. In Logan, W. W., editor: Breast carcinoma—the radiologist's expanded role, New York, 1977, John Wiley & Sons, Inc.

Holleb, A. I.: The technique of breast examination, CA **16:**7, 1966.

Holleb, A. I.: The technique of breast examination. In Holleb, A. I., editor: Breast cancer; early and late, Chicago, 1970, Year Book Medical Publishers, Inc.

Holleb, A. I.: Restoring confidence in mammography, CA **26:**376, 1976.

Horwitz, K. B., McGuire, W. L., Pearson, O. H., and others: Predicting response to endocrine therapy in human breast cancer; a hypothesis, Science **189:**726, 1975.

Huggins, C., and Bergenstal, D.: Inhibition of human mammary and prostatic cancers by adrenalectomy, Cancer Res. **12:**134, 1952.

Hunter, R. L., Ferguson, D. J., and Coppleson, L. W.: Survival with mammary cancer related to the interaction of germinal cancer hyperplasia and sinus histiocytosis in axillary and internal mammary lymph nodes, Cancer **36:**528, 1975.

Jensen, E. V., Block, G. E., Smith, S., and others: Estrogen receptors and breast cancer response to adrenalectomy: prediction of response in cancer therapy, Natl. Cancer Inst. Monogr. **34:**55, 1971.

Jensen, E. V., Smith, S., and DeSombre, E.: Hormone dependency in breast cancer, J. Steroid Biochem. **7:**911, 1976.

Johnson, R. E.: Treatment of breast cancer, N. Engl. J. Med. **291:**1188, 1974.

Jones, S. E., Durie, B. G. M., and Salmon, S. E.: Combination chemotherapy with adriamycin and cyclophosphamide for advanced breast cancer, Cancer **36:**90, 1975.

Kiang, D., and Kennedy, B.: Estrogen receptor assay in the differential diagnosis of adenocarcinoma, J.A.M.A. **238:**32, 1977.

Leis, H. P., Jr.: Diagnosis and treatment of breast lesions, New York; 1970, Medical Examination Publishing Co., Inc.

Leis, H. P., Jr.: Clinical diagnosis of breast cancer, J. Reprod. Med. **14:**231, 1975.

Leis, H. P., Jr.: Risk factors in breast cancer, AORN J. **22:**723, 1975.

Leis, H. P., Jr.: Breast lesions with malignant transformation potential. In Proceedings of the Nineteenth European Federation Congress of the International College of Surgeons, Amsterdam, 1976, American College of Surgeons.

Leis, H. P., Jr., Pilnik, S., and Black, M. M.: Diagnosis of breast cancer, Hosp. Med. **10:**33, 1974.

Lester, R. G.: Risk versus benefit in mammography, Radiology **124:**1, 1977.

Lipsett, M. B.: Hormones, nutrition, and cancer, Cancer Res. **35:**3359, 1975.

Logan, W. W.: Breast carcinoma—the radiologist's role in a non-screening situation, presented at the Radiological Society of North America, Chicago, December 1977.

Logan, W. W.: Overview of the radiologist's role in breast cancer detection. In Logan, W. W., editor: Breast carcinoma—the radiologist's expanded role, New York, 1977, John Wiley & Sons, Inc.

Logan, W. W., and Muntz, E. P. M., editors: Reduced dose mammography, New York, 1979, Masson Publishing USA, Inc.

Lyon, J. L., Klauber, M. R., Gardner, J. W., and others: Cancer incidence in Mormons and non-Mormons; Utah 1966-1970, N. Engl. J. Med. **294:**129, 1976.

Mammography Survey by American College of Radiology, September 1976.

Martin, J. W.: Xeromammography—an improved diagnostic method; review of 250 biopsied cases, Am. J. Roentgenol. **117:**90, 1973.

McGuire, W. L., Carbone, P. P., and Vokmer, E. P.: Estrogen receptors in human breast cancer, New York, 1975, Raven Press.

McGuire, W. L., Horwitz, K., Pearson, O., and Segaloff, A.: Current status of estrogen and progesterone receptors in breast cancer, Cancer **39:**2934, 1977.

Milbrath, J. R.: Does thermography aid in breast cancer detection? In Logan, W. W., editor: Breast carcinoma—the radiologist's expanded role, New York, 1977, John Wiley & Sons, Inc.

Milbrath, J. R.: Reduced dose xeromammography. In Logan, W. W., editor: Breast carcinoma—the radiologist's expanded role, New York, 1977, John Wiley & Sons, Inc.

Muntz, E. P.: Electrostatic imaging in mammography. In Logan, W. W., editor: Breast carcinoma—the radiologist's expanded role, New York, 1977, John Wiley & Sons, Inc.

Ostrum, B. J., Becker, W., and Isard, H. J.: Low dose mammography, Radiology **109:**323, 1973.

Rapp, F.: Viruses as an etiologic factor in cancer, Semin. Oncol. **3:**49, 1976.

Ravdin, R. G., Lewison, E. F., Slack, N. H., and others: Results of a clinical trial concerning the worth of prophylactic oophorectomy for breast carcinoma, Surg. Gynecol. Obstet. **131:**1055, 1970.

Roberts, J. G., Gravell, I. H., Baum, M., and others: Evaluation of radiography and isotopic scintigraphy for detecting skeletal metastases in breast cancer, Lancet **1:**237, 1976.

Schottenfeld, D.: Epidemiology of breast cancer, Clin. Bull. **5:**135, 1976.

Seidman, H.: Statistical and epidemiological data on cancer of the breast, New York, 1972, American Cancer Society, Inc.

Silverberg, E., and Holleb, A. I.: Cancer statistics 1975—twenty-five year cancer survey, CA **25:**2, 1975.

Simon, N., and Silverstone, S. M.: Radiation as a cause of breast cancer, Bull. N.Y. Acad. Med. **52:**741, 1976.

Stark, A. M.: The value of thermography as one modality in a screening project for breast cancer. In Logan, W. W., editor: Breast carcinoma—the radiologist's expanded role, New York, 1977, John Wiley & Sons, Inc.

Strax, P.: Results of mass screening for breast cancer in 50,000 examinations, Cancer **37:**30, 1976.

Tagman, H.: Antiestrogen in treatment of breast cancer, Cancer **39:**2959, 1977.

Tormey, D. C.: Combined chemotherapy and surgery in breast cancer; a review, Cancer **36:**881, 1975.

Torres, J. E., and Mickal, A.: Carcinoma of the breast in pregnancy, Clin. Obstet. Gynecol. **18:**219, 1975.

Wagai, T.: Ultrasound examination of the breast. In Logan, W. W., editor: Breast carcinoma—the radiologist's expanded role, New York, 1977, John Wiley & Sons, Inc.

Westberg, S. V.: Prognosis of breast cancer for pregnant and nursing women; a clinical statistical study, Acta Obstet. Gynecol. Scand. **25:**(4)1, 1946.

Wolfe, J. N.: Developments in mammography, Am. J. Obstet. Gynecol. **124:**312, 1976.

CHAPTER FIFTEEN

Cancer in pregnancy

One can hardly conceive of a more emotional set of circumstances than a pregnant woman discovered to have a malignancy. Many issues are immediately apparent. Is termination of the pregnancy necessary? Will malignancy or the therapy for the malignancy affect the fetus? Should therapy be deferred and initiated at the termination of the pregnant state? The answers to these questions are often arrived at with great difficulty. Fortunately, the peak incidence years for most malignant diseases do not overlap the peak reproductive years. Thus, as with any unusual situation that physicians rarely encounter, clear therapeutic decisions are not readily at hand. On the other hand, a significant number of well-studied reviews have been published and can provide some guidance in this dilemma. The largest series ever

376

reported was that of Barber and Brunschwig in 1968, which consisted of 700 cases of cancer in pregnancy. The most common malignancies in that series were breast tumors, leukemia and lymphomas as a group, melanomas, gynecologic cancer, and bone tumors, in that order.

The enormous physiologic changes of pregnancy suggest many possible influences on the malignant state. First, it has been assumed by many that malignancies arising in tissues and organs influenced by the endocrine system are possibly subject to exacerbation with pregnancy, and this has often been erroneously extrapolated to a recommendation for "therapeutic" abortion. Second, the anatomic and physiologic changes of pregnancy may obscure the subtle changes of an early neoplasm. Third, the increased vascularity as well as lymphatic dainage may contribute to early dissemination of the malignant process. Although all of these hypotheses are interesting, the validity of each is quite variable, even within the same organ.

PELVIC MALIGNANCIES
Malignancies of the vulva

Less than 50 cases of cancer of the vulva associated with pregnancy have been reported in the literature. The majority of these are invasive epidermoid carcinomas, with melanoma, sarcoma, and adenoid cystic adenocarcinoma being the next most common. The majority of patients have been between 25 and 35 years of age; the youngest patient diagnosed was 17. With the increasing frequency of the diagnosis of carcinoma in situ of the vulva, the occurrence of preinvasive disease with pregnancy is today not at all uncommon. As is the practice with cervical intraepithelial neoplasia, therapy for the vulvar counterpart is delayed until the postpartum period.

Vulvar malignancy diagnosed during the first and second trimesters is usually treated by radical vulvectomy with bilateral groin dissection some time after the fourteenth week of pregnancy When the diagnosis is made in the third trimester, many recommended a wide local excision with definitive surgery being postponed until the postpartum period. Since the disease occurs more frequently in the lower socioeconomic groups, where prenatal care is often not sought, many of these cases are diagnosed postpartum or at the time of delivery itself. In this group of patients definitive therapy should be commenced within 1 week of delivery in order to accomplish it during the same hospitalization as the delivery. The pregnant state does not appear to significantly alter the course of the malignant process; survival of these patients stage for stage is similar to that of nonpregnant patients.

There have been several reports of patients treated for carcinoma of the vulva with radical vulvectomy and bilateral inguinal lymphadenectomy who subsequently became pregnant and delivered normally. The decision on whether the patient should deliver vaginally or by cesarean section rests with the obstetrician but is heavily influenced by the state of the postsurgical vulva. In most instances the vulva is soft and would not impede a vaginal delivery. In other instances there may be a high degree of vaginal stenosis or other fibrosis that would suggest the advisability of cesarean section.

Vaginal tumors

The diagnosis of vaginal cancer during pregnancy is exceptionally uncommon, even with the recent rash of clear-cell adenocarcinoma of the vagina in DES-exposed offspring. Although all of these DES cancers have occurred in women under the age of 26, the appearance in association with pregnancy has been fortunately rare. Primary squamous cell carcinoma of the vagina discovered during pregnancy is exceptionally uncommon. A few scattered reports of sarcoma botryoides of the cervix and vagina in pregnancy are recorded. When these sarcomatous lesions occur in the upper half of the vagina with or without cervical involvement, the most appropriate therapy has been a radical hysterectomy, upper vaginectomy, and bilateral pelvic lymphadenectomy followed by postoperative adjuvant chemotherapy. Treatment of clear-cell adenocarcinoma of the cervix and upper vagina is surgically very similar. In both instances the pregnancy is disregarded if the patient is in the first or early second trimester. Should the pregnancy be further along, the decision for appropriate time of intervention would, of course, depend on the preferences of the patient and the physician. In instances where there is extensive involvement of the vagina by any lesion, including squamous cell carcinoma, one should seriously consider evacuation of the uterus via a hysterotomy or cesarean section and commencement of appropriate radiation therapy. Radical surgery appears to be appropriate only for the early lesions involving the upper vagina and/or cervix. Prognosis appears to be unaffected by the pregnancy.

Cervical cancer

A diversity of opinion abounds in the literature concerning the cause and effect of carcinoma of the cervix in the pregnant patient. It has been said by some that carcinoma of the cervix prevents pregnancy, whereas others claim that pregnancy prevents carcinoma of the cervix. Some reports emphasize the fact that pregnancy accelerates carcinoma of the cervix, whereas other authors believe that pregnancy actually slows the growth of carcinoma of the cervix. The younger a patient is when carcinoma of the cervix is found is thought to be a good prognostic indicator in some people's opinion, whereas others feel that youth is a detriment. High estrogen levels during pregnancy have been considered to predispose to cancer of the cervix by some, whereas others believe that the high estrogen content actually controls carcinoma of the cervix. Numerous articles in the literature state that radiotherapy is the treatment of choice for this lesion, whereas others feel that primary radical surgical therapy is the best treatment. These controversies have been well outlined by Waldrop and Palmer from the Roswell Park Memorial Institute and by Bosch and Marcial from the I. Gonzales Martinez Oncology Hospital in Puerto Rico. Unfortunately, these controversies have been perpetuated over the years. One reason for these different opinions may be that this lesion is somewhat infrequent; it is the unusual report in the literature that contains over 30 or 40 cases.

Since the peak age incidence for carcinoma of the cervix is in the mid-forties, one would not expect many cervical cancer patients to be concomitantly pregnant.

Reports in the literature show an overall incidence ranging from one to 13 cases in 10,000 pregnancies. Reports from large maternity hospitals give an average incidence of one cervical cancer per 2,500 pregnancies. Reports from large cancer centers reveal that about 1% of the women with carcinoma of the cervix are pregnant at the time of diagnosis. In the younger patients (under 50 years of age) with carcinoma of the cervix, however, Creasman and associates found that 9% were pregnant or had been pregnant within 6 months when a diagnosis of carcinoma of the cervix was established. This figure may be distorted by the referral nature of the institution from which they were reporting.

Carcinoma of the cervix is curable, particularly if it is diagnosed and treated in the early stages. The efficacy of the Pap smear in detecting early cervical disease is well documented and is an acceptable part of routine examination of the female patient. Since most women, and particularly young women, do not have an annual pelvic examination and Pap smear, pregnancy does offer an added opportunity for cancer surveillance.

Vaginal bleeding is the most common symptom seen in carcinoma of the cervix whether or not the patient is pregnant. Unfortunately, many times this symptom appears only with far advanced disease. Thirty percent of Creasman and associates' patients had no symptoms when the diagnosis of cervical cancer was established. When bleeding does occur during pregnancy, this symptom must be investigated and not automatically attributed to the pregnancy. Examination during the first trimester will not lead to abortion. Third-trimester bleeding can be adequately assessed in the oeprating room as a double set-up procedure.

The methods for diagnosis and treatment of this lesion in the pregnant or postpartum woman are the same as in the nonpregnant patient. Many times visual inspection is all that is needed for diagnosis of this malignancy.

The Pap smear is extremely accurate in detecting cervical lesions, particularly in the early nonclinical stages. In over half of the asymptomatic patients in the study by Creasman and associates, the only abnormality noted was that of an abnormal Pap smear. Colposcopically directed cervical biopsy is extremely accurate in diagnosing invasive squamous cell carcinoma of the cervix. The cone biopsy is needed only when a microinvasive lesion is found and a frankly invasive lesion must be ruled out.

The age range of patients was from 19 to 46 years with a mean of 33 years in Creasman and associates' series. In this group of patients, the age when the diagnosis of carcinoma of the cervix was made had no influence on the prognosis of the lesion within a given stage. This is compatible with other reported series previously mentioned.

For many years, parity has been considered to be an important factor in the cause of carcinoma of the cervix. Although early coital activity appears to be the important criterion as a possible etiologic factor, certainly early pregnancy and multiparity usually go hand in hand. The average parity of Creasman and associates' study group was 5.4. In the 1,307 patients in the same age group who had carcinoma of the cervix and were not pregnant, the average parity was only 3.5. It did not appear that a more advanced lesion was found with increasing parity, and prognosis was not related to parity as long as the patients were compared within a given stage.

Therapy for these lesions is outlined in Chapter 3. Choices for therapy depend on the stage of the pregnancy and the desires of the patient and the physician. In multiple reports there has been little difference in maternal survival rate if the pregnancy was terminated by cesarean section or vaginal delivery. This was borne out in the case experience from M. D. Anderson Hospital. The same appears to be true of fetal survival. This is not to be considered an endorsement of vaginal delivery as the delivery of choice in carcinoma of the cervix, because considerable difficulties can be encountered with this mode of delivery, particularly if there are large lesions. In most of the patients who do deliver vaginally, unfortunately, diagnosis of carcinoma is made several weeks postpartum. The major indications for cesarean section in patients with large cervical lesions are the bleeding and infection that can result from a vaginal delivery when the cervix is heavily involved with a malignant process.

As stated previously, intraepithelial neoplasia of the cervix should be treated expectantly during pregnancy. Adequate colposcopic examination with colposcopically directed biopsies is usually sufficient to rule out invasive disease (Fig. 15-1). Cone biopsy should be avoided if no more than preinvasive disease remains. The patient should then be reevaluated 6 weeks postpartum.

Surgical therapy can be instituted in the first trimester or in the early second trimester in the form of radical hysterectomy plus pelvic lymphadenectomy with the fetus in utero. In the late second trimester or early third trimester every consideration should be given to waiting until the baby is reasonably mature and then proceeding with a cesarean section, radical hysterectomy, and pelvic lymphadenectomy at the same operation. If the diagnosis is made during the post-partum period, a radical hysterectomy with bilateral node dissection is done 4 to 6 weeks after deliv-

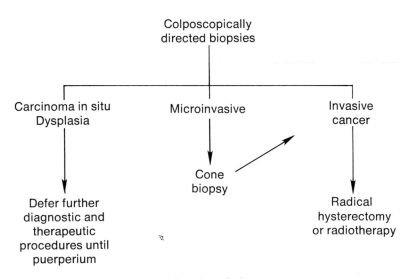

Fig. 15-1. Abnormal cytologic findings in pregnancy.

ery. The above recommendations are, of course, applicable only to stage I and early stage IIA lesions. In addition, an option for radiotherapy exists in these early lesions and in all more advanced lesions. The recommended treatment plan is outlined in Chapter 3.

Uterine cancer

Endometrial carcinoma in conjunction with pregnancy is extremely rare. In 1972, Karlen and associates reviewed the literature since 1900, summarized five acceptable cases, and added a sixth. Another case was added by Sandstrom and associates in 1979. This was noted as an incidental finding at therapeutic abortion. When endometrial carcinoma does occur with pregnancy it is usually focal, well differentiated, and minimally invasive or not invasive. In the report by Karlen and associates, four of the six women were over age 35. The recommended therapy is total hysterectomy with bilateral salpingo-oophorectomy and adjuvant radiotherapy where indicated.

Leiomyosarcoma and carcinosarcoma have also been reported during pregnancy. They are usually incidental findings noted in surgical specimens.

Fallopian tube cancer

The mean age of cancer of the fallopian tube is between 50 and 55 years. Thus, the possibility of its presence in pregnancy is extremely remote. There have been reported cases associated with pregnancy, and in those instances the neoplasm is usually unilateral and most often adenocarcinoma. The clinical presentation of carcinoma of the tube is quite variable and nonspecific even without an associated pregnancy. The usual watery, blood-tinged vaginal discharge would be obviated in pregnancy because at 12 weeks' gestation the communication between the uterine cavity and the fallopian tube is blocked. In most instances the diagnosis is established at laparotomy, and the treatment is total abdominal hysterectomy with bilateral salpingo-oophorectomy and postoperative radiation therapy or chemotherapy, depending on the operative findings and the residual disease following surgery. Several instances are reported in the literature of incidental findings of carcinoma in situ of the tube noted in specimens submitted following postpartum tubal ligation. In these instances a total abdominal hysterectomy with bilateral salpingo-oophorectomy has been recommended.

Ovarian cancer

Ovarian tumors are relatively infrequent complications of pregnancy, although when they do occur, they present challenging problems in diagnosis and management. The management of ovarian tumors in pregnancy is crucial because of the various complications that may develop, such as pelvic impaction, obstructed labor, torsion of the ovarian pedicle, hemorrhage into the tumor, rupture of the cyst, infection, and malignancy. Malignancy, although relatively infrequent and least acute of the complications in the pregnant patient, should always be foremost in the clinician's mind. Eastman and Hellman quoted an incidence of ovarian cysts in pregnancy of one in 81, and Grimes and associates stated that in one out of 328 pregnancies a cyst large enough to be hazardous is present.

Most cysts found in pregnant patients are follicular or corpus luteum cysts and are usually no more than 3 to 5 cm in diameter. Over 90% of these functional cysts will disappear as pregnancy progresses and are undetectable by the fourteenth week of gestation. If the cyst remains unchanged or increases in size the patient should be explored. Carcinoma of the ovary in pregnancy is relatively rare (the incidence is 2% to 5% of all ovarian neoplasms found in pregnancy).

The most pressing problems associated with ovarian tumors in pregnancy are the initial diagnosis and the differential diagnosis. When the tumor is palpable within the pelvis it must be differentiated from a retroverted pregnant uterus, a pedunculated uterine fibroid, carcinoma of the rectosigmoid, pelvic kidney, or a uterine congenital abnormality (e.g., accessory uterine horn). In the latter half of pregnancy, ovarian tumors are particularly difficult to diagnose (Fig. 15-2). As the tumor ascends into the abdominal cavity and beyond the reach of vaginal examination, abdominal palpation becomes the chief method of diagnosis. Ultrasonography is particularly helpful in this situation.

Torsion is particularly common in pregnancy, with a reported incidence of between 10% and 15% of ovarian tumors in pregnancy undergoing this complication. Most torsions occur when the uterus is rising at a rapid rate (8 to 16 weeks) or when the uterus in involuting (in the puerperium). About 60% of the cases occur at the beginning of the pregnancy and the remaining 40% in the puerperium. The usual sequence of events is sudden lower abdominal pain, nausea, vomiting, and, in some cases, shocklike symptoms. The abdomen is tense and tender, and there is rebound tenderness with guarding.

In many instances the presence of an ovarian tumor may not be suspected until delivery. The large uterus obscures the growth of the ovarian neoplasm. The tumor may be growing in the abdomen behind the large uterus and may not fall back into the cul-de-sac until it is very large. With a mechanical obstruction of the birth canal, exploratory laporotomy is indicated for both delivery of the baby and management of the ovarian neoplasm. Allowing labor to proceed with an ovarian neoplasm causing obstruction of the birth canal may result in rupture of the ovarian cyst. Even if the cyst is not ruptured, the trauma of labor may cause hemorrhage into the tumor followed by necrosis and suppuration.

Ovarian cancer in pregnancy is fortunately quite rare since the disease is most common in the age group over 50. The incidence for all pregnancies is from one in 8,000 to one in 20,000 deliveries. The diagnosis is usually fortuitous; the patient undergoes laparotomy for an adnexal mass that is subsequently found to be malignant. In many instances, the close observation of the pregnant patient has led to the discovery of a lesion in the earlier stages. If an ovarian malignancy is found at the time of abdominal exploration, the surgeon's first obligation is to properly stage the patient as outlined in Chapter 11. In the young pregnant patient one would expect

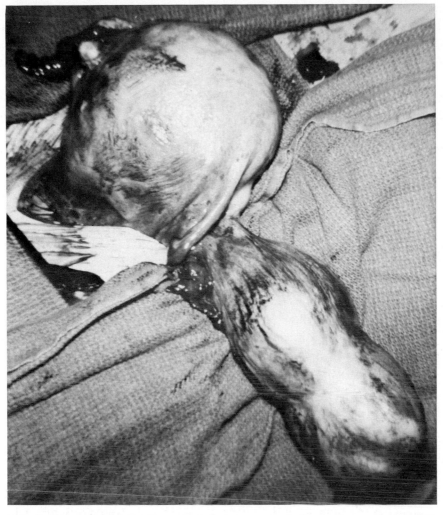

Fig. 15-2. Benign cystic teratoma, gross appearance at cesarean section (undiagnosed, preoperative).

to find germ cell tumors such as dysgerminoma, embryonal carcinoma, immature teratoma, and endodermal sinus tumor. Epithelial cancers such as papillary serous cystadenocarcinoma and papillary mucinous cystadenocarcinoma are more common as the patient approaches 40 and should be treated in the manner that is appropriate for the stage of the disease regardless of the pregnancy. Stage I lesions may be treated conservatively as outlined in Chapter 10. Patients with more advanced lesions should not be encouraged to follow a conservative treatment plan. The pregnant state does not appear to adversely affect the prognosis for the patient with an ovarian malignancy.

Fortunately, ovarian germ cell neoplasms occurring in pregnancy are usually benign. Dermoid cysts are by far the most common neoplastic cysts found in pregnancy. Attempts should be made to remove these in the early part of the second trimester whenever they are recognized early in pregnancy. Other ovarian germ cell neoplasms that are commonly found are malignant teratoma, endodermal sinus tumor, and embryonal carcinoma. Functioning ovarian tumors such as granulosa-stromal cell tumors and Sertoli-Leydig cell tumors are also found rarely. It is recommended that the management of these be similar to that in the nonpregnant patient.

In summary, the problem of ovarian tumor in pregnancy is quite simple. One must have a high index of suspicion, make the diagnosis early, and treat promptly. The difficulty arises when both patient and physician resist abdominal exploration during pregnancy because of fear of precipitating fetal wastage. However, the potential danger to the mother far exceeds the imagined danger to the child. Most of the difficulties seen with ovarian tumors are those of omission rather than commission. The probability of ovarian cancer must be kept foremost in the minds of physicians caring for these patients.

Other pelvic malignancies

Cancer of the bladder has been reported in pregnancy. About 95% of the cases are epithelial and start in the region of the trigone and spread by direct extension, by the lymphatics, and, less commonly, by the hematogenous route. Metastasis to the bone is common, mostly to the lumbar spine and pelvis. The prognosis depends on the extent of the disease. Superficial and well-differentiated tumors can be managed by local fulguration, whereas others require partial or total cystectomy for cure. Radiation therapy has also been used for lesions occurring in this area. It is obvious that the fetus in utero technically complicates the picture as far as radiation is concerned. In all cases the decision as to the mode of delivery must be individualized depending on the length of gestation as well as patient and physician preference.

Seventy percent of all colorectal cancer is found in the distal colon and rectum. Fortunately, this is a rare complication of pregnancy. Management of these tumors in pregnancy is the same as in the nonpregnant state. The gravid uterus will cause variations only in the mechanics of handling the bowel, not in the principle. Colorectal cancer found in the first trimester generally should be treated as if no pregnancy were present. Radical surgery at this stage is frequently followed by abortion. The tubes, ovaries, and uterus may be resected as dictated by the findings at the time of laparotomy. From 12 to 20 weeks, Barber and Brunschwig advocate routine hysterectomy to provide better exposure for an adequate margin of resection around the rectosigmoid tumors. Oophorectomy is recommended for all low-lying colonic tumors because of the high incidence of metastasis to the ovaries. The treatment of colorectal cancer during the third trimester is controversial. Some surgeons believe that with adequate exposure the neoplasm can be removed without disturbing the uterus and its content. Others believe that the resection should be carried out 2 weeks after cesarean section when the patient has regained her strength and when the uterus and the vasculature of the pelvis are less troublesome to the surgeon.

The malignant process (both bladder and bowel cancer) does not appear to be significantly influenced by pregnancy itself. The prognosis for the pregnant patient stage for stage is equivalent to her nonpregnant control.

Retroperitoneal sarcomas occur coincident with pregnancy and present technical difficulties for removal. Most of these lesions are neurofibrosarcomas or similar lesions, and their course is greatly dependent on the grade of the neoplasm. Therapy for low-grade sarcomas can be deferred to the postpartum period, when resection should be technically much easier. High-grade lesions have a very poor prognosis, and therapy must be individualized depending on the length of gestation and patient preference.

CHEMOTHERAPY

Many cytotoxic agents useful in chemotherapy for malignant neoplasms are teratogenic in both animals and humans receiving these drugs early in pregnancy. The use of these drugs often evokes moral and philosophical as well as medical and emotional decisions. Both mother and fetus are at risk. All antineoplastic drugs are theoretically teratogenic and mutagenic; their use can result in abortion, fetal death, malformations, and growth retardation. The long-term effect on the fetus is unknown. The problem of long-term observation has been dramatically emphasized by the occurrence of adenocarcinoma of the vagina in young women exposed to diethylstilbestrol in utero during the first trimester of pregnancy. A similar devastating long-term effect is possible with chemotherapeutic agents being used in pregnancy. These theoretical dangers to the fetus must be weighed against the possible detrimental effect to the mother of withholding these agents.

Most of the available data suggesting the teratogenicity and mutagenicity of chemotherapeutic agents has been derived from experiments in laboratory animals. These experiments only indicate potential danger to the human fetus. All chemotherapeutic agents profoundly affect rapidly growing tissues, and a high rate of cell division is characteristic of the fetus. Based on this reasoning, one would expect a much greater effect than is actually observed. Unquestionably, the first trimester of pregnancy is when the fetus is most vulnerable to cancer chemotherapeutic agents. There are two aspects to the problem of fetal damage: (1) death of the fetus, and (2) induction of fetal abnormalities inadequate to cause fetal death. Sokal and Lessman collected 50 reports of pregnant women who received anticancer chemotherapy. In their series there were 8 instances of fetal abnormalities, 16 spontaneous abortions, and 7 therapeutic abortions. They noted that no obvious fetal malformations were observed among those women who received chemotherapy only in the second and third trimesters of pregnancy. Although serious congenital anomalies and spontaneous abortions did occur in those patients receiving chemotherapy in the first trimester of pregnancy, such complications were not inevitable. The lack of adequate observation of the long-term status of the fetus or infant prevents any definite conclusions as to the relative safety or danger of anticancer chemotherapy during pregnancy, even in the second and third trimesters. It is surprising how often the detailed status of the fetus is not mentioned in available reports. Often the infant is described as being "normal" with few, if any, details on the physical or laboratory profile of the baby. Long-term observation is necessary in order to establish normalcy, since many of the defects may not be obvious on inspection and may emerge as derangements of growth, development, function, reproduction, and heredity.

Nicholson collected 185 cases of human pregnancies during anticancer chemotherapy. Of 110 women who received such treatment during the first trimester, the status of the fetus or infant was recorded in only 68 patients, where there were 15 instances of fetal abnormalities. Ten of these women received folic acid antagonists, two had taken busulfan, and one each had received 6-mercaptopurine, chlorambucil, and cyclophosphamide. No malformations were reported in the fetuses of 75 women who received chemotherapy during the second and third trimesters of pregnancy, although the status of the fetus or the infant is recorded in only 73 instances.

There is no doubt that the antifolics aminopterin and methotrexate, when given in the first trimester of pregnancy, almost invariably result in spontaneous abortion or an abnormal fetus. These drugs should not be given to the pregnant woman in the first trimester unless there is life-threatening disease that can be helped by the drug. If an antifolic is used and the mother does not have a spontaneous abortion, therapeutic abortion should be seriously considered. There is a small amount of data that would seem to indicate that aminopterin and methotrexate do not cause harm when given after the first trimester of pregnancy.

Although most of the other cancer chemotherapeutic agents, including 6-mercaptopurine, azathioprine, 5-fluorouracil, alkylating agents, vinca alkaloids, and procarbazine, are known to be teratogenic in animal experiments, surprisingly there have been very few case reports of fetal abnormalities resulting from the use of these agents in the first trimester of pregnancy other than the previously mentioned effects of antifolics. On the other hand, there have been isolated reports of fetal abnormalities with every drug. Thus, all cancer chemotherapeutic agents should be considered teratogenic and avoided in the first trimester of pregnancy if at all possible.

Although the alkylating agents are well-known teratogens in animal experiments, the dose regimen for treating humans is apparently such that the incidence of fetal abnormalities is low. However, since fetal abnormalities have occurred and are an ever present danger, alkylating agents should not be used in the first trimester of pregnancy unless the patient's life is threatened.

Of equal importance are the possible long-term gonadal effects of cytostatic agents, both on men and women. Some of the best evidence on the possible gonadal effects of these drugs can be found in the studies of reproduction following renal transplantation. These patients are maintained on immunosuppressive therapy with azathioprine (Imuran) and prednisone. The literature concerning the effects of this therapy on reproductive capacity and fetal outcome is mixed, with both optimistic and pessimistic reports. Mothers who become pregnant while on immunosuppression appear to deliver healthy babies barring prematurity and other obstetric problems. In addition, Penn and associates reported on 19 men on immunosuppressive therapies who fathered 23 children. Three were not delivered at the time of the report, one spontaneous abortion occurred, and there were 19 live births, only one of the infants having an anomaly (menigomyelocele).

Van Theil reported on 88 pregnancies in 50 women who had previously been treated for gestational trophoblastic disease with chemotherapeutic agents. No increase in fetal wastage, congenital anomalies, or complicated pregnancies were noted, suggesting that these drugs do not damage human oocytes in the doses and time period used. The possibility that recessive mutations were induced but were undetected could not be evaluated definitively and was recognized by the authors.

RADIATION THERAPY

The primary dilemma that faces both surgeon and obstetrician regarding radiation therapy during pregnancy is what the effect on the baby will be. Will irradiation of the fetal and maternal gonads contribute to reproductive difficulties in the future? The embryo undoubtedly represents the most radiosensitive stage in human life. This radiosensitivity is a combination of factors: (1) many of the cells in the embryo are differentiating, and differentiating cells are relatively more sensitive; (2) there is a high rate of mitotic activity in the cells of the embryo, and the mitotic phase of the cell is the most radiosensitive period in the life cycle of the cell; and (3) if the embryonic cell is genetically altered or killed during its development, the adult form will either be deformed or will not survive.

There are varying sensitivities within the variety of tissues in the human embryo. Various abnormalities have been attributed to irradiation of the embryo, with microcephaly and associated conditions being most often reported. Other abnormalities of the central nervous system, the eye, and the skeleton have also been ascribed to irradiation. However, an accurate prediction of incidence with regard to dose has not been possible. It is widely accepted that irradiation of human beings, especially their gonads, has certain undesirable effects. Any irradiation of gonadal tissue involves genetic damage, since the photons cause gene mutation or chromosome breakage with subsequent translocation, loss, deletion, and abnormal fusion of chromosomal material. Basically the effect is additive and cumulative, and generally the changes are in direct proportion to the total dose. Unfortunately there is no threshold for genetic damage, and even relatively small doses of irradiation can cause gene mutations, most of which can be harmful. It is estimated that 1 rad of radiation produces five mutations in every 1 million genes exposed. Fortunately, most mutants are recessive. Mutant effects are not seen in the first generation and may not be visible for many generations until two people with the same mutation mate. Most estimates of genetic damage are empirical, but it is estimated that to double the rate of gene mutation 25 to 150 rads must be given from birth to the end of reproductive age. Constant changes are being made in what is considered the permissible body dose of radiation. Some authorities cite 14 rads in the first 30 years of life, whereas others cite 10 rads or less as the maximum. This includes both medical and background sources.

From the standpoint of the fetus, the most sensitive period is day 18 through 38. After day 40, primary organ systems have developed and much larger doses of x-rays or gamma rays are necessary to produce serious abnormalities. There are three periods of fetal development that are highly significant from a radiologic point of view:

1. Preimplantation. In this phase, radiation produces an all-or-none effect in that it either destroys the fertilized egg or does not affect it significantly.

2. Organ system formation. This is the period from day 18 through 38, when doses of 10 to 40 rads may cause visceral organ or somatic damage. Microcephaly, anencephaly, eye damage, growth retardation, spina bifida, and foot damage are reported with doses of 4 rads or less. Cause and effect have not been proved with these lower dosages.

3. Period of fetal development after day 40, when larger doses are prone to produce external malformations but organ systems, especially the nervous system, may still be damaged. Doses over 50 rads may produce significant mental retardation and microcephaly even in the second trimester (Fig. 15-3).

Most radiologic diagnostic procedures should be avoided during the first and second trimesters of pregnancy. The exposure to the fetus and gonads will vary with the procedure performed and the precautions taken. A chest film will result in an

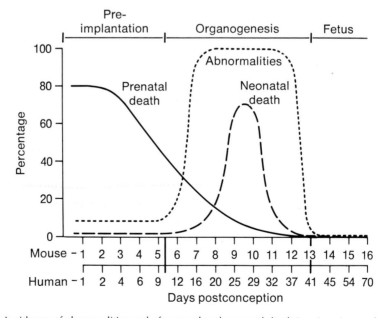

Fig. 15-3. Incidence of abnormalities and of prenatal and neonatal death in mice given a dose of 200 R at various times postfertilization. The lower scale consists of Rugh's estimates of the equivalent stages for the human embryo. (From Hall, E. J.: Radiobiology for the radiologist, New York, 1973, Harper & Row, Publishers, Inc.; adapted from Russell, L. B., and others: J. Cell Comp. Physiol. Suppl. 1, 1954, and Rugh, R.: Am. J. Roentgenol. **87:**559, 1962.)

1 CXR PLATE — 300 M RADS

exposure of 300 millirads per plate, whereas a barium enema will result in a total dose to the gonads and pelvis of 6 rads. In a pregnant patient, the barium enema is obviously a greater threat because of the greater dosage and the area irradiated. Any radiation therapy to the abdomen required during pregnancy should be postponed until after delivery if at all possible. There is evidence to suggest that even an exposure of 3 to 5 rads can result in an increase in benign or malignant tumors in the child after birth.

EXTRAPELVIC MALIGNANCIES
Hodgkin's disease

Hodgkin's disease commonly affects young people. It is now being cured and controlled for long periods with irradiation and chemotherapy. Hodgkin's disease in pregnancy occurs in approximately one in 6,000 deliveries. Barry and associates reported on 347 patients with Hodgkin's disease and yielded a total of 112 pregnancies. Many of the women in the study with active disease during pregnancy had disease activity above the diaphragm, and this was treated with external radiation while shielding the abdomen. Standard doses were given without apparent adverse effects to the fetus. Most reports have suggested that the onset of Hodgkin's disease during pregnancy does not adversely affect survival. Chemotherapy and radiation therapy to the abdomen can usually be postponed until the pregnancy has terminated. The drugs commonly used for Hodgkin's disease are contraindicated in the first and second trimesters of pregnancy and are preferably withheld until the postpartum period. The amazing successes recently achieved with early stages of this disease allow a lot more flexibility and improved regard for the fetus. Pregnancy itself does not appear to adversely affect the course of the disease, and interruption of pregnancy during the course of the disease is not strongly indicated.

The importance of staging in Hodgkin's disease was recognized by Peters as early as 1950, when he devised the first clinical staging classification. Then lymphography made possible the earlier detection of retroperitoneal lymph node involvement, and it became important to distinguish two subgroups: those with widespread disease confined to lymphatic organs and those with spread of disease beyond the lymph nodes, thymus, spleen, and Waldeyer's ring to one or more extralymphatic organs or tissues. The latter group is now recognized as stage IV disease (Table 15-1). Thorough staging of the pregnant patient is significantly compromised without termination of the pregnancy by one means or another (Table 15-2). The major difference in the workup of the pregnant patient lies with the last three diagnostic procedures given in Table 15-2. In recent years surgical staging has gained great popularity in Hodgkin's disease. Staging of the pregnant patient some time after the fourteenth week of pregnancy is quite feasible and often avoids the necessity of many of the diagnostic techniques that might be harmful to the fetus, such as lower extremity lymphangiogram, intravenous pyelography, and bone and liver scans. Splenectomy is often performed at these staging procedures, and no contraindication in pregnancy is presently known.

Table 15-1. Clinical staging of Hodgkin's disease

Stage I	Disease localized to a single lymph node, or a single lymph node–bearing area, either above or below the diaphragm
	IE Disease confined to a single focus in an extralymphatic organ other than liver or bone marrow
Stage II	Disease confined to two or more lymph node–bearing areas on the same side of the diaphragm
	IIE Involvement of one or more lymph node regions on either side of the diaphragm, plus a localized solitary area of contiguous spread to an extralymphatic organ other than liver or bone marrow
Stage III	Disease confined to lymph nodes, but involving both sides of the diaphragm
	IIIS Stage III involvement of the spleen
	IIIE Stage III with a solitary area of contiguous spread to an extralymphatic organ other than liver or bone marrow
	IIISE Stage IIIS plus IIIE
Stage IV	Disease with disseminated extranodal involvement, e.g., to liver, lung, bone marrow, skin

Table 15-2. Staging workup

1. Careful clinical history
2. Thorough physical examination with careful description of all superficial lymph node areas
3. Roentgenographic examination of chest, including tomograms if necessary
4. Liver function tests, particularly alkaline phosphatase and sulfobromophthalein (Bromsulphalein) excretion
5. Biopsy of bone marrow, needle or open
6. Complete blood counts and urinalysis
7. Serum electrophoresis
8. Lower extremity lymphangiograms
9. Intravenous pyelography
10. Bone and liver scans in symptomatic patients

The feature of the disease most helpful in selecting therapy and estimating the prognosis at the time of onset is its clinical extent. In general, the more widespread the disease, the poorer the prognosis, even if all apparent disease is confined to the lymphoid regions. The poorer prognosis of patients who present with involvement of sites beyond the usual lymphoid tissues is well known. Five-year survival rates of 50% are often reported for patients with widespread lymph node disease, and rates of 8% are reported for those with involvement of extranodal sites such as the lung, liver, bone, or bone marrow. Recently it has been shown that the prognosis of patients with limited disease, even if it is extranodal, is more favorable because radiotherapists have been able to adequately treat the limited extranodal disease. This

Table 15-3. The treatment of Hodgkin's disease

Stage	Recommended therapy	Estimated 5-year disease-free survival (%)	Experimental therapy
IA, I$_E$A IIA, II$_E$A	Total lymphoid radiotherapy	90	Limited radiotherapy ± combination chemotherapy
IB, I$_E$B IIB, II$_E$B	Total lymphoid radiotherapy	75	Total lymphoid radiotherapy + combination chemotherapy
IIIA, III$_E$A, III$_S$A II$_S$A, II$_S$B	Total lymphoid radiotherapy	60	Combination chemotherapy ± total lymphoid radiotherapy
IIIB, III$_E$B, III$_S$B	Total lymphoid radiotherapy or combination chemotherapy	40	Total lymphoid radiotherapy + combination chemotherapy
IVA, IVB	Combination chemotherapy or palliative approaches	25 0	Total lymphoid radiotherapy + combination chemotherapy Sequential chemotherapy

From Holland, J. F., and Frei, E. III: Cancer medicine, Philadelphia, 1973, Lea & Febiger.

extranodal disease must be limited to extranodal involvement adjacent to or contiguous with nodal disease. It has been well documented that females have a better prognosis than males. This is in part related to the greater frequency of a more favorable nodular sclerosis variety in women. Patients past the age of 40 have a poorer prognosis than younger patients, which tends to make the prognosis for patients with disease concomitant with pregnancy appear slightly more favorable than one would expect. In the past, pregnancy was thought to have an unfavorable effect on the course of Hodgkin's disease; this cannot be substantiated except inasmuch as diagnostic studies and therapy must be modified during pregnancy.

The treatment of Hodgkin's disease has undergone radical changes in the last 40 years (Table 15-3). Aggressive therapy has resulted in considerable improvement in overall survival rates for patients with Hodgkin's disease. The most successful and widely tested combination of drugs has been developed at the National Cancer Institute (DeVita and associates) and consists of six 2-week cycles of therapy with nitrogen mustard, vincristine, procarbazine, and prednisone, the so-called MOPP program. The major technical factors that determine the efficacy of radiation therapy in Hodgkin's disease are: the total radiation dose per field, the size, shape, and number of treatment fields, and the beam energy. Permanent eradication of any given site of involvement can be achieved consistently with doses of 3,500 to 4,500 rads delivered at a rate of 1,000 rads/week. The desirability of irradiating apparently uninvolved lymph node regions has long been advocated by experienced radiotherapists. This approach is based on the knowledge of the clinical behavior of Hodgkin's disease, the inadequacies of our diagnostic techniques to discover minute or microscopic foci

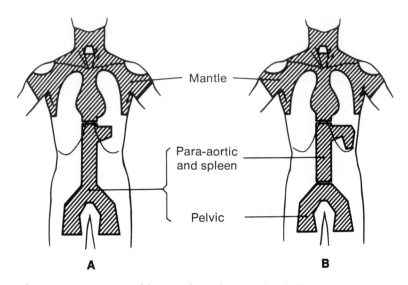

Fig. 15-4. Schematic representation of the "mantle" and "inverted Y" fields for total lymphoid irradiation. **A,** Two-field technique, with small extension to include the splenic pedicle, used in splenectomized patients. **B,** Three-field technique usually used when the spleen is still present. (From Rosenberg, S. A., and Kaplan, H. S.: Calif. Med. **113:**23, Oct. 1970.)

of the disease, the advantage and efficacy of avoiding patchwork and overlapping fields, and the possible reseeding of previously irradiated regions from unrecognized and untreated sites. Extended field irradiation, so-called total lymphoid or total radial therapy, is technically demanding and potentially hazardous (Fig. 15-4).

Proper, aggressive radiotherapy and chemotherapy for Hodgkin's disease require termination of pregnancy. One must individualize the application of aggressive diagnostic and therapeutic procedures in the pregnant patient with Hodgkin's disease. If she and her family absolutely refuse any intervention or treatment until the natural termination of the pregnancy, one has no choice but to wait. On the other hand, when one recognizes the potential curability of this disease, and not the concept of palliation prevalent 1 or 2 decades ago, one is less inclined to individualize or defer unless the pregnancy takes precedence. In patients with stage I or II disease with or without symptoms and irrespective of the length of gestation, vigorous therapy is strongly indicated. Delay should be minimal, and termination of pregnancy appears prudent unless the patient is well into her third trimester. Patients in the third trimester can begin the upper portion of the "mantle" technique of radiotherapy with proper shielding of the uterus (Fig. 15-4). Combination chemotherapy including the MOPP program is definitely contraindicated in the first trimester and relatively contraindicated in the second and third trimesters. Once again it should be emphasized that termination of the pregnancy before commencement of radiotherapy and combination chemotherapy is most desirable.

There are other diseases in the "malignant lymphoma" group that are closely related to Hodgkin's disease: lymphosarcoma, reticulum cell sarcoma, and giant follicular lymphoma. Fortunately, these tumors are more common in men and seem to predominantly occur in the fifth and sixth decades; thus, Hodgkin's disease remains the sole category of concern with regard to pregnancy.

A recent report by Holmes and Holmes addresses the reproductive prospects for Hodgkin's disease patients after therapy. Their study compared the outcome of 93 pregnancies in 48 patients with 228 pregnancies in 69 sibling controls. No statistically significant differences for spontaneous abortions or abnormal offspring were noted when all patients were compared with all controls or when 35 irradiated patients were compared with all controls. The pregnancy outcome of 13 patients who received both radiation and chemotherapy before pregnancy appeared to be compromised when compared with controls. Wives of male patients in this category were more likely to have spontaneous abortions than were wives of male controls; female patients in this category were significantly more likely to produce abnormal offspring than were female controls. Thus, in this series of patients therapeutic irradiation alone did not appear to jeopardize posttreatment reproduction in fertile Hodgkin's disease patients, but in the smaller group of patients who received both irradiation and chemotherapy the reproduction picture was statistically not as good. Trueblood and associates have emphasized surgical oophoroplexy when dealing with young women in whom preservation of ovarian function is desired and pelvic radiation is planned. This procedure is done at the time of staging laparotomy.

Leukemia

The average age of the patient with acute leukemia in pregnancy is 28 years. Premature labor is quite common in these women, and the average period of gestation is approximately 8 months. Postpartum hemorrhage occurs in around 10% to 15% of cases. The fibrinogen level in patients with acute leukemia in pregnancy may be reduced from the level anticipated at that stage of gestation. Frenkel and Meyers stated that pregnancy exerts no specific effect on the course of acute leukemia, except that early gestation poses an obstacle to vigorous treatment of leukemia. Other authors have observed that infants born of leukemic mothers are as well as normal controls. The following factors determine the delivery of a normal baby: (1) antimetabolite drugs are not administered, (2) radiotherapy to the uterus is not given during the first trimester of pregnancy, and (3) the fetus goes beyond the age of viability.

Chronic myelocytic leukemia comprises approximately 90% of all chronic leukemias in pregnancy. An additional 5% of the chronic leukemias in pregnancy are chronic lymphocytic leukemia. Several reports have recently shown that pregnant patients with chronic granulocytic leukemia treated during the first trimester with chemotherapy and radiation therapy to the spleen will usually deliver apparently healthy, viable babies if the uterus is protected with lead shields. Lee and associates reported 12 cases of leukemia associated with pregnancy. Six of seven women with chronic leukemia were treated with radiation therapy and chemotherapy and delivered apparently healthy infants. These authors stressed, however, that chemotherapy should be used with extreme caution, especially in the first trimester of pregnancy.

The decision on whether the pregnancy should be interrupted in pregnant patients discovered to have leukemia is really based on the desires of the patient. Prompt therapy is always most advisable with regard to the possibility of obtaining remission. However, the physician's advice to the patient should be influenced by the aggressiveness of the disease process. For instance, patients with chronic myelocytic leukemia are less likely to be harmed by deferring termination of pregnancy than patients with acute myelocytic leukemia demonstrating symptoms and a somewhat fulminating course.

Melanoma

Malignant melanoma may be one of the rare instances where pregnancy does adversely affect a malignant process. This has been suggested by many case reports in which pregnancy has been incriminated in the induction or exacerbation of a melanoma. Many observations have given support to this assumption concerning the adverse effect of pregnancy on malignant melanoma. Melanocyte-stimulating hormone (MSH) of the pituitary has been measured and noted to increase after the second month of pregnancy. Pregnancy is also associated with increased ACTH production, which results in heightened intrinsic MSH activity. Increased pigmentation is characteristic of pregnancy as evidenced in the nipple, vulva, and linea nigra and on occasion by changes in preexistent nevi. Estrogen itself (which is produced in enormous amounts during pregnancy) has been shown to control melanocyte activity in the guinea pig model. All melanomas masquerade as a nevus before their diagnosis. The average individual has 15 to 20 nevi, and removal of all these lesions prophylactically is hardly practical. Potentially dangerous nevi should be removed during childhood; these are the lesions on the feet, palms, genitals, and areas of persistent irritation from clothing.

In 1960 George and associates gave a comprehensive report of 115 cases of melanoma in pregnancy as compared with 330 controls from the same institution. In this report they disagreed with an earlier report from the same institution in that they found that spread to regional nodes appeared to be more rapid in the pregnant patient but that stage for stage there was no significant difference in the outcome for the patient. This was directly contradictory to an earlier philosophy popularized by Pack and Scharnagel that melanoma was indeed aggravated by the pregnant state.

The criteria for staging melanoma are presented in Table 15-4. Stage 0 primary melanoma is superficial, when invasion of the dermis is confined to the immediately adjacent subepidermal zone. Stage I primary melanoma extends deeper, and the greater the depth the more adverse the prognosis.

In 1961 White and associates reported a study of 71 young women (ages 15 to 39), 30 of whom were afflicted with melanoma during pregnancy. The 5-year survival rate in this group of 30 pregnant patients was 73%. The 41 patients not pregnant had a survival rate of 54%. They concluded that based on the 5-year survival rates in

Table 15-4. Criteria for staging melanoma

Stage 0	Superficial melanoma
Stage I	No metastases—primary melanoma only A. Intact primary melanoma B. Primary melanoma locally excised C. Multiple primary melanomas
Stage II	Local recurrence or metastasis All melanotic lesions within 3 cm of primary site (satellitosis)
Stage III	Regional metastases (3 cm from primary site) A. Intradermal (in transit metastasis) B. Regional lymph nodes AB. Intradermal and regional nodes
Stage IV	Distant hematogenous metastases A. Cutaneous B. Visceral C. Lymph nodes A-C. Combination of the above

pregnant and nonpregnant women with age and stage of disease taken into account, survival was equal in the two groups. No deleterious effect of pregnancy on survival of women with melanoma was demonstrated in this series.

The reported low incidence of metastasis of malignancies to products of conception is probably due to a number of factors. One factor is the unexplained resistance of the placenta to invasion by maternal cancer as demonstrated in many animal studies. Metastasis of maternal cancer to products of conception is rare despite the sizeable number of pregnancies at risk. Although melanoma accounts for only a small number of all cancers associated with pregnancy, almost half of all tumors metastasizing to the placenta and nearly 90% metastasizing to the fetus are melanoma.

Breast cancer

Cancer of the breast in pregnancy is a disaster for all involved. Both patient and physician find it difficult to accept this dread disease in a healthy, young pregnant woman. Since breast cancer is rare under the age of 35, this problem fortunately is a rare complication of pregnancy. Epidemiologically, it is known that there is an increased instance of breast cancer in certain families, the risk increasing five to ten times if a patient's mother or sister has had the disease. Although the overall survival rate for breast cancer is about 50%, with pregnancy the overall rate is reported by some to have dropped to 15% or 20%. Pregnant patients tend to have a higher incidence of positive nodes, and with positive nodes the prognosis is very bad and in all likelihood the neoplasm has metastasized at the time of the initiation of therapy. The advanced stage of the disease in the pregnant patient has been attributed to multiple factors. First and foremost, the engorged breast can successfully obscure a region for a much longer period. In addition, there may be increased vascularity and

Table 15-5. Haagensen clinical staging for breast cancer

Stage A	No skin edema, ulceration, or solid fixation to chest wall; axillary nodes clinically negative
Stage B	As in stage A, clinically involved nodes not more than 2.5 cm in transverse diameter and not fixed to skin or deeper structures; are palpable
Stage C	Any one of five grave signs present: 1. Edema of skin of limited extent (involves less than one third of breast surface) 2. Skin ulceration 3. Solid fixation to chest wall 4. Massive axillary nodes (more than 2.5 cm transverse diameter) 5. Fixation of axillary nodes to skin or deep structures
Stage D	All more advanced carcinomas including: 1. Any combination of 2 or more grave signs 2. Extensive edema (more than one third breast surface) 3. Satellite skin nodules 4. Inflammatory carcinoma 5. Clinically involved supraclavicular nodes 6. Parasternal tumor of internal mammary nodes 7. Edema of the arm 8. Distant metastases

From Haagensen, C. D.: Diseases of the breast, Philadelphia, 1971, W. B. Saunders Co.

lymphatic drainage from the pregnant breast, assisting the metastatic process. If a lesion is caught early (present less than 3 months, less than 2 cm, histologically nonanaplastic, and no positive nodes), the chance of survival for the pregnant or nonpregnant patient is the same, in the range of 70% to 80%. If, on the other hand, there is involvement of the subareolar region, diffuse inflammatory carcinoma, edema or ulceration of the skin, fixation of the tumor to the breast wall, or involvement of the high axillary, supraclavicular, or internal mammary nodes, the prognosis is very poor.

Staging of breast cancer is currently under a complicated system jointly recommended by the International Union Against Cancer and the American Joint Committee. The Haagensen clinical staging for breast cancer (Table 15-5) is more useful in pointing out the unfavorable prognostic indicators in this disease process.

Of all patients with breast cancer, 1% to 2% are pregnant at the time of diagnosis. The best evidence indicates that pregnancy does not augment the rate of growth or spread of breast cancer and that abortion for women with breast cancer does not improve the prognosis. Radical mastectomy is well tolerated during pregnancy, and the results of treatment during pregnancy are much the same, stage for stage, as they are in the nonpregnant woman. The treatment of the patient who has cancer of the breast during pregnancy is confused. Most reports have involved small numbers of patients and varying treatment plans. Most authorities recommend a radical mastectomy for patients with stage A and stage B disease. The extent of surgery in the treatment of cancer of the breast is being debated throughout the world, and that issue cannot be adequately addressed here.

Holleb and Farrow reported a series of 266 patients with carcinoma of the breast in pregnancy. There were 73 inoperable patients, and 93% of these patients died within 2 years of diagnosis. Seven of those patients had interruption of pregnancy, which did not seem to influence the course of the disease. The majority of patients in the series of 266 were treated by radical mastectomy and given postoperative radiation therapy. Twenty-eight patients were in the first trimester of pregnancy, and they had a 5-year survival rate of 25%. Half of the patients were allowed to deliver normally, and the other half underwent termination of pregnancy. The interruption of pregnancy did not seem to affect the clinical survival rate in the opinion of the authors. Indeed, the 5-year survival rate in the group that delivered normally was 33% as compared with 17% in the group in whom the pregnancy was interrupted.

Another report by Peters and Meakin of 70 cases of cancer of the breast occurring during pregnancy is worthy of review. All of these patients were treated by preoperative, postoperative, or palliative radiotherapy in conjunction with radical mastectomy. The overall survival rate in this series of patients was 32.9% at 5 years and 19.5% at 10 years. Three of twelve, or 25%, of those patients treated during the first and second trimesters survived 5 years. Only one of the nine patients treated during the third trimester survived 5 years, and she had active disease at the time of the report. Peters and Meakin suggested that delay should be considered in the treatment of carcinoma of the breast until after the baby is born.

Most clinicians feel that if the diagnosis is made in the first trimester, the pregnancy should be recommended for termination. Yet it has not been demonstrated that abortion increases the survival rate. The matter becomes more difficult when the patient is in the second or third trimester of pregnancy, and in most instances termination of pregnancy is not recommended since there is no clear evidence that this improves the survival rate despite the theoretical advantage in removal of a large estrogen source. In addition, several studies have now shown that prophylactic oophorectomy does not alter the course of the disease. The high probability of estrogen or progesterone dependency in a patient with carcinoma of the breast premenopausally suggests strongly that termination of pregnancy may be desirable. With estrogen-binding determinations now widely available, this decision may be made on a more scientific basis. One would be hard pressed to continue a pregnancy where positive estrogen binding has been demonstrated on the primary lesion in the breast and evidence of metastatic disease exists. If distant metastases occur after pregnancy, oophorectomy will produce a remission in 50% of patients. Interestingly, if a case does not respond to oophorectomy, it will not respond to androgen or estrogen administration. On the other hand, if there is a response and later relapse, androgen or estrogen will result in remission in about 25% of patients. A response to oophorectomy will also determine whether the patient will have a favorable result to a second or third procedure involving either adrenal or hypophyseal ablation.

The question of breast-feeding is another difficult issue. Many have postulated that breast cancer is of <u>viral origin</u>, and therefore the possibility exists that the contralateral breast will be contaminated with the etiologic agent, which will be passed on to the fetus. This theory has never been borne out in fact, but most surgeons recommend artificial feeding of the infant to avoid vascular enrichment in the opposite breast, which may also contain a neoplasm.

For very advanced disease, <u>chemotherapy</u> has been used <u>after the first trimester.</u> Alkylating agents, 5-fluorouracil, and vincrinstine are relatively safe and have been given with the fetus in utero. Methotrexate should be avoided if possible. Chemotherapy should be administered only when the patient is reluctant to have the pregnancy terminated and the disease appears to be progressing at an alarming rate. The issue of whether chemotherapy should be administered to patients with breast cancer in pregnancy is complicated by recent reports that suggest that both single-agent and combination chemotherapy may significantly improve survival in premenopausal patients when used in an adjuvant setting. Ten- and 15-year follow-ups are always necessary in breast cancer, but it would appear that the premenopausal patient is the best candidate for aggressive adjuvant chemotherapy and improved survival rate. This is especially pertinent to the patients in whom positive nodes are uncovered at the time of the initial procedure.

Bone tumors

Benign tumors of the bone rarely are a problem in pregnancy; however, two benign tumors can affect pregnancy and delivery: <u>endochondromas</u> and benign exostosis, which can develop at <u>the pelvic brim.</u> These may interfere with the progression of labor and the engagement of the head of the fetus by blocking the pelvic inlet and requiring cesarean section.

The most frequent primary tumors seen in the age group who may become pregnant are Ewing's sarcoma, osteogenic sarcoma, and osteocystoma. The usual areas attacked are the clavicle, sternum, spine, humerus, and femur, and these tumors are associated with local pain, mass, and disability. Signs and symptoms of myelitis can be produced by primary sarcoma of the spine, which is very painful when it involves the nerve roots. Fortunately, metastatic lesions to bone tend to occur in the lower thoracic and lumbar regions, with lesser incidence of involvement of the sacrum and pelvis. The malignancies that cause most of the metastatic disease in these areas are breast, uterus, thyroid, and adrenal cancers.

Primary bone cancer is treated by surgical excision, usually without regard for the pregnancy. X-ray examination and chemotherapy are often delayed until delivery if the neoplasm occurs in the pregnant patient. Pregnancy does not affect the growth of bone malignancy, nor does the tumor affect the pregnancy, so strong indications for termination of pregnancy are not present. Most recurrences from bone malignancy occur within the first 3 years following initial diagnosis, so the recommendation is often made that future pregnancies be deferred until that interval has passed.

BIBLIOGRAPHY

Allen, A. C., and Spitz, S.: Malignant melanoma; a clinicopathological analysis of the criteria for diagnosis and prognosis, Cancer **6:**1, 1953.

Barber, H. R. K., and Brunschwig, A.: Carcinoma of the bowel; radiation and surgical management and pregnancy, Am. J. Obstet. Gynecol. **100:**926, 1968.

Barry, R. M., and others: Influence of pregnancy on the course of Hodgkin's disease, Am. J. Obstet. Gynecol. **84:**445, 1962.

Beatson, G. T.: On the treatment of inoperable cases of carcinoma of the mamma; suggestions for a new method of treatment with illustrative cases, Lancet **2:**104, 1896.

Boronow, R. C.: Extrapelvic malignancy and pregnancy, Obstet. Gynecol. Surv. **19:**1, 1964.

Bosch, A., and Marcial, V. A.: Carcinoma of the uterine cervix associated with pregnancy, Am. J. Roentgenol. **96:**92, 1966.

Brodsky, I., Baren, M., Kahn, S. B., and others: Metastatic malignant melanoma from mother to fetus, Cancer **18:**1048, 1965.

Bunker, M. L., and Peters, M. V.: Breast cancer associated with pregnancy or lactation, Am. J. Obstet. Gynecol. **85:**312, 1963.

Byrd, B. F., Jr., and McGanity, W. J.: The effect of pregnancy on the clinical course of sarcoma of the soft somatic tissues, Surg. Obstet. Gynecol. **125:**28, 1967.

Cade, S.: Cancer in pregnancy, J. Obstet. Gynaecol. Br. Comm. **3:**341, 1964.

Carpenter, C. B., and Merrill, J. P.: Modification of renal allograft rejection in man, Arch. Intern. Med. **123:**501, 1969.

Cavell, B.: Transplacental metastasis of malignant melanoma, Acta Pathol. Suppl. **146:**37, 1963.

Cheek, J. H.: Cancer of the breast in pregnancy and lactation, Am. J. Surg. **126:**729, 1973.

Coates, A.: Cyclophosphamide in pregnancy, Aust. N.Z. J. Obstet. Gynaecol. **10:**33, 1970.

Cooper, D. R., and Butterfield, J.: Pregnancy subsequent to mastectomy for cancer of the breast, Ann. Surg. **171:**429, 1970.

Creasman, W. T., Rutledge, F., and Fletcher, G.: Carcinoma of the cervix associated with pregnancy, Obstet. Gynecol. **36:**495, 1970.

Daw, E. G.: Procarbazine in pregnancy, letter, Lancet **2:**984, 1970.

DeVita, V. H., Serpick, A. A., and Carbone, P. P.: Combination chemotherapy in the treatment of advanced Hodgkin's disease, Ann. Intern. Med. **73:**881, 1970.

Diamandopoulos, G. T., and Hertig, A. T.: Transmission of leukemia and allied diseases from mother to fetus, Obstet. Gynecol. **21:**150, 1963.

Donegan, W. L.: Breast cancer and pregnancy, Obstet. Gynecol. **50:**244, 1977.

Early, T. K., Gallagher, J. Q., and Chapman, K. E.: Carcinoma of the breast in women under thirty years of age, Am. J. Surg. **118:**832, 1969.

Eastman, N. J., and Hellman, L. M.: Ovarian tumors in pregnancy. In Eastman, N. J., and Hellman, L. M., editors: Williams' obstetrics, ed. 13, New York, 1966, Appleton-Century-Crofts.

Erwald, R.: Mammary carcinoma and pregnancy, Acta Obstet. Gynecol. Scand. **46:**316, 1967.

Frenkel, E. P., and Meyers, M. C.: Acute leukemia and pregnancy, Ann. Intern. Med. **53:**656, 1960.

Freckman, H. A., Fry, H. L., Mendex, F. L., and Maurer, E. R.: Chlorambucil and prednisone therapy for disseminated breast cancer, J.A.M.A. **189:**23, 1964.

George, P. A., Fortner, J. G., and Pack, G. T.: Melanoma with pregnancy; report of 115 cases, Cancer **13:**854, 1960.

Grimes, W. H., and others: Ovarian cysts in pregnancy, Am. J. Obstet. Gynecol. **68:**594, 1954.

Haagensen, C. D.: Cancer of the breast in pregnancy and during lactation, Am. J. Obstet. Gynecol. **98:**141, 1967.

Herbst, A. L., Ulfelder, H., and Poskanzer, D. C.: Adenocarcinoma of the vagina, N. Engl. J. Med. **284:**878, 1971.

Holmes, G. E., and Holmes, F. F.: Pregnancy outcome of patients treated for Hodgkin's disease; a controlled study, Cancer **41:**1317, 1978.

Holleb, A. I., and Farrow, J. H.: The relation of carcinoma of the breast and pregnancy in 283 patients, Surg. Gynecol. Obstet. **115:**65, 1962.

Holleb, A. I., and Farrow, J. H.: Significance of breast discharge, Cancer **16:**182, 1966.

Horsley, J. S. III, Alrich, E. M., and Wright, C. B.: Carcinoma of the breast in women 35 years of age or younger, Ann. Surg. **169:**839, 1969.

Karlen, J. R., Sternberg, L. B., and Abbott, J. N.: Carcinoma of the endometrium coexisting with pregnancy, Obstet. Gynecol. **40:**334, 1972.

Kasdon, S. C.: Pregnancy and Hodgkin's disease with a report of three cases, Am. J. Obstet. Gynecol. **57:**282, 1949.

Kempson, R. L., and Pokorny, G. E.: Adenocarcinoma of the endometrium in women aged forty and younger, Cancer **21:**650, 1968.

Kilgore, A. R.: Discussion of T. T. White and W. C. White; breast cancer and pregnancy; report of 49 cases followed five years, Ann. Surg. **144:**385, 1956.

Lee, R. A., Johnson, C. E., and Hanlon, D. G.: Leukemia during pregnancy, Am. J. Obstet. Gynecol. **84:**455, 1965.

Lee, W. T., and Hon, J. M.: Carcinoma of breast with ovarian metastasis, Cancer 27:1374, 1974.

Marinaccio, L., and Mazzarella, L.: Gravidanza con parto a termine in soggeto affetto da adenocantoma dell endometrio, Cancro 20:582, 1967.

Merkatz, I. R., and others: Resumption of female reproductive function following renal transplantation, J.A.M.A. 216:1749, 1971.

Miller, H. K.: Cancer of the breast during pregnancy and lactation, Am. J. Obstet. Gynecol. 83:667, 1962.

Nelson, J. H., Lu, T., Hall, J. E., and others: The effect of trophoblast on immune state of women, Am. J. Obstet. Gynecol. 117:689, 1973.

Nicholson, H. O.: Cytotoxic drugs in pregnancy, J. Obstet. Gynaecol. Br. Comm. 75:307, 1968.

Nieminen, U., and Remes, N.: Malignancy during pregnancy, Acta Obstet. Gynecol. Scand. 49:315, 1970.

O'Leary, J. A., Pratt, J. H., and Symmonds, R. E.: Rectal carcinoma in pregnancy, Obstet. Gynecol. 30:862, 1967.

Pack, G. T., and Scharnagel, I. M.: The prognosis for malignant melanoma in the pregnant woman, Cancer 4:324, 1951.

Penn, I., Makowski, E., Droegemueller, W., and others: Parenthood in renal homograft recipients, J.A.M.A. 216:1755, 1971.

Peters, M. V.: A study of survivals in Hodgkin's disease treated radiologically, Am. J. Roentgenol. 63:299, 1950.

Peters, M. V., and Meakin, J. W.: The influence of pregnancy in carcinoma of the breast, Prog. Clin. Cancer 1:471, 1965.

Raich, P. C., and Curet, L. B.: Treatment of acute leukemia during pregnancy, Cancer 36:861, 1975.

Ravdin, R. G., and others: Results of a clinical trail concerning the worth of prophylactic oophorectomy for breast carcinoma, Surg. Gynecol. Obstet. 131:1055, 1970.

Rissanen, P.: Carcinoma of the breast during pregnancy and lactation, Br. J. Cancer 22:663, 1968.

Robinson, D. W.: Breast carcinoma associated with pregnancy, Am. J. Obstet. Gynecol. 92:658, 1965.

Rodes, N. D., Blackwell, C. W., and Farrell, C.: Screening asymptomatic women for breast cancer, Mo. Med. 72:692, 1975.

Rosemond, G. P.: Management of patients with carcinoma of the breast in pregnancy, Ann. N.Y. Acad. Sci. 114:851, 1964.

Rosenberg, S. A.: A critique of the value of laparotomy and splenectomy in the evaluation of patients with Hodgkin's disease, Cancer Res. 31:1737, 1971.

Sandstrom, R. E., Welch, W. R., and Green, T. H.: Adenocarcinoma of the endometrium in pregnancy, Obstet. Gynecol. 53(S):73, 1979.

Schumann, E. A.: Observations upon the coexistence of carcinoma fundus uteri and pregnancy, Trans. Am. Gynecol. Soc. 52:245, 1927.

Shellito, J. G., and Bartlett, W. C.: Bilateral carcinoma of the breast, Arch. Surg. 94:489, 1967.

Shocket, E. C., and Fortner, J. G.: Melanoma and pregnancy; an experimental evaluation of a clinical impression, Surg. Forum 9:671, 1958.

Singleton, W. R., and Rutledge, F.: To cone or not to cone—the cervix, Obstet. Gynecol. 31:430, 1968.

Sokal, J. E., and Lessman, E. M.: The effects of cancer chemotherapeutic agents on the human fetus, J.A.M.A. 172:1765, 1960.

Taylor, S.: Endocrine ablation in disseminated mammary carcinoma, Surg. Gynecol. Obstet. 115:443, 1962.

Thomas, M. A., and McDonald, E. J.: Second thoughts on mammography, Med. Ann. D.C. 36:468, 1967.

Trueblood, W. H., Enright, L. P., and Nelsen, T. S.: Preservation of ovarian function with radiotherapy for malignant lymphoma, Arch. Surg. 100:236, 1970.

Urban, J. A.: Surgical therapy of primary breast cancer. In Barber, H. R. K., and Graber, E. A., editors: Gynecological oncology, Baltimore, 1970, The Williams & Wilkins Co.

Van Thiel, D. H., Ross, G. T., and Lipsett, M. B.: Pregnancies after chemotherapy of trophoblastic neoplasms, Science 169:1326, 1970.

Vitums, V. C., and Sites, J. G.: Leukemia in pregnancy, Med. Ann. D.C. 37:588, 1968.

Waldrop, G. M., and Palmer, J. P.: Carcinoma of the cervix associated with pregnancy, Am. J. Obstet. Gynecol. 86:202, 1963.

Wall, J. A., and Lucci, J. A., Jr.: Adenocarcinoma of the corpus uteri and pelvic tuberculosis complicating pregnancy, Obstet. Gynecol. 2:629, 1953.

Wallingford, A. J.: Cancer of the body of the uterus complicating pregnancy, Am. J. Obstet. Gynecol. 27:224, 1934.

Westman, A.: A case of simultaneous pregnancy and cancer of the corpus uteri, Acta Obstet. Gynecol. Scand. 14:191, 1934.

White, L. P., and others: Studies on melanoma; the effect of pregnancy on survival in human melanoma, J.A.M.A. 117:235, 1961.

White, T. T.: Cancer of the breast in the pregnant or nursing patient, Am. J. Obstet. Gynecol. 69:1277, 1955.

White, T. T., and White, W. C.: Breast cancer and pregnancy, Ann. Surg. 144:385, 1956.

I am convinced that during development and growth, malignant cells arise frequently, but that in the majority of individuals they remain latent due to the protective action of the host. I am convinced that this natural immunity is not due to the presence of antimicrobial bodies, but is determined purely by cellular factors. These may be weakened in the older age groups in which cancer is more prevalent.

PAUL EHRLICH (1909)

CHAPTER SIXTEEN

Tumor immunology

Historical review
Anatomy of the immune system
Mechanisms of immunity
Immunoprophylaxis
Principles of immunotherapy
Applications of immunotherapy in gynecologic
    oncology
Immunodiagnosis
Conclusions

HISTORICAL REVIEW

The word "immunity" means freedom from burden, and in its original application the burden was that of invasion by microorganisms. In modern times, the burden is much larger and also encompasses the reaction of the body to foreign tissue, such as an organ transplant, and to altered tissue, such as neoplastic growths. The nineteenth century saw the emergence of microbiology and immunology and witnessed the beginnings of vaccination in the prevention of disease. Edward Jenner successfully inoculated cowpox into human beings and was able to offer protection against smallpox. The practices of Jenner were extended by Pasteur, who established the value of preventive inoculation against a variety of animal and human diseases. It was because of Pasteur that the skepticism about the "germ theory" finally was dispelled, and Koch was able to lay down the fundamental laws regarding infectious agents with the "Koch postulates." The field of immunology was placed on a firm scientific foundation around the turn of the twentieth century with the recognition of immunolysis of foreign red cells by Bordet in 1898 and the description of the ABO blood groups by Landsteiner in 1904. In the early part of the twentieth century, the relative importance of phagocytosis and antibody production to host defense caused a sharp division of scientific opinion. One group of scientists led by a Russian, Elie Metchnikoff, held phagocytosis to be more crucial. Paul Ehrlich and his followers attributed greater importance to antibody attack upon the parasite. Ehrlich developed the theory of antigenic specificity, which depended, according to him, on chemical union between the antigen and side chains on the corresponding antibody. In 1908 the Nobel Prize was awarded to Ehrlich and Metchnikoff for their work on immunity.

Tumor immunology developed as an offshoot of transplantation immunology. The roots of transplantation immunology are found in the work of a Hungarian-born Viennese surgeon, Emerich Ullman, who successfully transplanted a kidney in a dog. His technique was perfected by Alexis Carrel, a graduate of the University of Lyon, who was working in Chicago between 1902 and 1904. Carrel applied the principles of vascular anastomosis to transplantation of a variety of organs. The techniques described by Carrel for developing vascular suture substances and his technique of vascular surgery have persisted to modern times. Carrel's work was to win him the Nobel Prize in medicine.

In 1923 and 1924, the pathology of transplantation rejection was described by Carol S. Williamson of the Mayo Clinic, and the phenomenon of first and second set rejection was documented by Holman, who worked with skin allografts on a burn victim. These findings laid the foundation for the classic work of Peter Gorer leading to the formulation of the theory of antigenic specificity of tissues from different individuals. The first clinical attempt at human kidney transplantation was performed at the Peter Bent Brigham Hospital in Boston by Charles A. Hufnagel, David A. Hume, and Ernest Landsteiner in 1947.

At about the same time, an interesting observation made in 1945 by R. Owen, a veterinary surgeon from Wisconsin, began to be widely appreciated by the scientific community. Owen noted that the in utero mixing of the circulation of monoplacental cattle led to the coexistence in the adult animal of two different blood groups, a condition called chimerism. In 1955, Billingham, Brent, and Medawar published their landmark paper on actively acquired tolerance of foreign cells in which they showed that if fetal mice were exposed to foreign cells in utero, then those mice, upon attaining adult age, would become tolerant to tissues from the original donor of the cells. In 1959, Macfarlane Burnet refined this concept and detailed the clonal selection theory of immunity. By 1960, teams of surgeons in the United States, France, and Britain were successfully transplanting kidneys, and their techniques have continued to the present. Drs. Burnet and Medawar were awarded the Nobel Prize in medicine in 1960 for their monumental work. The importance of cell surface antigens in transplantation immunity became well recognized and led to advances such as those of Paul Terasaki, who developed and popularized a method for matching tissues of organ donors and recipients to prolong transplantation survival.

As transplantation immunology (Table 16-1) became more thoroughly under-

Table 16-1. Tumor immunology is a form of transplantation immunology and the same terminology applies

| Genetic relationship | Antibody | Transplant | |
		Old term	New term
Identical, same individual	Auto	Auto	Syngeneic (autochthonous)
Identical twin	Iso	Iso	Syngeneic
Different individual, same species	Iso	Homo	Allogeneic
Different species	Hetero	Hetero	Xenogeneic

From DiSaia, P. J.: Tumor immunology; general aspects, Contemporary Ob/Gyn **4:**91, 1974, Medical Economics Co.

stood, some scientists referred back to the hypothesis of Paul Ehrlich, which stated that malignant neoplasms were antigenic and, as such, could be recognized by the host as foreign in much the same manner as allogenic tissue. Indeed, in 1908 Ehrlich indirectly suggested the theory of immunologic surveillance. Cancer-specific antigens were identified for the first time in experiments by Gross in 1943. He described the failure of mice to accept a transplant of a specific cancer after they had been immunized with material from the same cancer growing in pedigreed mice. Gross immunized mice by intradermal inoculation of tumor cells. The immunized animals rejected a subcutaneous transplant of the same tumor, but nonimmunized animals did not. His work was all but ignored until 1957, when Prehn and Main reported their experiments using syngeneic methylcholanthrene-induced fibrosarcomas. They observed that mice immunized against these fibrosarcomas by inoculation of living sarcoma tissue, following surgical removal of the growing tumor, were resistant to subsequent grafts of the same tumor. In addition, immunization with normal tissue did not confer resistance to the tumor graft. The mice that had become resistant to the tumors still accepted skin grafts from the primary host of these tumors. The rejection of the tumor tissue with simultaneous acceptance of normal tissue from the same donor to the same recipient proved Ehrlich's hypothesis to be correct. The malignant neoplasm appeared to have acquired an antigenic moiety during the malignant transformation of the mouse tissue that allowed that malignant tissue to now be recognized as "nonself," whereas corresponding normal tissue was still accepted as "self."

The experiments of Prehn and Main were repeated by many others in different tumor systems, and the following conclusions have been reached. Antigenic differences exist between cancer cells and their normal counterparts, and these differences are equivalent to weak transplantation antigens. It would appear that malignant tissues do (in most organisms in which they appear, including the human) evoke a measurable immunologic response. The specificity of the cell surface tumor antigens is, at present, somewhat in doubt, and therefore they have been termed tumor-associated antigens (TAA).

ANATOMY OF THE IMMUNE SYSTEM
Antigens

Tumor cells express most of the same cell surface antigens (e.g., transplantation or HLA antigens) as normal cells (Fig. 16-1). In addition, most tumor cells express specific antigens not found in similar normal cells. These antigens are termed tumor-specific antigens in animal studies and tumor-associated antigens in human malignancies. Experiments to demonstrate tumor-specific antigens involve a demonstration that pretreatment with a syngeneic tumor will influence the growth of a subsequent challenge with the same tumor. In animals this was possible after introduction of syngeneic inbred mouse strains, and in 1953 Foley produced the first such evidence. This was later followed by the studies of Prehn and Main. Such studies are not possible in humans; however, there are in vitro techniques for detection of tumor antigens, and these have been liberally applied to human tumors. Tumors vary widely in their immunogenicity. In general, those neoplasms induced experimentally in vivo with chemical or viral agents are highly immunogenic, whereas tumors arising spontaneously in vivo are poorly immunogenic.

Oncofetal antigens have also been described; these are antigens that are found in both fetal and malignant tissue. These normal antigens in the fetus are repressed as the process of intrauterine development proceeds toward birth and then de-repressed during the malignant transformation process. Their existence supports the concept that cancer represents a dedifferentiation to a more primitive cell type. The relationship between malignant neoplasms, specific tumor antigens, and fetal antigens is not clear. The most carefully studied oncofetal antigens in gynecologic cancer are carcinoembryonic antigen (CEA) and alpha-fetoprotein (AFP). The most apparent importance of these antigens is not in their possible protective value but in their ability to serve as tumor markers for various cancers. CEA initially stimulated great

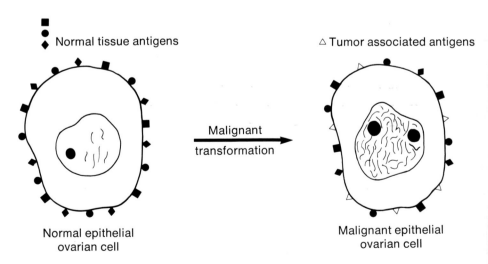

■
●
● Normal tissue antigens   △ Tumor associated antigens
◆

Malignant
transformation

Normal epithelial
ovarian cell

Malignant epithelial
ovarian cell

Fig. 16-1. Tumor-associated antigens (TAA) are additionally expressed on the tumor cell surface.

interest as a possible accurate diagnostic assay for gastrointestinal malignancies. However, with further study elevated levels were found in patients with benign disease (e.g., colonic polyps, severe cirrhosis, uremia, and inflammatory disease of the bowel). Indeed, CEA can be found in host of nongastrointestinal cancers, including several gynecologic malignancies (Fig. 16-2), and its value as a clinically usable tumor marker is very limited. AFP is detectable immunologically in serum from human fetuses. In the adult, it is found in patients with malignancies of endodermal origin, for example, liver tumors and gonadal tumors such as endodermal sinus tumor of the ovary. As with CEA, there does not appear to be a clear correlation between the level of AFP and the prognosis for the patient, and also like CEA, it is not disease specific. The presence of AFP with an ovarian neoplasm strongly suggests a diagnosis of endodermal sinus tumor, and the reappearance of detectable serum levels after a period of negative titers strongly suggests recurrent disease.

Lymphocytes

The lymphocyte was a little respected member of the family of circulating cells until recent recognition of its key role in immunity. It is the principal cell involved in recognizing an antigen as foreign and then initiating mechanisms to rid the host of the invader. The lymphocyte's recognition of "self" and "nonself" provides the host's key mechanism of homeostasis and is the starting point for all immune reactivity. These small cells with very large nuclei circulate into every tissue of the body, and when a processed antigen comes in contact with a lymphocyte, a series of events is triggered. The lymphocyte increases dramatically in size and undergoes lympho

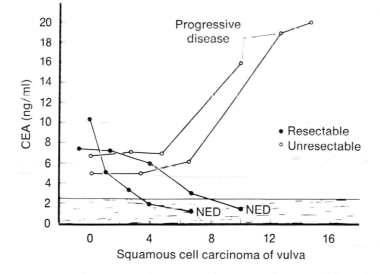

Fig. 16-2. Four patients with a positive plasma CEA value prior to therapy are followed subsequent to treatment. Progressive disease results in rising titers. (From DiSaia, P. J., and others: Obstet. Gynecol. **47**:95, 1976.)

blastogenesis, resulting in an immunoblast. The immunoblast proceeds toward development of humoral or cell-mediated immunologic effectors.

Activated lymphocytes can also produce a variety of soluble effector substances that participate in the complicated process called the immune response. These substances are called lymphokines and include among others the following:

1. Interferon, which blocks the replication of viruses and has antitumor activity
2. Cytotoxic factor, which is capable of killing foreign cells
3. Cell growth inhibitor, which can prevent cellular proliferation
4. Macrophage inhibition factor (MIF), which causes depression of macrophage activity
5. Chemotactic factors, which produce an attraction of macrophages, monocytes, and granulocytes
6. Lymphocyte activators, which stimulate lymphocyte activity
7. Transfer factor, which is an extract of lymphocytes capable of conferring specific antigen reactivity to the donor
8. Tumor necrosis factor, which is toxic in vitro for human neoplastic cells

Descriptions of new lymphokines produced by T-cells proliferate with every year of research; currently there are well over 25 known lymphokines.

Humoral factors

Some of the immunoblasts differentiate into plasma cells, which are largely responsible for humoral immunity. Antibodies are secreted by plasma cells into the

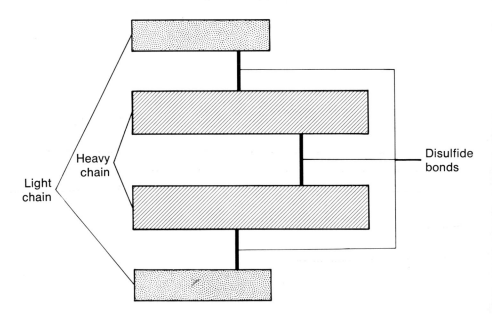

Fig. 16-3. Basic structure of an antibody molecule with two heavy chains and two light chains all connected by disulfide bonds.

vicinity of the antigenic stimulus, and there binding takes place with the inciting antigen. The basic unit of all antibodies is composed of four polypeptides, two light chains and two heavy chains linked to each other by several disulfide bridges (Fig. 16-3). There are five classes of antibodies: IgG, IgM, IgA, IgE, and IgD. It is estimated that 100,000 different antibodies can be produced by the human; specificity is a basic property of this system. An antibody directed toward a particular antigen will not confer protection against other antigens. This concept is termed the clonal selection theory, which states that each antibody-producing cell is committed to one particular antibody in production.

Macrophage

The macrophage is emerging as a major player in the host reaction to a tumor. Recent evidence has illustrated that the macrophage can be activated by lymphocytes and exert a killing effect on tumor cells on its own. The mechanism of this killing is unclear, but it would appear that direct contact with the target cell is necessary. The macrophage is derived from the circulating blood monocyte. The monocyte remains in the circulation for several days before coming to rest in the tissues, where it emerges as a highly active macrophage. In the tissues the macrophage has three key functions. First, it is a phagocyte clearing the tissue of foreign substances. Second, the macrophage functions in a chemotaxic capacity by following an increasing concentration gradient to the site of an immune reaction. Third and most important, the macrophage can process an antigen and express this antigen on its cell surface, where the antigen becomes immunogenic and capable of eliciting an immune response. Those antigens that escape this macrophage "processing" are weakly immunogenic and usually fail to evoke a significant response. Thus, the macrophage becomes an essential ingredient in the immune response. Phylogenetically, the macrophage is the first cell devoted primarily to defense against foreign substances so its recently recognized key role in the immune response should not be surprising.

MECHANISMS OF IMMUNITY

The immune mechanism consists basically of initial recognition and processing of foreign matter, an afferent mechanism leading to activation of the central immune system, and an efferent mechanism leading to the elimination of the offending material. The basic study of immunology concerns the reactions of the body to certain foreign materials presented to it, both living and nonliving. The immune reaction can be defined as an interaction between the invading foreign material and the defending host tissue. The cells of the afferent arm process the antigenic information and convey it to the central immune mechanism capable of reacting specifically to this information. The cells of the central mechanism are termed immunologically competent and are of the lymphoid series. This lymphoid tissue is present in peripheral lymph nodes, bone marrow, spleen, thymus, Peyer's patches of the intestine, thoracic duct, and the bloodstream itself. All antigens are recognized as either "self" or "nonself." It is known, however, that when recognition occurs, it is very specific and precisely directed against certain molecular configurations on the antigen. In addition, antigen and immunocompetent cells apparently must have physical contact to evoke a response.

Specific immune responses are mediated by two major categories of effectors, with considerable interaction between the two. One category of response can be transferred from one individual to another only by transferring living immunologi-

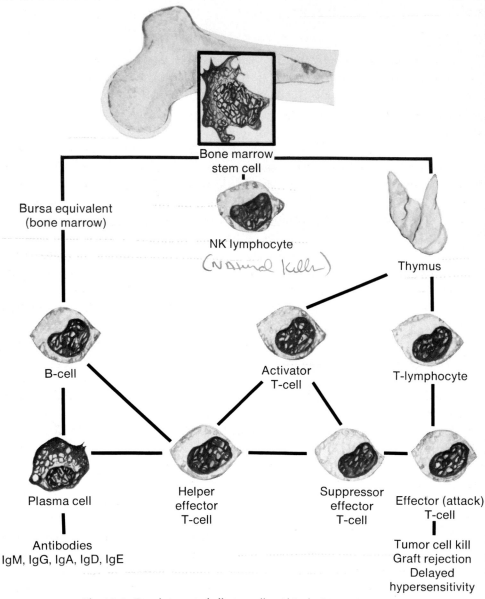

Fig. 16-4. Development of effector cells within the immune system.

cally competent cells or cultured products of these cells. This type of response is termed cell-mediated immunity. The second type of response can be transferred by cell-free serum and therefore is called humoral immunity (Fig. 16-4). The key to both of these responses is the small lymphocyte, which until recently was relegated to a position of relative obscurity in textbooks of physiology and hematology. The small lymphocyte is formed in the bone marrow from precursor stem cells and then released into the circulation, eventually coming to rest in the lymphoid organs. The small lymphocytes specialize early in their life by either passing through the thymus gland and differentiating into a cell that will participate in cell-mediated immunity or bypassing the thymus and undergoing differentiation into a cell that will mediate humoral immunity. Despite the crucial differences between these two types of cells, they are morphologically indistinguishable under the light microscope.

Cell-mediated immunity

Cell-mediated immunity (CMI, cellular immunity, transplantation immunity, or delayed hypersensitivity) is mediated by the lymphocyte that has passed through the thymus in its development. The exact mechanism of the thymic influence is not well understood in the human organism but is suspected of being hormonal. Once the lymphocyte has passed through the thymus in its development it remains under the influence of the thymus and is variously termed the thymic-dependent lymphocyte, T-lymphocyte, or simply T-cell (Fig. 16-5). These cells may also be involved in the pathogenesis of the more common autoimmune disorders. CMI is very commonly influenced by drugs, such as anesthetic agents and corticosteroids, or deficiencies in nutrition as well as by major injury or aging.

In recent years, techniques have been introduced that allow cellular migration to be followed. The techniques utilize either isotopic labeling of cells for short-term studies or chromosome markers for longer-term investigations. These experiments have demonstrated that the lymphocytes of the thymus arise by differentiation of cells that enter the thymic primordium from without, namely, from the bloodstream. In the adult these cells are derived from the bone marrow, and when these migrant stem cells enter the epithelial primordium of the thymus they proliferate and mature into small lymphocytes. As stated above, it is not known what is responsible for lymphocyte maturation within the thymus. Some have postulated a diffusible substance or a thymic hormone; others have postulated that cell contact and interaction within the thymic environment are the crucial factors (Fig. 16-6). Another complex issue for which we have little information is whether T-cell subpopulations represent separate lines of T-cell development or whether they are stages in a single differentiation pathway.

The thymus manufactures a large number of T-lymphocytes. These T-cells leave the thymus to enter the bloodstream, where they comprise about 60% of the peripheral blood lymphocytes. They then enter a unique pattern of recirculation, with many moving from blood to lymph node to thoracic duct, from whence they return to the blood. In the lymph node most T-cells reside in the deep cortex in areas in

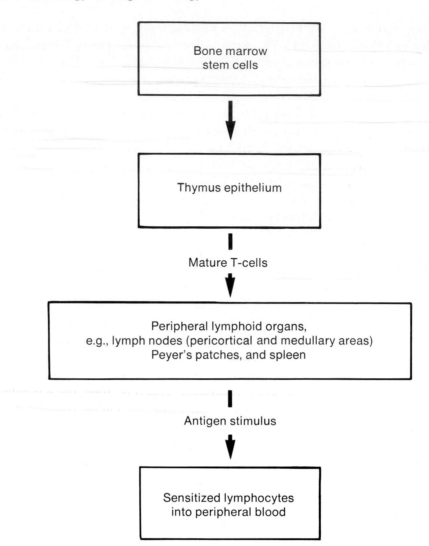

Fig. 16-5. Progress of T-cell lymphocyte maturation.

and between germinal centers. This pool of mature T-lymphocytes is often called the recirculating pool of long-lived T-lymphocytes (some undoubtedly memory cells), and some of these resting cells have been shown to live for over 20 years without dividing. It is important to note that the path of recirculation does not involve the thymus; for unknown reasons, once a T-cell leaves the thymus it does not appear to return to it.

Subpopulations of T-cells

There are several subpopulations of T-cells, each with different functions. There is substantial evidence for separate categories of functional T-lymphocytes, such as

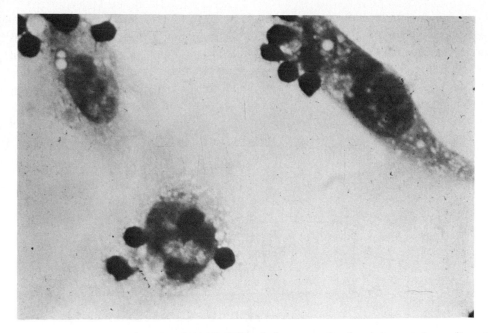

Fig. 16-6. Attack presensitized lymphocytes clustered about vacuolized and degenerating malignant squamous cells in vitro at 48 hours of co-cultivation.

the "helper" cell or "cytotoxic" or even "suppressor" cells (Fig. 16-4), but it is unclear whether these categories represent different functional states in the common differentiation pathway or whether they are quite separate pathways of maturation. Normal T-cells do not produce conventional immunoglobulin as is characteristic of B-cells. However, T-cells do have a crucial role in the regulation of immune responses by acting as potentiators or inhibitors of the B-cell transition into immunoglobulin-secreting plasma cells. The cells that potentiate this B-cell transition are classified as helper cells, whereas those that inhibit it are classified as suppressor cells. Suppressor cells have been identified in humans through a variety of circumstances. There is compelling evidence in mice and corroborating evidence in humans that help and suppression are mediated by distinct subsets of T-cells, each genetically committed to mediate only one of these two functions. In mice, helper T-cells and suppressor T-cells can be readily distinguished by their surface membrane antigen. Other evidence suggests that immunoregulatory T-cells may have an interim existence as inactive precursors, which might be referred to as pro-helper cells and pro-suppressor cells, which must react with a different set of activated T-cells before maturing into fully functional helper effector cells or suppressor effector cells. Physiologically, suppressor cells may terminate excessive immune responses after antigenic exposure, and they probably provide a safeguard against autoimmune reactions. It is not surprising, therefore, that recent evidence from a number of animal models of autoimmunity suggests that impaired suppressor T-cell function can lead to overt autoimmune disease.

An understanding of suppressor cell function in human neoplasia may alter the perspective and direction of oncologic researchers and clinicians. There is a real possibility that chemotherapy, radiation, and surgery might, in certain cases, benefit cancer patients by an indirect effect on suppressor cells as well as the obvious effect on the neoplasm itself. New immunotherapeutic strategies that incorporate recent insight regarding the suppressor cell network are nullifying suppressor cell systems that oppose tumoricidal immune effector mechanisms. In addition to switching off antibody production by B-cells, suppressor T-cells apparently are also capable of preventing lymphokine production by other T-cells.

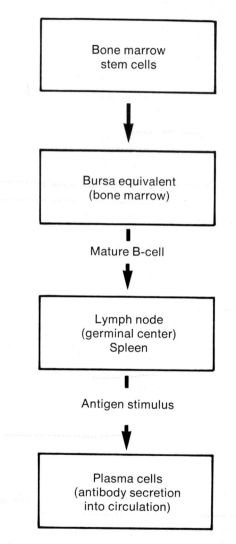

Fig. 16-7. Progress of B-cell lymphocyte maturation.

Humoral immunity

As the term suggests, humoral immunity is mediated by factors present in, and transferable by, serum; these include the classical antibody globulins. The cell responsible for the production of these antibodies is the second type of small lymphocyte, the B-cell (Fig. 16-7). In the chicken, these lymphocytes aggregate in a small organ called the bursa of Fabricius. Removal of the bursa was noted to render the chicken unable to produce antibodies, and the B-cells have thus come to be known as bursa-dependent cells. In humans there was a great deal of controversy as to the origin of these cells, but recent evidence has made it quite clear that these cells originate from the bone marrow and do not undergo maturation in the thymus. In humans (where there is no bursa of Fabricius), no one organ appears to have control of the B-cell production. Rather, B-cells are distributed in all areas of lymphoid tissue, including the spleen, lymph nodes, appendix, and Peyer's patches of the small intestine. With suitable stimulation, B-cells become metabolically active and begin to synthesize antibodies with great facility. The antibodies soon become detectable in the cytoplasm and then are secreted into the surrounding medium. It is at this point that the B-cell has undergone transformation into a plasma cell, which is the actual antibody producer. In a typical peripheral lymph node, B-cells occupy the germinal centers and T-cells the cortical areas; these areas are referred to, respectively, as the bursa-dependent and thymus-dependent areas of the node. Although the bone marrow appears to be the source of cells destined to make antibodies, the bone marrow itself is not the locus of large-scale antibody formation. Rather, it is the site of intense lymphocyte proliferation leading to the production of mature B-lymphocytes, which quickly leave the marrow and travel to peripheral lymphoid tissues. There they may meet the appropriate antigen, become stimulated to divide and differentiate into large lymphocytes and plasma cells, and actively manufacture

Table 16-2. Comparison of T- and B-cells

T-cells (thymus dependent)	B-cells (thymus independent)
Bone marrow origin	
Mature in thymus	Mature in lymph node
Concentrated in paracortical areas of the lymph node	Concentrated in germinal centers of the lymph node
Long-lived (months to years)	Short-lived (days to weeks)
Circulate widely	Less mobile, concentrated in lymph nodes and spleen
Sensitive to PHA	Insensitive to PHA
Sensitive to PWM	Sensitive to PWM
No immunoglobulins	Synthesize immunoglobulins
Cell-mediated immunity	Humoral immunity
Delayed hypersensitivity	Antibody production
Produce lymphokines	Do not usually produce lymphokines

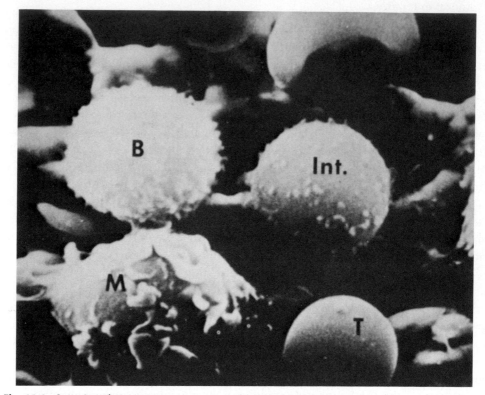

Fig. 16-8. Scanning electron microscopic view of peripheral blood leukocytes. (B, B-cell; M, macrophage; T, T-cell; Int., intermediate form, which may be of the "double cell" variety.)

antibodies. Resting B-lymphocytes are the typical small lymphocytes of the peripheral blood and, in fact, cannot be distinguished from resting T-lymphocytes under the usual light microscope (Table 16-2). Under the scanning electron microscope, typical B-cells have a hairy appearance with many small hairlike projections, whereas typical T-cells are smoother (Fig. 16-8). B-lymphocytes are particularly plentiful in areas where antibody production occurs, for example, in the germinal centers of the lymph nodes and in the diffuse lymphoid tissue of the gastrointestinal and respiratory tracts. They are less common in the blood, rare in the lymphatics and thoracic duct, and virtually absent from the thymus.

There is increasing evidence that the functional separation of T-cells and B-cells into two systems is not as clear-cut as formerly thought. An increasing number of biologically important responses are being discovered for which interplay of two systems is essential. This has been termed T-B cooperation. The presence of healthy T-cells is necessary for production by B-cells or many antibodies in response to antigenic stimulation and probably for the maintenance of immunologic memory for most antigens. The precise mechanism of this T-B cooperation is unknown; it may take the form of some messenger protein or actual physical contact and cytoplasmic bridging. Under suitable circumstances, B-cells are capable of secreting some of the non-immunoglobulin soluble products (lymphokines) that were formerly thought to be characteristic of T-cells, notably migration-inhibition factor. The biologic role of T-B cooperation is one of the most important areas for future research. There is a great deal of controversy regarding the order of production of immunoglobulins by the B-cell. Currently, it is thought that IgM is the first antibody produced, and then a switch to IgG production follows a signal possibly initiated by helper T-cells. Very recently, it has been theorized that IgD antedates the secretion of both IgM and IgG in embryonic life as well as in the adult. This is one of the many questions remaining to be settled.

Deficiencies of either or both of the thymic-dependent and bursa-dependent systems occur in a large variety of both congenital and acquired diseases. A list of the primary immunodeficiency syndromes includes chronic granulomatous disease, Chediak-Higashi disease, Bruton's syndrome, DiGeorge syndrome, ataxia-telangiectasia (Louis-Bar syndrome), and the Wiskott-Aldrich syndrome. The incidence of spontaneously occurring malignancy is increased appreciably in most of these conditions.

Suppression of the immunologic responses is a natural result of certain biologic processes such as pregnancy and aging. It also occurs in several systemic diseases, as a result of radiation or drug therapy, and following severe injuries. In most instances, CMI is suppressed more rapidly or profoundly than humoral immunity. With modern advances in immunologic techniques, the precise nature of the defect may be uncovered but is not known presently for many of these conditions. This kind of knowledge is essential if one is to treat these disorders effectively by immunologic means. Immunotherapy will be available in the near future, but its effectiveness will depend on the accurate diagnosis of the relevant immunologic defect and selective reversal. Conditions such as malnutrition, surgical trauma, burns, and accidental injuries will result in suppression of the host defense mechanism. This should be kept in mind in the design of an overall treatment plan for any patient.

Immunosurveillance

The mechanisms used by the host to mount a response against any antigens that are expressed by a neoplasm are called immunosurveillance. The primary function of the immune system is to recognize and degrade foreign ("nonself") antigens in the body that arise de novo or are inflicted upon the host. In tumor surveillance the assumption is made that the mutant cell will express one or more antigens that can be recognized as "nonself." A popular concept holds that mutant cells develop quite frequently in the human and are rapidly victimized by the ubiquitous and hopefully competent immunologic mechanisms. Mice deprived of CMI and exposed to an oncogenic agent will spontaneously develop more tumors. This is regarded as evidence of an immunosurveillance mechanism. Patients with advanced disease are often more immunosuppressed than patients with early disease (Fig. 16-9). Patients taking immunosuppressive drugs following renal transplantation have an increased incidence (100 times greater than matched controls) of malignancies. Nearly 50% of

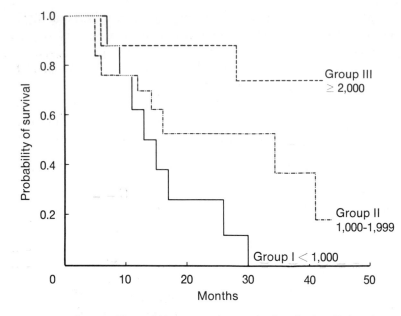

Fig. 16-9. Patients with stage III cervical cancer who received optimal radiation therapy. Survival (months) is correlated with initial peripheral blood lymphocyte counts. (Reprinted with permission from DiSaia, P. J., Morrow, C. P., Hill, A., and Mittelstaedt, L.: Immune competence and survival in patients with advanced cervical cancer; peripheral lymphocyte counts, J. Radiat. Oncol. **4:**449, 1978, Copyright 1978, Pergamon Press, Ltd.)

these tumors in immunosuppressed individuals are of mesenchymal origin (e.g., reticulum cell sarcomas), but a higher incidence of epithelial neoplasia, especially cervical intraepithelial neoplasia, has also been reported. Complementary evidence for the importance of tumor surveillance comes from the relationship between congenital or acquired immunodeficiency disease and tumor development; these patients also demonstrate an incidence of malignancy far in excess of matched controls.

Takasugi and others have called attention to a new subpopulation of lymphocytes called natural killer (NK) lymphocytes apparently active in the immunosurveillance of tumors. NK-cells from several species preferentially destroy malignant target cells in vitro and appear to need no prior sensitization. Indeed, NK-cells may be the effectors of tumor surveillance.

Escape from surveillance (Fig. 16-10)

There are several postulated mechanisms by which mutant cells might avoid an interaction with a potentially damaging immune system.

Lowered tumor antigenicity. Neoplasms that arise spontaneously are noted to be considerably less antigenic than those induced experimentally. Many human tumors may be weakly antigenic or nonantigenic.

Sneaking through. Old and others have reported neoplastic systems in which large inocula of immunogenic tumor cells fail to grow in a syngeneic recipient, but

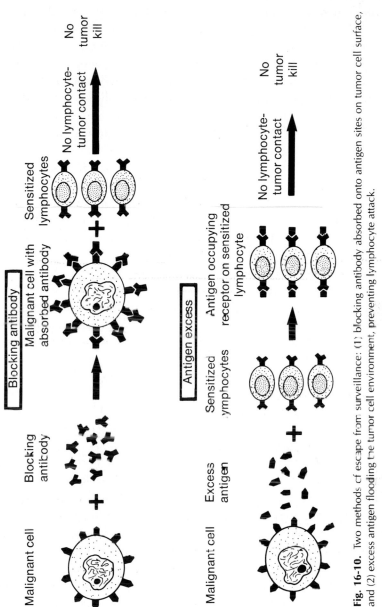

Fig. 16-10. Two methods of escape from surveillance: (1) blocking antibody absorbed onto antigen sites on tumor cell surface, and (2) excess antigen flooding the tumor cell environment, preventing lymphocyte attack.

smaller doses will grow and eventually overwhelm the host. The mechanism of "sneaking through" is unknown, but it may be related to the time of vascularization of the neoplasm.

Immunoresistance. Diminished sensitivity to rejection may develop in the same way that bacteria develop resistance to antibodies after repeated exposure. The cells may develop a decrease in cell surface antigenic sites (antigenic modulation) or relevant antibody-binding sites. Another mechanism that is easy to conceive calls for antigenic molecules on the surface of the tumor cell to be shed in large amounts into the surrounding extracellular fluid. The cell surface will then be rendered relatively immunoresistant as its locality becomes flooded with excess antigens. This may be classified then as a "blocking factor." Some have suggested that tumors that shed antigen rapidly are those of low immunogenicity which metastasize most rapidly.

Vascularization. Tumors probably reach to 1 to 2 mm in diameter before vascularization takes place. Folkman and Hochberg suggested that the vessels result from ingrowth of host cells, and thus the endothelium of the tumor vessels may be recognized as "self" and not rejected. Therefore, some neoplasms may proliferate with their antigens locked away behind a wall of "normal" endothelial cells unpenetrated by attack lymphocytes.

Immunosuppression. It has been well established that the presence of a cancer can significantly reduce an individual's capacity to mount a response to a great variety of antigens. Immunosuppressive factors have been described in the serum of cancer patients and confirmed in vitro. The mechanism by which these factors cause immunosuppression is currently not understood, but some authors have suggested that they suppress macrophage function. Some degree of immunosuppression has been found in almost all cancer patients studied. DNCB, DNFB, and a variety of skin test antigens have been used on patients with gynecologic malignancies. An increase in tumor burden is associated with a decreased percentage of patients responding to these tests, and both are associated with a poorer prognosis.

Blocking factors. Neoplasms may escape the immune mechanism by the development of systemic factors that abrogate the usual interaction with host defense capabilities. A number of serum factors have been identified in vitro: blocking antibodies, antigen-antibody complexes, and soluble antigen excess. When these blocking factors are operational, the state of the tumor-host relationship is one of tumor enhancement. The mechanisms involved may be quite similar to those described under immunoresistance. Excess free antibody may saturate antigenic sites on the cell surface, or conversely, excess free antigen may paralyze lymphocyte activity. In addition, recent studies suggest that the cellular factors of the immune system may be capable of causing tumor enhancement. In some animal and in vivo systems, small numbers of sensitized (tumor specific) lymphocytes can enhance tumor growth whereas larger numbers of the same cells will retard growth. This phenomenon has been referred to as immunostimulation, and if valid, it will help to explain the emergence of neoplasms beyond the subclinical stage where tumor cell numbers are very small and quite vulnerable. The puzzle is made more difficult by the fact that "deblocking" factors have also been described in the serum of cancer patients undergoing remission or following surgical debulking procedures. The mechanism involved in "deblocking" is unknown.

IMMUNOPROPHYLAXIS

Immunoprophylaxis is the induction of resistance to a tumor before its origination and should be clearly separated from immunotherapy, which is the treatment of established neoplasms and is a more difficult problem. Everyone interested in tumor immunology dreams of successes with immunoprophylaxis similar to those achieved with bacterial and viral illnesses. Immunoprophylaxis may be achieved by immunization either against the etiologic agent of the cancer (e.g., an oncongenic virus) or against the tumor specific cell surface antigens of the neoplasm. However, the oncogenic viruses of human cancer (if they exist) have not as yet been identified, and even if they exist we are unsure whether transmission is vertical or horizontal. The tumor specific cell surface antigens needed for the other approach have not as yet been adequately purified. Both pathways can be made to work in animal systems but have not been truly tested in humans. Some indirect evidence of a confirmatory nature comes from studies such as that of Rosenthal and associates, who reported a retrospective analysis of the leukemia death rate in an infant population from Chicago who received BCG compared with a similar population who had not received the vaccine. During the period 1964 to 1969, the death rate in the infants who were not vaccinated was six to seven times greater than the vaccinated group. At least one other study from Canada confirms the Rosenthal study, but others have not.

PRINCIPLES OF IMMUNOTHERAPY

It is obvious that the ultimate goal of immunotherapy is the complete destruction of all neoplastic cells. Short of obtaining that, the suppression of growth of tumor cells is desired. An expression of this therapeutic effect would be the prolongation of remission and the prevention of the appearance of metastatic disease. More often than not, the immunotherapist must be satisfied with evidence that the approach has achieved at least a reduction in the mass of tumor cells. Before the institution of immunotherapy, it is crucial to reduce tumor mass to a minimum, preferably less than 10^8 cells, by whatever means at hand—radical surgical procedures, chemotherapy, or irradiation therapy. It has been shown that immunotherapy can achieve little in the face of an overwhelming tumor burden, and immunotherapy by itself appears to be relatively ineffectual. At present it is always used with other cancericidal modalities, which are depended on to significantly reduce the tumor burden. As one would expect, immunotherapy has shown more effectiveness in neoplasms that are highly antigenic, e.g., Burkitt's lymphoma, malignant melanoma, and neuroblastoma. Most important, the reader should fully comprehend the embryonic nature of immunotherapy, and an attitude of cautious optimism must be maintained as this fetal area of research is brought to full term.

Nonspecific immunotherapy

A substance that increases response to an antigen is an adjuvant. Adjuvants may be effective by altering either the antigen itself or the immunologic reaction to the antigen. In the former instance, one can postulate a mechanism whereby the adjuvant would increase the release of antigen. Nonspecific immunotherapy directed toward the reaction to the antigen has focused on the cellular response. Recent studies suggest, however, at least two cellular cytotoxic mechanisms. One involves thymus-processed cytotoxic cells (T-cells), which recognize target antigens, and the other is controlled by a thymus-independent effector cell system, which is independent of the target antigen. The latter system is triggered to kill by recognition of antibody bound to the target, and it refutes our previously held simplistic view that stimulation of the cellular mechanism is beneficial whereas humoral immunity is of no aid. Present knowledge suggests four methods for stimulation of the host response mechanism: (1) increased or improved localization of cytotoxic antibody, (2) suppression of blocking factors, (3) more effective use of macrophage activity, and (4) heightened CMI.

The most widely used nonspecific immunotherapy has employed adjuvants such as bacillus Calmette-Guerin (BCG), *Corynebacterium parvum* (C-Parvum), levamisole, and MER. BCG is a live, attenuated strain of *Mycobacterium bovis*. *Corynebacterium parvum* is a gram-negative anaerobe given in a nonviable form. Levamisole is a synthetic antihelminthic drug that has been found to have significant effects on tumor immunity. MER is a methanol extraction of killed tuberculin bacilli.

The current era of experimentation with bacterial products began in 1959, when Old and associates demonstrated that injection of BCG was capable of inhibiting growth of tumors in mice. BCG had been introduced into clinical medicine in 1921 with its use as a vaccine against tuberculosis. Since 1921, many effects of BCG stimulating nonspecific immune responses in animals and humans have been demonstrated. Both humoral antibody synthesis and CMI are stimulated by BCG treatment. Mice injected with BCG show an increased resistance to infection with bacteria and are capable of clearing endotoxin and injected carbon particles far more rapidly than untreated mice. BCG injection leads to activation of macrophages as manifested by enhanced phagocytosis, increased microbicidal activity, increased macrophage metabolism, and increased ability of macrophages to kill tumor cell monolayer cultures. The most dramatic work with BCG was that of Rapp and associates with transplantable hepatoma in guinea pigs. They demonstrated that injection of BCG in growing intradermal tumor nodules was capable of eliminating the local nodule as well as eradicating tumor cells in draining lymph nodes. The dramatic response seen with guinea pig hepatoma may be due to cross-reactive antigens between BCG and this animal tumor. Recent evidence has shown that BCG may cross-react with antigens on human melanoma cells. In humans BCG has been used primarily in three ways: (1) intralesional injection, (2) systemic administration, generally by scarification or intradermal injection, and (3) mixed with cells and administered as a vaccine.

Intralesional use of BCG has largely been confined to treatment of cutaneous recurrences of malignant melanoma. In one series, approximately 90% of over 700 intracutaneously injected lesions in 36 patients could be made to undergo complete regression by BCG injection. Subcutaneous and visceral deposits of melanoma, however, are far more resistant to BCG treatment. Uninjected nodules surrounding the injected lesion that also undergo regression are always in the drainage area of the injected nodule. It would appear that direct contact between BCG and the tumor is essential for the therapeutic effect.

BCG administered intradermally by direct injection or by scarification techniques has been used in patients with leukemia and a variety of solid tumors. Most of the evidence for antitumor activity of BCG used systemically is derived from experiments involving pretreatment of animals. As immunotherapy in the treatment of established experimental tumors, it is remarkably ineffective. Mathé and associates reported success using BCG in children with acute lymphocytic leukemia, and Morton and associates reported improvement in survival using BCG after local excision and lymph node dissection in patients with stage II malignant melanoma. However, these studies have not been substantiated by prospective randomized trials. In acute lymphoblastic leukemia in childhood, two randomized control trials have failed to demonstrate any therapeutic effect. Others have studied BCG as an adjuvant to cyclophosphamide in a randomized control trail in patients with metastatic breast cancer. The objective response rate and the duration of response were unaffected by treatment with BCG in these breast cancer patients. Further prospective randomized trials are under way, but the enthusiasm once prevalent for solid tumor therapy appears to be weakening considerably.

Mathé and associates reported improvement in survival of patients with acute lymphoblastic leukemia treated with BCG plus allogeneic tumor cells. Morton and associates have also used BCG in conjunction with allogeneic tissue culture melanoma cells and reported this to be effective in patients with stage II and stage III malignant melanoma. However, convincing prospective studies of the value of such vaccines in the treatment of all solid tumors is currently lacking.

Corynebacterium parvum, like BCG, belongs to a group of bacterial agents that have stimulatory effects on the reticuloendothelial system, increase the phagocytic capacity of macrophages, and increase the resistance of animals to both infections and subsequent implantation or induction of experimental tumors. C-Parvum is also active by direct intralesional injection. In animal systems, C-Parvum given intravenously can induce regression of established local and pulmonary metastasis. C-Parvum was originally administered subcutaneously in combination with chemotherapy, and now several trials are under way utilizing this immunopotentiator intravenously. When used intravenously the drug produces high fever and shaking chills, and some patients have experienced thrombotic thrombocytopenic purpura. The potential of C-Parvum therapy, either subcutaneously or intravenously, has not been adequately investigated, although many clinical trials currently are under way. Unlike BCG, C-Parvum seems to act primarily by stimulating macrophage function; its effect on T-cell immunity is less clear.

Levamisole has been studied in animal systems, where it has been shown to potentiate the antibody and delayed hypersensitivity responses to a variety of antigens. It appears that levamisole can potentiate or permit expression of established delayed-type hypersensitivity reactions in previously immunocompetent individuals. One mechanism of levamisole action may be by causing maturation of thymus-derived immature lymphocyte precursors. It has been termed by some an "immunomodulator" in that it seems to reconstitute immunologic competence in patients who are immunosuppressed. Administration of levamisole before or concurrent with a bacterial adjuvant may augment the activity of the latter.

MER is the methanol extraction residue of BCG and was devised to overcome the problems associated with viable BCG preparations, including systemic BCG infection. This material, which is supplied as a particulate aqueous suspension, has shown both immunoprophylatic and immunotherapeutic activity comparable to that of BCG in a variety of animal models. It is administered intradermally or subcutaneously to humans. It produces rather severe local reactions characterized by inflammatory ulceration and/or sterile abscess formation. MER appears to be more immunopotentiating than BCG in humans and can restore established delayed hypersensitivity in approximately 20% of patients with widely metastatic solid tumors. A number of clinical trials with MER are currently under way, and additional data should be available soon.

A new category of substances that may have therapeutic value is the interferons. Interferons are inducible secretory glycoproteins that are produced both in vivo and in vitro by eukaryotic cells in response to viral infection and other stimuli. They induce a broad-spectrum resistance to viral infection. Interferon preparations have effects on tumor cells in vitro and antitumor activity in vivo by mechanisms that have not yet been identified but appear mediated in part through effects on several components of the immune response. These substances can be extracted from many cell types, but the leukocyte and lymphoblast appear to hold the most promise for therapeutic quality. Methods of production and purification are very expensive but available, and therapeutic trials are under way.

Various other factors (thymosins) have been identified that have thymic hormone-like activity. In general, these hormones can be expected to specifically increase host resistance through stimulation of the maturation of T-cells from precursor cells. This would represent an immunoaugmenting effect that should be helpful to patients with cancer, particularly those with T-cell deficiencies. A pilot study in patients with oat-cell carcinoma of the lung suggests that thymosin (fraction 5) given in conjunction with chemotherapy may prolong survival, especially of patients with relatively low immune reactivity before the beginning of therapy.

Specific immunotherapy

Tumor immunotherapy has been under study with extensive clinical trials, but less has been attempted using specific immunotherapy as compared with nonspecific modes. Specific immunotherapy can be active, passive, or adoptive.

Active specific immunotherapy calls for administration to the cancer patient of tumor cells, or their equivalent, bearing antigens that will cross-react with the neo-plasm. Tumor antigens are usually weakly antigenic, so that often immunostimulants (e.g., BCG) are administered jointly. Other attempts to heighten the immunoge-nicity of the tumor cells have been studied, such as surface changes by enzymes, viral incorporation, physical treatments, and chemical modifications. Although this remains an exciting field for future research, trials to date in humans have been disappointing.

An example of passive specific immunotherapy would be producing antisera to a patient's cancer in an animal (a great deal of absorption of foreign antigens would be necessary before use) or another cancer patient and then injecting the antisera into the patient. Passive transfer of antibodies has been attempted with no significant results. With further knowledge of the precarious role of antibodies, much less en-thusiasm has recently been noted, except in the area of "deblocking antibodies." Sjogren has reported on the existence of lymphocyte-dependent antibodies that ap-pear to arm cells and increase tumor kill. Others have described serum factors that appear to activate macrophages.

Adoptive specific immunotherapy would consist of the transfer of syngeneic, al-logeneic, or xenogeneic lymphoid cells from a specifically immunized donor to a tumor-bearing recipient. Unfortunately, in humans the recipient appears to rapidly reject the foreign cells, or even more disturbing, the donated immunocompetent cells may cause a graft-versus-host reaction in the immunodepressed cancer patient. Several other subcellular products have been studied as possible immunotherapeu-tic agents. They are the substances associated with states of delayed hypersensitivity, collectively known as lymphokines; the most widely studied substance is transfer factor. Parenteral administration of transfer factor in vivo converts nonsensitive re-cipient lymphocytes to a responsive state against specific antigens. The goal in using transfer factor is to provide patients with a means of instructing a clone of their own lymphocytes to recognize and reject the tumor. Although transfer factor could be manufactured in large amounts in animal systems, at present it has only been found in human systems, and its clinical use has been associated with only anecdotal re-sponses.

APPLICATIONS OF IMMUNOTHERAPY IN GYNECOLOGIC ONCOLOGY

Debois reported that patients receiving radiotherapy for stage IV cervical carci-noma had improved survival and response duration when they received levamisole immunotherapy concurrent with and subsequent to the radiotherapy as compared with a randomized group receiving placebo. A similar study is presently being con-ducted by the Gynecologic Oncology Group using C-Parvum as the immunoaug-menting agent. Jimi and associates administered BCG cell wall skeleton to patients with stage III and IV cervical carcinoma. The survival time in 28 cases was 12 months versus 4 months in 41 cases that were historical controls.

Juillard and associates conducted an interesting study of intralymphatic immu-notherapy for ovarian carcinoma using autologous or allogeneic ovarian tumor cells.

Irradiated ovarian tumor cells were injected into the lymphatics of the lower extremity monthly. One patient with ovarian cancer was treated in an optimum manner and showed significant regression of tumor after intralymphatic therapy. A similar study was conducted by Hudson and associates with patients receiving autologous and allogeneic tumor cell vaccine containing 2 x 10^7 irradiated tumor cells mixed with 2 x 10^5 viable BCG organisms on a monthly schedule. After surgical extirpation of ovarian cancer, four out of ten patients were alive and free of disease as compared with only four out of 25 historical controls after 2 years. In a study that was a follow-up to that reported by Hudson and associates, Crowther and Hudson reported that ten patients with ovarian cancer treated with tumor cell vaccine had a 21-month survival compared with 12 months in the historical controls. Wanebo and associates conducted a trial in advanced ovarian cancer patients who were given Cytoxan, Adriamycin, and 5-fluorouracil plus IV C-Parvum in escalating doses in a 14-day course. The C-Parvum was given subcutaneously between chemotherapy cycles. There was a 50% response rate in the patients who received the combination chemoimmunotherapy. This initial study was not a prospective randomized trial, but such a trial was carried out subsequently. The randomized trial had only 20 patients in each group, but response duration and survival were identical and did not confirm the impression derived from the pilot study. Creasman and associates conducted a similar pilot study using melphalan (Alkeran) in conjunction with intravenous C-Parvum for patients with advanced ovarian cancer. C-Parvum was given in a dose of 4 mg intravenously on day 7 in each chemotherapy cycle. The dose of melphalan was 1 mg/kg in divided doses over 5 days and repeated every 4 weeks. Responses were 53% in the chemoimmunotherapy group, which consisted of 45 patients, and 29% in 63 historical controls. The median survival duration was 24 months in the chemoimmunotherapy group versus 12 months in the chemotherapy controls. Another study using BCG in conjunction with Adriamycin and Cytoxan chemotherapy for disseminated ovarian cancer was reported by Alberts and associates. There were 118 evaluable patients in this prospective randomized study. After 36 months, the survival rate was 61% in the patients receiving Adriamycin-Cytoxan plus BCG and only 46% in the group receiving Adriamycin and Cytoxan alone. The median survival time was 23.5 months with Adriamycin-Cytoxan plus BCG and 13.1 months with Adriamycin and Cytoxan alone. Follow-up confirmatory studies are now under way.

IMMUNODIAGNOSIS

Immunodiagnosis is a field of investigative medicine largely based on the science of radioimmunoassay. Substances that are antigenic in animals or that can be bound to antigens can be measured in body fluids in very low concentrations. Tumor immunodiagnosis depends on the liberation by tumors of such substances into the bloodstream or other body fluids in a form or concentration not commonly found in healthy individuals. These substances, usually called tumor markers, are sometimes referred to as antigens, though they may not necessarily produce an immune response in the tumor-bearing host. Other substances may actually play a role in immunodiagnosis, e.g., hormones or the pregnancy-associated plasma proteins. Tumor-associated antigens and oncofetal antigens have been the major interest of tumor immunologists. In humans, evidence for the liberation of specific neoantigens is very scanty, and in ovarian cancer, early claims of the specificity of tumor extract antigenicity by Levi and Barber have awaited confirmation. Tumor-associated antigens have been roughly identified and characterized by Gall and associates and DiSaia. However, these antigens appear to have a unique ability to camouflage themselves among the normal proteins of the cell, defying attempts at refined isolation. Since the foundation of modern immunodiagnosis is the radioimmunossay, one must have an absolutely pure antigen to begin the process that will lead to a clinically useful tool. It is this purification of the tumor-associated antigen that has escaped investigators to date.

CONCLUSIONS

The field of tumor immunology has grown significantly in the last 2 decades, and it is impossible to address all aspects of this highly evolving area of scientific development in a chapter such as this. The reader is encouraged to obtain some of the references if additional information is desired. The two main objectives among those interested in clinical gynecologic tumor immunology continue to be methods of immunodiagnosis and immunotherapy. Immunodiagnosis is hampered at this point by the weakness of the tumor-associated antigens in gynecologic malignancies and the physicochemical and other technical problems associated with isolation of substances from the cell surface that vary only slightly from normal cellular molecules. The presence of tumor-associated antigens in gynecologic malignancies has been demonstrated by a number of indirect methods, and therefore the probability that an immunodiagnostic tool will be developed for the clinician is quite promising.

The status of immunotherapy in gynecologic cancer is similar to that in other human malignancies. Immunoprophylaxsis awaits identification of viral or other etiologic agents and/or purification of tumor-associated antigens. Both specific and nonspecific immunotherapeutic trials have been performed and are currently under way in various institutions, with rather mixed results. These less than optimum results are understandable if one takes into consideration the following factors. Most trials have used nonspecific immunotherapy, which relies on a generalized stimulation of the reticuloendothelial system with concomitant specific stimulation of clones directed toward the malignancy as a by-product. Specific immunotherapy has not been successful because of the weak immunogenic properties of the antigens involved. In addition, most clinical trials have been conducted in patients with a large tumor burden in whom reduction of that burden was assigned to surgery, chemotherapy, and/or radiotherapy. These cancericidal modalities are immunosuppressive in and of themselves and may abrogate the effectiveness of the immunopotentiator.

In 1980 the status of most immune monitoring techniques is quite disappointing. Indeed, most of the immune monitoring techniques that the immunotherapist formerly relied on to demonstrate an effect from immunotherapeutic agents have been demonstrated to be unreliable or inaccurate. Thus, the immunotherapist is forced to rely on clinical response as an endpoint, and clinical response is confused by the multiplicity of other factors involved in the patient's condition, such as other tumoricidal therapies, nutrition, and genetic make-up. In many ways, the cards have been stacked against the immunotherapist, and a certain amount of patience is appropriate among clinicians as these very complex issues are unraveled.

GLOSSARY

accessible antigens Antigens of self that are in contact with antibody-forming tissues and to a host that is normally tolerant.

active immunization Direct immunization of the intact individual or of immunocompetent cells derived from the individual and returned to him.

active immunotherapy May be divided into two groups: specific immunogens and nonspecific adjuvants. Active specific immunotherapy is attempted by the immunization of a tumor-bearing patient with autochthonous altered (radiation, chemical) tumor cells. Nonspecific immunotherapy attempts to augment antitumor immunologic activity with nonspecific stimulants such as BCG or C-Parvum.

adaptation A process whereby protection accorded a foreign graft from the immune reaction of the recipient renders it less vulnerable to immunologic attack by the host.

adjuvant A substance that when mixed with an antigen enhances its antigenicity.

adoptive immunization The transfer of immunity from one individual to another by means of specifically immune lymphoid cells or materials derived from such cells that are capable of transferring specific immunologic information to the recipient's lymphocytes.

agglutinin Any antibody that produces aggregation or agglutination of a particular or insoluble antigen.

allele An alternative gene acting at the same locus on the chromosome.

allergen A substance (antigen or hapten) that incites allergy.

allergy A state of specific increased reactivity to an antigen or hapten such as occurs in hay fever. The term is used to designate states of delayed sensitivity due to contact allergens.

alloantibody (isoantibody) Any antibody produced by one individual that reacts specifically with an antigen present in another individual of the same species. The term "isoantibody" is commonly used in hematology and "alloantibody" in tissue transplantation.

alloantigen (isoantigen) Any antigen that incites the formation of antibodies in genetically dissimilar members of the same species.

allogeneic Referring to genetically dissimilar individuals of the same species.

allogeneic disease Any systemic illness resulting from a graft-versus-host response when the graft contains immunologically competent cells and the host is immunologically incompetent (e.g., runt disease).

allograft (homograft) A graft derived from an allogeneic donor.

alloimmune Specifically immune to an allogeneic antigen.

alpha-fetoprotein (AFP) Synthesized in the fetus by perivascular hepatic parenchymal cells. It is found in a high percentage of patients with hepatomas and endodermal sinus tumor of the ovary or testes. It is a serum protein present in concentrations up to 400 mg/100 ml in early fetal life, falling to less than 3 μg/100 ml in adults. Increased levels may be detected in the serum of adults with hepatoma (80% positive) and endodermal sinus tumor (60% to 80% positive) and may be used to follow the disease progression.

anamnestic response (recall phenomenon, memory phenomenon) An accelerated response of antibody production to an antigen that occurs in an animal that has previously responded to the antigen.

anaphylaxis, acute Systemic shock (often fatal) that develops in a matter of minutes after subsequent exposure to a specific foreign antigen to which the host has already reacted.

anergy Absence of a hypersensitivity reaction that would be expected in other similarly sensitized individuals.

antibody (Ab) A substance (usually a gamma globulin) that can be incited in an animal by an antigen or by a hapten combined with a carrier and that reacts specifically with that antigen or hapten. Some antibodies can occur naturally without known antigen stimulation.

antibody reaction site (antigen binding site, antibody combining site) The inverted surface site on antibody that reacts with the antigen determinant site on antigen.

antibody response The production of antibody in response to stimulation by specific antigen.

antigen (Ag) A substance that can react specifically with antibodies and under certain conditions can incite an animal to form specific antibodies. Extrinsic: an antigen that is not a constituent or product of the cell. Intrinsic: an antigen that is a constituent or product of the cell.

antigen determinant A small, three-dimensional everted surface configuration on the antigen molecule that specifically reacts with the antibody reaction site on the antibody molecule.

antigenic paralysis See Immunologic tolerance.

Arthus reaction An inflammatory reaction characterized by edema, hemorrhage, and necrosis that follows the administration of antigen to an animal that already possesses precipitating antibody to that antigen.

atopy A hereditary predisposition of various individuals to develop immediate-type hypersensitivity on contact with certain antigens.

auto- Self or same.

autoantibodies Antibodies produced by an animal that react with the animal's own antigens. The stimulus is not known but could be the animal's own antigens or cross-reacting foreign antigens.

autoantigen A "self-antigen" that incites the formation of autoantibodies.

autochthonous (indigenous) Found in the same individual in which it originates, as in the case of a neoplasm; autochthonous tumor is a tumor borne by the host of origin.

autograft A graft derived from the same individual to whom it is transplanted.

autologous Derived from the recipient itself.

B-cell or B-lymphocyte A bone marrow cell. These cells mediate humoral immunity and are thymus-independent cells. In the avian species, these cells are derived from the bursa of Fabricius. In man, they originate in the bone marrow.

binding site A term used for the antibody-combining site and other sites of specific attachment of macromolecules to one another.

blocking factor A humoral antibody or an antigen-antibody complex or other factor that coats antigenic sites with a protective covering so that neither complement nor killer lymphocytes can attack the cell.

bursa of Fabricius A cloacal structure in Aves containing immature lymphoid elements (B-cells) and presumed to govern the production of humoral antibodies through these B-cells.

chimera An individual composed of genetically dissimilar tissues.

clone A population of cells derived from a single cell by asexual division.

committed cell A cell committed to the production of specific antibodies to a given antigen determinant. Committed cells include primed cells, memory cells, and antibody-producing cells.

complement (C') A multifactorial system of one or more normal serum components characterized by their capacity to participate in certain and specific antigen-antibody reactions.

complement activation Promotion of the killing or lytic actions of complement.

complement fixation The fixation of C' to an antigen-antibody complex.

cytophilic antibodies Antibodies with an affinity for cells that depend on bonding forces independent of those that bind antigen to antibody.

D-cell (double cell) Lymphocytes that appear to have characteristics of both T- and B-cells.

delayed hypersensitivity A specific sensitive state characterized by a delay of many hours in initiation time and course of reaction. It is transferable with cells but not with serum.

desensitization The procedure of rendering a sensitive individual insensitive to an antigen or hapten by treatment with that specific agent.

determinant group That part of the structure of an antigen molecule that is responsible for specific interaction with antibody molecules evoked by the same or a similar antigen.

enhancement factor See Blocking factor.

Fab (fragment antigen binding) That segment of the IgG antibody molecule, derived by papain treatment and reduction, containing only one antibody reaction site. Under oxidizing conditions, Fab fragments recombine to form the divalent molecule F(ab)$_2$ devoid of the Fc segment of the original molecule.

Forssman antigen An interspecies-specific antigen present in erythrocytes of many species, including some microorganisms, which is capable of inducing in animals devoid of such antigen the formation of lysin for sheep erythrocytes.

Freund's adjuvant Complete: Freund's emulsion of mineral oil, plant waxes, and killed tubercle bacilli used to combine with antigen to stimulate antibody production. Incomplete: Freund's mixture without tubercle bacilli.

hapten A substance that combines specifically with antibody but does not initiate the formation of antibody unless attached to a high molecular weight carrier.

helper factor Sensitized T-lymphocyte subpopulations release a helper factor that enables immunocompetent B-cells to respond to antigens that they otherwise are unable to recognize. The stimulated B-lymphocytes differentiate into plasma cells that produce antibody. The helper factor can also stimulate the B-lymphocyte to produce a variant of the B-cell, termed a killer cell (K), which is able to attack tumor cells only after the tumor cells have been exposed to specific antibody. Complement is not required for this action. *See also* Killer cell (K-cell).

hemagglutinin An antibody that reacts with a surface antigen determinant(s) on red cells to cause agglutination of those red cells.

hemolysin (amboceptor) An anti-red cell antibody that can specifically activate complement (C') to cause lysis of red cells.

hetero- Other or different; often used to mean "of a different species."

heterophil Pertains to antigenic specificity shared between species.

heterophile antigens Antigens common to more than one species.

heterozygosity The presence in a chromosome of dissimilar genes.

histocompatibility antigens (transplantation or HLA antigens) Antigens coded for by "histocompatibility genes" that determine the specific compatibility of grafted tissues and organs.

HLA antigens (human leukocyte antigen) A genetic locus containing two closely linked groups of several alleles (a subloci). They are present on the cell membranes of all nucleated cells and play a major role in determining graft take and rejection.

homologous See Allogeneic.

homologous disease See Allogeneic disease.

horizontal transmission of viruses Transmission of viruses between individual hosts of the same generation. *See also* Vertical transmission of viruses.

host The organism whose body serves to sustain a graft; interchangeable with the recipient.

humoral antibodies Antibodies present in body fluids.

humoral immunity Pertains to the body fluids, in contrast to cellular elements. It is initiated by the thymus-independent B-cells. These B-lymphocytes proliferate and differentiate into plasma cells that secrete immunoglobulins (IgG, IgM, IgA, IgD, and IgE).

immune The state of being secure against harmful agents (e.g., bacteria, virus, or other foreign proteins) or influences.

immune clearance Clearance of antigen from the circulation after complexing with antibodies.

immune response A specific response that results in immunity. The total response includes an afferent phase during which responsive cells are "primed" by antigen, a central response during which antibodies or sensitized lymphoid cells are formed, and an efferent or effector response dur-

ing which immunity is effected by antibodies or immune cells.

immunity The state of being able to resist and/or overcome harmful agents or influences. Active: Immunity acquired as the result of experience with an organism or other foreign substance. Passive: Immunity due to acquisition of antibody or sensitized lymphoid cells.

immunize The act or process of rendering an individual resistant or immune to a harmful agent.

immunocompetent cell (antigen-sensitive cell) Any cell that can be stimulated by antigen to either form antibodies or give rise to sensitized lymphoid cells including inducible cells, primed cells, and memory cells.

immunogen An antigen that incites specific immunity.

immunoglobulins (Ig) Classes of globulins to which all antibodies belong.

immunologic enhancement Enhanced survival of incompatible tissue grafts (tumor or normal tissue) due to specific humoral or other blocking factors.

immunologic paralysis Absence of normal specific immunologic response to an antigen, resulting from previous contact with the same antigen, administered in a quantity greatly exceeding that required to elicit an immunologic response. The normal capacity to respond to other unrelated antigens is retained.

immunologic surveillance Effective immunologic surveillance relies on the presence of tumor-specific antigenic determinants on the surfaces of neoplastic cells, which enable these altered cells to be recognized as "nonself" and to be destroyed by immunologic reactions.

immunologic tolerance (antigenic paralysis, immunologic suppression, immunologic unresponsiveness, antigen tolerance) Failure of the antibody response to a potential antigen after exposure to that antigen. Tolerance commonly results from prior exposure to antigens.

immunoreaction Reaction between antigen and its antibody.

interferon A protein released by cells in response to virus infection. It represents nonspecific immunity. This substance also appears to have nonspecific tumoricidal characteristics.

iso- Identical.

isoantibody The term used in blood grouping studies to designate an antibody formed by one individual that reacts with antigens of another individual of the same species. *See also* Alloantibody.

isoantigen See Alloantigen. The term "isoantigen" is commonly used in hematology.

isogeneic See Syngeneic.

isograft See Syngraft.

isoimmune See Alloimmune.

isologous See Syngeneic.

killer cell (K-cell) Sensitized T-lymphocytes produce a helper factor that acts on the immunocompetent lymphoid cell to produce a population of cells, probably variants of the B-cell, termed killer cells (K-cells), which are able to attack tumor cells that have been exposed to a specific sensitizing antibody. Unlike the usual humoral antibody (immunoglobulin) response, complement is not needed.

locus The precise location of a gene on a chromosome. Different forms of the gene (alleles) are always found at the same location on the chromosome.

lymphocyte A round cell with scanty cytoplasm and a diameter of 7 to 12 μ. The nucleus is round, sometimes indented, with chromatin arranged in coarse masses and without visible nucleoli. Lymphocytes may be actively mobile.

lymphoid cell(s) Any or all cells of the lymphocytic and plasmacytic series.

lymphokine Substances released by sensitized lymphocytes when they come in contact with the antigen to which they are sensitized; examples include transfer factor (TF), lymphocyte-transforming activity (LTA), migration inhibition factor (MIF), and lymphotoxin (LT).

macrophage Large mononuclear phagocyte; in the tissues, this cell may be called a histiocyte and in the blood a monocyte. An antigen must come in contact with or pass through a macrophage before it can become a processed antigen with the ability to encounter and then sensitize a small lymphocyte.

macrophage-activating factor (MAF) Sensitized T-lymphocytes can release a nonspecific macrophage activating factor that creates a cytotoxic population of macrophages that appears to distinguish malignant from normal cells, killing only malignant ones.

memory cells Cells that can mount an accelerated antibody response to antigen.

migration inhibition factor (MIF) A lymphokine produced when a sensitized lymphocyte is exposed to an antigen to which it is sensitized. MIF inhibits the migration of these lymphocytes.

mitogen A substance that induces immunocompetent lymphocytes to undergo blast transformation, mitosis, and cell division (causing mitosis or cell division).

mosaic An individual composed of two or more genetically dissimilar cell lines but from the same species. This can come about either by somatic mutation or by grafting cells between individuals of very close genetic constitution, such as dizygotic twins.

natural antibodies Antibodies that occur naturally without deliberate antigen stimulation.

natural killer lymphocytes (NK-cells) Lymphocytes that are active in the immune surveillance of tumor. NK-cells can lyse malignant target cells in vitro and appear to need no prior sensitization.

nonspecific immunization Refers to stimulation of the general immune response by the use of materials (e.g., BCG or PHA) that are not antigenically related to the specific tumor.

nude mice Mice born with a congenital absence of the thymus. The blood and thymus-dependent areas of the lymph nodes and spleen are depleted of lymphocytes.

oncogenic An agent capable of causing normal cells to acquire neoplastic characteristics. The term is often applied to viruses, such as adenoviruses.

passive transfer of immunity The transfer of specific antibody from one individual to another.

phytohemagglutinins Lectins extracted from the red kidney bean, *Phaseolus vulgaris* or *P. communis;* the extract can be purified to yield a glycoprotein mitogen that stimulates lymphocyte transformation and causes agglutination of certain red cells; provides a method for calculating the pool of thymus-dependent lymphocytes (T-cells).

pokeweed mitogen (PWM) A mitogen extracted from the pokeweek plant; it can be purified to yield a specific glycoprotein. PWM stimulates blast formation of both B- and T-cells.

precipitin An antibody that reacts specifically with soluble antigen to form a precipitate.

prophylactic immunization Represents preimmunization of an individual against a causative agent (e.g., oncogenic virus) or tumor-specific antigen, in advance of any natural encounter with the agent or tumor.

runt disease A condition of dwarfing that follows the injection of mature allogeneic immunologically competent cells into immunologically immature recipients. It is characterized by failure to thrive, lymph node atrophy, hepato- and splenomegaly, anemia, and diarrhea.

sensitize The process of increasing the specific reactivity of a subject or cell to an agent. Commonly used to designate the process of increasing reactivity due to specific antibodies or "immune cells."

Shwartzman reaction A local nonimmunologic inflammatory reaction with hemmorrhage and necrosis produced by the injection of a bacterial endotoxin.

suppressor T-cells Represent an important set of feedback controls, centered around sensitized T-lymphocytes, through which inhibitory populations of these T-cells suppress the production of sensitized lymphocytes and antibody-forming cells.

syngeneic (isogeneic) Pertaining to genetically identical or nearly identical animals, such as identical twins or highly inbred animals.

syngraft (isograft) A graft derived from syngeneic donor.

T-lymphocyte (T-cell) Lymphocytes that have matured and differentiated under thymic influence, termed thymic-dependent lymphocytes. These cells are primarily involved in the mediation of cellular immunity, as well as tissue and organ graft rejection.

transfer factor A heat labile, dialyzable extract of human lymphocytes (a lymphokine) that is capable of conferring specific antigen reactivity to the donor.

tumor angiogenesis factor (TAF) Represents the induction of the growth of blood vessels due to this stimulant released by tumor cells. The growth of a tumor appears to parallel the development of new blood vessels.

tumor necrosis factor (TNF) A lymphokine released by the macrophage that is toxic for neoplastic cells.

vaccination Injection or ingestion of an immunogenic antigen(s) for the purpose of producing active immunity.

vaccine A suspension of dead or living microorganisms that is injected or ingested for the purpose of producing active immunity.

vertical transmission of viruses Transmission from one generation to another. Can include transmission from one generation to the next via milk or through the placenta.

xenogeneic (heterologous) Pertaining to individuals of different species.

xenograft (heterograft) A graft derived from an animal of a different species than that of the one receiving the graft.

BIBLIOGRAPHY

Alberts, D. S.: Adjuvant immunotherapy with BCG of advanced ovarian cancer; a preliminary report. In Salmon, S. E., and Jones, S. E., editors: Adjuvant therapy of cancer, Amsterdam, 1977, Elsevier/North-Holland Biomedical Press.

Alberts, D. S., Moon, T. E., O'Toole, R. and others: BCG as an adjuvant to Adriamycin-Cytoxan for advanced ovarian cancer; a Southwest Oncology Group study. In Jones, S., and Salmon, S. E., editors: Second International Conference on Adjuvant Therapy of Cancer, New York, 1979, Grune & Stratton, Inc.

Bansal, S. C., and Sjogren, H. O.: "Unblocking" serum activity in vitro in the polyoma system may correlate with antitumour effects of antiserum in vivo, Nature [New Biol.] **233**:76, 1971.

Barber, H. R.: Immunobiology for the clinician, New York, 1977, John Wiley & Sons, Inc.

Barlow, J. J., and Bhattacharya, M.: Tumor markers in ovarian cancer; tumor associated antigens, Semin. Oncol. **11**:203, 1975.

Billingham, R. E., Brent, L., and Medawar, P. B.: Acquired tolerance of skin homografts, Ann. N.Y. Acad. Sci. **59**:409, 1955.

Boronow, R. C., Barber, H. R., Cohen, C., and DiSaia, P. J.: Symposium; immunologic diagnosis of ovarian cancers, Contemp. Ob/Gyn **4**:53, 1974.

Braun, W., and Ungar, J., editors: Nonspecific factors influencing host resistance, Basel, 1973, S. Karger.

Broder, S., and Waldmann, T. A.: The suppressor-cell network in cancer, N. Engl. J. Med. **229**:1281, 1335, 1978.

Creasman, W. T., Gall, S. A., DiSaia, P. J., and Whisnant, J. K.: Chemoimmunotherapy in the management of primary stage III carcinoma of the ovary, Cancer Treat. Rep. **63**:319, 1979.

Crowther, M. E., and Hudson, C.: Experience with a pilot study of active intralymphatic immunotherapy, Cancer **41**:2215, 1978.

Currie, G. A.: Eighty years of immunotherapy; a review of immunological methods used for the treatment of human cancer, Br. J. Cancer **26**:141, 1972.

Currie, G. A.: Cancer and the immune response, London, 1974, Edward Arnold (Publishers) Ltd.

Currie, G. A., and Alexander, P.: Spontaneous shedding of TSTA by viable sarcoma cells; its possible role in facilitating metastatic spread, Br. J. Cancer **29**:72, 1974.

Debois, J. M.: Five-year experience with levamisole in cancer patients. Third interim report. Clinical Research Report on R 12564/69, 1978, Janssen Research Productive Information Service.

DiSaia, P. J.: Studies in cell-mediated immunity in two gynecologic malignancies, Cancer Bull. **23**:65, 1971.

DiSaia, P. J.: Tumor immunology; general aspects, Contemp. Ob/Gyn **4**:91, 1974.

DiSaia, P. J.: Immunological aspects of gynecologic malignancies, Reprod. Med. **14**:17, 1975.

DiSaia, P. J.: Overview of tumor immunology in gynecologic oncology, Cancer **38**:566, 1976.

DiSaia, P. J., Haverback, B. J., Dyce, B. J., and Morrow, C. P.: Carcinoembryonic antigen in patients with gynecologic malignancies, Am. J. Obstet. Gynecol. **121**:159, 1975.

DiSaia, P. J., Morrow, C. P., Haverback, B. J., and Dyce, B. J.: Carcinoembryonic antigen in cancer of the female reproductive system; serial plasma values correlated with disease state, Cancer **39:**1265, 1977.

DiSaia, P. J., Morrow, C. P., Hill, A., and Mittelstaedt, L.: Immune competence and survival in patients with advanced cervical cancer; peripheral lymphocyte counts, J. Radiat. Oncol. **4:**449, 1978.

DiSaia, P. J., Morrow, C. P., and Townsend, D. E.: Synopsis of gynecologic oncology, New York, 1975, John Wiley & Sons, Inc.

DiSaia, P. J., Nalick, R. H., and Townsend, D. E.: Antibody cryotoxicity studies in ovarian and cervical malignancies, Obstet. Gynecol. **1:**314, 1973.

DiSaia, P. J., and Rich, W. M.: Value of immune monitoring in gynecologic cancer patients receiving immunotherapy, Am. J. Obstet. Gynecol. **135:**907, 1979.

DiSaia, P. J., and Rutledge, F. N.: Cell-mediated immunologic response to two gynecologic tumors, Cancer **23:**1129, 1971.

Eilber, F. R., and others: Immunotherapy as an adjunct to surgery in the treatment of cancer, World J. Surg. **1:**547, 1977.

Folkman, J., and Hochberg, M.: Self-regulation of growth in three dimensions, J. Exp. Med. **138:**745, 1973.

Gall, S. A., Walling, J., and Pearl, J.: Demonstration of tumor-associated antigens in human gynecologic malignancies, Am. J. Obstet. Gynecol. **115:**387, 1973.

Goodnight, J. E.: Immunotherapy for malignant disease, Ann. Rev. Med. **29:**231, 1978.

Gutterman, J. U., Mavligit, G., Gottlieb, J. A., and others: Chemoimmunotherapy of disseminated malignant melanoma with DTIC and BCG, N. Engl. J. Med. **291:**592, 1974.

Halpern, B.: Corynebacterium parvum; applications in experimental and clinical oncology, New York, 1975, Plenum Publishing Corp.

Hudson, C. N., Crowther, M. E., Poulton, T., and others: Experience of a pilot study of active specific immunotherapy in advanced ovarian cancer. In Davis, W., and Harrap, K. R., editors: Characterization and treatment of human tumours, Proceedings of the Seventh International Symposium on the Biological Characterization of Human Tumours, Amsterdam, Excerpta Medica Foundation, Advances in Tumour Prevention, Detection and Characterization **4:**332, 1978.

Jimi, S., Watanabe, Y., Mashiba, H., and others: Immunotherapy of uterine cervical cancer with BCG cell-wall skeleton, Proc. Jap. Cancer Assoc., Abstract No. 257, 1977.

Juillard, G. J., Boyer, P. J., and Yamashiro, C. H.: A phase I study of active specific intralymphatic immunotherapy, Cancer **41:**2215, 1978.

Lawrence, H. S.: Immunotherapy with transfer factor, N. Engl. J. Med. **287:**1092, 1972.

Levi, M. M.: Antigenicity of ovarian and cervical malignancy in a view toward possible immunodiagnosis, Am. J. Obstet. Gynecol. **109:**689, 1971.

Maserang, V. L., and others: Immunodiagnosis of human malignancy, South. Med. J. **70:**222, 1977.

Mathé, G.: Active immunotherapy, Adv. Cancer Res. **14:**1, 1971.

Mathé, G., and others: Attempts at immunotherapy of 100 patients with acute lymphoid leukemia; some factors influencing results, Natl. Cancer Inst. Monogr. **36:**361, 1972.

Morton, D., Eilber, F. R., and Malmgren, R. A.: Immunological factors which influence response to immunotherapy in malignant melanoma, Surgery **68:**158, 1970.

Morton, D. L., and Goodnight, J. E.: Clinical trials of immunotherapy, Cancer **42:**2224, 1978.

Nalick, R. H., DiSaia, P. J., Rea, T. H., and Morrow, C. P.: Immunocompetence and prognosis in patients with gynecologic cancer, Gynecol. Oncol. **2:**81, 1974.

Nalick, R. H., DiSaia, P. J., Rea, T. H., and others: Immunologic response in gynecologic malignancy as demonstrated by the delayed hypersensitivity reaction; clinical correlations, Am. J. Obstet. Gynecol. **118:**393, 1974.

Old, L. J., and others: The role of the reticuloendothelial system in the host reaction to neoplasia, Cancer Res. **21:**1281, 1961.

Old, L. J., and others: Antigenic properties of chemically-induced tumors, Ann. N.Y. Acad. Sci. **101:**80, 1962.

Pilch, Y., Myers, G. H., Sparks, F. C., and Golub, S. H.: Prospects for the immunotherapy of cancer. In Current problems in surgery, Chicago, 1975, Year Book Medical Publishers, Inc.

Rao, B., Wanebo, H. J., Ochoa, M., and others: Intravenous Corynebacterium parvum; an adjunct to chemotherapy for resistant advanced ovarian cancer, Cancer **39:**514, 1977.

Rapp, H. J., and others: Antigenicity of new diethylnitrosamine-induced transplantable guinea pig hepatoma, J. Natl. Cancer Inst. **41:**1, 1968.

Rosenthal, S. R., Crispen, R. G., Thorne, M. G., and others: BCG vaccination and leukemia mortality, J.A.M.A. **222:**1543, 1972.

Sadler, T. E., and Castro, J. E.: Treatment of a metastasizing murine tumour with Corynebacterium parvum, Br. J. Cancer **63:**292, 1976.

Sinkovics, J. G., DiSaia, P. J., and Rutledge, F. N.:

Tumour immunology and evolution of the placenta, Lancet **2:**1190, 1970.

Sjogren, H. O.: Blocking and unblocking of cell-mediated tumour immunity. In Busch, H., editor: Methods in cancer research, New York, 1973, Academic Press, Inc.

Smith, R. T.: Potentials for immunologic intervention in cancer. In Amos, B., editor: Progress in immunology, New York, 1971, Academic Press, Inc.

Smith, R. T.: Possibilities and problems of immunologic intervention in cancer, N. Engl. J. Med. **287:**439, 1972.

Streilein, J. W.: Immunotherapy of cancer, Surg. Gynecol. Obstet. **147:**769, 1978.

Takasugi, M., Mickey, M. R., and Terasaki, P. I.: Reactivity of lymphocytes from normal persons on cultured tumor cells, Cancer Res. **33:**2898, 1973.

Wanebo, H. J., Ochoa, M., Gunther, U., and others: Randomized chemoimmunotherapy trial of CAF and intravenous C. parvum for resistant ovarian cancer—preliminary results, Proc. Am. Assoc. Cancer Res. **18:**225, 1977.

Ziegler, J. L., and Magrath, I. T.: BCG immunotherapy in Burkitt's lymphoma; preliminary results of a randomized clinical trial, Natl. Cancer Inst. Monogr. **39:**199, 1973.

APPENDIX A

Staging

STAGING OF CANCER AT GYNECOLOGIC SITES
CERVIX UTERI, CORPUS UTERI, OVARY, VAGINA, AND VULVA

In 1976 the AJC adopted the classification of the International Federation of Gynecology and Obstetrics (FIGO), which is the format used in the "Annual Report on the Results of Treatment in Carcinoma of the Uterus, Vagina and Ovary." Published every 3 years, this report has utilized the FIGO classification with periodic modifications since 1937. Numerous institutions throughout the world contribute their statistics for inclusion in this voluntary collaborative presentation of data.

Since 1966 the TNM Committee of the International Union Against Cancer (UICC) has promulgated its recommendations for the classification of gynecologic tumors. From time to time, often in concert with representatives of FIGO, these recommendations also have been modified. The most recent revision in 1976 has brought the TNM and FIGO definitions into full conformity with each other. At this time, therefore, all systems are substantially in full agreement both as to categories and details.

Anatomy and classification by sites of malignant tumors of the female pelvis
Cervix uteri
1.0 anatomy

1.1 PRIMARY SITE: The cervix is the lower third of the uterus. It is roughly cylindrical in shape, projects through the upper, anterior vaginal wall and communicates with the vagina through an orifice called the external os. Cancer of the cervix may originate on the vaginal surface or in the canal.

1.2 NODAL STATIONS: The cervix is drained by preureteral, postureteral, and uterosacral routes into the following first station nodes: parametrial, hypogastric (obturator), external iliac, presacral, and common iliac. Para-aortic nodes are second station and juxtaregional.

From Manual for staging of cancer 1978, Chicago, 1978, American Joint Committee for Cancer Staging and End Results Reporting.

433

1.3 METASTATIC SITES: The most common sites of distant spread include the lungs and skeleton.

2.0 Rules for classification

2.1 CLINICAL-DIAGNOSTIC STAGING: Careful clinical examination should be performed in all cases, preferably by an experienced examiner and with anesthesia. The clinical staging must not be changed because of subsequent findings. When there is doubt as to which stage a particular cancer should be allocated, the earlier stage is mandatory. The following examinations are permitted: palpation, inspection, colposcopy, endocervical curettage, hysteroscopy, cystoscopy, proctoscopy, intravenous urography, and x-ray examination of the lungs and skeleton. Suspected bladder or rectal involvement should be confirmed by biopsy and histologic evidence. Optional examinations include: lymphangiography, arteriography, venography, laparoscopy, and others. Because these are not yet generally available and also because the interpretation of results is variable, the findings of optional studies should not be the basis for changing the clinical staging.

2.2 SURGICAL-EVALUATIVE STAGING: Surgical evaluation is applicable only after laparotomy and examination of tumor and nodes. Conization or amputation of the cervix is regarded as a clinical examination. Invasive cancers so identified are to be included in the reports (see 4.0).

2.3 POSTSURGICAL TREATMENT-PATHOLOGIC STAGING: In cases treated by surgical procedures, the pathologist's findings in the removed tissues can be the basis for extremely accurate statements on the extent of disease. These findings should not be allowed to change the clinical staging but should be recorded in the manner described for the pathologic staging of disease. The pTNM nomenclature is appropriate for this purpose. Infrequently, it happens that hysterectomy is carried out in the presence of unsuspected extensive invasive cervical carcinoma. Such cases cannot be clinically staged or included in therapeutic statistics, but it is desirable that they be reported separately. Only if the rules for clinical staging are strictly observed will it be possible to present comparable results between clinics and by differing modes of therapy.

2.4 RETREATMENT STAGING: Complete examination using the procedures cited in 2.1, including a search for distant metastases, is recommended in cases known or suspected to have recurrence. Biopsy and histologic confirmation are particularly desirable when induration and fibrosis from previously treated disease are present.

3.0 Staging classification

FIGO NOMENCLATURE

Stage 0   Carcinoma in situ, intraepithelial carcinoma
Stage I   The carcinoma is strictly confined to the cervix (extension to the corpus should be disregarded)

Stage IA   Microinvasive carcinoma (early stromal invasion)

Stage IB   All other cases of stage I; occult cancer should be marked "occ."

Stage II   The carcinoma extends beyond the cervix but has not extended to the pelvic wall. The carcinoma involves the vagina, but not as far as the lower third

Stage IIA   No obvious parametrial involvement *(vagina)*

Stage IIB   Obvious parametrial involvement *parament.*

Stage III   The carcinoma has extended to the pelvic wall. On rectal examination, there is no cancer-free space between the tumor and the pelvic wall. The tumor involves the lower third of the vagina. All cases with hydronephrosis or nonfunctioning kidney are included, unless they are known to be due to other cause   *(A) — vagina*

Stage IIIA   No extension to the pelvic wall

Stage IIIB   Extension to the pelvic wall and/or hydronephrosis or nonfunctioning kidney

Stage IV   The carcinoma has extended beyond the true pelvis or has clinically involved the mucosa of the bladder or rectum. A bullous edema as such does not permit a case to be allotted to stage IV

Stage IVA   Spread of the growth to adjacent organs

Stage IVB   Spread to distant organs

Notes about the staging. Stage IA (microinvasive carcinoma) represents those cases of epithelial abnormalities in which histologic evidence of early stromal invasion is unambiguous. The diagnosis is based upon microscopic examination of tissue removed by biopsy, conization, portio amputation, or removal of the uterus. Cases of early stromal invasion should thus be allotted to stage IA.

The remainder of stage I cases should be allotted to stage IB. As a rule these cases can be diagnosed by routine clinical examination.

Occult cancer is a histologically invasive cancer that cannot be diagnosed by routine clinical examination. As a rule it is diagnosed on the basis of a cone, the amputated portio, or on the removed uterus. Such cancers should be included in stage IB and should be marked "stage IB, occ."

Stage I cases can thus be indicated in the following ways:

Stage IA   Carcinoma in situ with early stromal invasion diagnosed on tissue removed by biopsy, conization, portio amputation, or on the removed uterus

Stage IB   Clinically invasive carcinoma confined to the cervix

Stage IB, occ   Histologically invasive carcinoma of the cervix which could not be detected at routine clinical examination but which was diagnosed on the basis of a large biopsy specimen, a cone, the amputated portio, or the removed uterus

As a rule, it is impossible to estimate clinically whether a cancer of the cervix has extended to the corpus or not. Extension to the corpus should therefore be disregarded.

A patient with a growth fixed to the pelvic wall by a short and indurated but not nodular parametrium should be allotted to stage IIB. It is impossible, at clinical examination, to decide whether a smooth and indurated parametrium is truly cancerous or only inflammatory. Therefore, the case should be placed in stage III only if the parametrium is nodular to the pelvic wall or if the growth itself extends to the pelvic wall.

The presence of hydronephrosis or nonfunctioning kidney due to stenosis of the ureter by cancer permits a case to be allotted to stage III even if, according to the other findings, the case should be allotted to stage I or stage II.

The presence of bullous edema, as such, should not permit a case to be allotted to stage IV. Ridges and furrows into the bladder wall should be interpreted as signs of submucous involvement of the bladder if they remain fixed to the growth at palposcopy (i.e., examination from the vagina or the rectum during cystoscopy). Finding malignant cells in cytologic washings from the urinary bladder requires further examination and a biopsy from the wall of the bladder.

TNM NOMENCLATURE

3.1 PRIMARY TUMOR (T)

TIS   Carcinoma in situ
         See Stage 0

T1, 1a, 1b, 2a, 2b, 3a, 3b, 4
         See corresponding FIGO stages

3.2 NODAL INVOLVEMENT (N)

NX   Not possible to assess the regional nodes
N0   No involvement of regional nodes
N1   Evidence of regional node involvement
N4   Involvement of lumbo-aortic nodes

3.3 DISTANT METASTASIS (M)

MX   Not assessed
M0   No (known) distant metastasis
M1   Distant metastasis present
         Specify _____
         Specify sites according to the following notations:
            Pulmonary—PUL
            Osseous—OSS
            Hepatic—HEP
            Brain—BRA
            Lymph nodes—LYM
            Bone marrow—MAR
            Pleura—PLE
            Skin—SKI
            Eye—EYE
            Other—OTH

4.0 Postsurgical treatment residual tumor (R)

R0   No residual tumor
R1   Microscopic residual tumor
R2   Macroscopic residual tumor
        Specify _____

5.0 Stage grouping (correlation of AJC, TNM, and FIGO nomenclatures)

Stage 0	TIS		
Stage IA	T1a	NX	M0
IB	T1b	NX	M0
Stage IIA	T2a	NX	M0
IIB	T2b	NX	M0
Stage IIIA	T3a	NX	M0
IIIB	T3b	NX	M0
Stage IVA	T4a	NX-0-1	M0
Stage IVB	Any T	Any N	M1

6.0 Histopathology

Cases should be classified as carcinoma of the cervix if the primary growth is in the cervix. All histologic types must be included. Grading by any of several methods is encouraged but is not a basis for modifying the stage groupings. When surgery is the primary treatment, the histologic findings permit the case to have pathologic staging as described in 2.3. In this the pTNM nomenclature is to be used. It is desirable that all tumors be microscopically verified but cases that clinically are likely to be cancer without such confirmation should be included with special attention to descriptive detail. The number should be kept to a minimum.

7.0 Data form for cancer staging

The data collecting form that follows has been designed for use by institutions in summarizing the described information on individual cases. One should be on file in the registry for each accession. An additional checklist is recommended whenever a patient arrives at a new point for staging such as postsurgical, pathologic, etc.

The checklist includes the relevant items of information desirable at all gynecologic sites but only those need be used which apply in a given case. However, as complete a record as possible is necessary for accuracy in staging and analysis of results.

The diagrams are most helpful to those who review cases subsequently. Individuals are urged to mark in contrasting color (red) the location of tumor and satellites on the relevant diagrams at the time of initiation of the form.

Corpus uteri
1.0 Anatomy

1.1 PRIMARY SITE: The upper two-thirds of the uterus above the level of the internal cervical os is called the corpus. The fallopian tubes enter at the upper lateral corners of a pear-shaped body. That portion of the muscular organ which is above a line joining the tubo-uterine orifices is often referred to as the fundus.

1.2 NODAL STATIONS: The major lymphatic trunks are the utero-ovarian (infundi-bulor-pelvic), parametrial, and presacral, which drain into the hypogastric, external iliac, common iliac, presacral, and para-aortic nodes.

1.3 METASTATIC SITES: The vagina and lung are the common metastatic sites.

2.0 Rules for classification

2.1 CLINICAL-DIAGNOSTIC STAGING: Careful clinical examination should be performed, preferably by an experienced examiner and with anesthesia, before any definitive therapy. The clinical staging must not be changed because of subsequent findings. When there is doubt as to which stage a particular cancer should be allocated, the earlier stage is mandatory. The following examinations are permitted: palpation, inspection, colposcopy, endocervical curettage, hysteroscopy, cystoscopy, proctoscopy, intravenous urography, and x-ray examination of lungs and skeleton. Optional examinations include lymphangiography, arteriography, venography, and laparoscopy. Sounding and determination of the depth of the uterine cavity is an important step. Fractional curettage is essential with separation of endometrial and endocervical curettings. Careful inspection and palpation of the vagina should be carried out to assess the entire length of the vaginal tube from the apex to the urethra.

2.2 SURGICAL-EVALUATIVE STAGING: Biopsy proof is advised for suspected vaginal, bladder, or rectal invasion. Laparotomy is needed for evaluation and examination of pelvic and para-aortic lymph nodes.

2.3 POSTSURGICAL TREATMENT-PATHOLOGIC STAGING: Hysterectomy with or without pelvic node dissection provides the basis for surgical-pathologic staging and should not be substituted for clinical staging.

2.4 RETREATMENT STAGING: Utilization of available procedures noted above is required, particularly since induration and necrosis can occur after irradiation; scarring and nodularity to a vaginal cuff can occur after surgery. A reevaluation for distant metastases, as well as T and N compartments, is recommended.

3.0 Staging classification
FIGO NOMENCLATURE

Stage 0   Carcinoma in situ. Histologic findings are suspicious of malignancy; cases of stage 0 should not be included in any therapeutic statistics

Stage I   The carcinoma is confined to the corpus

        Stage IA   The length of the uterine cavity is 8 cm or less

        Stage IB   The length of the uterine cavity is more than 8 cm

        It is desirable that the stage I cases be subgrouped with regard to the histologic type of the adenocarcinoma as follows:

        G1   Highly differentiated adenomatous carcinoma

        G2   Moderately differentiated adenomatous carcinoma with partly solid areas

G3   Predominantly solid or entirely undifferentiated carcinoma

Stage II   The carcinoma has involved the corpus and the cervix but has not extended outside the uterus

Stage III   The carcinoma has extended outside the uterus but not outside the true pelvis

Stage IV   The carcinoma has extended outside the true pelvis or has obviously involved the mucosa of the bladder or rectum. A bullous edema as such does not permit a case to be allotted to stage IV

Stage IVA   Spread of the growth to adjacent organs

Stage IVB   Spread to distant organs

Notes about the staging. Studies of large series of cases of endometrial carcinoma limited to the corpus have shown that the prognosis is related to some extent to the size of the uterus. However, an enlargement of the uterus may be caused by fibroids, adenomyosis, and other disorders. Therefore, the size of the uterus cannot serve as a basis for subgrouping stage I cases. The length and the width of the uterine cavity are related to the prognosis. The great majority of cases of corpus cancer belong to stage I. A subdivision of these cases is desirable. Therefore, the Cancer Committee recommends a subdivision of stage I cases with regard to the length of the sound used and to the histologic examination of the curettings.

Extension of the carcinoma to the endocervix is confirmed by fractional curettage, hysterography, or hysteroscopy. Scraping the cervix should be the first step of the curettage and the specimens from the cervix should be examined separately. Occasionally, it may be difficult to decide whether the endocervix is involved by the cancer. In such cases, the simultaneous presence of normal cervical glands and cancer in the same section will give the final diagnosis.

Extension of the carcinoma outside the uterus should refer a case to stage III or stage IV. The presence of metastases in the vagina or in the ovary permits allottment of a case to stage III.

TNM NOMENCLATURE

3.1   PRIMARY TUMOR (T)

TIS   Carcinoma in situ

T1, 1a, 1b, 2, 3, 4

See corresponding FIGO stages

3.2   NODAL INVOLVEMENT (N)

NX   Not possible to assess the regional nodes

N0   No involvement of regional nodes

N1   Evidence of regional node involvement

3.3   DISTANT METASTASIS (M)

MX   Not assessed

M0   No (known) distant metastasis

M1   Distant metastasis present

Specify _____

Specify sites according to the following notations:

Pulmonary—PUL	Bone marrow—MAR
Osseous—OSS	Pleura—PLE
Hepatic—HEP	Skin—SKI
Brain—BRA	Eye—EYE
Lymph nodes—LYM	Other—OTH

4.0 Postsurgical treatment residual tumor (R)

R0	No residual tumor
R1	Microscopic residual tumor
R2	Macroscopic residual tumor
	Specify _____

5.0 Stage grouping (correlation of AJC, TNM, and FIGO nomenclatures)

Stage 0	TIS		
Stage IA	T1a	NX	M0
IB	T1b	NX	M0
Stage II	T2	NX	M0
Stage III	T3	NX	M0
	T1-3	N1	M0
Stage IVA	T4a	NX-1	M0
IVB	Any T	Any N	M1

6.0 Histopathology

It is desirable that stage I cases be subgrouped according to the degree of differentiation described on microscopic examination. The predominant lesion is adenocarcinoma, but all histologic types should be reported. However, choriocarcinomas, sarcomas, mixed mesodermal tumors, and carcinosarcomas should be presented separately.

7.0 Data form for cancer staging

The form presented is suitable for tumors at all gynecologic sites. One should be filled out on each new case entered into the registry.

Ovary

1.0 Anatomy

1.1 PRIMARY SITE: Ovaries are a pair of solid bodies, flattened ovoids 2.0 to 4.0 cm in diameter, that are connected by a peritoneal fold to the broad ligament and by the infundibulo-pelvic ligament to the lateral wall of the pelvis.

1.2 NODAL STATIONS: The lymphatic drainage occurs by the utero-ovarian and round ligament trunks and an external iliac accessory route into the following regional nodes: external iliac, common iliac, hypogastric, lateral sacral, and para-aortic nodes, and, rarely, to inguinal nodes.

1.3 METASTATIC SITES: The peritoneum including the omentum and pelvic and abdominal viscera are common sites for seeding. Diaphragmatic involvement and liver metastases are common. Pulmonary and pleural involvements are frequently seen.

2.0 *Rules for classification*

It is desirable to have a clinical stage grouping of ovarian tumors similar to those already existing for other malignant tumors in the female pelvis. Sometimes it is impossible to come to a final diagnosis by inspection or palpation or by any of the other methods recommended for clinical staging of carcinoma of the uterus and vagina. Therefore, the Cancer Committee of FIGO has recommended that the clinical staging of primary carcinoma of the ovary should be based on clinical examination, that is, curettage, and roentgen examination of the lungs and skeleton, as well as on findings by laparoscopy or laparotomy.

2.1 CLINICAL-DIAGNOSTIC STAGING: Although clinical studies similar to those for other sites may be used, the establishment of a diagnosis most often requires a laparotomy, which is most widely accepted in surgical-pathologic staging. Clinical studies, if carcinoma of the ovary is diagnosed, include routine radiography of chest and abdomen, liver studies, and hemograms.

2.2 SURGICAL-EVALUATIVE STAGING: Laparotomy and biopsy of all suspected sites of involvement provide the basis for this type of staging; this staging is often identical to postsurgical staging. The role of laparoscopy needs to be better defined. Histologic and cytologic data are required.

2.3 POSTSURGICAL TREATMENT-PATHOLOGIC STAGING: This should include laparotomy and resection of ovarian masses, as well as hysterectomy. Biopsies of all suspicious sites, such as the omentum, mesentery, liver, diaphragm, and pelvic and para-aortic nodes, are required.

2.4 RETREATMENT STAGING: Second-look laparotomies and laparoscopy are being evaluated due to the limitation of routine pelvic and abdominal examinations in detecting early recurrence. Other optional and investigative procedures include ultrasound and computerized axial tomography. All suspected recurrences need biopsy confirmation.

3.0 *Staging classification*
FIGO NOMENCLATURE

Staging is based on findings at clinical examination and surgical exploration. The final histologic findings (and cytologic when available) after surgery are to be considered in the staging.

Stage I   Growth limited to the ovaries

        Stage IA   Growth limited to one ovary; no ascites

                IAi   No tumor on the external surface; capsule intact

                IAii   Tumor present on the external surface, or capsule(s) ruptured, or both

Stage IB   Growth limited to both ovaries; no ascites

IBi   No tumor on the external surface; capsule intact

IBii   Tumor present on the external surface, or cap-
sule(s) ruptured, or both

Stage IC   Tumor either stage IA or IB, but with ascites* present
or with positive peritoneal washings

Stage II   Growth involving one or both ovaries with pelvic extension

Stage IIA   Extension and/or metastases to the uterus and/or tubes

Stage IIB   Extension to other pelvic tissues

Stage IIC   Tumor either stage IIA or stage IIB, but with ascites*
present or with positive peritoneal washings

Stage III   Growth involving one or both ovaries with intraperitoneal metastases
outside the pelvis, or positive retroperitoneal nodes, or both. Tumor
limited to the true pelvis with histologically proven malignant extension to small bowel or omentum

Stage IV   Growth involving one or both ovaries with distant metastases. If pleural
effusion is present there must be positive cytology to allot a case to
stage IV. Parenchymal liver metastasis equals stage IV

Special
cate-
gory   Unexplored cases that are thought to be ovarian carcinoma

TNM NOMENCLATURE

3.1   PRIMARY TUMOR (T)

T1ai, 1aii, 1bi, 1bii, 1c, 2a, 2b, 2c, 3

See corresponding FIGO stages

3.2   NODAL INVOLVEMENT (N)

NX   Not possible to assess regional nodes

N0   No involvement of regional nodes

N1   Evidence of regional node involvement

3.3   DISTANT METASTASIS (M)

MX   Not assessed

M0   No (known) distant metastasis

M1   Distant metastasis present

Specify _____

Specify sites according to the following notations:

Pulmonary—PUL

Osseous—OSS

Hepatic—HEP

---

*Ascites is peritoneal effusion that, in the opinion of the surgeon, is pathologic, or clearly exceeds normal
amounts, or both

Brain—BRA
Lymph nodes—LYM
Bone marrow—MAR
Pleura—PLE
Skin—SKI
Eye—EYE
Other—OTH

4.0 Postsurgical treatment residual tumor (R)

R0   No residual tumor
R1   Microscopic residual tumor
R2   Macroscopic residual tumor
      Specify _____

5.0 Stage grouping (correlation of AJC, TNM, and FIGO nomenclatures)

Stage IAi	T1ai	N0	M0
IAii	T1aii	N0	M0
IBi	T1bi	N0	M0
IBii	T1bii	N0	M0
IC	T1c	N0	M0
Stage IIA	T2a	N0	M0
IIB	T2b	N0	M0
IIC	T2c	N0	M0
Stage III	T3	N0-1	M0
	T1-2	N1	M0
Stage IV	Any T	Any N	M1

6.0 Histopathology

The task force of the AJC endorses the histologic typing of ovarian tumors as presented in the WHO publication no. 9, 1973, and recommends that all ovarian epithelial tumors be subdivided according to a simplified version of this. The types recommended at the present time are as follows: serous tumors, mucinous tumors, endometrioid tumors, clear cell (mesonephroid) tumors, undifferentiated tumors, and unclassified tumors.

  A) Serous cystomas
    1) Serous benign cystadenomas
    2) Serous cystadenomas with proliferating activity of the epithelial cells and nuclear abnormalities, but with no infiltrative destructive growth (low potential malignancy)
    3) Serous cystadenocarcinomas
  B) Mucinous cystomas
    1) Mucinous benign cystadenomas
    2) Mucinous cystadenomas with proliferating activity of the epithelial cells

and nuclear abnormalities, but with no infiltrative destructive growth (low potential malignancy)

   3) Mucinous cystadenocarcinomas

C) Endometrioid tumors (similar to adenocarcinomas in the endometrium)

   1) Endometrioid benign cysts

   2) Endometrioid tumors with proliferating activity of the epithelial cells and nuclear abnormalities, but with no infiltrative destructive growth (low potential malignancy)

   3) Endometrioid adenocarcinomas

D) Clear cell (mesonephroid) tumors

   1) Benign clear cell tumors

   2) Clear cell tumors with proliferating activity of the epithelial cells and nuclear abnormalities, but with no infiltrative destructive growth (low potential malignancy)

   3) Clear cell cystadenocarcinomas

E) Unclassified tumors which cannot be allotted to one of the groups A-D

F) No histology

G) Other malignant tumors

Malignant tumors other than those of the common epithelial types are not to be included with the categories listed above. However, the more common ones such as granulosa cell tumor, immature teratoma, dysgerminoma, and endodermal sinus tumor may be collected and reported separately by institutions so desiring, particularly those with a pediatric population among their patients.

In some cases of inoperable widespread malignant tumor, it may be impossible for the gynecologist and for the pathologist to decide the origin of the growth. In order to evaluate the results obtained in the treatment of carcinoma of the ovary, it is, however, necessary that all patients are reported on, as well as those who are thought to have a malignant ovarian tumor. If clinical examination cannot exclude the possibility that the lesion is a primary ovarian carcinoma, a case should be reported in the group "special category"and will belong to either histologic group E or F. Cases where exploratory surgery has shown that obvious ovarian malignant tumor is present, but where no biopsy has been taken, should be classified as ovarian carcinoma, "no histology."

7.0 Data form for cancer staging

The form presented is applicable to tumors of all gynecologic sites. One should be filled out on each new case as it is entered into the registry. The diagrams are particularly useful in ovarian cancer.

Vagina

The rules for classification are similar to those for the cervix uteri and should be referred to accordingly.

1.0 Staging classification

Stage 0   Carcinoma in situ; intraepithelial carcinoma

Stage I   The carcinoma is limited to the vaginal wall

Stage II   The carcinoma has involved the subvaginal tissue but has not extended
            to the pelvic wall

Stage III   The carcinoma has extended to the pelvic wall

Stage IV   The carcinoma has extended beyond the true pelvis or has involved the
            mucosa of the bladder or rectum. Bullous edema as such does not
            permit a case to be allotted to stage IV

            Stage IVA   Spread of the growth to adjacent organs

            Stage IVB   Spread to distant organs

TNM NOMENCLATURE

1.1   PRIMARY TUMOR (T)

        TIS   Carcinoma in situ

        T1, T2, T3, T4

                See corresponding FIGO stages

1.2   NODAL INVOLVEMENT (N)

        NX   Not possible to assess the regional nodes

        N0   No involvement of regional nodes

        N1   Evidence of regional node involvement

1.3   DISTANT METASTASIS (M)

        MX   Not assessed

        M0   No (known) distant metastasis

        M1   Distant metastasis present

                Specify _____

                Specify sites according to the following notations:

                    Pulmonary—PUL

                    Osseous—OSS

                    Hepatic—HEP

                    Brain—BRA

                    Lymph nodes—LYM

                    Bone marrow—MAR

                    Pleura—PLE

                    Skin—SKI

                    Eye—EYE

                    Other—OTH

Vulva

The rules for classification are similar to those at the other gynecologic sites.
Tumors present in the vulva as secondary growths from either a genital or extragenital site should be excluded. Malignant melanoma should be separately reported.

The femoral, inguinal, external iliac, and hypogastric nodes are the sites of regional spread.

1.0 Staging classification

FIGO NOMENCLATURE

Stage 0   Carcinoma in situ

Stage I   Tumor confined to vulva—2 cm or less in diameter. Nodes are not palpable or are palpable in either groin, not enlarged, mobile (not clinically suspicious of neoplasm)

Stage II   Tumor confined to the vulva—more than 2 cm in diameter. Nodes are not palpable or are palpable in either groin, not enlarged, mobile (not clinically suspicious of neoplasm)

Stage III   Tumor of any size with (1) adjacent spread to the urethra and any or all of the vagina, the perineum, and the anus, and/or (2) nodes palpable in either or both groins (enlarged, firm, and mobile, not fixed but clinically suspicious of neoplasm)

Stage IV   Tumor of any size (1) infiltrating the bladder mucosa or the rectal mucosa or both, including the upper part of the urethral mucosa, and/or (2) fixed to the bone or other distant metastases. Fixed or ulcerated nodes in either or both groins

TNM NOMENCLATURE

1.1   PRIMARY TUMOR (T)
        TIS, T1, T2, T3, T4
                See corresponding FIGO stages
1.2   NODAL INVOLVEMENT (N)
        NX   Not possible to assess the regional nodes
        N0   No involvement of regional nodes
        N1   Evidence of regional node involvement
        N3   Fixed or ulcerated nodes
        N4   Juxtaregional node involvement
1.3   DISTANT METASTASIS (M)
        MX   Not assessed
        M0   No (known) distant metastasis
        M1   Distant metastasis present
              Specify _____
              Specify sites according to the following notations:
                    Pulmonary—PUL
                    Osseous—OSS
                    Hepatic—HEP
                    Brain—BRA
                    Lymph nodes—LYM
                    Bone marrow—MAR

Pleura—PLE
Skin—SKI
Eye—EYE
Other—OTH

Stage grouping

Stage I	T1	N0	M0
	T1	N1	M0
Stage II	T2	N0	M0
	T2	N1	M0
Stage III	T3	N0	M0
	T3	N1	M0
	T3	N2	M0
	T1	N2	M0
	T2	N2	M0
Stage IV	T1	N3	M0
	T2	N3	M0
	T3	N3	M0
	T4	N3	M0
	T4	N0	M0
	T4	N1	M0
	T4	N2	M0

All other conditions containing M1a or M1b

Data form for cancer staging

Use of the form is recommended in every new case entered into the registry regardless of site.

Basic principles in gynecologic radiotherapy

All life on our planet has evolved in a milieu in which the major source of all energy essential for biologic processes has been in the form of radiant energy, or radiation. Various forms of irradiation influence living material in a variety of ways. Sunlight provides heat, light, and energy for plant photosynthesis, while radio waves provide a means of communication (Table B-1). In general, most radiations are not harmful in ordinary quantities but actually are helpful to life processes. However, certain types of high-energy, or "ionizing," radiation are not entirely harmless but provide useful tools in gynecology, both for diagnostic and therapeutic purposes. These high-energy radiations are injurious to biologic material, and their use in oncology depends on the ability of these energy sources to provide an injury from which normal tissue may recover more effectively than malignant tissue. They can produce deleterious effects in all forms of life, from the relatively simple unicellular plants and animals to the complex higher organisms.

The change produced by these radiations may be grossly apparent soon after exposure of the living organism, but more often the radiation changes do not appear (on cursory examination) to have affected the organism at all. At this time there may be small cellular changes that can only be detected by careful chemical or microscopic study and may not be apparent for many years or indeed may manifest themselves only in the offspring of the irradiated organism. The attitude concerning radiation exposure should always be that diagnostic tests, therapeutic radiation, and

Table B-1. Electromagnetic spectrum

X-ray	124 ev-124 Mev	Wavelength 100 Å-0.001 Å
Ultraviolet	3-124 ev	Wavelength 4,000 Å-100 Å
Visible	2-3 ev	Wavelength 7,000 Å-4,000 Å
Infrared	0.01-1 ev	Wavelength 0.01 cm-10^4 cm
Radio waves	10^{10}-10^4 ev	Wavelength 3 × 10^5-1 cm

radiation acquired incidentally from the environment can all be detrimental. Although in many instances the chance of injury from diagnostic or environmental radiation is slight, the possibility of damage from a known exposure must always be weighed against the importance of the information to be gained or the effect desired. Certainly, incidental exposure must be avoided through control of environmental hazards wherever possible.

The radiation emission of isotopes such as radium and cesium is now used for therapeutic purposes in the treatment of a wide variety of human malignancies. In addition, over the past 3 decades a variety of machines capable of producing radiant energy of high intensity have become available and are also used extensively in the treatment of human malignancies. Those machines that emit energies greater than 1 million electron volts (1 Mev) are the most commonly used at present and constitute the so-called supravoltage-megavoltage era; among these pieces of equipment are the cobalt generators, betatron, and linear accelerator (Table B-2).

PHYSICAL AND CHEMICAL NATURE OF RADIATION

The physical forces of concern are termed ionizing radiations because of their characteristic ability to transfer their energy to matter by separating orbital electrons from their atoms, thus forming physical ion pairs. The term is an inclusive one, since the phenomenon may be caused by particulate radiations as well as electromagnetic waves (photons). Those radiations that originate from decay of an atomic nucleus are termed gamma rays; those that originate outside the atomic nucleus are termed x rays and are emitted when high-energy charged particles (electrons) bombard a suitable target such as tungsten. When these fast-moving electrons approach the fields around the nuclei of the atoms of the target material, they are deflected from their path and energy is emitted in the form of electromagnetic radiation (photons). These emitted x-rays may have any energy from zero to a maximum that is determined by the kinetic energy of the bombarding electrons. Machines such as the betatron and linear accelerator are capable of generating electrons at high accelera-

Table B-2. Modalities of external radiation

Modality	Voltage	Source
Low voltage (superficial)	85-150 kv	X-ray
Medium voltage (orthovoltage)	180-400 kv	X-ray
Supervoltage	500 kv-8 mv	X-ray (linear accelerator) ^{60}Co ^{137}Cs ^{226}Ra
Megavoltage	Above supervoltage energy	Betatron Synchrotron Linear accelerator

tions, and therefore the x-rays generated by these machines are quite high in energy. A continuous spectrum of x-rays of various energies can be produced when a large number of impinging electrons are involved. Other x-rays are produced when a high-speed electron impinging on a target material knocks out an orbital electron (ionization) from a target atom. When this electron is from an outer shell and comes to rest in another orbit, it is during this latter transition that an x-ray is given off. The photon energy of that x-ray represents the difference in energies of the inner and outer orbital electron levels. It should be remembered that gamma rays and x-rays can be collectively termed photons, and what is of medical importance is the energy of the photon and not the source.

The interaction of photons with matter is accomplished through three mechanisms: the photoelectric effect, Compton's scattering, and pair production. All of these processes result in either ionization of molecules within the target or possible free radical formation. Free hydrogen atoms and free hydroxyl radicals are a frequent product of the bombardment of water by high-energy photons. About half of the H atoms encounter OH radicals and reform stable H_2O molecules. The other half encounter other hydrogen atoms and form H_2. The OH radicals may react in a similar way, meeting other OH radicals and forming H_2O_2 in about half the instances. In reality, the irradiation of pure water by electrons or photons results in very few H atoms before they diffuse away. The addition of soluble O_2, however, causes the H atoms to react so as to form the radical HO_2. This is less reactive than the OH radical and permits the decomposition of water to H_2O_2 to proceed. These excited and ionized molecules are very unstable and react with proteins and other key substances within the cell. Many other events may occur with photon bombardment: long-chained molecules may be split and regrouped, aggregates may be produced, and ring forms may be disrupted indiscriminately. Certainly, chemical bonds may be vulnerable to inactivation by oxidation, resulting in loss of functional capacity. All of the chemical changes may ultimately be translated into biologic injury at a cellular level.

BIOLOGIC EFFECTS OF RADIATION

The selective destruction of tissues forms the basis of therapeutic radiology. Neoplastic cells are usually more easily killed by radiation than are their parent cells in the surrounding normal tissues. The magnitude of the differences in radiovulnerability between normal and cancerous tissues determines in large part whether the particular neoplasm considered for radiation can be eradicated. This relative difference in local radiovulnerability is referred to as a difference in radiosensitivity or the therapeutic ratio. It is essential that it be understood that radiosensitivity and radiocurability are not identical in meaning. Relatively radioresistant tumors accessible to high-dose local radiation therapy are curable, whereas radiosensitive tumors that are widely metastasized at the start of therapy, or shortly thereafter, can only be controlled locally. An excellent example of a relatively radioresistant tumor is squamous cell carcinoma of the cervix, and yet this malignancy remains one of the most curable tumors of humans because of its accessibility to high-dose irradiation and the relatively radioresistant nature of the hosting normal tissues (e.g., cervix and vagina). The ability to place radium or cesium in juxtaposition to the malignancy within dose ranges tolerable to the surrounding normal tissue is the key to success.

As a result of the chemical changes that have been described above, very large molecules (common in biologic systems) will undergo a variety of structural changes that may lead to altered function. "Degradation," or breaking into smaller units, has been shown to occur when large molecules are radiated. "Cross-linking" is another common structural change. A long molecule that is somewhat felxible in structure can undergo intramolecule cross-linking when a chemically active locus is produced on it and when this spot can come in contact with another reactive area. If the cross-linking is extensive, not only are the molecules incapable of normal function but they may no longer be soluble in the system. Many macromolecules are held in a rigid configuration by intramolecular cross-linking bonds, that is, specific chemical groups are linked together, frequently by hydrogen atoms, to form a three-dimensional structure. The hydrogen bonds are among the weakest in the molecule and thus are the first to be broken by radiation. Such structural changes can lead to severe alterations in the biochemical properties of the molecule.

In this manner, radiation effects on molecules such as proteins, enzymes, nucleic acids, and certain lipids can have profound effects on the cell that in turn can alter the organ and the organism. The initial chemical change occurs in a fraction of a second and is rarely detected directly. Some of these chemical changes are repaired almost immediately, and others that occur within less important structures may result in alterations that are rarely recognizable. The majority follow the pattern in which transition between a chemical change in a system and the biologic manifestation of this change is complicated and often obscure. Absorption and utilization of energy by a cell entail a complex chain of events in which multiple proteins are involved; radiation damage to these vital proteins can result in loss of cell membrane integrity and even cell death.

Although a variety of morphologic and functional changes have been described that occur in irradiated cells, the bulk of both direct and indirect evidence suggests that cell nuclei are the major site of radiation damage leading to cell death. For example, it has been calculated that 1 million rads is required to inactivate certain cytoplasmic enzymes systems in the cell, and doses of 1,000 roentgens or more are usually required to damage cell membranes. In contrast, chromosomal aberrations and mutations can be produced by very low radiation doses. Since only a few hundred rads are needed to produce a high degree of lethality in most proliferating cells in tissue culture, it seems most logical that the nuclear changes produced by the low doses are responsible for the cell death.

GENETIC EFFECTS OF RADIATION

It is not possible to generalize and assign a specific mutation rate to a specific dose of radiation. Gene loci differ markedly in their mutability, and the rather random damage exerted by irradiation on any particular chromosome makes predictability exceedingly difficult. Certainly the mitotic stage, cell type, sex, species, and dose rate all influence the rate of mutation production as studied in lower animals and bacteria. Data accumulated in lower animals are difficult to extrapolate to humans, and therefore prediction of mutation rates cannot be expected from the evidence that has been accumulated from various types of radiation exposure; direct evidence of radiation-induced mutation in humans is lacking. The largest group of humans available for study are descendents of those exposed to radiation in Hiroshima and Nagasaki, and while there has been no detectable effect on the frequency of prenatal or neonatal deaths or on the frequency of malformations in subsequent generations, this does not mean that no hereditary effects were produced by the irradiation. The number of exposed parents was small, and for many the dosages were so low that it would have been surprising if an increase in mutation had been detected in such a brief period. There just has not been sufficient time for the several generations needed to reveal recessive damage.

It is perfectly logical to expect that radiation exposure will increase the mutation rate in humans. This is based largely on experiments in mice, where it is estimated that the doubling dose (that which will double the spontaneous mutation rate) for humans probably lies between 10 and 100 rads. For an acute exposure to irradiation the probable value is between 15 and 30 rads, and for chronic irradiation it is probably around 100 rads. The Committee on Genetics of the Nuclear Regulatory Commission has recommended that no individual from conception to the age of 30 years be subjected to more than 10 rads of man-made irradiation to the gonads. Cosmic radiation, estimated to total approximately 4 rads in this same span of years, is not

Table B-3. Average radiation dose to fetus and to maternal gonads from various diagnostic examinations (first trimester)

Examination	Dose to fetus and maternal gonads (millirads)
Lower extremity roentgenography	1
Cervical spine roentgenography	2
Skull roentgenography	4
Chest roentgenography	8
Pelvic roentgenography	40
Chest fluoroscopy	70
Cholecystography	200
Lumbar spinal roentgenography	275
Abdominal roentgenography	290
Hip roentgenography	300
Intravenous or retrograde pyelography	400
Upper gastrointestinal roentgenography	500
Lower gastrointestinal roentgenography	800

From DiSaia, P. J., Nolan, J. D., and Arneson, A. P.: Gynecological radiotherapy. In Danforth, D. N., editor: Obstetrics and gynecology, ed. 3, New York, 1977, Harper & Row, Publishers, Inc.

included in this 10-rad permissible dose. With the use of image intensifiers, improved x-ray film, appropriate shielding to prevent scatter, and the like it is possible to attain satisfactory x-ray visualization of internal structures with reduced exposure. The average dose of irradiation to the gonads of some common diagnostic techniques is given in Table B-3.

EFFECTS OF RADIATION ON THE FETUS

The classical effects of radiation on the mammalian embryo are (1) intrauterine and extrauterine growth retardation, (2) embryonic, fetal, or neonatal death, and (3) gross congenital malformations. The structure most readily and consistently affected by radiation is the central nervous system. If the acute in utero exposure is below 25 rads these classic effects of radiation are never observed in experimental animals nor, in all likelihood, in humans. Not only are the absorbed dose and the stage of gestation important in interpreting the effect of irradiation of a mammalian embryo but the dose rate must also be taken into consideration. Most embryonic pathologic effects are reduced significantly by decreasing the dose rate to allow a recovery process to function. The peak incidence of gross malformations occurs when the fetus is irradiated during the early organogenesis period (10 to 40 days of gestation in the human), although cellular, tissue, and organ hypoplasia can be produced by radiation throughout organogenetic, fetal, and neonatal periods if the dose is high enough. There is no stage of gestation during which an exposure of 50 rads is not associated with a significant probability of an observable embryonic pathologic effect: increased incidence of death during the preimplantation period, malformations during the early organogenetic stage, and cell deletions and tissue hypoplasia during the fetal stages. Animal experiments indicate that all embryos exposed to 100 rads or more after implantation will exhibit some degree of growth retardation. Finding and recognizing radiation-induced deleterious effects in offspring irradiated in utero becomes increasingly difficult with decreasing doses (less than 10 rads) because of their low probability of occurrence and the high natural incidence of defects. From the clinical point of view, an absorbed dose of 10 rads to the fetus at any time during gestation can be considered a practical threshold for the induction of congenital defects, below which the probability of producing adverse effects becomes exceedingly small. Diagnostic x-ray procedures (Table B-3) should be avoided in the pregnant woman unless there is overwhelming urgency. In women of childbearing age, possible damage to an early conceptus can be prevented by performing such tests immediately after the commencement of a menstrual period.

Some concrete information is available from the Japanese survivors of the A-bomb attacks in 1945. Plumer reported on 205 children, aged 4½ years, who were exposed at Hiroshima during the first half of intrauterine life. Of the 11 who were within 1,200 meters of the hypocenter, seven had microcephaly with mental retardation, a diagnosis not made in any of the 194 children exposed at greater distances. At Nagasaki, 30 mothers were exposed within 2,000 meters of the hypocenter and showed major signs of having received a large radiation dose, such as alopecia, purpura, oral pharyngeal lesions, or petechiae. There were 7 fetal deaths, 6 neonatal or infant deaths, and 4 instances of mental retardation among the 16 surviving children. Hall has reached the following conclusions:

1. Moderately large doses of radiation (greater than 200 rads) delivered to the human embryo before 2 to 3 weeks' gestation is not very likely to produce severe abnormalities in most children born, although a considerable number of embryos may be resorbed or aborted (all or none phenomenon).
2. Irradiation between 4 and 11 weeks' gestation would lead to severe abnormality of many organs in most or all children.
3. Irradiation between 11 and 16 weeks' gestation may produce few eye, skeletal, and genital organ abnormalities, but stunted growth, microcephaly, and mental retardation are frequently present.
4. Irradiation of the fetus between 16 and 30 weeks' gestation may lead to a mild degree of microcephaly, mental retardation, and stunting of growth.
5. Irradiation after 30 weeks' gestation is not likely to produce gross structural abnormalities leading to a serious handicap in early life but could cause functional disabilities.

GENERAL CONCEPTS OF CLINICAL RADIATION THERAPY

The technical modalities used in modern radiation therapy may be divided into two major categories:

1. External irradiation. This applies to irradiation from sources at a distance from the body (e.g., teletherapy with cobalt 60, linear accelerator, betatron, or standard orthovoltage x-ray machines).
2. Local irradiation. This applies to irradiation from sources in direct proximity to the tumor.
   a. Intracavitary irradiation with applicators loaded with radioactive materials such as radium or cesium (e.g., vaginal ovoids, vaginal cylinder, intrauterine tandem, or Heyman capsules).
   b. Interstitial irradiation usually delivered in the form of removable needles containing radium, cesium, or iridium. Also applies to permanent isotope implants, e.g., ^{125}I seeds.
   c. Direct therapy usually delivered by means of cones from an orthovoltage machine (e.g., transvaginal).
   d. Intraperitoneal or intrapleural instillation of radioactive colloids, e.g., ^{32}P.

External irradiation

The energy and penetrating power of ionizing radiation increase as the photon wavelength decreases (Table B-1). Thus, differences in the physical characteristics of the radiation used are of great importance in therapeutic radiology. The clinically important changes occur with radiation generated in the range of 400 to 800 kv (kilovolts). Above this energy, the advantages are reduced absorption of radiation in bone, less damage to the skin at the portal of entry, better tolerance of the vasculo-

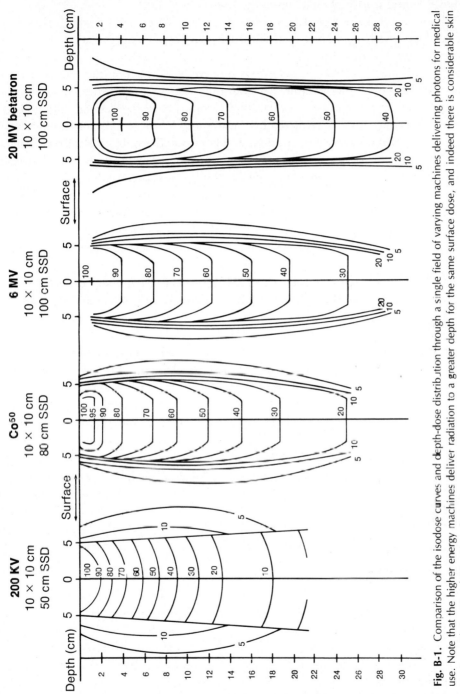

Fig. B-1. Comparison of the isodose curves and depth-dose distribution through a single field of varying machines delivering photons for medical use. Note that the higher energy machines deliver radiation to a greater depth for the same surface dose, and indeed there is considerable skin sparing with 6 mV and 20 mV equipment.

connective tissue, greater radiation at the depth relative to the surface dose, and reduced lateral scatter of radiation in the tissues (Fig. B-1).

The reduced skin effect of supervoltage radiation as compared with orthovoltage radiation is based on the physical fact that with higher energy radiation, forward scattering (in the direction of the primary beam) of radiation in the absorber is greater and lateral scattering less. With supervoltage radiation the maximum ionization occurs below the level of the epidermis. For example, with cobalt 60 teletherapy, maximum ionization occurs about 5 mm below the surface, although the surface dose may be only 40% of this maximum. As the energy of irradiation increases, it becomes more penetrating; as photons and resultant electrons become more energetic, they travel a greater distance into absorbing material. Therefore, the percentage of irradiation at any specific depth, compared with the surface dose, increases as the energy increases. This advantage of supervoltage and megavoltage is of clinical importance in the treatment of tumors that are located deep within the human organism (e.g., carcinomas of the bladder and endometrium), where the introduction of a sufficiently high dose with medium voltage radiation is difficult or impossible.

In the supervoltage range, absorption of radiation in bone approximates that in water or soft tissue per unit density whereas with medium voltage, radiation absorption is considerably greater in bone than in soft tissue. The vasculoconnective tissue immediately adjacent to the bone around the haversian channels receives a sufficiently higher dose because of static irradiation. This higher dose increases the risk of bone necrosis by destruction of the osteoblastic elements and damage to the vascular system. Furthermore, preferential bone absorption leads to a reduction in the dose at the point of interest when thick bone must be traversed by the radiation. In addition, it has been observed clinically that as irradiation energy increases, similar tumor effects can be produced with less damage to important adjacent normal structures. The incidence of severe mucosal and skin reactions is reduced, and apparently there is less damage to the vasculoconnective tissue. This greater tolerance of vasculoconnective tissue to a higher dose of properly protracted supervoltage radiation therapy is one of the factors that permits the planned combination of radical preoperative radiation with surgery without appreciably increasing the surgical risks beyond those associated with surgery alone.

Local irradiation

Local application of radiation permits very high doses to restricted tissue volumes. It is in this situation that the physical principle (inverse square law) that the intensity of irradiation rapidly decreases with distance from the radiation source is used to advantage. One needs a small tumor with well-defined limits and a clinical situation where it is desirable to restrict the volume of tissue irradiated. Larger volumes of tissue that need radiation therapy are best treated with external irradiation. Radium has been the most frequent element used for local application both in the form of tubes and needles. In recent times, other materials (^{60}Co, ^{137}Cs, ^{192}Ir, ^{182}Ta) have been available for local application (Table B-4). The major disadvantage of these materials compared with radium is the appreciably shorter half-life. Several of these materials have advantages over radium in that they may be incorporated in solid materials such as ceramics and need not be used in the form of a powder-gas substance as is the case with radium. Radium tubes and needles contain radium powder, and many of its decay products are in gas form within the same container. Other substances that have been used as implants in the tumor are gold (^{198}Au) and iodine (^{125}I) seeds; these are permanent implantations and are difficult and awkward because of the difficulty of preparation, the rather rapid radioactive decay, and the difficulty in obtaining homogeneity of dosimetry.

The term dosimetry is applied to the measurement and calculation of dose that the patient receives, and if the radiation intensity decreases rapidly with increasing depth in tissue, as is the case with local irradiation (Fig. B-2), that tissue adjacent to the radiation source may theoretically be treated adequately without harmful irradiation to the underlying structures. The effectiveness of this distribution of irradiation is, of course, dependent on careful application of these sources. Interstitial application of radioactive sources is a great deal more difficult than intracavitary application. A system of multiple discrete sources often results in a less homogeneous isodose pattern than irradiation from external sources or from a well-placed intracavitary source (Fig. B-3).

Some of the high cure rates obtained by gynecologic oncologists are due to the accessibility of vaginal and uterine cancer to local irradiation. This accessibility allows relatively high doses of irradiation to be delivered to the neoplasm with relatively safe amounts of normal tissue exposure. Indeed, meticulously applied local irradiation is often the factor that distinguishes institutions with low morbidity and high cure rates.

Table B-4. Isotopes commonly used in radiation therapy

Isotope	Energy (Mev)	Half-life
^{137}Cs	0.662	30 years
^{60}Co	1.173, 1.332	5.3 years
^{198}Au	0.411	2.69 days
^{192}Ir	0.47	74 days
^{226}Ra	0.8	1,620 years
^{222}Rn	0.8	3.83 days
^{182}Ta	1.18	115 days
^{125}I	0.027-0.035	60 days
^{252}Ct Cf	0.8 (photons) 2.09 and 2.35 (neutrons)	265 days

From DiSaia, P. J., Nolan, J. D., and Arneson, A. P.: Gynecological radiotherapy. In Danforth, D. N., editor: Obstetrics and gynecology, ed. 3, New York, 1977, Harper & Row, Publishers, Inc.

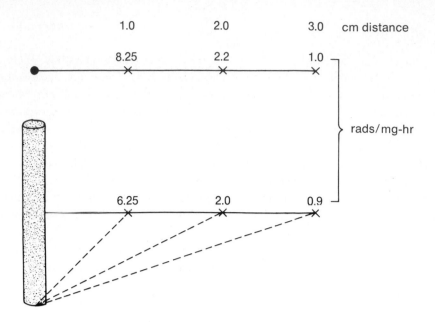

Fig. B-2. Radiation effects at various distances from 1-mg point source of radium. (From Danforth, D. N., editor: Obstetrics and gynecology, ed. 3, New York, 1977, Harper & Row, Publishers, Inc.)

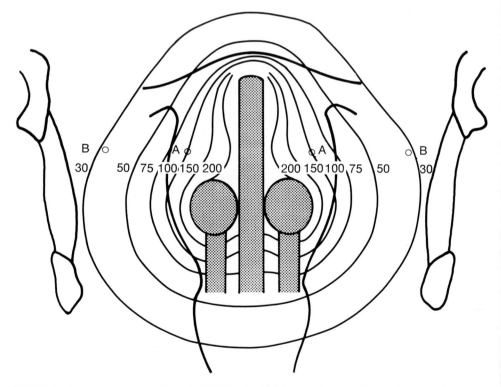

Fig. B-3. Isodose curves surrounding a typical Fletcher-Suit intracavitary application (tandem plus ovoids) for cervical cancer. Note the location of points A and B and the relative dose rates at distances from the system.

TOLERANCE OF PELVIC ORGANS

The tolerance of any tissue to irradiation therapy is dependent on several characteristics of the radiation, including (1) the fractionation technique, (2) the total dose given, (3) the dose rate, and (4) the volume irradiated. Fractionation is a function of the number of treatments. With external irradiation, the patient is usually treated 4 to 5 days per week. Fractionation is closely tied to dose rate, which is the quantity of irradiation given in each of these sessions, usually expressed as dose per week. Pelvic radiation delivered to a patient for a total dose of 5,000 rads given in five daily fractions each week for 5 weeks is well tolerated in most instances. However, if that same total dose of 5,000 rads were given in five fractions of 1,000 rads each Monday for 5 consecutive weeks, very few if any of the patients would tolerate that kind of fractionation or dose rate. The lower the dose rate and the higher the fractionation, the better the normal tissue tolerance of the irradiation given. Obviously there has to be a balance because excessive fractionation or very low dose rates will not accomplish tumor kill. The volume of tissue irradiated becomes an integral factor in tolerance and is difficult to separate from dose rate or fractionation. As an example, a 1-cm circular field of skin would easily tolerate the fractionation and dose rate of 1,000 rads each Monday for 5 consecutive weeks. However, for a larger volume, such as whole-pelvis radiation, such a treatment plan could not be tolerated. The greater the volume of tissue irradiated, the more difficult the normal tolerance.

Irradiation tolerance of organs of the pelvis varies slightly from patient to patient and is, of course, subject to the factors mentioned above, such as volume, fractionation, and energy of irradiation received. The administration of radium by one technique or another may also result in different dose distributions and considerably affect tolerance. As is illustrated in many areas of oncology, the more advanced the lesion, the greater the dose necessary for eradication and the greater the incidence of morbidity (Table B-5). With advanced disease, higher risks of injury are not only present but justified. This, coupled with the fact that advanced cancer is often already compromising the integrity of the bladder and rectum, means that serious sequelae often develop in patients with advanced cervical, vaginal, and corpus lesions.

The tissues composing the cervix and the corpus of the uterus can tolerate very high doses of radiation. In fact, they withstand higher doses than any other compa-

Table B-5. Squamous carcinoma dose-tumor volume relationships (90% control)

Subclinical disease	5,000 rads
<2 cm	6,000 rads
2-4 cm	6,800 rads
4-6 cm	7,300 rads
>6 cm	7,890 rads

From Wharton, J. T., Jones, H. W. III, Day, T. G., Jr., and others: Preirradiation celiotomy and extended field irradiation for invasive carcinoma of the cervix, Obstet. Gynecol. **49:**333, 1977.

rable volume of tissues in the body; doses of 20,000 to 30,000 rads in about 2 weeks are routinely tolerated. This remarkable tolerance level permits a large dose and allows a very high percentage of central control of cervical cancer. It is the unusual radiation tolerance of the uterus as well as the vagina that accounts for the success of radium in the treatment of cervical lesions. It would appear that the epithelium of the uterus and vagina have unusual ability to recover from radiation injury.

The sigmoid, rectosigmoid, and rectum are more susceptible to radiation injury than other pelvic organs. The frequency of injury to the large bowel is often dependent on the relationship of the structure of the distribution of radium as well as on the total dose administered by both external beam and the intracavitary radium system. With external beam alone the large bowel is the most sensitive of pelvic structures to irradiation. The bladder tolerates slightly more radiation than the rectum according to most authorities. Fletcher has proposed a rule of thumb that gives the upper limits of pelvic irradiation and indirectly gives the tolerance of the bladder and rectum. The rule is that the sum of the central dose by external beam plus the number of mg-hours of radium or cesium administered by intracavitary techniques should never exceed 10,000. This rule of thumb may not be valid unless the Fletcher-Suit brachytherapy systems are used. Most of this is applicable to therapy for the uterus, cervix, and vagina. In general, if a heavy dose of intracavitary irradiation is applied centrally for a small lesion, the amount of external beam applied centrally must be kept to a minimum. Conversely, if a lesion is large and the vaginal geometry poor, a minimum intracavitary dose can be given and the dose administered centrally by external beam may be quite high (6,000 to 7,000 rads).

Pelvic radiation usually spares the small bowel since that structure is normally in constant motion. This tends to prevent any one segment from receiving an excessive dose. However, if loops of small bowel are immobilized as a result of adhesions due to previous surgery, they may be held directly in the path of the radiation beam and thus be injured. The result of such an injury is usually not manifested for at least a year or more after completion of radiation and is accompanied by narrowing of the lumen associated with mucosal ulceration of that segment of bowel.

It is extremely important that students of this subject comprehend the concept of permanent injury to normal tissue (Fig. B-4). When any area of the body is subjected to tumoricidal doses of radiation, the normal tissues of that area suffer an injury that is only partially repaired. The tumor tissue will disappear, but the normal tissue bed remains, and the injury that is only partially repaired must be seriously considered should other disease processes affect that area in subsequent decades. Radiobiologists estimate that in the case of injury to normal tissues, only 5% to 20% of the damage is repaired. Thus, the normal tissue in the irradiated area can retain a very considerable handicap. Should a second malignant neoplasm arise in that same area many years later, additional tumoricidal radiation is not possible because of the lingering injury. In addition, any surgical procedures performed within a previously irradiated field will be associated with a higher risk for poor healing, fistula formation, etc.

CONCEPT of PERMANENT Injury to Normal Tissue.

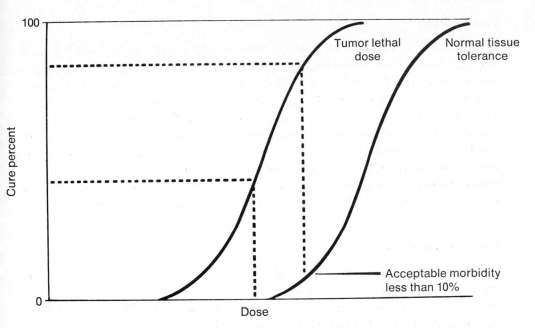

Fig. B-4. Diagrammatic representation of the parallel of tumor response and normal tissue tolerance curves demonstrating the relationship between increasing dose, increasing cure rate, and increasing morbidity. Under ideal circumstances (as depicted here), an 80% to 90% cure rate can be achieved with 5% to 10% morbidity. Pushing the cure rate carries with it an increase in morbidity. On the other hand, attempts to avoid all morbidity significantly reduce the ability to cure. Although the shape of these curves will vary for various tumor types and dose rates, the general concepts are valid whenever radiotherapy is used to treat malignant lesions.

NEW RADIATION MODALITIES

Hypoxic cells are more resistant to gamma ray and x-ray than are oxygenated cells. Whereas the cells in most normal tissues are well oxygenated, most solid tumors have regions of hypoxic cells. In order to get adequate coverage of the tumor, radiation portals necessarily must include adjacent normal, well-oxygenated tissue. Therefore, during treatment a point may be reached when all the well-oxygenated cells in the surrounding tissues have received a tolerance dose of radiation beyond which severe damage would result yet the hypoxic cells in the tumor are still viable and will subsequently cause regrowth of the tumor.

Conventional radiation (x-rays or gamma rays) deposits energy in tissues via electrons that lose their energy slowly, resulting in a low linear energy density along the electron track, or low linear energy transfer (LET). High LET radiations (fast neutrons or negative π mesons) are more effective against hypoxic cells than are low LET radiations. This means that for the same reaction produced in the healthy cells by all radiation modalities, the high LET types have a higher probability (1.5 to 2.5 times that of x-rays) of killing the hypoxic tumor cells.

Fast neutrons

Although the rationale for neutron radiotherapy is well established, treatment considerations are currently limited by the availability of suitable neutron sources. There are two practical sources of a fast-neutron beam for radiotherapy, the cyclotron and the D-T generator. the D-T generator derives its name from the fact that a deuteron beam (D) is accelerated into a tritium target (T), resulting in the release of a neutron and a helium The neutron is emitted with an energy of 14 Mev, which results in a depth-dose distribution similar to that of ^{60}C0 gamma rays. In the cyclotron the neutrons are generally produced by bombarding deuterons onto a beryllium target. In general, the average neutron energy will be a little less than half the deuteron energy, and with some of the larger machines this is approximately 15 to 16 Mev.

Negative π mesons

Negative π mesons, or pions, as they are often called, are negatively charged particles that have a mass 273 times that of an electron. Pions can be produced in any nuclear interaction if the energy of the primary particle is sufficient to create the rest mass of the pion. For radiotherapy, pions with energies between 40 and 70 Mev are of interest, since these particles have a depth range in tissue of approximately 6 to 13 cm. The production of pions involves a large and expensive accelerator facility. The dose delivered by a beam of negative pions to a tissuelike medium increases very slowly with depth in the beginning but gives rise to a sharply defined maximum near the end of the range. This is known as the Brogg peak and is a property that pions have in common with all other heavy charged particles. The unique characteristic of negative pions is that when they come to rest they are captured by the nuclei of the medium, which causes these nuclei to disintegrate, or to explode, into short-range and heavily ionizing fragments; this has been called the "star" effect. Thus, this radiation has a high biologic effectiveness and a low dependence on oxygen.

GLOSSARY

central axis depth dose The plot of the dose along the central axis from the point of beam entry into the patient.

dosimetry The term applied to the measurement and calculation of dose that the patient receives.

electron volt (ev) The energy of motion acquired by an electron accelerated through a potential difference of 1 volt.

excitation The moving of an electron to a more distant orbit within the same atom.

gamma rays (originate inside the nucleus) Electromagetic irradiation emitted by excited nuclei. The gamma rays from an isotope will have one or several sharply defined energies.

half-life The time required for half the atoms of a radioactive species to disintegrate.

HVL Half-value layer; of a beam of x-rays or gamma rays this is the thickness of a given material that will reduce the radiation intensity to one half.

inverse square law The intensity of radiation from a point varies inversely as the square of the distance from the source. Thus, the dose rate at 2 cm from a source is one fourth that at 1 cm. At 3 cm the dose rate is one ninth that at 1 cm.

ionization The removal of an electron from an atom, leaving a positively charged ion.

ionizing radiation Radiation capable of causing ionization.

isotope Nuclides having an equal number of protons but a different number of neutrons (excitable situation).

kev 1,000 ev.

LET Linear energy transfer; the energy lost by the

particle or photon per micron of path depth. High LET radiations are more effective against hypoxic cells.

maximum permissible dose The dose of whole-body irradiation that has been calculated as being within the limits of safety and expressed as 5(n − 18) rads, where n is the age in years of the individual.

Mev 1,000,000 ev.

penumbra The radiation outside the full beam. Often caused by scatter or incomplete collimation.

rad A unit of absorbed dose of ionizing radiation equivalent to the absorption of 100 ergs per gram of irradiated material.

roentgen (R) An internationally accepted unit of radiation quantity; that quantity of "x-ray or gamma irradiation such that the associated corpuscular emission per 0.001293 grams of air produces, in air, ions carrying 1 esu of quantity of electricity of either sign."

X-rays (originate outside the nucleus) X-rays emitted by a particular generator will emit a spectrum of energies.

BIBLIOGRAPHY

Danforth, D. N., editor: Obstetrics and gynecology, New York, 1977, Harper and Row, Publishers, Inc.

Fletcher, G.: Textbook of radiotherapy, Philadelphia, 1975, Lea & Febiger.

Hall, E. J.: Radiobiology for the radiobiologist, New York, 1973, Harper and Row, Publishers, Inc.

Plumer, C.: Anomalies occurring in children exposed in utero to the atomic bomb in Hiroshima, Pediatrics **10:**687, 1952.

APPENDIX C

Gynecologic Oncology Group adverse effects criteria

System	0	1 = Mild	2 = Moderate	3 = Severe	4 = Life-threatening
Hematologic					
WBC (/mcl)	≥4,000	3,000-3,999	2,000-2,999	1,000-1,999	≤1,000
Granulocytes (/mcl)	≥1,500	1,000-1,499	500-999	250-499	<250
Platelets (/mcl)	≥150,000	100,000-149,999	50,000-99,999	25,000-49,999	<25,000
Anemia/blood loss (cumulative)	No transfusion	Drop in HGB of <2 gms not requiring transfusion	Transfusion 1 or 2 units	Transfusion 3 or 4 units	Reexploration to control bleeding, transfusion 5 units or hypovolemic shock
Genitourinary					
Renal					
BUN	<20 mg%	21-40 mg%	41-60 mg%	>60 mg%	Irreversible; requiring dialysis
Creatinine	<1.0 × N	1.1-2 × N	2.1-5 × N	5.1-10 × N	>10.0 × N
Creatinine clearance	0-33% ↓	↓ 33%-50%	↓ 50%-80%	↓ 80%-90%	> ↓ 90%
Proteinuria	None	1+ <300 mg%	2-3 + 300-1,000 mg%	4 + >1,000 mg%	Renal failure
Bladder and ureter					
Acute	No problems	Dysuria, frequency and/or micro-scopic hematuria; injury of bladder with primary repair	Bacterial infection; gross hematuria not requiring transfusion (less than 2 gms% decrease in HGB); injury requiring reanastomosis or	Gross hematuria requiring transfusion (greater than 2 gms% decrease in HGB); sepsis, obstruction, or fistula requiring secondary operation;	Life-threatening hematuria or septic shock; obstruction of both kidneys or vesicovaginal fistula requiring diversion

		minimal telangiectasia with edema on cystoscopy	tion; moderate telangiectasia; gross hematuria less than 2 gms% decrease in HGB); bladder volume less than 150 cc	vere pain; gross hematuria requiring transfusion (greater than 2 gms% decrease in HGB); permanent unilateral loss of function of kidney	volume requiring diversion or catheter drainage; fistula; necrosis, permanent bilateral obstruction or loss of renal function requiring dialysis
Gastrointestinal					
Motility problems					
Nausea and vomiting	None	Nausea only	Vomiting controlled by drugs	Vomiting 6x/day in spite of antiemetics requiring IV and tube	Life-threatening dehydration or bleeding
Diarrhea	<3 BM/day	3-4 liquid stools	4 liquid stools requiring medication	Bloody diarrhea; needs IV and/or blood	Life-threatening dehydration or bleeding
Constipation	None	Oral therapy	Enemas required	Impaction	Obstruction
Mechanical problems	None	Temporary ileus of 3 days or fewer duration	Ileus requiring tube decompression; narrowing of intestinal segment on x-ray, or moderate mucosal edema on procto exam	Surgically correctable defect—no stoma	Fistula, perforation, chronic bleeding requiring diversion
Stomatitis	None	Erythema and/or exanthema	Ulcers—able to eat	Ulcers—unable to eat	Life-threatening dehydration; hemorrhage; sepsis

Continued.

Produced by the Gynecologic Oncology Group, George Lewis, Jr., M.D., Chairman, a national cooperative group funded by the National Cancer Institute.

Gynecologic Oncology Group adverse effects criteria—cont'd

System	0	1 = Mild	2 = Moderate	3 = Severe	4 = Life-threatening
Hepatic (N = Normal)					
SGOT	Normal	Up to 2N	2.1-5N	5.1-10N	>10N
Alkaline phosphatase	Normal	Up to 2N	2.1-5N	5.1-10N	>10N
Bilirubin	Normal	Up to 2N	2.1-5N	5.1-10N	>10N
Pulmonary					
X-ray findings	None	Segmental atelectasis or blunted costophrenic angle	Lobar atelectasis or effusion occupying up to half of one hemithorax	Effusion occupying more than half of one hemithorax	Life-threatening total lung atelectasis
Functional problems	None	Pulmonary functions impaired but patient asymptomatic	Pulmonary symptoms requiring therapy but not assisted ventilation	Assisted ventilation needed	Shock lung
Cardiovascular					
Dyspnea/fluid accumulation/energy/pain	Normal	Asymptomatic	Transient symptomatic dysfunction requiring no therapy	Dysfunction not responsive to therapy	Symptomatic dysfunction responsive to therapy
Cardiac rhythm, inflammation or performance (cardiac output or pressures) or peripheral resistance	Normal	Abnormal sign or test	Transient symptomatic dysfunction requiring no therapy	Dysfunction not responsive to therapy	Symptomatic dysfunction responsive to therapy; cardiac arrest
Venous problems	None	Superficial phlebitis	Pelvic or deep vein thrombophlebitis	Pulmonary embolus	Pulmonary embolus requiring embolectomy or caval lectomy

			ing surgical treatment	requiring resection with anastomosis	tion; resection of organ (bowel, limb, etc.)
Peripheral neurologic					
Reflex	Normal	Decreased DTRs	Absent DTRs		
Strength	Normal	Mild weakness	Moderate weakness	Severe weakness, paresis; cannot squat or sit up in bed unassisted	Paralysis; transverse myelitis
Sensory	Normal	Mild pain; mild paresthesia	Moderate pain; moderate paresthesia	Severe pain; severe paresthesia	
Central neurologic					
Mental status; mood, ideation, memory, consciousness	Normal	Transient alteration and/or minimal lethargy	Alteration substantially affecting function < 50% of time or of function	Alteration substantially affecting function > 50% of time or of function	Comatose
Motor paresis	None	Mild or transient	Substantially affects function, < 50% decrement in baseline capabilities	Substantially affects function, > 50% decrement in baseline capabilities	Paralysis
Cerebellar	Normal	Mild or transient alteration	Substantially affects function, < 50% decrement in baseline capabilities	Substantially affects function, > 50% decrement in baseline capabilities	Confined to bed
Seizure disorder	Normal	Transient, not requiring therapy	Transient or satisfactorily controlled medical therapy	Seizure disorder not controlled by medical therapy	Status epilepticus

Continued.

Gynecologic Oncology Group adverse effects criteria—cont'd

System	0	1 = Mild	2 = Moderate	3 = Severe	4 = Life-threatening
Cutaneous					
Skin (NOTE: If related to sun exposure or within radiation site)	None	Erythema	Dry desquamation; vesiculation; pruritus	Moist desquamation; ulceration; surgical debridement	Exfoliative dermatitis; necrosis; requiring grafting
Alopecia	None	Thinning	Bald patches	Total reversible	Total nonreversible
Wound	None	Wound seroma; cuff hematoma	Abscess or superficial separation	Fascial disruption with evisceration	Necrotizing fasciitis
Lymphatics	None	Mild lymphedema	Moderate lymphedema requiring compression	Severe lymphedema limiting function	Severe edema limiting function with ulceration
Fever (NOTE: If drug induced)	< 38° C	38-40° C less than 24 hours duration	38-40° C greater than 24 hours duration	> 40.1° C	Fever with hypotension
Allergic	None	Dermatitis or urticaria	Bronchospasm, oral therapy required	Bronchospasm, parenteral therapy required; serum sickness	Anaphylaxis

Index*

A

Actinomycin D; *see also* Dactinomycin
  and nonmetastatic trophoblastic disease,
    175–176
  uterine sarcoma and, 164
Adenocarcinoma
  cervical, 59
  clear-cell, *40*
    age-specific incidence rates of, *39*
    drug therapy and, 42
    of genital tract, 38–42
    recurrences of, 42
    suggested management of, 41T
  fallopian tube; *see* Fallopian tube, carcinoma of
  ovarian; *see also* Ovary, neoplasms of
    endometrioid, 271–272
    mucinous, 269–270
    papillary serous, *267 268*
  uterine, 128–152
    causes of, 128
    diagnosis of, 130–131
    epidemiology of, 129–131
    incidence of, 128–129
    prognostic factors in, 131–138
    risk factors in, 129T
    vaginal, 217–218
Adenomatous hyperplasia, 109–110, *110*
  atypical, 110–111, *111*
  premalignant potential of, 112–113
Adenosis, vaginal, 40
  adenocarcinoma and, 42–44
Adnexa, anatomy of, 223
Adnexal mass, 223–233
  differential diagnosis of, 224T, 224–231
  of gynecologic origin, 225–230
  management of, 231–233
  nongynecologic, 230–231

Adolescent, cervical cancer and, 6
Adrenalectomy, breast cancer and, 371–372
Adriamycin; *see also* Doxorubicin
  uterine sarcoma and, 164–165
Alkeran, *see* Melphalan
Alkylating agents, 288
Alopecia, chemotherapy and, 294–295
Alpha-fetoprotein (AFP), 404
  in endodermal sinus tumor, 325
Antibiotics in chemotherapy, 288
Antigen(s)
  carcinoembryonic (CEA), 404
  oncofetal, 404
  tumor-associated, *404*, 404–405
Antigenicity, lowered tumor, 416
Antimetabolites, 288
Antineoplastic agents in exploratory laparotomy,
    309
Arrhenoblastoma, *341*, 341–342
Ataxia-telangiectasia, 415

B

Bacillus Calmette-Guerin (BCG), 420
Bagshawe chemotherapy and poor prognosis
    GTN, 181T
Barium enema, squamous cancer of vagina and,
    211
Bartholin's gland carcinoma, vulvar, 204
Basal cell carcinoma, vulvar, 205
Basal cell hyperplasia, 4
B-cell lymphocyte, maturation of, *412*, 413
B-cells, compared with T-cells, 413T, 414
Biopsy
  cone, 22
    in pregnancy, 12
  Kevorkian-Young cervical, 12
  outpatient, 363
Bladder, cancer of, in pregnancy, 384
Bleeding, rectal, and cervical cancer, 57
Blenoxane; *see* Bleomycin

---

*Italicized numbers indicate illustrations; T
following page number indicates table.

469